To Doug,

A true Clinician Scientist!

Min & Don

A Biographical History of Endocrinology

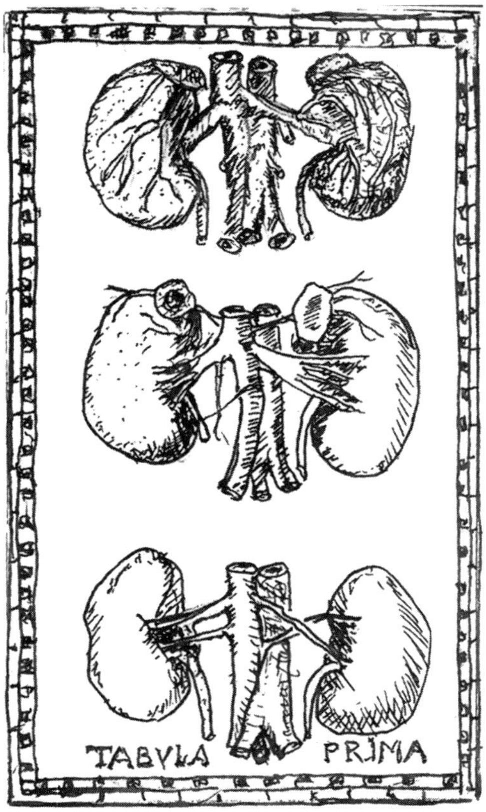
TABVLA PRIMA

A Biographical History of Endocrinology

D. Lynn Loriaux

This work is a co-publication between the Endocrine Society and John Wiley & Sons, Ltd.

WILEY Blackwell

ENDOCRINE SOCIETY

This work is a co-publication between the Endocrine Society and John Wiley & Sons, Ltd.

Editorial Offices
1606 Golden Aspen Drive, Suites 103 and 104, Ames, Iowa 50010, USA
The Atrium, Southern Gate, Chichester, West Sussex, P019 8SQ, UK
9600 Garsington Road, Oxford, OX4 2DQ, UK

Endocrine Society Office
2055 L Street NW Suite 600, Washington, DC 20036, USA

For details of our global editorial offices, for customer services and for information about how to apply for permission to reuse the copyright material in this book please see our website at www.wiley.com/wiley-blackwell.

Library of Congress Cataloging-in-Publication Data

Names: Loriaux, Lynn, author.
Title: A biographical history of endocrinology / D. Lynn Loriaux, MD, PhD.
Description: Ames, Iowa : John Wiley & Sons, Inc., 2016. | Includes bibliographical references and index.
Identifiers: LCCN 2015044547 (print) | LCCN 2015045716 (ebook) | ISBN 9781119202462 (cloth) | ISBN 9781119202479 (pdf) | ISBN 9781119202554 (epub)
Subjects: LCSH: Endocrinology–History–Biography.
Classification: LCC QP187 .L57 2016 (print) | LCC QP187 (ebook) | DDC 612.4–dc23
LC record available at http://lccn.loc.gov/2015044547

A catalogue record for this book is available from the British Library.

Wiley also publishes its books in a variety of electronic formats. Some content that appears in print may not be available in electronic books.

Set in 9.5/12pt Meridien by SPi Global, Pondicherry, India

1 2016

Frontispiece

It was in 1977 or 1978 when Mort Lipsett, my scientific mentor, found me at work in the laboratory and told me that in 3 weeks I would be going to Rome to give a series of lectures for him. He could not go because he had to give testimony to congress about the NIH budget and could not leave town. It was very bad timing, but it was evident that I could not say no. He said,

"Call Mario Andreoli. He is in charge of the program, he will give you what you ask, within reason, to cover my absence."

Caught off guard, I said, "Mort, there is a book I want to see, *Eustachius Anatomy*. There are only two known copies, one in London, and one in the Vatican. I want to see that book."

He said, "Tell Mario."

I called Mario and told him what I wanted in return for making the trip.

He said, "I will get back to you," and the next day he called. "One of my associates here, Gaetano Fraiese, has an uncle who is a Cardinal in the Vatican. Gaetano said it can be arranged. So, are you coming?"

"Yes."

With considerable difficulty, I found my way to the Polyclinico Umberto where the meeting was to be held, and to the right building, and then to the right lecture hall, and the lectures began. The meeting was about a week long, as I recall, and I asked once or twice about the book. Responses were vague, shrouded with the "veil of impossibility" for such a request. I became convinced that it would not happen, but that the trip had been well worth the effort.

The last day and the last lecture rolled around and, about 10 minutes before the end of that lecture, one of the doors that stood to either side of the lectern opened and a middle-aged man, in an impeccably pressed blue suit and sunglasses, stood there and watched the last few slides. When the lecture ended, and the desultory applause died down, he motioned me to come with him. I had no idea who this person was and I motioned to my friend, Giancarlo D'Agata, to find out what was going on. He said he didn't know either, but that he would come with me. Thus emboldened, I packed up my slides and baggage (I had a flight back to the USA that evening) and we went with the man, through the corridors to a black limousine, idling at the curb on a narrow side street. He motioned us into the car, and the journey began, with *cavalieri* fore and aft, sirens wailing. We didn't stop until we reached the long outside wall of the Vatican where people line up to get into the museums. We pulled up to the only entrance on that street. The Swiss guards snapped to attention and the gate opened. We drove, ultimately, into a large courtyard, completely paved with brick, with high walls on all sides. No windows. There was only one door, and we stopped in front of it. The door opened and a smallish man in tweed wearing very thick lenses motioned us in. We entered a small anteroom with a library table up against one wall. There were four books, bound in vellum, lying on a white cloth. There were four pairs of white gloves.

"Opuscula Anatomica."

There were four of them, seemingly in perfect shape. The chapters on the adrenal gland were marked with a slip of white paper, as were the copper plates that were not supposed to be in the book. They were present in every one. I asked if I could take a few pictures and the librarian said no, but that I could mark pages that I wanted with slips of paper, and they would photograph them for me. I thought the likelihood that I would ever see any of those slides was low, but I marked as many pages as I thought reasonable. We were in there for an hour or more. It was getting late, and I had a plane to catch. We left and made our way to the airport exactly as we had gone to the Vatican. When we reached the airport, I got my bag, and the man in the blue suit walked me to the front of the customs line, made a small bow with a nod of the head, and was gone.

Three weeks later, a white cardboard box arrived in the mailbox. It contained about 100 slides, everything I had marked. It was an adventure.

The prevailing dogma of the day was that the copper plates produced by Eustachius and Pier Matteo Pini, illustrating Eustachius' dissections of the adrenal gland, were not included in the *Opuscula*. There are 47 known copper plates. The first nine were included in the *Opuscula*. The remaining 38 plates were intended for a major anatomy text by Eustachius, but he died before the book could be written. The plates stayed with the Pini family.

Lancisi, the Papal Physician to Pope Clement XI, found the plates with the help of Pini's heirs, the Rossi family, and published them in 1714 with his own commentary. There were 38 of them; one plate was engraved on both sides. Eustachius' commentary accompanies the plates that were reprinted from the *Opuscula*. Lancisi describes the other 39. The plates illustrating the adrenal gland, among other things, the first nine, were all included in the *Opuscula* in 1563. They were rejoined with the others and reprinted by Lancisi in 1714. Thus the confusion and the explanation.

The copper plates, from which the freehand drawing shown on page ii was made, are the works of Eustachius and his relative, Pier Matteo Pini, of Urbino. Each Tabula has two or three figures. There are three in this one. The adrenal glands (*glandulae reni incumbentes*) can be seen behind the upper poles of the kidneys in figure 1, and in front of upper poles of the kidney in figure 2. They are also prominently displayed in Tabula II, figures 1, 2 and 3, and Tabula III, figures 2 and 3.

Eustachius' copper plates are often described as "stiff" and overly differentiated, more like a blueprint than an anatomical drawing. On the other hand, what he describes and shows is clear and unambiguous, clearer than most anatomical drawings of the time. Most helpful are the margins of the plates which are "scaled" with 1–35 units on the x axis (probably centimeters) and 1–60 units on the y axis. His descriptions are accompanied by "coordinates," allowing the reader to focus on the exact place that he is discussing. This was a major improvement, replacing arrows to, and letters on, the organs themselves. The calibrated margins did not catch on, and are seen only on the Eustachius copper plates.

Sources

Choulant L, Garrison FH: *History and Bibliography of Anatomic Illustration In Its Relation to Anatomic Science and the Graphic Arts*. Chicago, IL: The University of Chicago Press, 1920.

Lancisi GM: Tabulae Anatomicae Bartholomaei Eustachii. Rome, 1714.

Dedications

Life passes at an ever increasing pace, and I bruxate over all of the things I should have done and did not. One of those things was to thank the mentors in my life for all that they did for me. They are all dead now. Still, I need to acknowledge them. There were four.

Robert Packard Martin

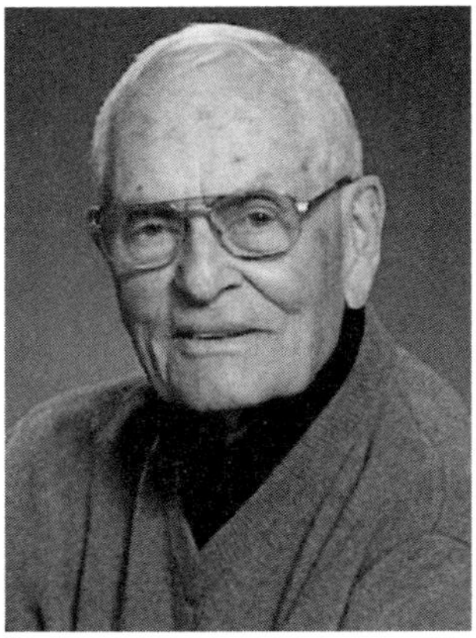

Robert Packard Martin
Used with permission from Lois Martin.

Robert Packard Martin was Professor of Biochemistry at Colorado State University. I began college as an animal husbandry major. I soon realized that the major made sense only if I had animals to husband. I had none, nor was I likely ever to have any. I changed my major to pre-vet, and signed up for organic chemistry, among other things. To make ends meet, I had several jobs. I had a jazz quartet that played Saturday nights in the little saloons that dot the front range, south to north. I worked weekends swamping out the stalls and the small animal rooms in a gnotobiotic facility. I worked every week night in the Department of Biochemistry, washing the scientific glassware, usually between the hours of midnight and one or two in the morning. One night a stranger walked into the washroom.

> "Are you Lynn?"
> "I am. What did I do?"
> "Nothing. Rogan sent me."

Rogan was the Organic Chemistry Professor, and I had done well in his class.

> "How would you like to come work with me in the laboratory? We can meet two afternoons a week, and I will pay you the same as you make here. Someone else can do this job."
> "What would I have to do?"
> "Work in a lab. If I don't miss my mark, you know nothing about gas chromatography, buffers, electrobalances, spectrophotometers, and scintillation counters. Am I right?"

His assumption was correct. I took the job, and soon we were doing experiments and published a few papers.

"Do you like this stuff?" he asked one day.
"I love it," I said.
"Then you have to go to medical school."
"Not possible. My father is an artist."
"MD/PhD. It can happen." And it did.

During World War II, Dr. Martin was a fighter pilot instructor at Kirkland Airforce Base in Albuquerque. One morning, July 16, 1945, he was flying out of the airbase with four other planes when, at about 10,000 feet (the ground there is 6,000 feet), at 5.29 a.m., the southern New Mexico sky over the Jornada del Muerto turned instantly from dark to a brighter than midday. It lasted two seconds, then faded to a red and purple, and the night returned.

It is remembered that Bob Martin said to his flight, "I don't know what that was, but if we show two of them to the enemy, the war will be over!"

Robert Martin taught me the basics of steroid chemistry.

Matthew W. Noall

Matthew W. Noall had just moved to Baylor College of Medicine in the Departments of Pathology and Biochemistry when I arrived. That he would be my PhD advisor and mentor had already been arranged by Dr. Martin. They had both received their PhD degrees in the pre-eminent Steroid Chemistry and Biochemistry Unit under Leo Samuels at the University of Utah. As I began my work with Dr. Noall, it became clear that his approach was considerably more "basic" than what I had grown accustomed to. For example, he insisted that I understood, and could teach, the chemistry of every steroid derivatization we did, the physics of every instrument I depended upon, and how the instrument could be optimized for the projected task. I should be able to perform the routine maintenance. No steroid was considered pure until it had been re-crystallized to constant specific activity or isotopic ratio. Every reaction had to be conducted in a fume hood, and the safety techniques used with radioisotopes had no "wobble room." I couldn't move on to actual experiments until I had written a computer program in Fortran. He checked my lab books at least weekly. It was just what I needed, not what I wanted. We did it his way. Trial by fire.

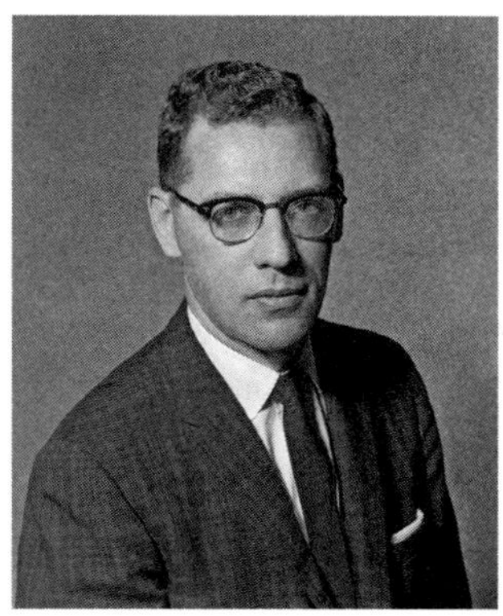

Matthew W. Noall
Photo courtesy of Baylor College of Medicine Archives.

I learned about the NIH Clinical Associate Program from Vernon Knight, Chief of Infectious Diseases at Baylor. As I learned more about it, it seemed like the perfect place for me. I applied and was invited for an interview. I was scheduled for a visit. The round trip ticket on Eastern Airlines, Houston to Washington, DC and back, was US$300. After the MD graduation ceremony, I discussed the plan with my father, including the US$300 request. He thought about what I had told him, and he asked,

"What are the chances you will get in?"

I said they were slim, only 50 were chosen out of thousands of applicants.

"Too slim," he said. "Save your requests for something reasonable."

Crestfallen, I told Noall about the predicament. He said, "Cheer up! I'll give you the money. I believe that you will get in!"

He was right. I did get in. It would not have happened without him, in more ways than one. When I left Houston for Boston, I still had no money to pay him back. I suggested I leave with him my reloading press, dies, and powder measure to cover the US$300. He said, "Just what I had hoped for. Call it even." It was worth US$50 at most. He was that way.

George Widmer Thorn

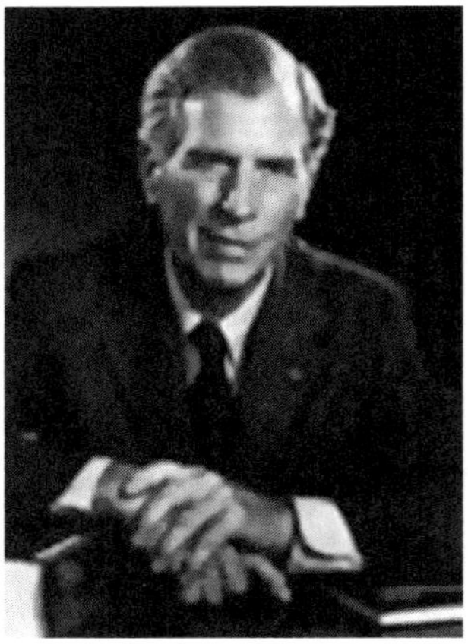

George Widmer Thorn
Used with permission from the Karsh Foundation.

George Widmer Thorn was the Chief of Medicine at the Peter Bent Brigham Hospital when I was a medicine house officer there, 1968–70. Thorn was one of the leading figures in medicine in the world. He had developed the treatment regimen for adrenal insufficiency using desoxycorticosterone acetate. He was a founding editor of *Harrison's Textbook of Medicine*. He was the first Director of the Howard Hughes Foundation. He was on everybody's list of "Greatest" doctors.

Thorn was available to the house staff, and got to know most of us through Grand Rounds presentations, Christmas parties, and the annual banquet. That was usually the sum of it. He and I, however, through the medium of a catastrophe (see Chapter 82) got to know each other better than most. I talked with him often during my house staff years and the NIH years that followed. We exchanged greetings every Christmas until he died. He was a mentor for life.

What he did for everybody who worked with him "on the wards," was to show them, by example, what a complete physician was. Many of his patients had adrenal insufficiency, and their management was straightforward. Most of his patients, however, were ill, often invalids, and had been to the "best places" with no benefit. They were referred to Thorn as the last resort. He would start with a careful history and physical examination. He would find out their worst fear, and invite the relevant specialists to visit. He would see them every day. He would teach them in small increments that there were many more diseases than we had ever dreamed of. He would tell them that we did know the ones that can kill, and "you don't seem to have any of those." For most doctors, this would be the end of the line. Thorn, however, would treat them. They were ill. Vitamins were a favorite, as were minerals and essential amino acids. Everything passed the risk/benefit ratio test. He would alter the combinations much like an optometrist asks, "which is better, 1 or 2?" They would get better. They would get out of bed. They would begin to "work" from the hospital, and then agitate to go home. He would keep them longer, until they would insist he let them go. They would leave, better, often much better than when they had come. Sometimes they never needed to come back. Sometimes they needed repeat visits to "stay well." It was a remarkable thing to see. The only other doctor I have seen do this was Michael DeBakey. He "made" his patients get well, and they did better than those of the other surgeons. George Thorn taught us that illness is sometimes caused by a disease, sometimes not. The "illness," however, always deserves to be treated. He was the kindest man I have known.

Mortimer B. Lipsett

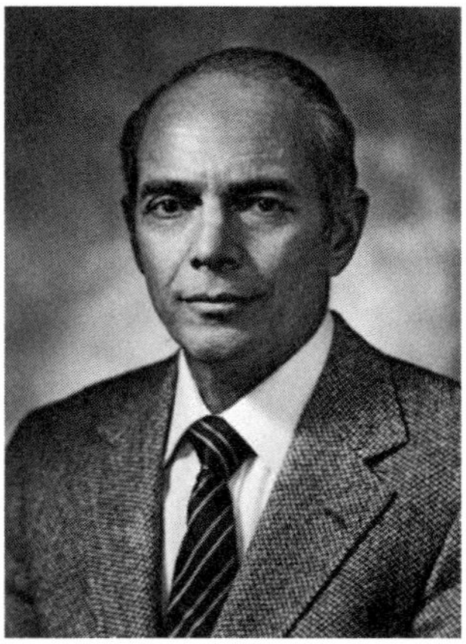

Mortimer B. Lipsett
Used with permission from Loriaux, D. Lynn: In Memoriam, Mortimer B. Lipsett. *Endocrinology* 1987; 120(2): 841–3.

Everybody who ever met Mort Lipsett will tell you that he was the smartest man they have ever encountered (see Chapter 100). His facility with facts and figures, and his knowledge base and the accuracy with which he could use it was simply incomparable. Nobody, in my experience, comes close. Meetings with Mort were like a cage fight; somebody had to win before you could get out, and somebody usually got hurt. My first experience with this happened at the very beginning of my years at the NIH.

I was presenting a complicated patient to the assembled endocrine host at a weekly "combined" conference. It was a "small print" disease for me, and I knew what I didn't know. I knew I was on thin ice most of the time. When I finished, however, the questions were mostly "soft balls." Nobody had much to say. Mort said nothing. As an afterthought, I added that the man was a type 2 diabetic and I had prescribed an ADA diet.

Mort woke up.

"Why did you do that?" he asked.
"Well," I said. (Who could object to this? I thought.)
"Do you know what this will do to his grocery bills? Can he afford it? What will it cost his wife in time and effort? Is there any evidence that this can help him as an outpatient? Could that even be measured?"

Mort stood up and started walking toward the door, shaking his head. Just as he got the door open, I blurted this out:

"Well, this is the way we did it at Mecca."

Halfway out of the door, Mort stopped in his tracks, pivoted 180 degrees, fixed me with his gaze, and said,

"You are at the NIH now. We don't do anything to our patients that we don't fully understand and can defend in the sense of cost and benefit."

He turned to go out, but pivoted again,

"By the way," he said, "This is Mecca."

The door closed behind him as he left the room. You could hear a pin drop. Nobody moved, everyone looking at the floor for what seemed a very long time.

Mort and I worked together until his death 14 years later. He did not have a lot of friends, probably by design. They take up a lot of time. I am sure of only three, counting me. We met when there was something to meet about. No dogma was safe. No non-sequitur survived. No assumption went unexamined. It was not until many years later that I thought we could just have conversation. It is one of the best things that ever happened to me.

When Odysseus left Ithaca to fight the Trojan War, he asked his friend Mentor to oversee the education and development of his son, Telemachus, while he was away. Mentor was the surrogate father, trusted by Odysseus to do the right things. These four were my mentors. They told me when I did well, but more importantly, when I did not. It was pro bono, a necessary quality. None of them would ever let me say "thank you!"

Contents

Preface

The beginning of this book can be linked to a telephone call I received from Mr. John Gardner, a Senior Editor at Williams and Wilkins Publishing Company in Baltimore. The year was 1989. He asked if I could come to Baltimore to meet with him, and a time was set. The purpose of that meeting turned out to be the development of a new clinical journal in endocrinology. We mapped out on that day what became *The Endocrinologist.* One of its main features was the "Historical Vignette." I told John that I could not move forward with the project until I had offered to let the Endocrine Society be involved in some way. I was invited to the 1990 Endocrine Society Council meeting to present my case. Jack Groski was the president. My main points were that, compared to other subspecialty societies, the Endocrine Society did little for the endocrinologists in practice. A bona fide clinical journal would help. Second, the journal could become another "money maker" for the society. Jean Wilson spoke for the society in thanking me for coming to them, but that they were happy with the current structure and wished me well. So, I went ahead with Williams and Wilkins. We had the Journal up and running within the year.

In the beginning, I wrote all of the Historical Vignettes, and Clark T. Sawin did the book reviews. With time, I had to have help with the Vignettes, so Clark stepped in and we began to alternate issues until his untimely death in 2004, after which I wrote all of them again. The Journal had a run of 20 years, six issues a year, 120 Vignettes. Of these, Clark wrote 45, and I wrote the rest except for a few; Michael Bliss wrote about J.J.R. MacLeod, Jim Magner wrote about Emil Fischer, Leon Speroff wrote about Soranus of Ephesus and Gregory Pincus, Ron Rosenfeld wrote about Henry Turner, and Harry K. Ziel co-wrote about Frederick L. Hisaw. In the table of contents, the author of each chapter is identified.

When the Journal ended for lack of advertising funds in 2010, I wanted to ensure that the Vignettes would not be lost. I was fortunate to get the copyrights to all of them, with the idea of putting together a Biographical History of Endocrinology. It has been a steady grind since then but, with the help of the Endocrine Society and Wiley, the Publisher, it finally came together.

There is already an outstanding book on the history of endocrinology written by Victor Medvei. It is encyclopedic and beautifully written. My guess is that not many have read it. Most use it as a reference source which can be counted on for fidelity. *A Biographical History of Endocrinology* is written to be read. Each chapter is only a few pages long and illustrates the role of the subject in the progress of our medical specialty. I expect there will be some controversy about who I included in the book and who I did not. Hopefully, somewhere down the line there will be a second edition and these shortcomings can be remedied.

I would like to acknowledge the following people who played an important role in the creation of this book. First, to John Gardner and his staff at Williams and Wilkins for supporting the concept in the beginning. Terri Loriaux, Jennifer Loney, and Patricia Hastart prepared all of the manuscripts for editing, over and over again. Stacey Lipps retrieved all of the manuscripts from Lippincott and reformatted them in a book format. Taryn Aab has typed it all again, downloaded the chapters to at least four different sites, coordinated all of the copyright issues, including tough ones like the Vatican, and kept the entire operation on track. Her input was essential to the successful completion of this project. Giancarlo D'Agata, an old friend from Catania, stepped in to help with permissions from the Vatican when the English language was not up to the task.

Finally, I want to emphasize again the contributions to this work made by Clark T. Sawin. His influence is found on every page.

Sine Qua Non

CHAPTER 1

Diabetes and the Ebers Papyrus (1552 B.C.E.)

The Ebers Papyrus was found between the legs of a mummy in the Assissif district of the Theben Necropolis. The exact tomb of origin is unknown, and it is not recorded that the tomb suggested the occupant was a physician. The Papyrus was purchased in Luxor by Edwin Smith in 1862, who sold it to George Ebers, a well-respected Egyptologist in 1872. Ebers published a facsimile in English and Latin in 1875 dating from 1552 B.C.E. It is believed to be the oldest preserved medical document. The Papyrus is 30 cm in height and 20.23 m (66 feet 4 inches) in length and is divided into 110 pages. It is written in the Hieratic script. It contains chapters on helminthiasis, ophthalmology, dermatology, gynecology, obstetrics, dentistry, and surgery. There is a short section on psychiatry, describing a "despondency" that seems very close to our concept of depression. More than 700 magical formulas are described, including incantations and folk remedies [1]. Of great interest to endocrinologists is the opinion that the first known medical reference to diabetes mellitus is in the Ebers Papyrus. The reference is a single phrase: "to eliminate urine which is too plentiful."

> Unfortunately, the crucial word, Asha, can mean both "plentiful" and "often," and it is unclear whether the condition described was polyuria (increased volume of urine) or increased frequency of micturition, very often due to cystitis. The latter condition is much more common and therefore the more likely interpretation [2].

The medicine of the Egyptians was referred to by the Greeks as conservative and unchanged from the medicine of the early dynasties. Herodotus wrote that "medicine is practiced among them on a plan of separation; each physician treats a single disease, and not more; thus the Country abounds with physicians, some undertaking to cure the diseases of the eyes, others of the head, others again of the teeth, and others of the intestine and some of those which are internal" [3].

Galen and Hippocrates both refer to a period of study at the temple of Imhotep in Memphis. Interestingly, in their subsequent writings, neither refers to diabetes in a

A Biographical History of Endocrinology, First Edition. D. Lynn Loriaux.

This work is a co-publication between the Endocrine Society and John Wiley & Sons, Ltd.

way we would consider sufficient to describe the disease. Their descriptions do not go beyond that contained in the Ebers Papyrus.

The first convincing description of diabetes appears in about 100 C.E. by Aretaeus of Cappadocia:

> Diabetes is a wonderful affliction, not very frequent among men, being a melting down of the flesh and limbs into urine. The patients never stop making water, but the flow is incessant, as if the opening of aqua ducts. Life is too short, disgusting, and painful, thirst unquenchable, excessive drinking, which, however, is disproportionate to the large quantity of urine, for more urine is passed; and one cannot stop them either from drinking or making water; or, if for a time they abstain from drinking, their mouth becomes parched and their body dry, the viscera seems as if scorched up; they are affected with nausea, restlessness, and burning thirst, and at no distant term they expire [4].

This is truly the first accurate description of the disease and, at least for me, represents the first clear recognition of the disease. Nonetheless, the Ebers Papyrus is a riveting document revealing an astonishing medical sophistication in the Nile River Valley, 3500 years ago.

References

1. Sanders LJ: From Thebes to Toronto and the 21st century. *Diabetic Spectrum* 2002; 15: 56–60.
2. Nunn JF: *Ancient Egyptian Medicine*. Norman, OK: University of Oklahoma Press, 1996, p. 91.
3. Herodotus: "The Persian Wars." In JE Schadle, History of Medicine. *The St Paul Medical Journal*, November 1904, p. 807.
4. *Aretaeos of Kappadokia: The Extant Works*, edited and translated by Francis Adams. London, 1806, pp. 338–40.

This chapter has been reproduced from Loriaux, D. Lynn: Diabetes and the Ebers Papyrus: 1552 B.C. *The Endocrinologist* 2006; 16(2): 55–6.

CHAPTER 2
The Greek Myths and the First Physicians (1100 B.C.E.)

Greek mythology surrounds the beginnings of western medicine, culminating in the cult of Asclepius. A short version of the Olympian creation myth follows.

In the beginning there was only the void. Ether began to fill the void and with the introduction of Eros, attraction, the chaos of the beginning began to organize. Gaea, our Earth, was formed. In the beginning all was dark. Night was the darkness of earth, and Erebus was the darkness of the underworld. At the edge of creation, Night and Erebus came together and produced heavenly light in the ether, stars, and Earthly light creating day.

Earthly light revealed Uranus, the sky. Uranus showered earth with fertile rain and mountains and the sea, Pontus, came into being. This was followed by grass, flowers, and trees, and then the beasts, all in their proper places. Uranus and Gaea (sky and earth) continued to procreate. Among the first creations were the twelve Titans, the three Cyclops, and the three Hecatoncheires, 100-handed creatures. Uranus disliked the Cyclops, and banished them to the underworld. He also disliked the Hecatoncheires, and forced them back into Gaea's womb. She cried out for help, and Cronus, the last born Titan, killed Uranus by castration. He grasped the genitalia with his left hand, and severed them with his right. It is said that this is the beginning of the "left is sinister" myth.

Cronus, with his sister Titan, Rhea, had six progeny, the original Olympian Gods. Before his death, Uranus had prophesied that Cronus would be usurped by one his children, so Cronus ate them all (Saturn eating his children). Rhea protected the last of her children, Zeus, by giving Cronus a stone wrapped in swaddling clothes instead of Zeus and Cronus swallowed it. Zeus, thus spared, was raised on the island of Crete. With time, he met and married Metis, a Titan. She prepared an emetic potion which Zeus, disguised as a cup bearer, gave to Cronus. Cronus promptly vomited up the stone and all of Zeus' brothers and sisters, the Olympian Gods.

Zeus gathered the Olympian Gods together and a protracted and brutal war ensued. The Olympian Gods prevailed, and all of the Titans were banished to Tartarus except

A Biographical History of Endocrinology, First Edition. D. Lynn Loriaux.

This work is a co-publication between the Endocrine Society and John Wiley & Sons, Ltd.

for a few. These included Prometheus and Epimetheus, who were rewarded for their neutrality in the Olympian Titan wars.

The Olympian Gods now reigned supreme. They divided up creation among themselves. Zeus was the supreme God and God of the Sky. Hera, his sister, was his wife, and created the galaxy with a spray of milk from her right breast. Neptune was Lord of the Sea. Hades was Lord of the Underworld. Demeter was Goddess of Fertility and Agriculture.

Now the Gods began to procreate with each other seemingly at random. There were many children born of God–Titan unions. Athena was one such God, born of a complex union between Zeus and Metis. Gods also could create lesser Gods from whole cloth, such as Aphrodite, who was created from sea foam.

One striking example of this kind of creation was man. Zeus instructed Prometheus, the forward-thinking Titan, to create a creature in the image of the Gods, a mortal, to be a competitor with the other creatures that now populated the Earth. Prometheus began his assignment by molding his concept of what Zeus wanted out of clay. He showed it to Athena, the Goddess of Knowledge and Courage. She was so taken with the clay figurine that she cradled it in her arms and blew her breath into its nostrils, thus giving it life. It was the first man. The relationship between Athena and man seemed to Zeus to be too close and getting closer. To discourage it, he ordered Haphaestus, the crippled God of Smiths, to create a woman of unparalleled and arresting beauty in the image of the Goddesses. Thus, the first woman was born. She was called Pandora.

Zeus sent Pandora to Prometheus with a sealed box containing all of the good and bad things that could beset man and many of the other creatures as well. Zeus gave her instructions never to open the box. Prometheus did not want to be bothered by this new creature, so he gave her to Epimetheus, the hedonist Titan. He immediately told Pandora to open the box, which she did. All of the ills and the advantages that could accrue to man were thus loosed upon the world, all except for hope. Pandora closed the box before hope could escape. Thus only man is plagued with hope, ensuring his misery for all time.

The other of Zeus' two loves was Leto. Born on the island of Kos, she was one of the most beautiful Titans. With Zeus she had the twins Apollo and Artemis. After that, she fades from the scene.

Apollo becomes one of the foremost of the Gods. He was revered for his genius. He was the first physician. His abilities to heal almost everything with the root of the peony plant were legendary. Physicians of antiquity often were called "Sons of Paean." Apollo, as his father before him, had many loves that spanned the possible spectrum: nymphs, humans, Titans, demigods, and other Gods. One of these was Coronis, a beautiful human, the daughter of the King of Lapiths in Thessaly. Apollo fell in love with her. When Apollo was traveling and could not be with her, she remained at her castle on the shores of Lake Boebeis, guarded by a white crow. But Coronis had a secret passion for Ischys, a handsome Arcadian, and one time, when Apollo was absent, she admitted Ischys to her couch. The white crow flew immediately to inform Apollo, who was so enraged that his glare singed the crow's feathers. They have been black ever since.

Apollo told his twin sister Artemis, the Huntress, of the deceit, and she killed Coronis with a quiver of arrows. On her funeral pyre, it was discovered that Coronis harbored a living child in her womb. The child was surgically released by Hermes, alive and well, and Apollo named the boy Asclepius. He took the infant to the cave of Cheiron, the Centaur, and instructed him to raise the boy and teach him the "healing arts."

As a young man, Asclepius was exceptionally skilled in surgery and the application of the medical arts. As he became more mature, he developed the ability to restore people to life. Hades strongly resented this, and complained to Zeus. He caught Zeus at a bad moment and, in a fit of pique, Zeus killed Asclepius with a lightning bolt. With time, Zeus regretted this hasty gesture, and restored Asclepius to life as a full God, Immortal, and Olympian. Asclepius carried a hefty staff, symbolic of his connection to Olympus, and curled around the staff was a snake. Snakes were thought to be immortal because they renewed themselves each year when they shed their skin. Snakes became the messengers to all the Gods, carrying information back and forth on the omphalos (umbilicus). The staff symbolizes the umbilicus and cord that connects all Gods to Mount Olympus.

Asclepius had eight children with Epione, five daughters (Hygeia, Panacea, Aceso, Iaso, and Agiaea) and three sons (Machaon, Podaleirios, and Telesphoros). Telesphoros is often depicted with Asclepius as a dwarf. He became the demigod of convalescence, his name meaning "bringer of completion."

All of this became formalized into the cult of Asclepius, and his temples, the Asclepions, became the medical centers of the day. It is in this setting that Hippocrates, son of a temple priest, first recognized disease entities. He showed that diseases could be grouped according to three traits, and that a triad defined a syndrome. Syndrome means traveling together down "the road." Patients with the same syndrome followed the "same road." Since the road went to a known destination, the physicians could now, with some certainty, predict the course and the probable outcome in a given patient: prognosis. Western medicine begins here.

Sources

Graves R: *The Greek Myths*. New York: Penguin Books, 1960.

Hamilton E: *The Greek Way*. New York: W.W. Norton & Co, 1942.

CHAPTER 3
Kos and Alexandria (400 B.C.E.–400 C.E.)
The First Human Anatomy

The history of western medicine is tightly interwoven with the histories of Kos and Alexandria.

Kos is the second largest island in the Dodecanese group. This group of 12 islands is in the southeast reach of the Aegean Sea, the eastern limit of the Sea of Crete, and the point where east met west in the classical period of 500–300 B.C.E. The largest island in the group is Rhodes, and there are over 150 other islands, 26 of which are uninhabited.

The earliest history of the island group identifies a Minoan culture. Mycenaean Greeks occupied in about 1400 B.C.E., followed by the Dorians in 1100 B.C.E. By 600 B.C.E., Rhodes and Kos were the dominant islands. Three main cities emerged on Rhodes: Lindos, Kamiros, and Ialyssos. Kos City flourished on the island of Kos, as did Knidos and Halicarnassus on the mainland. Together, these six cities are known as the Dorian Hexapolis. With the first defeat of the Persians in 478 B.C.E., the Hexapolis joined with the Athenaean Delean league and came to define the eastern limit of Greece.

Kos became the gateway for transshipment of all things "eastern" into Greece, including culture, art, cuisine, mythology, and, importantly, silk. Silk weaving became the major industry on Kos. Kos silk was famous for its unique transparency and is featured prominently in many artistic treatments of feminine beauty. The primacy of Kos silk endured for centuries. Wine was the second industry. The third was a burgeoning as a center of learning that energized everything around it. The Ptolemaic pharaohs developed a provincial branch of the Museum of Alexandria on Kos and the island became a favorite spot for the education of Ptolemaic princes and intellectuals.

The cult of Asclepius came to Kos with the Dorians, and one of the most famous Asclepions (healing temples) in the Grecian world was built on the outskirts of Kos City. Its fame spread far and wide, and its infrastructure was supported by a strong Kos economy. It was in this Asclepion that the transformative changes that defined western medicine occurred.

A Biographical History of Endocrinology, First Edition. D. Lynn Loriaux.

The Asclepion of Kos covered 5.7 hectares (14.3 acres) and was arranged on three levels. The entryway opened into a large courtyard surrounded by a stone wall with an interior loggia, under which most of the primary care such as cuts, abrasions, fractures, and the self-limited diseases of children were managed. If the complaint was not obvious, the patient was referred to "Internal Medicine." The patient ascended to the second level, usually with a domestic animal in tow: sheep, pig, goat, or cow. The animal would be sacrificed by exsanguination, and the entrails spread out on the marble alter. The nature of the ailment would be read in the peristalsis of the large and small bowels, accompanied by an analysis of the concurrent flight of nearby birds, the winds, gathering storms, etc. This "augury" would often identify the offended God and offerings to the appropriate God could be prescribed accordingly.

The most stubborn cases were referred to the third and highest temple level. Here, temple sleep ("incubation") was prescribed. Through the night, the priests would walk their "rounds", and when periods of rapid eye movement sleep were detected in a sufferer, they would awaken the patient and listen to the description of the dream. This would usually allow a final dispensation. It was in this place that the temple snakes lived out their lives, slithering over and between the sleeping sufferers and serving to move the latest intelligence between the patients and the Gods via the staff of Asclepius.

The occupation of "temple priest" was an hereditary one, passed from father to son. Hippocrates' father, Heraclides, was a temple priest. Together, they made the "temple rounds". With time, Hippocrates began to recognize patterns of signs and symptoms in the sick. He found that patients who shared three or more signs or symptoms usually followed the same clinical course and outcome. Thus, the "triad" was born. Recognizing a syndrome allowed for prognosis–successful prediction of the eventual outcome. This was achieved without magic or incantation, augury or revealed truth. Western medicine emerged. Students and patients flocked to Kos to work with the priests of the Asclepion. With time, it was written down in the Hipprocratic Corpus. The "Oath" was created to give the profession a code of behavior. Kos remained the center of medical evolution for the next 300 years.

Alexander III (Alexander the Great) was born in Pella, Macedonia in July of 356 B.C.E. His father was Philip II of Macedon and Alexander was the first among a number of claimants to the throne. In 336 B.C.E., Philip was assassinated by Pausanias, the captain of his personal bodyguard and Alexander was proclaimed king. He was 26 years old. He was short of stature at 5 foot 7 inches, sturdy, with one blue eye and one brown one. He probably had a right fourth cranial nerve palsy as well: he held his head, at rest, with his nose pointing toward his left shoulder. He was smart. He was educated. His tutor was Aristotle, believe it or not. He was ruthless in the Homeric sense of the word. He eliminated all potential pretenders to the throne. He had his cousin, Amyntas IV, executed. He had two princes from the region murdered. His mother, Olympia, had her own daughter Europia, Alexander's sister, burned alive.

News of Philip's death led to a host of uprisings in the nascent Empire. Alexander would have none of it. At the head of Philip's army, he crushed Thessaly, Thebes, Athens, and Corinth. He crossed the Aegean Sea and subdued the Thracians, then the Illyrians. He crossed the Hellespont in 334 B.C.E., and routed the Persians at the battle of Granicus. He then subdued Halicarnassus and the other cities of the region. He slashed the Gordian knot. In his next encounter with the Persians, Darius fled the battlefield leaving behind his wife, two daughters, and his mother. Alexander stormed Tyre and killed all men of military age. He sold the women and children into slavery. The same fate awaited Gaza. He conquered Egypt, where he was feted as a liberator.

Before leaving Egypt, Alexander developed the plans for a new city, Alexandria. It would become the new capital of Egypt, and the conduit through which all of the riches of the Nile would flow to Greece. The site was at the westernmost extremity of the Nile delta, behind a low "island of the Pharos" that protected the city from attack by sea, and defended from North Africa by the estuarial waters of Lake Marotis. The Canopic branch of the Nile was channeled into the city as an abundant supply of fresh water.

Alexander left the site within a year to subdue the remnants of the Persian Empire. He died in Babylon, and his body was returned to Alexandria in 303 B.C.E., where his body was lain in a gold sarcophagus filled with honey and placed in a mausoleum at the highest point in the city.

The city had been under construction for 8 years, the project being directed by Cleomenes, the viceroy appointed by Alexander. In his "will," however, he gave the Egyptian realm of his Empire to Ptolemy, his most loyal general. Ptolemy became the first Pharoah in the Ptolemaic dynasty that lasted until Cleopatra's death in August of 30 B.C.E. In the 300 years of the Ptolemaic era, Alexandria became the largest city in the world.

The Ptolemies were committed to a Hellenic City, rich in culture and learning. The center of learning became the library of Alexandria and its associated museum, which consisted of an observatory, lecture halls, and laboratories that nurtured a growing scientific community. Philosophers, poets, artists, mathematicians, astronomers, and physicians all made their way to Alexandria.

There was an associated medical school. Human dissection was a part of the curriculum. It was the only government-sanctioned program of human dissection in the world. Human anatomy reached its apogee with the work of two men: Herophilus of Chalcedon (335–254 B.C.E.) and Erasistratus of Kos (304–259 B.C.E.).

> It is a cruel misfortune that not a single complete treatise of any of the works of these great Alexandrian pioneers of human dissection has survived. As a consequence of the loss, we are dependent for our knowledge of them upon isolated quotations and reports of their work found in later medical authors such as Rufus of Ephesus [1].

Galen quotes their work four centuries after they lived. He remarks that Erasistratus' account of the valves of the heart made it redundant for him to do it again.

> The phenomenon how membranes adhere to the mouths of the vessels which the heart employs in the service of introducing and expelling its material is examined by Erasistratus in his work *On Fevers*. Some have had the effrontery to deny the existence of these membranes and claim that they were invented by a follower of Erasistratus to establish his doctrine. But knowledge of them is now so widespread amongst doctors that anyone who was not aware of them would seem to be utterly out of date. There are at the mouth of the vena cava three

> membranes which in their arrangement are very like the barbs of arrows – whence, I imagine, some of the Erasistrateans called them "tricuspid". At the mouth of the vein-like artery; (which is what I call the divided vessel leading from the left ventricle of the heart into the lungs) the membranes, though very similar in shape, are unequal in number. For to this mouth alone, only two membranes, adhere.
>
> Each of the other two mouths have three membranes, all of them sigmoid. As Erasistratus says in his explanation of the phenomenom, each of the two mouths evacuates material, the one evacuates blood to the lung, and the other pneuma into the whole living creature. These membranes, in his opinion, perform a reciprocal service for the heart, by alternating at the appropriate times – those which adhere to the vessels which lead matter into the heart from the outside, are tripped by the entrance of the material and, falling back into the cavities of the heart, by opening their mouths, give an unimpeded passage to what is being drawn into their cavity.
>
> For, he says, material does not rush in spontaneously, as into some inanimate vessel; but heart itself, dilating like a coppersmith's bellows, draws the material in, filling itself in diastole. Membranes, which, he said, lie on the vessels which lead material out of the heart, are considered by Erasistratus to behave in the opposite way. For they incline outwards from within and, being tripped by the material passing out, open their mouths in proportion [2].

Anyone who has butchered a domestic animal or dissected a cadaver that has not had its vascular system filled with colored latex, blue for veins and red for arteries, will know that in death, the veins contain blood and the arteries are empty. Arteries contain air. The scientists of the time called this air the "pneuma" and gave it the function of distributing the "animal spirit" extracted by venous blood from air inspired into the lungs.

Galen codified the concept of the "pneuma" into his philosophy, which held strong for 1500 years until William Harvey sorted the issue out.

> The venous blood passed through the vena cava into the right side of the heart, where impurities were discharged through the pulmonary artery into the lungs and were thus exhaled through the trachea. This purified blood then ebbed back into the venous system. Part of the venous blood in the right ventricle passed through small channels in the interventricular septum, where it came in contact with the air which had passed into the left ventricle from the lungs through the pulmonary vein [3].

Galen spent 11 years in Alexandria. It was there that he developed his theory of the pneuma and the vital animal spirits which, in fact, was taken directly from the work of Diascorides and Erasistratus 400 years before.

Vesalius, in the early Renaissance, became convinced that Galen had never dissected the human body. It might be true, but what he drew from the works of the Alexandrians was of the first order, and dominated anatomical thinking for 2000 years.

We think of the "Dark Ages" as beginning with the Barbarian invasions of Rome. In medicine, however, there was an earlier "Dark Age" that began with the decline of Alexandria beginning with the burning of the library by Julius Caesar and ending with the murder of Hypatia in 415 B.C.E.

Kos provided the Asclepion and the curiosity to recognize diseases as entities, syndromes with a natural history. Alexandria provided the setting in which the anatomy and physiology of the human body could be studied. Galen did what he could with both, 400 years later, but by then, Alexandria had been razed at least five times, the library burned and scattered and the glory that was Kos and Alexandria, as far as medicine is concerned, was gone forever. The new homes for medical progress were Baghdad and Cordoba.

References

1. Penfield W: The Asclepiad Physicians of Cnidus and Cos, with a note on the probable site of the Triopion Temple of Apollo. *Proc Am Philos Soc* 1957; 101(5): 393–400.
2. Major RH: *A History of Medicine*. Springfield, IL: Charles C. Thomas, 1954.
3. Longrigg J: Anatomy in Alexandria in the third century BC. *Br J Hist Sci* 1988; 21: 455–88, pp. 477–8.

CHAPTER 4

Hippocrates
(400 B.C.E)
Western Medicine Begins

> Medicine is the most distinguished of all the arts,
> but through the ignorance of those who practice it,
> and of those who casually judge such practitioners,
> it is now of all the arts by far the least esteemed.

This unflattering summation of the medical profession, one that could have been written today, was penned more than 2000 years ago in the short treatise, *Law*, in the Hippocratic Corpus [1]. Of all physicians, Hippocrates did more than any other to change this opinion of medicine and its practitioners. The medicine of Hippocrates developed in the fourth century B.C.E. Before Hippocrates, Greek medicine was dominated by physician priests. The primary god of healing in the Greek pantheon was Apollo. Arrows from his bow could visit plagues and pestilence upon mortal men. He was the physician to the Gods of Mount Olympus, whom he treated with the root of the peony (hence his name "Paean," and the common reference to physicians as "sons of Paean"). Apollo taught the art of medicine to the Centaur Chiron, son of Saturn, and Chiron was tutor to the heroes Jason, Hercules, Achilles and, most importantly, Asclepius, son of Apollo by the nymph Coronis. Asclepius became so skilled in medicine that Pluto accused him of depopulating Hades, and Zeus killed him with a thunderbolt. Thus, he became the patron of healing, and the temples of his cult were known as Asclepions. In these temples, Asclepius was represented as a handsome god-like figure attended by the sacred snake, entwined around a staff, the familiar "staff of Asclepius." Hygieia and Panacea, two of Asclepius' many children, were responsible for the care of the sacred snakes. Asclepius was usually accompanied by a tiny hooded dwarf, Telesphorus, the god of convalescence. The most famous of the Asclepions were at Kos, Epidauros, Cnidus, and Pergamon. The sick made pilgrimages to these "medical centers" from all over the ancient world. Patients were received by the priests of the temple and regaled with the deeds of Asclepius, followed by prayers to specific gods associated with the "chief" complaint and the sacrifice of a cock or ram.

A Biographical History of Endocrinology, First Edition. D. Lynn Loriaux.

Treatment consisted, in the main, of mineral water baths, massage, inunction with oils and unguents, and the special rite of "incubation" or "temple sleep." If the patient slept, curative advice came in the form of a dream, frequently interpreted by a priest making "rounds" in the night. If the patient improved, a votive in the form of a terra-cotta or waxen image of the diseased part was presented to the temple for display, a form of "outcomes" advertising. In addition to the temple priests, "alternative" forms of medicine were practiced by "philosophers" who would dispense medical advice, and by the gymnasts who treated disease with baths and prescriptions for a healthful lifestyle. Greek medicine before Hippocrates was a mélange of religion, philosophy, and some science. Hippocrates turned all of this upside down.

Hippocrates was born on the island of Kos about 400 B.C.E. He was the son of a physician priest. In fact, this is all we know about Hippocrates from contemporary historical sources. He is alluded to in a play by Aristrophanes, and mentioned in two of Plato's dialogues, *Protagoras* and *Phaedrus.* The traditional story of his life is derived mostly from the account given by Soranus of Ephesus in the second century A.D., a source far removed from its subject and likely to be corrupted to some degree [2]. Soranus tells us that Hippocrates was born at the beginning of the 80th Olympiad, that he received his medical education from his father, a priest in the Asclepion of Kos, that he traveled extensively, and that he practiced medicine in Thrace, Macedonia, and Thessaly. The date of his death is unknown, but he is thought to have lived to an age somewhere between 85 and 109 years. What is not in dispute is that Hippocrates' life spanned the window in time that was associated with a spectacular efflorescence of the human intellect. "The list of Hippocrates contemporaries includes Sophocles, Plato, Euripides, Aristophanes, Pindar, Socrates, Herodotus, Thucydides, Phydias and Polygnotus" [2]. Athenian democracy reached its peak and the seeds of free inquiry took root here. "Never before or since have so many men of genius appeared in the same narrow limits of space and time" [3].

Hippocrates' seminal contributions to medicine are three. He divorced the concept of etiology from divine intervention, he defined an ethical code of conduct for the physician, and he based the growth of medical knowledge upon observation and analysis rather than mysticism and conjury. These innovations define modern medicine as we know it today. Although we attribute these advances to Hippocrates, they are in fact the product of a school of thought and practice built and recorded by many. What we know of these contributions comes to us in a collection of writings known as the Hippocratic Corpus.

> In medicine, substantial amounts of the more ancient pre-aristotelian medical material were collected in the early days of the Alexandrian school, around 300 B. C. It has come down to us under the name of Hippocrates, the "father of medicine" and is known to scholars as the Hippocratic Collection. It has not reached us without considerable alteration and accretion. Many have been worked over by later hands. Some have been translated into the ionic dialect to bring them into line with more "authentic" works. Many have been annotated and interpolated. Some of a much later date have been inserted into the collection. In spite of these defects and mishaps the Hippocratic Collection is of priceless value. It contains by far the largest body of prearistotelian science that has survived. It contains the earliest complete scientific treatises that have reached us from any source or in any language.

> Each individual treatise of the Hippocratic Collection – and there are at least seventy – requires separate and individual treatment from the point of view of style, authorship, philosophical associations, language, sources, doctrine, and interpretation. We are, in fact, in the presence of not one book, or even a collection of books, but of a whole library, the items of which are separated by many centuries of time [4].

Many scholars have attempted to identify the works in the collection that were actually penned by Hippocrates. These attempts are generally subjective and based primarily on style and the acceptability of the conceptual content to the modern medical mind. W.H.S. Jones, in the 1923 Loeb Classical Library Edition, chose six treatises that he thought most likely to be "authentic": *Prognostics; Regimen in Acute Diseases; First and Third Books of the Epidemics; Aphorisms; Airs, Waters, and Places*; and three surgical works, *Fractures, The Articulations*, and *Injuries of the Head*. He skillfully summarized the medical philosophy contained in these works and, by so doing, distilled the Hippocratic approach into medical practice:

1. Diseases have a natural course, which the physician must know thoroughly so as to decide whether the issue will be favorable or fatal.
2. Diseases are caused by a disturbance in the composition of the constituents of the body. This disturbance is connected with atmospheric and climatic conditions.
3. Nature tries to bring these irregularities into a normal state by the action of innate heat which "concocts" the "crude" humors of the body.
4. There are critical days at fixed dates, when the battle between nature and the disease reaches a crisis.
5. Nature may win, in which case the morbid matters in the body are evacuated or carried off ... or the "coction" of the morbid elements may not take place, in which case, the patient dies.
6. All that the physician can do for the patient is to give nature a chance to remove by regimen all that may hinder nature in her beneficent work [5].

You will detect much that is modern here. First is the emphasis on correct diagnosis through the recognition of *syndromes* endowing the physician with foresight, *prognosis*. Second is a complete rupture with dogma-based concepts of pathophysiology. Disease is caused by an imbalance in the constituent parts of the body, a *dyscrasia*. These imbalances can be understood by careful study of the sick. Third is the concept of a natural tendency to healing. It is the physician's role to promote this tendency by removing all possible obstacles to it. In fact, if we cleave away the concept of the four humors and the notions of "coction" and "critical days," we are left with the first premises of modern medical thought.

The *Aphorisms* is the most widely read treatise in the collection. There are 422 aphorisms in the book. The most famous is the first, Section 1, Number 1 [6]:

> Life is short; art is long; opportunity fugitive; experience delusive; judgment difficult. It is the duty of the physician not only to do that which immediately belongs to him, but likewise to secure the cooperation of the sick, of those who are in attendance, and of all the external agents.

Several aphorisms are of interest to the endocrinologist:

- "If a woman who is neither pregnant, nor lately delivered, have milk in her breasts, she labors under obstructed menstruation" (Section 5, Number 39).
- "If the catamenia are suppressed, without being followed by rigor or fever, but by disinclination for food, pregnancy may be suspected" (Section 5, Number 61).
- "Eunuchs are not affected by gout, nor do they become bald" (Section 6, Number 28).

Others are not so impressive:

- "The male fetus is situate chiefly on the right, and the female on the left of the womb" (Section 5, Number 48).
- "When the pregnant uterus contains twins, if one breast becomes flaccid, one of the twins is expelled, if the right breast, the male, but if the left, the female" (Section 5, Number 38).

The Hippocratic Corpus contains a section "On the Glands" (Peri Adenos) [11]. The key passages are these:

> They do not suffer very much trouble, but when they do suffer they make the rest of the body suffer through their own ailment. But, they in turn suffer little with the rest of the body. Their ailments: pustules arise, scrofulous swellings erupt and fever grips the body. They are subject to these when they are filled with moisture from the rest of the body flowing into them.
>
> This flows from the rest of the body through the vessels, which are hollow and extend through the glands in great numbers, with the result that whatever moisture they (the vessels) draw proceeds readily into them (the glands). And, if the stream is copious and diseased, the glands become taut within themselves. In this way, fever is kindled and the glands become swollen and inflamed.

He is talking about lymph nodes.

The now classic description of the "face of death", the "Hippocratic Facies," is found in the *Prognostics* [7]:

> A sharp nose, hollow eyes, collapsed temples; the ears cold, contracted, and their lobes turned out; the skin about the forehead being rough, distended, and parched; the color of the whole face being green, black, livid, or lead colored.

Other signs of impending death include: "If he be found with his feet naked and not sufficiently warm, and the hands, neck, and legs tossed about in a disorderly manner and naked, it is bad, for it indicates aberation of the intellect."

> When ... the hands are waved before the face, hunting through empty pace, as if gathering bits of straw, picking the nap from the coverlet, or tearing chaff from the wall, all such symptoms are bad and deadly.

Shakespeare's description of the death of Falstaff in *Henry V* draws directly from the Hippocratic description:

> Hostess: Nay, sure he's not in hell: He's in Arthur's bosom, if ever a man went to Arthur's bosom. A' made a finer end, and went away, an it had been any christom child; a' parted even just between twelve and one, even at the turning o' the tide: for after I saw him fumble with

> the sheets, and play with flowers, and smile upon his fingers' ends, I knew there was but one way; for his nose was as sharp as a pen, and 'a babbled of green fields. ... a' bade me lay more clothes on his feet: I put my hand into the bed and felt them, and they were as cold as any stone; then I felt to his knees, ... and so upward and upward, and all was as cold as any stone [8].

The greatest contribution of the Hippocratic School, by all accounts, is the oath [9].

> I swear by Apollo the physician, and Asclepius, and Hygiea and Panacea, and all the gods and goddesses, that, according to my ability and judgment, I will keep this oath and this stipulation-to reckon him who taught me this art equally dear to me as my parents, to share my substance with him, and relieve his necessities if required; to look upon his offspring in the same footing as my own brothers, and to teach them this art if they shall wish to learn it, without fee or stipulation; and that by precept, lecture, and every other mode of instruction, I will impart a knowledge of the art to my own sons, and those of my teachers, and to disciples bound by a stipulation and oath according to the law of medicine, but to none others. I will follow that system of regimen which, according to my ability and judgment, I consider for the benefit of my patients, and abstain from whatever is deleterious and mischievous. I will give no deadly medicine to anyone if asked, nor suggest any such counsel; and in like manner, I will not give to a woman a pessary to produce an abortion. With purity and holiness I will pass my life and practice my art. I will not cut persons laboring under the stone, but will leave this to be done by men who are practitioners of this work. Into whatever houses I enter, I will go into them for the benefit of the sick, and will abstain from every voluntary act of mischief and corruption and, further, from the seduction of females or males, freemen and slaves. Whatever, in connection with my professional practice, or not in connection with it, I see or hear, in the life of men, which ought not to be spoken of abroad, I will not divulge, as reckoning that all such should be kept secret. While I continue to keep this Oath unviolated, may it be granted to me to enjoy life and the practice of the art, respected by all men in all times. But should I trespass and violate this Oath, may the reverse be my lot!

In this short document, Hippocrates differentiates the "profession" of medicine from a trade, defines the relationship between physician and patient, recognizes and provides for the limits of individual expertise, establishes a standard of conduct that permits only benevolent acts, and establishes a code of confidentiality. More than any other factor, the precepts in this pledge, put into action, modernized the ethics of medical practice and, as a consequence, the perception of the medical profession. Thus, Robert Louis Stevenson could write in the preface to *Underwoods*, 2400 years later:

> There are men and classes of men that stand above the common herd: the soldier, sailor and shepherd not infrequently; the artist rarely; rarer still, the clergyman; the physician almost as a rule. He is the flower (such as it is) of our civilization; and when that age of man is done with, and only to be marvelled at in history, he will be thought to have shared as little as any in the defects of the period, and most notably exhibited the virtues of the race. Generosity he has, such as is possible to those who practice an art, never to those who drive a trade; discretion, tested by a hundred secrets, tact, tried in a thousand embarrassments; and what are more important, Heraclean cheerfulness and courage. So that he brings air and cheer into the sick room, and often enough, though not so often as he wishes, brings healing.

The greatness of modern medicine is, in large measure, due to the precept that the physician works for the patient, and always in the best interest of the patient.

The current trend is for the physician to work for the best interest of a health maintenance organization, and not necessarily for the best interest of the patient. It is a system in which, often enough the physician cannot be selected, hired, or fired by the patient. The extent to which we survive this regressive step and avoid anew the characterization of physicians that began this chapter will depend upon an objective and dispassionate analysis of the effects of the coming change. Again, Hippocrates has shown us the way.

> I have written this down deliberately, believing it is valuable to learn of unsuccessful experiments and to know the causes of their failure [10].

References

1. Jones WHS: *The Works of Hippocrates*, Vol. 2. Cambridge, MA: Harvard University Press, 1957, p. 263.
2. Major RH: *A History of Medicine*, Vol. I, Springfield, IL: Charles C. Thomas, 1954, p. 188.
3. Garrison FH: *History of Medicine* (3rd edn.). Philadelphia, PA: WB Saunders, 1922, p. 86.
4. Singer C: The father of medicine. *Times Literary Supplement*, April 3, 1924, pp. 197–8.
5. Jones WHS: *The Works of Hippocrates*, Vol. 1. Cambridge, MA: Harvard University Press, 1957, p. XVI.
6. *The Genuine Works of Hippocrates*, edited by F. Adams. Special Edition, The Classics of Medicine Library. Birmingham, AL: Gryphon Editions, pp. 697ff.
7. *The Genuine Works of Hippocrates*, edited by F. Adams. Special Edition, The Classics of Medicine Library. Birmingham, AL: Gryphon Editions, pp. 236–9.
8. Shakespeare W: *The Life of King Henry V*, Act II, scene III.
9. *The Genuine Works of Hippocrates*, edited by F. Adams. Special Edition, The Classics of Medicine Library. Birmingham, AL: Gryphon Editions, pp. 779–80.
10. *The Genuine Works of Hippocrates*, edited by F. Adams. Special Edition, The Classics of Medicine Library. Birmingham, AL: Gryphon Editions, pp. 119–20.

This chapter has been reproduced from Loriaux, D. Lynn: Hippocrates. *The Endocrinologist* 1994; 4(1): 3–6.

CHAPTER 5
Aristotle
(384–322 B.C.E.)
Experiments of Nature

Aristotle was the first to describe the consequences of an endocrine ablation: castration. He and Plato were the leading intellects of Classical Greece.

Aristotle was born in 384 B.C.E. in the town of Stagira on the Aegean Sea near the Macedonian border and the modern city of Thessaloniki. His mother was from Chalcis, a town to the north of Athens on the island of Euboea. His father, Nicomachus, was a physician, a member of the "Sons of Aesclepius." He was the court physician to Amyntas II, the father of Philip of Macedon. The Hippocratic movement was well ingrained at this time. Many diseases had been recognized, and the concepts of diagnosis, syndrome, and prognosis were well established. It is thought that Aristotle studied medicine for a time. Some claim that he practiced medicine when he first went to Athens in 367 B.C. at the age of 17, but the evidence is fragmentary. Since Nicomachus died when Aristotle was 10 years old, his hopes for a career in medicine were likely thwarted without a father in the profession.

When Aristotle arrived in Athens, he enrolled in Plato's "Academy." Plato was 61 years old when Aristotle began his work with him. The focus of the Academy in this period was politics, legislation, and a growing interest in mathematics and astronomy. Aristotle stayed at the Academy for 20 years.

He modeled his writings on those of Plato, which were famous for a flowing yet lucid style with great economy of expression. Aristotle and Plato, although intellectual rivals, were on good terms and had a healthy mutual respect. When Plato died in 347 B.C.E. his nephew, Speusippus, became head of the Academy. Aristotle left soon after the appointment for a new "colonial" academy in the city of Assus, near the ancient city of Troy. Hermias, the tyrant of the region, became a pupil of Aristotle, and then a friend. Aristotle married Hermias' adopted daughter. Theophrastus, another pupil, lived on the nearby island of Lesbos and persuaded Aristotle to move to Mytilene, the capital city of Lesbos. He moved there in 344 B.C.E. and spent 2 years studying marine biology.

A Biographical History of Endocrinology, First Edition. D. Lynn Loriaux.

This work is a co-publication between the Endocrine Society and John Wiley & Sons, Ltd.

Aristotle returned to Macedonia in 342 B.C.E. as tutor to the young Alexander. Aristotle was known and respected at the Macedonian Court for his great intellect and skills as a teacher. His association with Hermias, who at the time was planning an expedition against the Persians with Philip, facilitated the appointment. Aristotle remained in Macedonia for 7 years, 3 of which were spent as mentor to Alexander, who was 13 years old when his studies with Aristotle began. When Philip left for the Persian campaign in 340 B.C.E., Alexander became regent of Macedonia and Aristotle saw less of him. Alexander admired Aristotle to the extent that he took Aristotle's nephew, Callisthenes, with him as his historian on the great expedition to the east. He sent many specimens of flora and fauna to Artistotle for study. When Alexander became king in 336 B.C.E., Aristotle returned to Athens.

In Athens, Aristotle's friend Xenocrates had become head of the Academy. Aristotle established a new school, the Lyceum. The Lyceum was also known as the peripatetic school after the habit of the headmaster to teach while walking with students around the school on a path that wound through the gardens. The mornings were devoted to the difficult subjects in philosophy, and the afternoons to rhetoric and dialectic. It is believed that the bulk of Aristotle's writings represent lectures he prepared for his courses at the Lyceum.

His works of "compilation" almost certainly belong to these years. He drew up lists of the victors in the Pythian and Olympic Games. He made a chronology of Athenian drama which remains the basis for dating Greek plays. He organized the collection of 58 Greek "constitutions," and his work "On the Athenian Constitution," is the only extant contemporary study of the subject. He also wrote an account of the "Customs of Barbarians" and a treatise on "Cases of Constitutional Law." The results of his work on natural history are, however, his greatest legacy, and are remarkable for their modernity, especially his "History of Animals." It is in this work we find a passage of great interest to endocrinologists:

> Some animals change their form and character, not only at certain ages and at certain seasons, but in consequence of being castrated; and all animals possessed of testicles may be submitted to this operation. Birds have their testicles inside, and oviparous quadrupeds close to the loins; and of viviparous animals that walk some have them inside, and most have them outside, but all have them at the lower end of the belly. Birds are castrated at the rump where the 2 sexes unite in copulation. If you burn this twice or thrice with hot irons, then, if the bird be full-grown, his crest grows sallow, he ceases to crow, and foregoes sexual passion; but if you cauterize the bird when young, none of these male attributes or propensities will come to him as he grows up. The case is the same with men: if you mutilate them in boyhood, the later-growing hair never comes, the voice never changes but remains high-pitched; if they be mutilated in early manhood, the late growths of hair quit them except the growth on the groin, and that diminishes but does not entirely depart. The congenital growths of hair never fall out, for a eunuch never grows bald [1].

Alexander died in 323 B.C.E. While he was alive, Aristotle enjoyed the protection of Antipater who oversaw Alexander's affairs in Greece. With the news of Alexander's death, the Athenian party staged an uprising directed at Antipater and, through him, at Aristotle. Aristotle was charged with impiety because of a eulogy he had written for Hermias many years before. Fearing for his life, he fled Athens to his mother's property in Chalcis. He lived only a few months more, dying in 322 B.C.E.

Aristotle determined, in great measure, the form and direction of western intellectual growth. His range of erudition stretches credulity. He worked in physics, chemistry, zoology, biology, botany, psychology, politics and ethics, logic and metaphysics, history, literary theory, rhetoric, and dialectic. He created formal logic (Aristotelian logic) and began the formal study of zoology. In the latter case, the fragment cited above gives us a glimpse of his remarkable insight and attention to detail. His father was a physician, and many believe that by training, he was too. His historical importance in the development of western culture stands first in the universe of scholars.

Reference

1. *Aristotle: History of Animals*, edited by DM Balme. Cambridge, MA: Harvard University Press, 1991, p. 157.

This chapter has been reproduced from Loriaux, D. Lynn: Aristotle (384–322 BC). *The Endocrinologist* 2005; 15(4): 197–8.

CHAPTER 6
Soranus of Ephesus (98–138 C.E.)
Obstetrics and Gynecology

In 1936, Dr. Norman E. Himes published a scholarly and well-researched book on the history of contraception, which remains unparalleled for its descriptions of the attempts of various civilizations to control population growth. The book, called *Medical History of Contraception*, has an unusual dedication [1]:

To
Soranos
(98–138)
Most brilliant gynecologist of antiquity,
whose originality and distinguished career
illuminated a future path of medicine
for nearly two thousand years.

Soranus is considered to have been the first specialist in obstetrics and gynecology. He was born of Greek parents, in Ephesus in 98 C.E. He studied medicine in Alexandria and practiced in Rome at the time of Trajan and Hadrian. Although his main interests were obstetrics, gynecology, and pediatrics, he wrote on everything. His major text, *Gynecology*, was written in the first half of the second century. He died about 40 years before Galen wrote his major works.

Ephesus is located near the modern city of Izmir, Turkey. It was a port city founded in the eleventh century B.C.E. by Ionian Greeks. Possession of the city changed with each century's latest conqueror. After the Persians were driven out by Alexander in 333 B.C.E. Ephesus flourished under Macedonian rule. The city became Roman in 189 B.C.E. and remained a commercial center until it declined under the Byzantine Empire. The harbor filled with silt and it was abandoned in the fourteenth century.

At the time Soranus came to Rome, there were two principal medical schools of thought. The Methodists were followers of Asclepius and promoted the Hippocratic belief that disease was a problem separate from the body and the soul (i.e., it resided within the patient and was influenced by all that the individual did). The Methodists

A Biographical History of Endocrinology, First Edition. D. Lynn Loriaux.

believed that the body was composed of "atoms" and that if these became too constricted they should be treated with laxatives, and if too relaxed, they should be treated with astringents. That some disorders seemed to be a mixture of the two extremes and required simultaneous opposing treatments was a vexing problem. The Methodists were probably good physicians, largely because they advocated fresh food, exercise, and rest to let the atoms work out their own problems.

The other school, the Empiricists, believed in observation and experimentation. By noting what worked on one patient, the same treatment could be applied to similar cases. The Empiricists used everything at their disposal, including bleeding and purging, and tended to overtreat their patients [2].

Soranus was a Methodist. He brought a new intelligence to contemporary medical writing. He wrote treatises "On Acute and Chronic Disease," "On the Signs of Fracture" and, most importantly, "Diseases of Women." He would begin his chapters with a review of the literature before he went on to describe the causes, symptoms, and treatment. He was one of the first physicians who refused to accept blindly the beliefs held by his predecessors. His text was in Greek and it continued to be an important resource for 1500 years, at which time it was lost. It was rediscovered in 1838 and translated into Latin, German, French, and English, continuing to influence the practice of medicine until the early twentieth century.

Soranus described human dissections and noted several differences between humans and "dumb beasts." He knew that the uterus was not essential to life, and he observed that amenorrhea was linked to lactation. He further observed that amenorrhea could occur in the young, the aged, the pregnant, in singers, and in those who take too much exercise. He advocated taking a careful history, and cautioned that not all cases of amenorrhea required treatment. His treatment consisted of rest, warmth, and quiet.

He wrote an entire chapter on "The Debilitated or Atonic Uterus." This condition was associated with abnormal menstruation, abortions, and premature labor. He did not approve of treating a prolapsed uterus by giving the patient cold barley-water to drink after being suspended head down on a ladder for a day and a night. Nor did he approve of using a bellows to blow the uterus back into position. He did, however, use half a pomegranate soaked in vinegar as a pessary [3].

He recorded many observations of interest to endocrinologists, commenting on the melasma of pregnancy, the association of amenorrhea with women who were masculine in appearance, and clitoral enlargement in women who had the characteristics of what we now recognize as congenital adrenal hyperplasia.

Population control was a problem that received considerable attention by Greek physicians and writers. Plato and Aristotle both argued in favor of "zero" population growth. It was Soranus who first taught specific techniques of contraception, some of which were based on an inadequate understanding of the menstrual cycle.

> People should abstain from coitus at the times we have indicated as especially dangerous, that is, the time directly before and after menstruation. Further, the woman ought in the moment during coitus when the man ejaculates his sperm, to hold her breath, draw her body back a little

so that the semen cannot penetrate into the os uterus, then immediately get up and sit down with bent knees, and in this position, provoke sneezes.

Conception is prevented by smearing the mouth of the womb with old (sour) oil or honey or cedar gum or opobalsam (balm Gilead), either alone or mixed with ceruse (white lead), or with an ointment prepared with myrtle oil and ceruse, or with alum, which is likewise to be watered before coitus, or galbanum in wine. Soft wool introduced into the mouth of the womb or the use of astringent or occlusive pessaries before coitus are also effective. For, if such means operate astringently and cooling, they close the mouth of the womb before the moment of coitus and prevent the entrance of the sperm into the os uteri [4].

Soranus seems to have been the first to emphasize that the best way to avoid repeated therapeutic abortions was to prevent conception. He scoffed at the use of magic in the form of amulets and talismans. He gave explicit directions on how to make concoctions that combined a barrier with a spermicidal preparation. He favored making pulps from nuts and fruits (probably very acidic and spermicidal) and described 40 different combinations. He warned about using potions to be taken orally, noting that this attempt to prevent conception causes considerable damage. Soranus compared a woman made old before her time by multiple pregnancies to an exhausted agricultural field.

In Rome, unmarried citizens could not inherit property, and married citizens without children could receive only half of their inheritance. Citizens with three children were not taxed, but to have more than three children was exceptional (the economic burden of a large family was well-recognized). The citizens of Rome were interested in limiting family size and providing optimum birthing and care of children, especially in the face of high infant mortality rates. These were important reasons for the success of Soranus' writings.

Soranus' observations on pediatric nutrition and hygiene include the first recognizable account of rickets. He was the first to describe "version" (turning) of the fetus during delivery. More importantly, he discouraged the use of brute force and other dangerous treatments.

References

1. Himes NE: *Medical History of Contraception*. Baltimore, MD: Williams & Wilkins, 1936.
2. Graham H: *Eternal Eve. The History of Gynaecology & Obstetrics*. Garden City, NY: Doubleday & Company, 1951.
3. Medvei VC: *A History of Endocrinology*. Lancaster: MTP Press, 1982.
4. Temkin O (trans.): *Soranus' Gynecology*. Baltimore, MD: Johns Hopkins Press, 1956.

This chapter has been reproduced from Speroff, Leon: Soranus of Ephesus. *The Endocrinologist* 1994; 4(4): 230–2.

CHAPTER 7

Aretaeus of Cappadocia (First and Second Centuries C.E.)

The most remarkable thing about Aretaeus is the disparity between the quality of writing that characterizes all of his extant works, and the abject paucity of what we know about him. The only fact that is uniformly agreed is that his roots were in Cappadocia. Cappadocia is an arid highland in the east of Turkey. The Euphrates River marks its eastern extent before it bends to the south and flows through Mesopotamia. It is an area famous for its underground cities. More than 200 have been excavated. Cappadocia was a Roman province and a buffer to the East for 800 years beginning in 17 C.E.

It is generally thought that Aretaeus and Galen were contemporaries. It is said that Aretaeus studied at the Asclepion of Pergamon and spent time studying anatomy and physiology in Alexandria, as did Galen. He is also thought to have practiced medicine in Rome, as did Galen. The "Rome" conclusion is based entirely one of Aretaeus' prescriptions for wines known only to be available in Rome: Falernian, Jundau, Signine, and Surrentine. Flimsy evidence.

If it is true that Aretaeus lived in Rome at the same time as Galen, however, it is most remarkable that he never mentions Galen, and that Galen never mentions Aretaeus. For me, this confirms that they were not contemporaries. Other more erudite scholars of the period, however, have a different view. Francis Adams, who translated Aretaeus' works from Latin to English in 1856 for the Sydenham Society, wrote the following in his Editor's Preface [1]:

> Nothing definite can be determined respecting the age in which Aretaeus flourished, beyond a probable approximation to the period. When we take into account how eminent both Galen and he were, as professional authorities, it appears singular that neither of them should have made the slightest allusion to the other. For, on the one hand, considering how voluminous the works of Galen are, and the frequency with which he refers to the names of almost every author at all distinguished in the literature of medicine, from Hippocrates down to his own day, one cannot but think it improbable that he would have neglected to mention Aretaeus if the latter had acquired his mature reputation at the time when Galen was engaged with the

A Biographical History of Endocrinology, First Edition. D. Lynn Loriaux.

This work is a co-publication between the Endocrine Society and John Wiley & Sons, Ltd.

composition of his own works. And, on the other hand, Galen, both in his lifetime, and for many centuries afterward, was so indisputably regarded as the *facile princeps* of medical authorities, that one cannot conceive it at all likely that a subsequent writer would have treated in an elaborate and critical manner of the same subjects, without making any allusion to doctrines which were then commanding such universal applause. We cannot, then, reconcile these difficulties otherwise than by supposing that the two authors must have been contemporaries; and that whether from a concealed feeling of rivalry, or in accordance with the established usage of living authors to one another, the one had avoided to mention the other. It is deserving of remark that we have a still more extraordinary example of two contemporary authors under similar circumstances, mutually neglecting to quote one another, in the case of two writers who lived a short time before Galen, namely Dioscorides and the Elder Pliny; both of whom are most voluminous and accurate writers, and both handle the same subjects critically, yet, as we have stated, neither of them takes the slightest notice of the other. In this instance, indeed, there are various circumstances which lead us to infer that the Roman writer, who is merely a great compiler on all subjects, was indebted to the Greek authority on the Materia Medica, and hence the learned are pretty generally agreed that the work of Dioscorides must have preceded that of Pliny, although both were productions of the same age. One thing, at least is indisputable respecting them, as every person familiar with their productions must be convinced, that there is such a congeniality and accordance between their opinions on various subjects which they treat of in common, that we can have no hesitation in setting them down as authors who had lived about the same time. And I am clearly of opinion from my long familiarity with the works of Galen and Aretaeus, that one can decidedly detect a corresponding coincidence between the literary and professional views of these authors. Both had chosen Hippocrates for their model, and had their minds thoroughly imbued with his opinions. Both show an intimate acquaintance with the true spirit of the Platonic philosophy, as manifested in the first and succeeding centuries. Both display a great acquaintance with Sphygmology, and use the same identical terms in describing the varied conditions of the arterial pulse. Both possess a more intimate knowledge of Anatomy than any of the other authorities on ancient medicine. In Therapeutics, also, there is a striking coincidence between them; and, in regard to the Materia Medica, both not only prescribe the same simples, but also, in many instances, the same compound medicines. Altogether, then, there is such a conformity between both their theoretical and practical views in their profession as we never find to exist except between authors who lived in or about the same period. It is true there is one striking difference between them – one writes modern Attic in a style worthy of Xenophon or Theophrastus, whereas the other uses Ionic or old Attic, bearing a considerable resemblance to the language of Hippocrates and Herodotus. This, however, when attentively considered, will be found to be a confirmation of my views regarding the identity of the age in in which the two authors in question flourished; for it would appear to have been the practice of learned men in the second century, from some unexplained taste, to write sometimes in the one dialect and sometimes in the other. Thus Arrian, who flourished in the earlier part of that century – that is to say, immediately before Galen – although in most of his historical philosophical works he uses very pure Attic, has made use of Ionic, or at least a modified imitation of it, in one of his works, the *Indica*. In like manner his contemporary Lucian, whose general style is chaste and elegant Attic, has left among his books two tracts written in the Ionic dialect, namely *de dea Syria* and de *Astrologia*. In the same way we can account for a difference between the practice of our two authors in regard to the class of poets which they familiarly quote, our author always quoting Homer, and Galen the dramatic poets; for this difference of taste is obviously the necessary consequence of the style affected by each of them, since the Ionic dialect is inseparably connected with the Homeric poems, and the Attic with the Athenian drama.

From what has been stated it will be seen there is a large amount of probabilities that our author must have been a contemporary of Galen, respecting who it is satisfactorily ascertained that he was born AD 131, and that he died about the end of that century. We cannot then be far from the truth if we assume it as a settled point in the chronology of medical literature that Aretaeus flourished about the middle of the second century of the Christian era."

What everyone agrees upon is the efficiency, economy, and clarity of Aretaeus' prose when compared to Galen. Galen can be stiff. Aretaeus flows. There is an explanation for this. Galen's writings resurfaced after the Dark Ages by making the "grand circuit:" Rome to Constantinople, Constantinople to Edessa to Jundi Shapur, Jundi Shapur to Baghdad, and finally to the translators in Toledo and Monte Casino. Greek to Latin, Latin to Farsi, Farsi to Syrine, Syrine to Latin. Aretaeus, on the other hand, was translated only once, from Greek to Latin, by Paulus Crassus, in Venice in 1552. Aretaeus avoided the grand circuit and all of the literary corruption associated with it. Aretaeus reached Venice when the Byzantine scholars fled Constantinople as it fell to the Turks in 1453. They took the manuscripts to Italy. Aretaeus' original Greek edition was published for all to see and read in 1554. When we read Aretaeus in English, there have been, at most, two translations. It makes all the difference. Here are some of Aretaeus' writings for you to judge yourself, starting with the most celebrated.

On diabetes

Diabetes is a wonderful affliction, not very frequent among men, being a melting down of the flesh and limbs into urine. Its cause is of a cold and humid nature, as in dropsy. The course is the common one, namely, the kidneys and bladder; for the patients never stop making water, but the flow is incessant, as if from the opening of aqueducts. The nature of the disease, then, is chronic, and it takes a long period to form; but the patient is short-lived if the constitution of the disease be completely established; for the melting is rapid, the death speedy. Moreover, life is disgusting and painful; thirst, unquenchable; excessive drinking, which, however, is disproportionate to the large quantity of urine, for more urine is passed; and one cannot stop them either from drinking or making water. Or if for a time they abstain from drinking, their mouth becomes parched and their body dry; the viscera seem as if scorched up; they are affected with nausea, restlessness, and a burning thirst; and at not distant term they expire [2].

On tetanus

Tetanus, in all its varieties, is a spasm of an exceedingly painful nature, very swift to prove fatal, but neither easy to be removed. They are affections of the muscles and tendons about the jaws; but the illness is communicated to the whole frame, for all parts are affected sympathetically with the primary organs. There are three forms of the convulsion, namely, in a straight line, backwards, and forwards. Tetanus is in a direct line, when the person laboring under the distention is stretched out straight and inflexible. The contractions forwards and backwards have their appellation from the tension and the place; for that backwards we call Opisthotonos; and that variety we call Emprosthotonos in which the patient is bent forwards by the anterior nerves. For the Greek word τόνος is applied both to a nerve, and to signify tension.

The causes of these complaints are many; for some are apt to supervene on the wound of a membrane, or of muscles, or of punctured nerves, when, for the most part, the patients die. Spasm from a wound is fatal. And women also suffer from this spasm after abortion; and, in this case, they seldom recover [2, p. 246].

On rabies

But likewise a man will be seized with rabies, from respiring of the effluvia of the tongue of a dog, without ever having been bitten [2, p. 250].

On the paroxysm of epilepsy

But, if it be near the accession of the paroxysm, there are before the sight circular flashes of purple or black colors, or all mixed together, so as to exhibit the appearance of the rainbow expanded in the heavens; noises in the ears; a heavy smell; they are passionate, and unreasonably peevish. They fall down, some from any such cause as lowness of spirits, but others from gazing intently on a running stream, a rolling wheel, or a turning top [2, p. 243].

On melancholy

A story is told, that a certain person, uncertainly affected, fell in love with a girl; and when the physicians could bring him no relief, love cured him. But I think that he was originally in love, and that he was dejected and spiritless from being unsuccessful with the girl and appeared to the common people to be melancholic. He then did not know that it was love; but when he imparted the love to the girl, he ceased from his dejection, and dispelled his passion and sorrow; and with joy he awoke from his lower of spirits, and he became restored to understanding, love being his physician [2, p. 300].

There are no words for these descriptions of disease other than "the best." He is in a league of his own. No one else comes close. I save the best for last.

On the stomachic affections

It is familiar to such persons as from their necessities live on a slender and hard diet; and to those who, for the sake of education, are laborious and persevering; whose portion is the love of divine science, along with scanty food, want of sleep, and the meditation on wise sayings, whose lot is the contempt of a full and multifarious diet; to whom hunger is for food, water for drink, and watchfulness in place of rest; to whom in place of a soft couch, is a hammock on the ground without bed-clothes; a mean coverlet, a porous mantle, and the only shelter to whose

> head is the common air; whose wealth consists in the abundant possession and use of divine thought for all these things they account good from love of learning; and, if they like any food, it is of the most frugal description, and not to satisfy the palate, but solely to preserve life; no quaffing of wine to intoxication, no recreation, no roving or jaunting about; no bodily exercise nor plumpness of flesh; for what is there from which the love of learning will not allure one? – from country, parents, brothers, oneself, even unto death. Hence, to them, emaciation of the frame; they are ill-complexioned; even in youth they appear old and dotard in understanding; in mind cheerless and inflexible; depraved appetite, speedy satiety of the accustomed slender and ordinary food, and from want of familiarity with a varied diet, a loathing of all savory viands; for it they take any unusual article of food, they are injured thereby and straightway abominate food of all kinds. It is a chronic disease of the stomach [2, p. 349].

The person Aretaeus describes is himself. Galen was a physician to the emperors of Rome and Aretaeus was an itinerate physician to the poor, the hoi polloi. Galen and Aretaeus lived in the same time, but far apart in station. They never crossed paths. They never knew of each other. What we have is probably all that Aretaeus ever wrote. He wrote it himself, no secretaries. His material was mostly unknown and, hence, did not go with Nestorians to Jundi Shapur. Lucky for us that some poor scholar, fleeing Constantinople, gathered scrolls on his way out, and sold them to the first interested person in Venice to get enough money to live. Luckily, it was translated, and only once, from Greek to Latin. It gives us our best chance to see clearly the life of one of history's greatest physicians, Aretaeus of Cappadocia.

References

1. *The Extant Works of Aretaeus, the Cappadocian,* edited and translated by Francis Adams. London: Sydenham Society, 1856.
2. *The Extant Works of Aretaeus, the Cappadocian.* Special Edition. Birmingham, AL: Gryphon Editions, 1990.

CHAPTER 8
Galen
(130–200)
The First "Human Anatomy"

Galen was the greatest physician of antiquity after Hippocrates. His anatomical texts and system of medicine dominated the profession during his lifetime and for 1500 years thereafter.

From the fifteenth century on, Galen is usually referred to as "Cl. Galen." This was assumed to mean that his first name was Claudius, but the Cl. is now known to refer to Clarisimus, "most brilliant." His first name remains unknown.

Galen was born about 130 C.E. on a farm on the outskirts of the Greek city of Pergamon [1]. The ruins of this city are near present-day Bergama in western Turkey. Pergamon was situated atop a 1000-foot prominence overlooking the confluence of three rivers in a beautiful and fertile valley. One of the most striking cities of antiquity, its architecture and school of sculpture were among the best of the Hellenistic period. ("The Dying Gaul," in the Capitoline Museum in Rome, is a surviving example of the brilliance of Pergamene sculpture.)

Galen's mother was said to be a difficult woman who was "quarrelsome, frequently bit her servants, and fought with her husband worse than Xantippe with Socrates" [2]. His father, a prominent architect in Pergamon, was intelligent and nurturing and had an intense interest in Galen's intellectual development. He ensured that the young Galen had a broad and liberal education. He studied all of the four leading "systems" of the time: Platonism, Aristotelianism, Stoicism, and Epicureanism. When he was 17, he began his studies at the Asclepion of Pergamon. The Asclepion, a precursor of the modern "medical center," was the most important building in Pergamon. It was a healing center, a medical school, a religious sanctuary, and a "recreation center" where rhapsodists, musicians, and thespians entertained [3]. In the second century, the Asclepion of Pergamon was a magnet for pilgrims in need of healing. In the Byzantine era, it was one of the "wonders of the world." Pergamon was perhaps the leading medical center of its time and it was here that Galen began the study of anatomy under the tutelage of Satyros, the leading anatomist of the day.

A Biographical History of Endocrinology, First Edition. D. Lynn Loriaux.

This work is a co-publication between the Endocrine Society and John Wiley & Sons, Ltd.

Four years later, after the death of his father, Galen left Pergamon for Alexandria, which was the scientific center of the Empire, with the largest library in the world. Alexandria had nurtured many of the greatest scientists of antiquity: Hipparchus, Ptolemy, Herophilus, and Dioscorides, among others. Galen stayed there at least 5 years. He focused on the study of anatomy, but also began the study of medicine in earnest. He said he was disappointed by medical education in Alexandria: "The art of medicine was taught by ignoramuses in a sophistical fashion in long illogical lectures to crowds of 14-year-old boys who never got near the sick." Critical of the careless use of medical terms, Galen began his extraordinary career as a medical writer with a general dictionary in 45 books, and a medical dictionary in 5. Neither survives.

Galen returned to Pergamon as a physician, and was promptly appointed "physician to the gladiators." This was a desirable appointment because, in a social climate that discouraged dissection of human subjects, Galen could study human anatomy *in vivo* as it was displayed by his grievously injured patients. A sudden and unexpected war between Pergamon and the Galatians put an end to the gladiatorial games, and Galen left for Rome to "try his luck." He quickly established a successful medical practice among the upper classes and the nobility and, with time, became physician to the Emperor. Suddenly, he was one of the most prominent persons in the "Eternal City." All was abandoned after only 4 years, however, with the appearance of the "Plague of the Antonines." This plague, probably typhus or smallpox, induced many to leave the capital city, Galen among them. He returned to Pergamon, but was soon ordered to the Roman imperial camp at Aquileia where Marcus Aurelius appointed him chief court physician and sent him back to Rome to oversee the health of the royal family. He continued as court physician through the reign of Marcus Aurelius, the reign of Commodus, his despotic son, and into the reign of Septimus Severus.

Galen remained in Rome for more than 20 years, years of almost unbelievable productivity. He left for the last time in 192 C.E. following the catastrophic fire that destroyed the Temple of Peace on the Via Sacra and, with it, many of Galen's most important philosophical treatises in manuscript form. He returned to his place of birth to spend the remainder of his life in study and meditation interspersed with travel. He died on one such trip, probably in Sicily, at the age of 70 years.

"No physician, before or since, has exercised so great an influence on medical history. For 14 centuries, physicians followed his words with the same veneration and feeling for infallibility as the theologians followed the teachings of the church fathers" [2]. Galen wrote in Greek. He wrote 125 books on the general topics of philosophy, mathematics, grammar, and law. We know of 126 medical texts, 43 of which are lost. In addition, 19 book fragments and 15 commentaries have been published. There are 80 fragments as yet unpublished. The works on medicine alone exceed 2.5 million words. It is likely that this represents less than two-thirds of what he wrote. The standard edition of Galen's works (published by Carolus Kuhn, Leipzig, 1821) is 22 volumes in length. Of Galen's works, three were most influential: the *Ars Medica*, a general abridgment of his encyclopedic text of medicine, the *Megatechne* or *Ars Magna*; his anatomical text, *De Usu Partium Corporis Humani* (the use of the parts of the human body); and his guide to dissection in 15 volumes, *De Anatomicis Administrationibus*.

Galen's medicine was based on the theory of temperaments. The theory derived from the tradition of the four elements (earth, air, fire, and water), the four qualities (dry, wet, cold, and hot), and the four humors (blood, yellow bile, black bile, and phlegm). Galen believed that there were four "healthy" dispositions: sanguine (hot and wet), phlegmatic (cold and wet), choleric (hot and dry), and melancholic (cold and dry). Deviations from one's fundamental disposition indicated an improper mixing of the humors (dyscrasia) and provided a rational basis for therapy. The theory, first alluded to in the Hippocratic treatise on the nature of man, was powerfully expanded and embellished by Galen (Pericrasion, *De Temperamentis*) and it became the foundation of medical thought for 1500 years. Without a thorough understanding of the theory, diagnosis and rational therapy were believed impossible.

Galen's osteology was based on study of the human skeleton. He divided the bones into long bones and flat bones, distinguishing between the apophyses, epiphyses, and diaphyses. He also distinguished diarthroses (articulations with movement) from synarthroses (articulations without movement). The rest of his anatomy, however, was based largely on dissections of animals, primarily swine and the Barbary ape, a macaque indigenous to northern Africa. Nonetheless, he described much that accurately reflects the human anatomy. His descriptions of the large muscles of the body are still used in textbooks of anatomy. He also described the dura and pia mater, the corpus callosum, the third and fourth ventricles, and all of the cranial nerves. He noted that the heart has four cavities and four orifices, three with valves of three leaves, one with a valve of two.

Galen's most serious error was his concept of the circulation of the blood. He believed that the liver was the center of the venous system and that it introduced a natural spirit into the blood that was then distributed to the rest of the body. The venous blood entered the lungs via the right side of the heart and discharged impurities into exhaled air. His theory was that the arterial blood extracted a "vital spirit" from a "world spirit" in inhaled air and, in turn, transmitted it to the rest of the body. This spirit was transformed into the "animal spirit" in the brain, and the waste products of the reaction gravitated down through the pituitary stalk into the pituitary gland, where they were discharged through ducts in the ethmoid and sphenoid bones into the nasopharynx, appearing as nasal mucus, or "pituita" [4]. This concept of pituitary function prevailed for more than 1500 years until Schneider [5] and Lower [6] showed in the seventeenth century that no connections exist between the ventricles of the brain and the nasopharynx. Galen's concept of the three spirits and the movement of the blood to and fro dominated physiological thought until William Harvey dispelled the idea in 1628.

Galen was among the first to recognize the ductless glands:

> The neck has two glands in which moisture is generated, as in the epiglottis a thick and viscid humor is secreted for the moistening of that organ. But from the true glands which are in the neck and from the substance of the epiglottis there are no ducts through which the humor may flow, as in the case of the two glands of the tongue. But those which are in the neck are of a spongy nature and from them the humor oozes out and trickles down, there being no necessity for ducts (which the others need) whereby the fluid may be carried [7].

Following the collapse of the Western Roman Empire, Galen's written works survived in Constantinople and continued as the basis of Byzantine medicine. With the decline of that culture, the works were translated into Arabic. The process seems to have begun in earnest in the ninth century in Baghdad. These translations formed the backbone of Arabic medicine and reached their full influence in the *Canon of Avicenna*, which was "the most famous medical textbook ever written" according to William Osler. With the expansion of the Islamic empire, Galen's writings followed its advance and were re-introduced into Europe in Spain and southern France. The immense task of re-translation into Latin was begun in monasteries like Monte Casino in the latter half of the eleventh century. Three hundred years were required to complete the effort. These translations provided the theoretical core of medieval European medicine and remained unchallenged until the Renaissance.

With the death of Galen, innovation in medicine fell into a state of suspended animation. The next great innovator was Vesalius in the sixteenth century, followed by William Harvey in the seventeenth. There are many explanations for the durability of Galen's anatomy, physiology, and medicine. These include the debilitating effects of the ongoing assault on civilization by the armies of the Khans, the proscriptions against human dissection in the Arabic culture, and the natural tendency to seek and accept authority by the Christians of medieval Europe. All play some role, but the primary reason probably resides in the exceptional quality and immense breadth of Galen's written legacy. He was a giant among men. For such people, an "incidence" of one in every 1500 years is not unreasonable.

References

1. Garrison FH: *History of Medicine* (3rd edn.). Philadelphia, PA: Saunders, 1922, p. 103.
2. Major RH: *A History of Medicine*. Springfield, IL: Charles Thomas, 1954, p. 188.
3. Sarton G: *Galen of Pergamon*. Lawrence, KS: University of Kansas Press, 1954, p. 12
4. Harris GW: Humours and hormones. *J Endocrinol* 1971; 53: ii–xxiii.
5. Schneider CV: *Liber Primus de Catarrhis*. Wittebergae: T. Mevii and E. Schumacheri, 1660.
6. Lower R: *Tractatus de Corde. Dissertatio de Origine Catarrhi in qua Ostenditur Ilium non Provenire a Cerebro*. Londini: J. Redmayne, 1670, pp. 221–39.
7. Medvei VC: *A History of Endocrinology*. Lancaster: MTP Press, 1982, p. 64.

This chapter has been reproduced from Loriaux, D. Lynn: Galen. *The Endocrinologist* 1993; 3(3): 163–5.

CHAPTER 9
Avicenna (980–1037 C.E.)
Preservation of "Classical" Medicine

The medicine of Classical Greece and Rome, Hippocrates and Galen, is the foundation on which the renaissance in western medicine, marked by the publication of Vesalius' *De Humani Corporis Fabrica* in 1543, is based. These classics, however, were nowhere to be found in medieval Europe between the years of 410 C.E., when Rome was sacked by Alaric, and 1080 C.E., when Constantinus Africanus published the *Canon of Avicenna* as his own work in Salernum. Where were these classics in this period and how did they return?

Galen died in 200 C.E., the high water mark of the classical period. Rome fell to Alaric and the Visigoths in 410, followed by repeated ravages by the Goths and the Huns. Its strength was undermined by the rise of Christianity, which challenged its religion, by disease (malaria and plague), which sapped its strength, and by the barbarian horde, which shook its confidence. Constantine, in 326, changed the official religion of Rome to Christianity and moved the capital to Byzantium, a Greek city on the Bosphorus. This denervated eastern remnant of Roman glory lasted until 1453, when Constantinople was swept away by Muhammad II. The darkness that was the medieval period, however, had long since descended upon the continent.

The Council of Ephesus, in 431 C.E., deposed Nestorius as patriarch of Constantinople and excommunicated him and all of his followers. The cause of this was the Nestorian heresy: Mary was the mother of Jesus but was not the mother of God. The Nestorians were banished and fled, first to the city of Edessa in Asia Minor. There they established one of the great universities of the time, based on Greek and Roman science, literature, and medicine. Within 20 years, however, the Nestorians were again displaced, and many of the academics escaped to the city of Jundi Shapur in Persia. There a university was built around them, and the formidable work of translating the classics into Persian and Syriac began.

Mohammed and a small band of followers fled to Medina-Hejira in 622 C.E., marking the first year of the Muslim calendar. One hundred years later, the Muslim empire extended from Asia Minor across Egypt and Northern Africa and Spain to the Pyrenees.

A Biographical History of Endocrinology, First Edition. D. Lynn Loriaux.

This work is a co-publication between the Endocrine Society and John Wiley & Sons, Ltd.

Charles Martel ended the advance at the battle of Tours in 732. Baghdad became the capital of the Eastern Caliphate, Cordoba in the west. The University of Jundi Shapur, now part of Islam, was encouraged, supported, and ultimately moved to Baghdad a century later. In Baghdad, the translation of the classics from Persian, Syriac, Greek, and Latin into Arabic began. The first of the great translators was Yuhanna Ibn Musawayh, Mesue, a Nestorian Christian (777–857). He was physician to four caliphs and president of the College of Translators for 50 years. One of his students, Johannitius, a Christian from Hira, was dismissed by Mesue for disturbing his lectures with too many questions. Several years later, a former classmate recognized him as a street person. Johannitius said that after his dismissal he had decided to suspend the study of medicine while he learned Greek. Johannitius showed his friend his translation of the Aphorisms of Hippocrates. When the translation was shown to Mesue, a reconciliation was effected and one of the most important academic collaborations of all time ensued. Together, all of the works of Galen, Oreibasios, the seven books of Paul of Aegina, the *Materia Medica* of Dioscorides, the entire *Corpus Hippocraticum*, the *Organon*, *Metaphysics*, *Ethics*, and *Physics* of Aristotle, the *Politics*, *Laws*, and *Timaeus* of Plato, the *Mathematics* of Menelaus, Autolycus, and Archimedes, Porphyry's *Isagoge*, the Quadripartitum of Ptolemy, and the Septuagint (the Greek Old Testament).

These two men saved the core of classical learning from almost certain extinction, and their work provided the foundation of Arabic learning, including Arabic medicine. This body of knowledge was codified into the most famous medical textbook of all time, the *Canon of Avicenna*. Avicenna was born in Afshana, Persia. His father was a tax collector. At the age of 10, he had memorized the Koran. In succession, he devoted himself to the study of law, mathematics, physics, and philosophy. He began the study of medicine at 16. When he was 18 years of age, his reputation as a physician was such that he was summoned to court to treat a favorite son of the Caliph. The prince's recovery gained Avicenna access to the royal libraries and other academic resources. Three years later, Avicenna completed his encyclopedia of all sciences but mathematics.

Leclerc writes that "Avicenna is an intellectual phenomenon. Never, perhaps, has an example been seen of so precocious, quick, and wide an intellect, extending and asserting itself with so strong and indefatigable an activity" [1]. This energy produced 20 books on religion, philosophy, astronomy, and poetry. His poetry was written in Persian and is believed by some scholars to be the finest ever written in that language. Some quatrains attributed to Omar Khayam now are believed to be from the pen of Avicenna.

Major describes Avicenna thus:

> Avicenna's philosophical writings have placed him at the pinnacle of Arabic philosophy with only one possible rival, Averrhoes. His philosophy was in the main the cool, intellectual view of Aristotle, tempered by the mysticism of Plotinus and the Neo-Platonists.
>
> Avicenna's works on mathematics are striking and original. In physics, he studied motion, contact, force, vacuum, heat and light, suggesting that the speed of light was capable of being measured. He studied the physics of musical tones and of harmony and wrote extensively on mineralogy and chemistry, refuting the theory of the transmutation of metals and holding that

differences between metals were fundamental, a view in opposition to the prevailing theories of the alchemist.

His 100 odd books are overshadowed by his great Canon (Al Qanun) "the most famous medical text book ever written" and "a medical bible for a longer period than any other work". Five hundred years after it was written, the Canon was a required textbook at the University of Vienna.

In this work, a huge tome containing more than 1,000,000 words, Avicenna attempted to codify all existing medical knowledge, just as a jurist might attempt to codify and bring into harmony all existing legal knowledge. Avicenna attempted to write an all-embracing book on medicine following the exact rules of logic and attempting to fit each bit of anatomy, physiology, diagnosis and treatment into its proper niche with mathematical accuracy. This final massive structure had many imperfections since its foundation of anatomy and physiology was faulty. Anatomy itself was largely a closed book to the Islamic physicians who, with a possible exception of a few adventurous souls, practiced no dissection since it was forbidden by their religion. The celebrated Yuhanna ibn Masawayh is said to have dissected apes, but this was an isolated instance, and Yuhanna was a Christian. Avicenna's anatomy, like that of his Muslim colleagues, was based on the writings of the Greeks. As for physiology, Erasistratus and, later, Galen, had broken the path 700 years before, but no one else had ventured on it.

These great defects do not imply that the work possessed little merit, quite the contrary. No unworthy book could have dominated medicine for centuries, as the Canon did, without possessing extraordinary merit [2].

Osler notes:

It is safe to say that the "Canon" was a medical bible for a longer period than any other work. It stands for the epitome of all precedent development, the final codification of all Graeco-Arabic medicine. It is a hierarchy of laws liberally illustrated by facts which so ingeniously rule and are subject to one another, stay and uphold one another, that admiration is compelled for the sagacity of the great organizer who, with unparalleled power of systematization, collecting his material from all sources, constructed so imposing an edifice of fallacy. Avicenna, according to his lights, imparted to contemporary medical science the appearance of almost mathematical accuracy, whilst the art of therapeutics, although empiricism did not wholly lack recognition, was deduced as a logical sequence from theoretical (Galenic and Aristotelian) premises. Is it, therefore, matter for surprise that the majority of investigators and practitioners should have fallen under the spell of this consummation of formalism and should have regarded the "Canon" as an infallible oracle, the more so in that the logical construction was impeccable and the premises, in the light of contemporary conceptions, passed for incontrovertible axioms? [3]

In short, Avicenna codified all that was known of medicine from the classical era and melded it with the medicine of the early medieval period using the tools of Aristotelian logic. Classical medicine was thus preserved.

The Arabic translations of the classics found their way back into continental Europe via two paths. First, a North African Christian monk, Constantinus Africanus (1020–1087), came to the University at Salernum about the middle of the eleventh century. He was a native of Carthage and gained fluency in several oriental languages through extensive travel. He translated Avicenna, Hippocrates, and Galen into Latin and set the stage for the Salernitanum curriculum based on the authority of Hippocrates and Galen. Constantinus Africanus ended his days as a translator in Monte Casino. Second, and perhaps the more important source, was the group of Latin translators in Spain, particularly in Toledo:

> From the middle of the twelfth until the middle of the thirteenth century, an extraordinary number of Arabic works in philosophy, mathematics, and astronomy were translated. Among the translators, Gerard of Cremona is prominent, and has been called the "Father of Translators." He was one of the brightest intelligences of the Middle Ages, and did a work of the first importance to science, through the extraordinary variety of material he put in circulation [3].

Thus the great circle–Greek and Latin to Persian, Persian to Syriac, Syriac to Arabic, and Arabic to Latin–was closed. That some corruption of content and emphasis occurred in this journey is certain, but that we have anything classical is one of the triumphs of the academic enterprise. The enabling link was the Islamic Empire, and its most distinguished luminary was Avicenna. After Leonardo, he is thought by many scholars to be the second of the world's universal geniuses. He was the greatest physician of his day.

References

1. Leclerc L: *Histoire de la Médecine Arabe*. Paris, 1876, Vol. 1, p. 139.
2. Major RH: *A History of Medicine*. Springfield, IL: Charles C. Thomas, 1954, Vol. 1, p. 244.
3. Osler W: *The Evolution of Modern Medicine*. Birmingham, AL: The Classics of Medicine Library, 1982, p. 98–101.

Source

Neuburger M: *History of Medicine*. London: Oxford University Press, 1910, Vol. 1, pp. 346–84.

This chapter has been reproduced from Loriaux, D. Lynn: Avicenna. *The Endocrinologist* 1998; 8(5): 319–22.

CHAPTER 10
Andreas Vesalius (1514–1564)
The Renaissance in Medicine

Andreas Vesalius ushered western medicine into the Renaissance in 1543. He was born in Brussels on New Year's Eve, 1514. He came from a distinguished medical family. His great grandfather, Johannes, was physician to Maria, wife of Emperor Maximilian 1. His grandfather, Eberhardt, was a court physician, and his father, Andreas, an apothecary to Charles V. The family, originally called Witting, had its roots in Wesel in the Duchy of Cleves, and the family name was changed to recognize this origin. Wesel, Flemish for weasel, accounts for the three weasels in the family coat of arms, and the Latinized form of the name, Vesalius.

As a child, Vesalius was fascinated by anatomy, and is recorded to have dissected many small animals: mice, cats, rats, and moles. He began his formal education at Louvain, from whence he went to Paris to begin his medical studies at 17 years of age. Here, he studied with the famous Jacques DuBois, Latinized to Sylvius, who described the Sylvian fissure, among other things. He was a charismatic teacher who drew students from all over the continent. The professor would sit at his desk and lecture from the anatomical text while a surgeon dissected the cadaver and a demonstrator indicated with a wooden pointer the parts described. Sylvius often had as many as 400 students in a class. He stated that "progress in knowledge beyond Galen is impossible"[1].

When he was 21, Vesalius assisted Guinterius in preparing an anatomical text, *Institutiones Anatomica*, that was an epitome of Galen's anatomy. Vesalius then journeyed to Venice, where he met and befriended Johann Stephan Kalcar (Calcar), a Flemish student of Titian. Together they went to Padua, where Vesalius received his doctor's degree on December 5, 1537. Vesalius and Calcar then collaborated on the famous *Six Anatomical Tables (Tabulae Anatomicae Sex)*. This was a sensation, primarily because of the beautiful illustrations by Calcar. The text, however, still carried many Galenic errors such as the five-lobed liver and the hepatic origin of the venous system. An immediate result of this success was Vesalius' appointment as professor of surgery and anatomy at the University of Padua. He was 23 years of age.

A Biographical History of Endocrinology, First Edition. D. Lynn Loriaux.

This work is a co-publication between the Endocrine Society and John Wiley & Sons, Ltd.

The next 5 years were ones of extraordinary effort. Vesalius began his academic career by dispensing with the surgeon and demonstrators in his lectures and doing all of the dissections himself (*"Tangitis res vestries minibus, et his credite* [Touch with your own hands, and trust in them]") [2]. His demonstrations and lectures were enthusiastically received, and as he proceeded with the work, he recognized the many errors in Galen's human anatomy. At length, he realized that Galen often was not describing human beings, but animals, and he concluded that Galen had never dissected a human body. He resolved to write an authoritative work on human anatomy and, 5 years later, at the age of 28, *De Humanis Corporis Fabrica* was finished. The illustrations, 300 in number, were done by his friend Calcar. Not trusting the quality of the printing in Venice, Vesalius packed the blocks for these illustrations onto mules and personally took them over the Alps to Basle. Thus, in 1543, the same year that Copernicus published his new theory of the Universe, *De Revolutionibus Orbium Coelestium*, Vesalius' great book appeared. It contained 663 folio pages in addition to the 300 illustrations just mentioned. An epitome, designed for classroom use, was published simultaneously. A second edition, improved but not materially changed, appeared in 1555.

De Fabrica is a landmark in the history of medicine. The illustrations by Calcar are far superior in artistic quality and anatomic fidelity to anything that had gone before and, for the first time, Vesalius' observations gave a comprehensive and accurate picture of the human anatomy.

He described in great detail the thyroid gland, "Glandes Laryngis Radici Adnatae," [1] and the pituitary gland, "Glandula Pituitam Cerebri Excipiens." In the 1555 edition he described the ovaries:

> The testes of women contain, besides blood vesicles, some sinuses full of this watery fluid which, if the testis has not been previously damaged, but is squeezed and makes a noise like an inflated bladder, will spurt out like a fountain to a great height during dissection. As this fluid is white and like a milky serum in healthy women, so I have found it to be a wonderful saffron yellow color and a little thicker in two well-bred girls who were troubled before death with a strangulation of the womb; the testis of one of the girls, or at any rate one of the sinuses in it, protruded like a rather large pea full of yellow fluid [3].

Later, two students of Vesalius, Fallopius and Eustachius both critics of Vesalius' work, were to carry the study of endocrine anatomy beyond the *Fabrica*. Fallopius described the corpus luteum, and Eustachius the adrenal glands, "Glandulae Renis Incumbentes."

Upon his return to Padua, Vesalius was cruelly attacked by established authority, by some of his most respected students and, most painfully, by his teacher Jacobus Sylvius. Sylvius continued to accept Galen as the ultimate authority and glibly justified the differences between the Galenic and Vesalian descriptions of human anatomy: "man had changed, but not for the better!" [4]. Distressed and melancholy, Vesalius burned his remaining manuscripts and, following his father's example, left Padua to become a court physician to Charles V of Spain.

When Charles V left public life and took refuge in a cloister, Vesalius became physician to his son, the famous Philip II. Vesalius married, settled down, and gave up anatomic investigation completely. Equal fame as a physician, however, was quickly established. When Henry II of France sustained a mortal head injury in a joust, as an example, it was Vesalius who was called from Spain to attend the French King [5]. In 1564, 20 years after joining the Spanish court, Vesalius became embroiled in a complicated and dangerous event that led, indirectly, to his untimely death. The facts in the case remain vague, but the event centers about the death of a Spanish nobleman entrusted to his care. With the death of the man, Vesalius requested permission for a post-mortem examination, which was granted. Upon entering the chest cavity, apparently in the presence of the family, the heart was observed to beat. The family, understandably distressed, denounced Vesalius before the inquisition, and his execution by *auto-da-fé* was narrowly averted by Philip II on the condition that Vesalius would "expiate his crime by a pilgrimage to Jerusalem and Mount Sinai" [6]. On the return voyage, the ship was assailed by contrary winds and, after prolonged hardship, landed on the Greek isle of Zante. Here, in the town of Zakynthos, Vesalius died of a fever and was buried by a visiting Venetian goldsmith to prevent him from becoming "food and nourishment for wild beasts" [7].

Thus ended the life and career of one of the pivotal figures in western medical history. Hippocrates, Galen, Vesalius, and Harvey are its early milestones. Vesalius' career reached its apogee when he was 28 years of age. His achievement struck down dogma and opened the way for medical science as we know it. All that follows can be traced, in some way, to this moment in time. The subsequent events of Vesalius' life are all too familiar, and serve to reaffirm the power of a confederation of the mediocre. "To have completed, before his 29th year, a task of this magnitude at a period when dissection was difficult to make and authority difficult to resist," wrote William Osler [8], "is a feat to which the literary efforts of medicine offer no parallel." It remains so today.

References

1. Major RH: *A History of Medicine*, Vol. 2. Springfield, IL: Charles C. Thomas, 1954, p. 404.
2. Boerhaave H, Albini BS: *Opera Omnia Anatomica et Chirurgia*. Lugduni: Du Vivie et Ver beek, Folio, 2 Vols, 1725.
3. Medvei VC: *A History of Endocrinology*. Boston: MTP Press, 1982, p. 105.
4. Garrison FH: *History of Medicine*. Philadelphia, PA: W.B. Saunders 1922, p. 216.
5. Norwich I: A consultation between Andreas Vesalius and Ambroise Pare at the deathbed of Henri II, King of France, 15 July 1559. *South African Med J* 1991; 80: 245–7.
6. Lasky II: The martyrdom of Doctor Andreas Vesalius. *Clin Orthop* 1990; 259: 304–11.
7. O'Malley CD: *Andreas Vesalius of Brussels, 1514–1564*. Berkeley, CA: University of California Press, 1964.
8. Garrison FH: In defense of Vesalius. *Bull Soc Hist Med* 1916; 4: 47.

This chapter has been reproduced from Loriaux, D. Lynn: Andreas Vesalius (1514–1564). *The Endocrinologist* 1993; 3(1): 3–4.

CHAPTER 11
Bartolomeo Eustachi (Eustachius) (1520–1574)
The Adrenal Gland

Little is known of the life of Eustachius. He comes to light in most biographical material as a professor of anatomy in Rome at the College Della Sapienza. He was a contemporary of Vesalius but never worked with him. In fact, Eustachius, Realdo Colombo (who was Vesalius' prosector in Padua), and Gabriele Falloppio were Vesalius' most effective contemporary critics. The other committed critic was Sylvius, Vesalius' former mentor. Sylvius' criticisms of Vesalius were based wholly in Sylvius' belief in the infallibility of Galen. Eustachius, Columbus, and Fallopius, however, based their criticisms on dissection and careful study. Together, they rectified many of the minor errors in the "Fabrica" and did much to finalize a complete and accurate anatomy of the human body in the sixteenth century.

In his early years, Eustachius was a devoted Galenist. But he was also observant and able to see the fidelity in Vesalius' dissections and to recognize the extraordinary advance that Vesalius' work had given the medical world. Eustachius had planned to produce his own "opus magnum" on the human anatomy. He died before it was completed. He did, however, produce 47 illustrations on copper plates for the text, created with the aid of the Roman artist Pier Matteo Pini of Urbano. The first eight deal with the study of the kidneys, the azygos vein, and the auditory organ. The eighth plate deals with the veins of the arms and the heart. The studies of the kidney clearly show, for the first time, the adrenal gland as an organ independent of the kidney. This is best illustrated on the first plate, Tabula Prima. These eight plates were published in Eustachius' first anatomy book, *Opuscula Anatomica*, written with Fallopius, in 1563. Eustachius says of these glands, "Nihilominus ne aliquid in hac tractione praetermissum esse quispiam mihi jure objiciat: consentaneum esse duxi de quibusdam renum glandulis ab aliis anatomica practermissus hoc loco scribere" (roughly: Nevertheless, nobody has previously shown the adrenal glands to be a separate anatomic entity as described here).

Eustachius was the physician to the Cardinal Giulio della Rovere, who called Eustachius to come see him at his summer place because of illness. Eustachius died on

A Biographical History of Endocrinology, First Edition. D. Lynn Loriaux.

This work is a co-publication between the Endocrine Society and John Wiley & Sons, Ltd.

the way. His Opus Magnum was never written. Pini kept the remaining plates in his family. They finally found their way to the Vatican library and were given to Pope Clement XI (1649–1721). Pope Clement, in turn, gave them to his personal physician, Giovanni Lancisi.

Lancisi was born in Rome in 1654 and educated at the Collegio Romano and the University of Rome. He became an assistant physician to the Hospidale di Santo Spirito, where he spent the rest of his professional life. He was, at the same time, the prosector of anatomy at the Collegio della Sapienza, thus following in the footsteps of Eustachius. Lancisi published the plates with his own notes in 1714 in book form: *Tabulae Anatomicae Clarissimi viri Bartholomaei Eustachii*. To make the collection complete, he reprinted the first eight plates in *Opuscula*, leading to all of the confusion about the first description of the adrenal gland. It is generally believed that the world had to wait 140 years for *Tabula Prima* to be rejoined with the text. In fact, they were together from the beginning.

Eustachius is better remembered for the Eustachian valve in the right auricle and the Eustachian tube that he rediscovered. He also described the cochlea and the ligaments of the malleus and stapes. He was the first to use the term "isthmus" to describe the portion of the thyroid gland connecting its two lobes. He was the first to describe the thoracic duct, the abducens nerve, and he wrote the best treatise of his time on the structure of the teeth, *Libellus de dentibus*.

Although Eustachius was greatly overshadowed in his lifetime by Vesalius, Columbus, Fallopius, and Fabricius, he is now recognized as one of the "giants" of the anatomic renaissance of the sixteenth century.

Sources

Choulant L, Garrison FH: *History and Bibliography of Anatomic Illustration in its Relation to Anatomic Science and the Graphic Arts*. Chicago, IL: University of Chicago Press, 1920.

Bartolomeo Eustachii and Gabriele Fallopio: *Opuscula Anatomica*. Venetis, 1563.

Giovanni Lancisi: *Tabulae Anatomical*. Rome, 1714.

This chapter has been reproduced from Loriaux, D. Lynn: Bartolomeo Eustachi (Eustachius) (1520–1574). *The Endocrinologist* 2007; 17(4): 195.

CHAPTER 12
Santorio Santorio (1561–1636)
Insensible Loss

Santorio Santorio (latinized as Sanctorius Sanctorius) was born March 29, 1561 in Capodistria, a pleasant little town on an island in the Adriatic, 15 miles distant from Trieste. At the time, it was the capital city of the district of Istria, hence its name. His father was Chief of Ordnance in the district and his family well to do. He was taken to Venice for his schooling and, at 14, entered the University of Padua where he studied philosophy and then medicine. He received his medical degree at 21 years of age.

Maximilian, King of Poland, wrote to the faculty of Padua in 1587 asking that they recommend to him an excellent physician. The vicar wrote back "We have a very excellent man, name and surname, Santorio, native of Justinopolis (the Latin name for Capodistria). His learning, fidelity and industry is most highly esteemed by all of us, it is possible he can easily be induced to take this journey" [1]. Santorio went to Poland where he remained for 14 years and where he was known as a skillful physician and was consulted throughout Eastern Europe. It was while in Poland that Santorio wrote his first book, *Methodus Vitandorum Errorum Omnium qui in Arte Medica Contingent* (Method of combating all errors that occur in the art of Medicine) published in Venice in 1602. It was, in the main, a work on differential diagnosis drawing mainly from Hippocrates, Galen, and Avicenna. A favorable response to the book led to his appointment as professor of medicine at Padua in 1611. According to the records of the University, Santorio

> made his entrance into the school in our company and with an extraordinarily numerous audience treating this most honorable subject in a most elegant and learned oration, to the complete taste of everyone, gave proof of his ability and especially of his great intelligence [1].

One year later, Santorio published his *Commentary on the Medicine of Galen*. In the second edition of this book is the first clear description of the use of the thermometer:

> We by a glass instrument then determined the temperature, by this method we knew the extremes and the mean: we apply snow to the glass sphere of the instrument so that water ascends to the highest point. Next we apply the flame of a candle so that the water descends to

A Biographical History of Endocrinology, First Edition. D. Lynn Loriaux.

This work is a co-publication between the Endocrine Society and John Wiley & Sons, Ltd.

> the lower point. Knowing the extremes we immediately determine the mean and the temperature, so that no matter how much any portion recedes, it will be easily perceived [2].

The thermometer that Santorio used consisted of a glass globe connected to a glass tube that was immersed into a bowl of colored water. The globe was heated before the tube was immersed and, as the air cooled, water was drawn up into the tube. The height of the water in the tube was then marked when the globe was cooled with snow, heated with a flame, and at room temperature. It is believed that Santorio became aware of the thermometer through his friendship with Galileo. He realized its potential clinical utility and explored this in some detail in his *Commentaria in Primam Fen Primi Libri Canonis Avicenna* (Commentaries on the first part of the first book of the Canon of Avicenna).

It was also in this book that Santorio described the "pulsilogium." Santorio used Galileo's innovation of timing the swing of a pendulum with his pulse to time the pulse with a pendulum. To do this, he used a cord with swinging weight and lengthened the cord until the pendulum and the pulse were coincident. The pulse rate was then measured as the length of the cord. This is also discussed in his commentary on Avicenna.

Santorio's greatest achievement, however, was the discovery of insensible water loss. This was accomplished by the simple means of living for days at a time on a balance. His weight, all that he consumed, and all that he excreted were carefully measured and revealed conclusively that there was an insensible loss of water that could not be accounted for even by perspiration. Santorio concluded that there was abundant water in exhaled air, as revealed by a cold mirror. These findings were reported in his next book, *Ars Sanctorii Sanctorii de Statica Medicina*. This book, published in 1614, passed through 28 Latin editions and was translated into Italian, English, and German. The sensation it created in the medical world was due to its innovative application of the experimental method of Galileo, Santorio's friend, to human physiology in carefully planned prospective experiments.

Santorio sent a copy of *Statica Medicina* to Galileo, who had meanwhile gone to Florence. The accompanying letter, which bears the date of February 9, 1615, has been preserved. It states that his work is based on two certain principles. "The first, enunciated by Hippocrates, that medicine is addition and subtraction, adding that which is deficient and taking away that which is superfluous; the second principle is experiment." Boerhaave wrote that "no book on medicine is written with such perfection." Santorio is now regarded as the father of the science of metabolism [1].

Santorio was appointed President of a new University in Padua in 1616, the Collegia Veneto. Because of ongoing faculty strife, however, he resigned in 1624 to return to Venice and the practice of medicine. His practice flourished, particularly among the wealthy and influential. He ultimately became President of the Venetian College of Physicians and, in 1630, was appointed Chief Health Officer of Venice to fight the plague that was devastating the city.

Santorio died in February 22, 1636, from some undiagnosed urinary tract disease. His skull is preserved in the Anatomical Museum at Padua.

Castiglioni says of Santorio and his life; "He was, in the field of medicine, the first and most happy innovator, the most courageous initiator of that method of exact investigation, to which medical science owes its greatest successes: the foundation stone upon which has been constructed the entire structure of modern medicine" [3].

References

1. Major RH: Santorio Santorio. *Ann Med History* 1938; 10: 369–81.
2. Mitchell SW: *The Early History of Instrumental Precision in Medicine*. New Haven, CT: Tuttle, Morehouse & Taylor, 1892.
3. Castiglioni A. *La Vita e l'opera di Santorio Capodistriano*. Bologna: Cappelli, 1920.

This chapter has been reproduced from Loriaux, D. Lynn: Santorio Santorio (1561–1636). *The Endocrinologist* 2005; 15(2): 63–4.

CHAPTER 13
William Harvey (1578–1657)
The First Great Experiment, "*De Motu Cordis*"

William Harvey was the first to show that the heart pumps blood into arteries, then into veins, and back to the heart again. It is one of the great discoveries in the history of medicine. The development of this concept, culminating in Harvey's discovery, had a long gestation. Galen (130–200 C.E.) showed that arteries carry blood, not air, and that venous blood is darker than arterial blood. He believed that the pulse was an ebb and flow of blood to and from the heart and that the right and left ventricles were connected by pores in the interventricular septum. This galenic concept was dogma until challenged by Vesalius 1400 years later. Vesalius showed convincingly that there were no interventricular pores. Michael Servetus (1509–1533) then described the minor (pulmonary) circulation. He wrote in his *Christianisimi Restitutio* that the blood passes from the right ventricle to the left, not "through the septum ... as commonly believed, but by another admirable continuance, the blood being transmitted from the pulmonary artery to the pulmonary vein by a lengthened passage through the lungs in the course of which it is elaborated and becomes a crimson color" [1, p. 491]. Servetus never completed his study of the circulation. "Eccentric" views on the trinity (Mary is the mother of Jesus, but not of God) and his position on the "fallacy of infant baptism" led to his arrest and trial for heresy. He was burned at the stake in Geneva on October 27, 1533. His concept of the pulmonary circulation remained unnoticed for another 144 years.

Realdo Colombo was born in Cremona in 1516. He was a colleague of Vesalius in Padua. He also understood the minor circulation. In his *De re Anatomica* he states that:

> Between the ventricles there is a system by which it is thought that the blood from the right ventricle passes to the left, but they are very much in error, for the blood is carried by the pulmonary artery to the lungs, from which it passes with the air, by the pulmonary vein to the left ventricle of the heart [1, p. 492].

Andrea Cesalpino, anatomist and physician to Pope Clement VIII, wrote in 1571 (*Quaestionum Peripateticarum*) that "the circulation of the blood which takes place from the right ventricle to the left ventricle, in passing through the lungs, agrees quite

---

A Biographical History of Endocrinology, First Edition. D. Lynn Loriaux.

This work is a co-publication between the Endocrine Society and John Wiley & Sons, Ltd.

exactly with the following facts, which are apparent from dissection. There are two vessels which end in the right ventricle, two in the left. One of the two is afferent, the other efferent" [1, p. 494].

Finally, Fabricius of Acquapendente noted in 1574 that veins have valves that permit flow only toward the heart. This was published as a slim folio titled *De Venarum Ostiolis* in 1603. Fabricius was Harvey's mentor while in Padua. Thus was Harvey prepared when, in 1615, he began a series of vivisections in dogs in association with the Lumlian lectures. In these vivisections he was able to show that a ligature around the femoral artery emptied the artery and the veins distal to the tie, and a release of the ligature filled the artery and all of its associated veins. The idea was complete:

> First of all, the auricle contracts, and in the course of its contraction throws the blood (which it contains in ample quantity as the head of the veins, the store house and cistern of the blood) into the ventricle, which being filled, the heart raises itself straightway, makes all its fibers tense, contracts the ventricles, and performs a beat, by which beat it immediately sends the blood supplied to it by the auricle into the arteries; the right ventricle sending its charge into the lungs by the vessel called vena arteriosa (pulmonary artery) which, in structure and function, and all things else, is an artery; the left ventricle sending its charge into the aorta, and through this by the arteries to the body at large [2, p. 31].

William Harvey was born in 1578 in Folkestone, near Dover, one of the Cinque Ports of east Kent, England. William's father, Thomas, was in the "carrying trade" as might be expected of a businessman from this region. He was a prominent citizen, serving as mayor of Folkestone in 1586, 1599, 1601, and 1611. William's mother, Joan, was Thomas' second wife. A brass plate in the parish church says of her:

> A. D. 1605, Nov 8th dyed in ye 50th yeere of her age, Joan, wife of Tho. Harvey, mother of 7 sones and 2 daughters. A Godly Harmless Woman: A chaste loveing wife: A charitable quiet neighbour; a comfortable friendly matron: A provident diligent housewife; a careful tenderhearted mother: Deere to her husband: Reverensed of her children; Beloved of her Neighbours; Elected of God Whose Soule rest in Heaven: her body in this Grave: To her a happy Advantage: to hers, an Unhappy loss [3, p. 5].

William was the eldest child. His six brothers (John, Thomas, Daniel, Eliab, and the twins, Michael and Mathew) all became prominent citizens, pursuing careers at court or in the business world of London. None of the children received a consistent education, getting the rudiments haphazardly from occasional itinerant schoolmasters. Nonetheless, William learned enough to gain admission to the King's School in Canterbury when 9 years of age.

The statutes stated that "if any of the boys be remarkable for extraordinary slowness and dullness or for a disposition repugnant to learning, we will that after much trial by the Dean, or in his absence by the vice-dean, he be expelled and another substituted, that he may not, like a drone, devour the honey of the bees" [3, p. 7]. All students were required to know by heart the Lord's Prayer, the Angelus, the Apostle's Creed, and the Ten Commandments. William was admitted to Gonville and Caius College of Cambridge University when he was 15 years old. John Caius, who endowed the college, was an eminent physician and anatomist who had been a schoolmate of Andreas Vesalius at Padua. On his return to Cambridge, he applied for and received a *Charter of Anatomie* from Queen Elizabeth, allowing the dissection of the bodies of two criminals each year. For this reason, Caius College was a magnet for English students interested in medicine. A Matthew Parker Scholarship, the first medical scholarship in England, allowed Harvey to finish his medical training in Padua, then at the apogee of its fame as the greatest medical center in the world. This fame was due largely to a long tradition of excellence in anatomy, the professors at that time being Vesalius, Columbus, Fallopius, and Fabricius. In addition, the clinical school at Padua, under the direction of Montanus, was greatly esteemed. Harvey stayed for 2 years, leaving with his medical degree in 1602. To commemorate his graduation, Harvey was allowed to have his "stemma" (a coat of arms) painted on the cloister ceiling. It can be seen there still.

> The symbol, presumably chosen by Harvey himself, was a white sleeved arm holding, against a red background, a lighted candle entwined by two green serpents. If the serpents are to be regarded as the symbols of Esculapius, the lighted candle seems prophetic of Harvey's achievement in illuminating medical art with the truths of scientific discovery [3, p. 23].

Harvey returned to London in 1602 and obtained a license to practice medicine in 1604. In that same year, he married Elizabeth Brown, daughter of Dr. Lancelot Brown, physician to Queen Elizabeth and, later, to King James. Brown was a powerful promoter of Harvey but died in 1605, too early to significantly alter the events of Harvey's career.

Harvey's first professional opportunity came in 1609 when he was appointed physician to St. Bartholomew's Hospital; he was the sixth person to hold this post. He was physician to the poor of the hospital: "one day in the week at least through the year, or oftener as need shall require, you shall come to this hospital, and cause the hospitler, Matron, or Porter, to call before you in the hall of this hospital such and so many of the poor harbored in this hospital as shall need the counsel and advice of the physician" [3, p. 53].

In 1615, Harvey was given the important responsibility of the Lumlian Lectures, a series of public lectures on the subject of surgery, delivered at 10.00 a.m. every Wednesday and Friday over a 6 year curriculum. As part of these lectures, a series of anatomical demonstrations was required; the demonstrations were given in alternation with a Fellow of the College of Physicians. It was in these dissections and vivisections that Harvey correctly deduced the nature of the circulation. In the notes of one lecture in 1616, added as an addendum at a later date, is the following passage:

> William Harvey demonstrates by the structure of the heart that the blood is constantly passed through the lungs into the aorta.... He demonstrates by ligature the passage of blood from artery to veins. Thus is proved a perpetual motion of the blood in a circle caused by the pulsation of the heart [3, p. 490].

Twelve years elapsed before his views were published in the landmark book *Exercitatio Anatomica de Motu cordis et Sanguinis in Animalibus.*

Harvey was a contemporary of William Shakespeare (1564–1616). He probably saw Shakespeare and the King's men act at court in his role as physician to the King. There is no record, however, that they ever met. There is an active controversy focusing on the "true" author of Shakespeare's plays. Did Shakespeare really write them, or was he merely a convenient "cover" for another who did not wish to be directly associated with the thespian life? There are two leading candidates for this distinction: Edward de Vere, 17th Earl of Oxford, and Francis Bacon. Whomever it was, that person had an almost perfect grasp of the circulation before 1608 when *Coriolanus* was written. Menenius Agrippa, in his discourse on the importance of the belly in the body politic says (Act 1, Scene 1):

> True it is my Incorporate Friends (quotes he) That I receive the general food at first which you do live upon; and fit it is, Because I am the store-house, and the shop of the whole body. But if you do remember I send it through rivers of your blood, even to the court, the heart, the seat of the brain and through the crankes and offices of man [3, p. 10].

How could Shakespeare know this 20 years before the publication of *de Motu* and 8 years before the first Lumlian Lecture? He could have known William Harvey. Interestingly, William Harvey saw Francis Bacon as a patient at least twice, May 24, 1617 and March 6, 1619, both seemingly for gout. Both visits were long after the 1608 publication of *Coriolanus*.

Edward de Vere was a favorite of Queen Elizabeth, perhaps even her lover for a time. He died in 1604, 2 years after Harvey returned from Padua. Harvey's father-in-law was physician to the Queen during the 2 years in question. He could have been the "go-between" if the concept of the circulation was mature in Harvey's mind at the time, which it appears not to have been.

There is another possibility; Edward de Vere, in 1575, set out upon a tour of the continent that was to last more than a year. Notably, the tour included a five month sojourn in Padua. The purpose of the stay must have been to visit the University, perhaps the greatest in the world at that time. A highlight would have been the anatomy amphitheater and the lectures of Fabricius. These lectures certainly would have included a demonstration of the venous system and its valves because it was newly discovered by Fabricius and a focus of his attention at the time. Could Edward de Vere have formulated the concept independently? By all accounts, he had the intellectual power for such a leap: "Oxford was the most eligible of all young bachelors at Elizabeth's court-brilliant, gallant, witty, artistic, athletic, pedigreed, rich, the observed of all observers" [4, p. 112].

William Harvey went on to more triumphs, being among the first to bring rigor to the study of embryonic development. He spent his last years living with his brother Eliab. It is said that he retained all of his mental faculties to the last. On the morning of his death, about 10:00, he

> went to speak, and found he had the dead palsy in the tongue; then he saw what was to become of him, he knew there was then no hopes of his recovery, so presently sends for his young nephews to come up to him, to whom he give one his watch (twas a minute watch with which he made his experiments); to another, another remembrance, etc., made sign to Sambroke, the apothecary, to let him blood in the tongue, which did little or no good; and so he ended his dayes [3, p. 411].

The renaissance in medicine took two great steps. The first was made by Vesalius, who challenged authority based on personal experience and scholarship. The second was made by William Harvey, who, by application of careful observation, deduction, and the use of experiment, solved the riddle of the heart. Modern medicine begins at this place.

References

1. Major RH: *A History of Medicine*. Springfield, IL: Charles C. Thomas, 1954.
2. Willis R (trans.): An anatomical disquisition on the motion of heart and blood in animals. In *The Works of William Harvey, M.D.* London: Sydenham Society, 1847.
3. Keynes G: *The Life of William Harvey*. Oxford: The Clarendon Press, 1966.
4. Sobran J: *Alias*. New York: The Free Press, 1997.

This chapter has been reproduced from Loriaux, D. Lynn: Historical Note: William Harvey (1578–1657). *The Endocrinologist* 1998; 8(4): 237–40.

CHAPTER 14
Thomas Wharton (1614–1673)
Codifying the Glands

Thomas Wharton is credited with the first description of the submaxillary salivary duct, hence "Wharton's duct," and the eponym, "Wharton's jelly," which comes from Wharton's noting the mucinous material in the umbilical cord. In 1656 he wrote the first book devoted entirely to glands, titled *Adenographia,* and in it he named the thyroid gland with the name that we use today. Wharton created the first true delineation of the body's glands and synthesized what was then known about these organs.

Wharton was a London physician who lived through one of England's most turbulent times. Charles I was overthrown and beheaded after the English Civil War between the Royalists and the Parliamentarians. Oliver Cromwell and the Parliamentarians ran the country for over a decade (1649–1660) before the Restoration of Charles II in 1660 [1]. These were the terrible years of 1665–1666 when London was afflicted with both the Great Plague and the Great Fire. Through all this, Scotland and Ireland were hardly settled or quiet. They were more or less continually at war with England. Wharton managed to avoid the warring factions and carried on his practice in London as an elite physician. More importantly, he studied and worked with a group of like-minded colleagues at the College of Physicians (later, the Royal College; though chartered by Henry VIII in the previous century, the "Royal" was added only after Cromwell's rule ended).

Wharton was born in Durham. Little is known of his early life except that his father died when he was 15 years old and he had a serious febrile illness at 19. We then see him at age 23 as a student at Cambridge where he was a "sizar," a title unique to Cambridge and Trinity College, Dublin, that signifies a student whose expenses were paid by the college in return for work as a servant. His area of study is unknown. He received no degree. He transferred to Trinity College, Oxford, in 1642, and may have been influenced by William Harvey, who was a major supporter of science at London's Royal College of Physicians. Harvey was the discoverer of the circulation of the blood and he was in Oxford that year because of his attendance as one of the physicians to Charles I, who had been forced to Oxford in the early part of the Civil

A Biographical History of Endocrinology, First Edition. D. Lynn Loriaux.

This work is a co-publication between the Endocrine Society and John Wiley & Sons, Ltd.

War. Wharton left Oxford almost immediately, perhaps because Oxford had become a Royalist stronghold. He went to Bolton where he spent the next 3 years as a tutor for the illegitimate son of the Earl of Sunderland. Again, he got no degree from Oxford nor did he become a cleric as most at Oxford had done before the war. To become a cleric might well have been hazardous when one considers the deep religious basis of the war itself.

It was during these years, the early 1640s, that Wharton seems to have become interested in chemistry. In those days, chemistry included alchemy, medicine, and astrology. He moved to London, which was in Parliamentary hands, in 1645 and studied medicine under the tutelage of John Bathurst (1614–1659). Bathurst was both a Fellow of the College of Physicians and Oliver Cromwell's physician. When the First Civil War ended in 1646 with Charles I's capture by, and Oxford's surrender to, the Parliamentarians under Cromwell, Wharton returned briefly to Oxford to receive his MD. Wharton then returned to London where, in 1657 he became physician to St. Thomas' Hospital. He remained in London for the rest of his life.

Wharton was admitted to the College of Physicians in 1647. He was a full Fellow by 1650. This was an important honor because, at the time, the college was limited to 30 or 40 members, including Harvey who had returned to London after Oxford fell in the war. The members were not only elite physicians but also investigators. Despite the political differences between London and Oxford, the physicians and those we might now call scientists at Oxford and the physicians at the London College worked together, under Harvey's influence, to investigate nature and medicine. The College of Physicians was probably the main focus of scientific investigation in England at the time. The Royal Society was not started until the Restoration in 1660. In 1648 the College had a laboratory as well as a museum and a study area donated by Harvey himself. All of this was lost in the Great Fire a few years later.

Francis Glisson (1597–1677), an active disciple of Harvey and the describer of Glisson's capsule (the fibrous envelopment of the porta hepatis), was a leading investigator in the College [2]. Despite the fact that he was a professor of medicine at Cambridge for the last half of his life, he was at the same time quite active in the College. His first book in 1650 set the collaborative tone. *On Rickets* was the work of a group at the College rather than Glisson's alone, although the others working with him agreed to have Glisson write the final text and take the credit. Glisson's books were written in English. Harvey's were published in Latin which helped to increase their readership.

Glisson's disciples were scientists in the College. Some of their work was Harveian in that it included physiologic studies akin to Harvey's studies of the circulation. But it was thought equally good science to dissect the human body or, for that matter, any animal. One of the goals of the new science was a comparative analysis of the anatomy of mammals. Knowledge was what was sought, rather than the application of a particular method. One of these disciples was Wharton and his method was anatomic (with a bit of early microscopy) rather than physiologic.

Glisson was undoubtedly the stimulus for Wharton's work on glands. The full title of his book is *Adenographia, Glandularum, Totius Corporis Descriptio* (Adenographia, or the description of the glands of the entire body) [3]. It was written in Latin and appeared in print in London in 1656. The book itself was derived from the Gulstonian Lectures that Wharton gave in 1652 [4]. These lectures were supported by the will of Dr. Goulston in 1632 and have been given, more or less continually, since 1639. Wharton's will specified that they would be given by one of the four newest members of the College (as they still are today) and that, if possible, they were to be accompanied by the dissection of a human body. This has not been done for some time. Wharton's presentation was, in fact, done with a dissection. The College, usually its President, chose the speaker and the topic. The speaker was expected to present original work, often with the collaboration of several members of the College. There was a penalty to be paid if the lectures were not given when required [5,6].

When Harvey established the facts of the circulation of the blood, the liver, previously thought to be the organ of blood production, suddenly had no known function. Glisson's Gulstonian Lecture in 1641 attempted to clarify this impasse. As Glisson worked, he developed a physiologic theory that attempted to explain the functions of various organs in light of Harvey's discoveries. It should be clear at this point that in the seventeenth century it was respectable science to make an anatomic observation and then offer a physiologic function in the absence of what we would now consider supporting physiologic evidence.

Glisson mulled over the newly discovered lymphatic system [7]. The lymphatic vessels, hard to see but, once seen, easy to follow, had tiny valves just as did the veins. Harvey had shown that valves in veins directed the flow of blood away from organs; so, Glisson thought, valves in lymphatics did the same thing. He saw lymphatics coming from many organs, including glandular structures, and thought that they were the "venous" part of another circulatory system. But, if lymph flowed from these organs, by analogy with the circulation of the blood, something had to bring fluid to them. Glisson decided that the "something" was nerves. The hypothesis implied that nerves have invisible channels in them through which the fluid flowed. Thus, nerves brought the fluid to various organs and lymphatics took it away. His theory was more complex than this because he had to deal with the problem of where the fluid was made. He decided that some nerves took up fluid from mesenteric glands (mesenteric lymph nodes or glands) or the spleen. The fluid taken up by nerves was then distributed throughout the nervous system, and thence through the nerves to various organs of the body, including many other glands. The nerves must have a "twoway" fluid flow and the glands of the body are critical to the functioning of this complex circulation that nourished the body's tissues.

Glisson attributed two other functions to glands. One was the ability to secrete material extracted from the nerve fluid (e.g., the testis, breast, pancreas, and submaxillary gland) (Wharton had just found the submaxillary's duct – but still thought the parotid had no duct, which was not found until Stensen uncovered it). Another was the capacity to extract useful substances from the nerve fluid (e.g., the parotid, axillary or thyroid glands) and put the lymph back into the lymphatics. Sometimes, this type of gland purified the fluid. For example, the "kidneygland" or (adrenal) did this. Here, both Wharton and Glisson implied a theory that we would find quite modern. The gland had a positive attraction for the important substance in the nerve fluid. Some of the glands' actions were to change the quality of the fluid before releasing it back to the lymphatics, which could be seen as a kind of "internal secretion."

The upshot of all this theorizing was that the glands, rather than being oddities of unknown function scattered throughout the body, became functionally quite important and were now seen as a system rather than a random collection. Because of the newly perceived importance of the glands, Glisson probably influenced the College President, Francis Prujean (1593–1666), to assign the topic to Wharton. Glisson's interest was also high enough that he personally worked with Wharton for some of the time while Wharton was dissecting and thinking in preparation for his lectures.

Wharton's first step was to state that glands "are parts whose sole function is secretion." Then he decided what "was" and "was not" a gland. He excluded the tongue, the brain, and the spleen (this last in part because it was not necessary for life). He included all we now call endocrine glands, which is the first time these had been considered as part of a system, and included every other organ we call a "gland" (e.g., all of the body's lymph glands, all the exocrine glands, and the breast, placenta, seminal vesicles, and tonsils). He was thorough. He and his colleagues studied a wide range of animals, including cattle, sheep, and shrews.

He provided an accurate description of the adrenal gland and realized that it was relatively larger in embryos than in adults. He thought there was a cavity in the center of the adrenal which we now know is the result of post-mortem changes. He did not know "what matter they secrete" but thought that whatever it was, it was "useful, because it is continually taken into the veins." An aspect of his reliance on the past is when he speculated on the diseases that might affect adrenal glands: "you will find nothing about them in the authorities. Therefore it will be very difficult to come to any definite conclusion."

He was aware of the pineal gland, named by the Greeks for its pinecone shape. He rejected the Cartesian argument that the pineal gland is the seat of the rational soul or *anima*. How could such a function be served by an organ with "no communication with the external organs?" He decided, because of its location, that the pineal served to get rid of excremental by-products of the nearby parts of the brain.

He modified the ancient view that the pituitary gland was simply a way station for central nervous system mucus as it was discharged through the cribriform plate into the nose. Such a function needs a conduit, he reasoned, and this gland has a parenchyma. Because there is a parenchyma, it must do something in addition to acting as a conduit: "the superfluous fluids of the brain ... may contain within themselves some juice that is nutritious with regard to other parts and that the duty of this parenchyma is to separate that nutritious juice ... doubtless it is transmitted into the ... plexuses of the nerves that are connected to it."

Wharton devoted 70 pages, or about one-quarter of his book, to various reproductive glands. The testes in men are well-described and their secretion, the seminal fluid, is described as a mixture of arterial extract and the "noblest" fluid from the nerves. Whatever the testes produced, Wharton thought that procreation did not occur unless the fluid from the testis was combined with that from the seminal vesicles and the prostate. The testes in women, as they called ovaries, were of uncertain function but it was clear that they are needed for reproduction. Removing the female testis leads to sterility – "we must come to the conclusion that women's testicles do produce sperm and have vessels to ejaculate it." Sperm was the term for seminal or other reproductive fluid, not for the spermatozoon or ovum. He did not know about gametes but did conclude that fertilization occurred near the ovary and that the mixture of men's and women's sperm went through the ovary's "ejaculatory vessel (Fallopian tubes) onto the wall of the womb, so that the foetus may be fashioned from it." A good description, particularly when Harvey himself thought that the ovary had no role whatsoever in reproduction.

Chapter 18 covers the thyroid gland or, as Wharton said, glands. He gave them this name because of the shield-shaped cartilage nearby. He noted the weight in man (about 55 grams in a 28-year-old man) as well as in several other animals. As for substance, it is "rather glutinous ... its parts are firmly attached to each other, and even resist when cut repeatedly with a knife." He thought that this gland had four functions. One fits with his and Glisson's theory: to take up fluid from the recurrent nerve and convey it "through its lymph ducts, back into the vessels classed as veins." Another is to "heat the cartilages to which it is fixed, which would otherwise be somewhat cool"; he reasoned this function from his observation of numerous thyroid arteries. He also thought that the thyroid gland would "effect the lubrication of the larynx with its vapour, and so make the voice more smooth, melodious, and pleasant." Wharton seems to believe, as did many for the next century and a half, that there was a thyroid duct. Finally, he adopts an ancient proposed function: "to make a large contribution to the roundness and beauty of the neck ... for this reason, they occur larger in women, and make their necks more even and beautiful." The idea that goiter is beautiful lasted for another two centuries [8].

Wharton addressed the problem of disease only in passing. He mentions goiter but does not clearly tie its occurrence to the thyroid gland, although Girolamo Fabrici (1533–1619) made the connection a generation before Wharton's lectures. Wharton was similarly vague about the difference between scrofula and struma but that is understandable as the confusion between tuberculous lymphatic glands in the neck and goiter lasted well into the eighteenth century.

Wharton's work was influential in its time but the influence faded after two or three generations. Glisson praised it highly [9]. However strange some of Wharton's interpretations may seem to us now, he was in fact the organizer of "the glands."

After the Restoration of Charles II in 1660, and the beginning of the Royal Society that same year, the scientific activities of the College of Physicians fell into eclipse, worsened by the destruction of its property in London's Great Fire of 1666. Wharton refused to join the Royal Society as did Glisson and others in the College, although he could easily have done so. He disagreed with the Society's approach to investigation. They were too mechanistic for him [10]. He did well in his practice and continued as physician to St. Thomas' Hospital. When the bubonic plague struck London in 1665, he was tempted to leave the city as did many of his colleagues. He did not go. His patients at the hospital included some of the King's Foot Guards. In return for caring for them, Wharton was promised an appointment as physician to the King. However, as often happens when the crisis is over, the King did not deliver. Instead, Wharton was allowed to add a field to his family's coat of arms as an honor, for which he had to pay £10! He wrote little else and practiced medicine, particularly at St. Thomas', until his death in 1673 at age 59.

Wharton's memorial in the Church of St. Michael was moved when the church was torn down in 1897. His portrait, said to be painted by Van Dyck, survives. It was presented to the Royal College of Physicians by his physician grandson, George, in 1729. Christopher Wharton, an eighth-generation descendant and also a physician and member of the College, was the final stimulus to get Thomas Wharton's book translated from Latin into English, 340 years after it first appeared. So Wharton lives – we have his book and can see at last his influence on our specialty.

References

1. *Encyclopaedia Britannica* (11th edn.). New York: The Encyclopaedia Britannica Co. 1910 (for articles on Oliver Cromwell and English kings).
2. Frank RG Jr: *Harvey and the Oxford Physiologists. Scientific ideas and social interaction.* Berkeley, CA: University of California Press, 1980.
3. Freer S: *Thomas Wharton's Adenographia* (translated from the Latin). Oxford: Clarendon Press, 1996.
4. Freer S: Introduction. In *Thomas Wharton's Adenographia* (translated from the Latin), edited by S Freer. Oxford: Clarendon Press, 1996, p. xii.
5. Munk W: *Roll of the Royal College of Physicians of London: Comprising biographical sketches* (2nd edn.), Vol. I, 1518 to 1700. London: College of Physicians 1878 (contains short biographies of Harvey, Glisson, and Wharton).
6. Munk W: *Roll of the Royal College of Physicians of London: Comprising biographical sketches* (2nd edn.), Vol. III, 1801 to 1825. London: College of Physicians, 1878 (contains information on the origin of the College, Gulstonian Lectures).
7. Cunningham A: The historical context of Wharton's work on the glands. In *Thomas Wharton's Adenographia* (translated from the Latin), edited by S Freer. Oxford: Clarendon Press, 1996, p. xxvii.
8. Sawin CT: Goiter. In *Cambridge History and Geography of Human Disease*, edited by KF Kiple. Cambridge: Cambridge University Press, 1993.
9. Wharton T: *Adenographia: sive, glandularum totius corporis descriptio*. London, 1656.
10. Webster C: The College of Physicians: "Solomon's House" in Commonwealth England. *Bull Hist Med* 1967; 41: 393.

This chapter has been reproduced from Sawin, Clark T: Historical Note: Thomas Wharton (1614–1673) and the glands of the body. *The Endocrinologist* 2000; 10(5): 283–8.

CHAPTER 15

Marcello Malpighi (1628–1694)

The Capillary

Malpighi supplied the final link in understanding the circulation of the blood. Galen described the four chambers of the heart and the connecting valves. He believed that arterial blood and venous blood communicated via pores in the interventricular septum. Other anatomists, in particular Servetus and Colombo, described the pulmonary circulation in anatomic terms, but how the system functioned still remained a mystery. Fabricius of Aquapendente discovered the venous valves, allowing blood to flow only in the direction of the heart, and William Harvey put it all together in *De Motu Cordis*. He described the circulation as efferent from the left side of the heart, afferent into the right side of the heart, the two sides communicating through the pulmonary or minor circulation. It was still uncertain, however, how arterial blood made its transit into the venous system, a question conveniently ignored by Harvey. Malpighi squared the circle with his histological description of capillaries in frog and tortoise lungs and in the toad bladder. He observed the transit of "red globules" from artery to vein in *in vivo* preparations. He founded the science of microscopic anatomy, and is generally thought of as the "father of histology."

Malpighi was born in Crevalcore, near Bologna, on March 10, 1628. He was raised on a farm. He entered the University of Bologna at 17 years of age, but was forced to abandon his studies for more than 2 years to settle family affairs when his father, mother, and paternal grandmother all died within months of each other. He was granted doctorates in medicine and in philosophy in 1653. Upon graduation, he applied for a position as lecturer at Bologna, but it was 3 years before the post was awarded. He became a lecturer in logic. Contemporaneously, he was offered the first chair in Theoretical Medicine at the University of Pisa, which he accepted. He remained in Pisa for 3 years. It was in Pisa that Malpighi met and befriended Giovanni Borelli, a mathematician and polymath interested in animal movement among other more abstract things. Borelli exerted a powerful effect on Malpighi's scientific outlook and became a mentor for, and collaborator with, Malpighi for the remainder of his life.

A Biographical History of Endocrinology, First Edition. D. Lynn Loriaux.

This work is a co-publication between the Endocrine Society and John Wiley & Sons, Ltd.

After 3 years in Pisa, Malpighi returned to Bologna, claiming family pressures and poor health as the reasons. Three years later, on the recommendation of Borelli, he was again offered a professorship at another university, Messina. Again, Malpighi took the job and was appointed as a Professor Primus in Medicine. He remained there for 4 years and then returned to Bologna for the last time. He remained there for the next 25 years until, in 1691, in failing health, he was appointed as the personal physician to Pope Innocent XII. He died of a stroke in Rome on September 30, 1694.

During his student years in Bologna, Malpighi was one of a few select students invited to attend private dissections and vivisections by Bartolomeo Massari, university professor and leading anatomist of his time. In 1654, Malpighi married Francesca Massari, the younger sister of the great anatomist. She died a year later, but Malpighi's life as an anatomist was ensured. Malpighi's first article appeared in 1661. It was published as two letters to his friend Borelli, "De pulmonibus." In this landmark article, Malpighi described the anatomy of the frog lung, bronchioles, alveoli, and the pulmonary capillary bed. In these capillaries (capilla means scalp hair) he could see, *in vivo*, "red globules" moving from arterioles to venules. The capillary bed was the final insight required to solidify the concept of the circulation of the blood. This and other articles were noticed by Henry Oldenburg, Secretary of the Royal Society of England. Oldenburg asked if Malpighi would correspond with him, and Malpighi became the first Italian fellow of the Royal Society. From this time forward, most of his discoveries were published in the *Proceedings of the Royal Society*.

Malpighi studied the development of the chicken embryo. He was convinced that he could see the form of the chick in unfertilized eggs. This became an important force in the "predelineation" movement. This was one of Malpighi's scientific errors. Malpighi's study of the liver, spleen, and kidney convinced him that organs are composed of glandular structures, corpuscles, that in aggregate, constitute the organ. He described the renal corpuscle (nephron), the splenic corpuscle (lymphoid centers), and the hepatic secretory unit. He studied insects and described the trachea through which insects breathe. He made a comprehensive study of the silkworm (*De Bombyce*). He studied the clotting of blood (*De Polypo Cordis*). He was the first person to describe the erythrocyte. He studied neuroanatomy and concluded that the brain is an endocrine organ. He studied plants and described the annular rings and deduced their cause. The great Swedish botanist Linnaeus named a family of plants after Malpighi, the Malpighiaceae.

The last decade of Malpighi's life was accompanied by challenge and criticism as is often the case for scientific pioneers. Pope Innocent XII intervened and invited him to Rome in 1691 as papal archiater (first physician) to the Pope. He was further honored by election to the College of Doctors in Medicine and a teaching appointment in the Papal Medical School. He died September 30, 1694. He is buried in the church of Santi Gregorio e Siro in Bologna. The inscription on the marble tablet over his tomb reads "Summum Ingenium, Integerrimam Vitam, Fortem Strenuamque Mentem, Audacem Salutaris Artis Amorem" (great genius, honest life, strong and tough mind, audacious love for the medical profession).

Sources

Major RH: *A History of Medicine*. Springfield, IL: Charles C. Thomas, 1954.

Meli DB: *Mechanism, Experiment, Disease; Marcello Malpighi and Seventeenth Century Anatomy*. Baltimore, MD: Johns Hopkins University Press, 2011.

This chapter has been reproduced from Loriaux, D. Lynn: Marcello Malpighi: 1628–1694. *The Endocrinologist* 2010; 20(2): 45.

CHAPTER 16
Richard Lower (1631–1691)
The Pituitary Gland

Richard Lower was the son of a country gentleman. He was born on a family estate near St. Tudy, Cornwall, England. He attended the Westminster School of St. Peter's College, probably the most celebrated British preparatory school of the era. The headmaster of Westminster saw great promise in Lower and arranged for his admission to Christ Church College at Oxford University. At Oxford, Lower earned an MA degree in 1655 and Bachelor of Medicine and Doctor of Medicine degrees in 1665. He studied chemistry under Peter Stahl, and became the protégé and assistant to Thomas Willis, then renowned as one of the greatest medical scientists in England. An informal group of scientists known as the "Oxford Physiologists" formed about the same time. Members included Thomas Willis, Ralph Bath, Robert Boyle, Robert Hooke, John Locke, John Mayow, Thomas Millington, Walter Needham, William Petty, Henry Stubbe, John Wallis, John Ward, and Christopher Wren. Lower, Millington, and Wren were key collaborators with Willis in his monumental *Cerebri Anatome*. It was Lower that developed the syringes that were capable of perfusing the cerebral venous and arterial circulations of the brain and who did most, if not all, of the dissections.

This was a time of great tension between the traditional "Galenists" and the new physiologists led by William Harvey. One of the more prominent of the "Galenists," Edmond Meara, attacked Willis, Lower, and the rest of the Oxford Physiologists in a book titled *Examen dia Thomae Willisii de Febriobus* (Examination of the Discourse of Thomas Willis on Fever). At issue was the strong support Willis professed for the scientific method of William Harvey. Lower rose up in defense of Willis, and single-handedly published *Diatribe Thomae Willsii de Febriobus Vindicato* (Vindication of the Discourse of Thomas Willis on Fever). The *Diatribe* vigorously defended Willis, Harvey, and Boyle, and proposed a fruitful research agenda for the future.

Lower married Elizabeth Billing in 1666 and had three daughters by her. Willis moved to London in 1666, and Lower followed him soon after. He set up a practice of medicine, but continued to collaborate with Willis until Willis died in 1675. Lower was

A Biographical History of Endocrinology, First Edition. D. Lynn Loriaux.

This work is a co-publication between the Endocrine Society and John Wiley & Sons, Ltd.

made a Fellow of the Royal Society in 1667, and a Fellow of the Royal College of Physicians in 1675, the year that Willis died.

With the death of Willis, Lower became one of the leading physicians in London and the physician to King Charles II, who he attended in his last illness. Lower was a Whig and a strong protestant. With the rise of King James II, Lower lost favor at court and his position as physician to the king was terminated.

Lower's scientific contributions can be thought of in three phases. The first was work done in association with Thomas Willis. Lower played a critical role in the research that went into the publication of Willis' famous text, *Cerebri Anatome* [1]. As noted, Lower developed the metal syringes that allowed for the perfusion of the venous and arterial systems of the brain, and his skills with dissection of the brain were legendary.

In *Cerebri Anatome,* Willis says of Lower:

> But for the more accurate performing this work, as I had not leisure, and perhaps not wit enough of myself, I was not ashamed to require the help of others. And here I made use of the Labours of the most Learned Physician and highly skilful Anatomist, Doctor *Richard Lower*, for my help and Companion; the edge of whose Knife and Wit I willingly acknowledge to have been an help to me for the better searching out both the frame and offices of before hidden Bodies. Wherefore having got this help and Companion, no day past over without some Anatomical administration; so that in a short space there was nothing of the Brain, and its Appendix within the Skull, that seemed not plainly detected, and intimately beheld by us. After this, we entered upon a far more difficult task, the Anatomy.

It was Lower who showed that ligation of three of the four arteries supplying the brain can be survived because of the collateral circulation provided by the circle of Willis.

Lower's first independent scientific work was published in 1669, *Tractatus de Corde* [2]. In this work he showed that the color change of venous blood, blue, to arterial blood, red, was not caused by the motion of the lungs, but by the exposure of lung tissue to air. Through careful dissection, he revealed the sustentacular scaffolding of the heart and he showed that all of the lymph from the small intestine and ileum flowed into the Cisterna Chylie, and thence through the thoracic duct and into the left subclavian vein. Intertwined with this work were his studies on blood transfusion. Lower showed for the first time that blood could be transfused from animal to man, and from man to man.

One chapter in *Tractatus* eventually became an independent publication, *De Catarrhis* [3], published in 1672. Since the time of Galen, it was believed that the "natural spirit" was converted into the "vital," or "animal," spirit in the brain and that the by-product of this conversion, *pituita* (Latin for phlegm), was expelled by the pituitary gland through the cribriform plate, and into the nasal cavity as catarrh. Dogma held that any fluid overload was managed by the ventricles of the brain and that normal fluid balance was maintained by the excretion of pituita, again expressed as nasal and pulmonary catarrh. Lower examined these concepts in detail, finding through careful dissection no pores connecting the nasal cavity with the pituitary gland or with the sella turcica. He did several experiments using milk and tiny carbon fragments suspended in an aqueous solution that were introduced into the subdural space or into the lateral ventricles. He found no evidence for the transmission of these substances into the nasal cavity, thus ending the Galenic concept of pituitary function. He did conclude, however, that the first cranial nerve was responsible for the sense of smell. These studies were among the first in medicine to extend the scientific method into the experimental method, a very important transition.

Lower died on January 17, 1691, from pneumonia, presumably initiated by smoke inhalation that occurred when he helped to extinguish a house fire in London several days before.

References

1. Willis, Thomas: *Cerebri Anatome: cui accessit nervorum descriptio et usus.* Amsterdam: Gerbrandum Schagen, 1664.
2. Lower, Richard: *Tractatus de Corde: Item De Motu & Colore Sanguinis, Et Chyli in eum Tranfitu.* Amsterdam: Danielem Elzevirium, 1669.
3. Lower, Richard: *De Catarrhis.* London: Dawsons of Pall Mall, 1672.

This chapter has been reproduced from Loriaux, D. Lynn: Richard Lower: 1631–1691. *The Endocrinologist* 2010; 20(4): 147–8.

CHAPTER 17

Regnier de Graaf (1641–1673)

The Graafian Follicle

De Graaf was a Dutch physician who was born in Schoonhoven, Holland, and practiced in Delft, about 30 miles away. He studied medicine in Utrecht (1660) and Leiden (1663), then a major medical center. A fellow student of de Graaf's was Jan Swammerdam, an excellent anatomist and biologist who never practiced medicine and who was later involved in a priority dispute with de Graaf. Another contemporary was Niels (Nils) Stensen, also called Steno, the Danish anatomist who described the parotid duct in 1660. He worked with Sylvius, van Horne, and Swammerdam in the 1660s and received his MD at Leiden in 1664 [1, 2].

As a student at Leiden, de Graaf was encouraged in research. De Graaf's first research work, while a student, was on the pancreas. He was able to cannulate both the pancreatic duct and one of the salivary gland ducts and do simple studies on the fluids he obtained. Sylvius suggested that he write up his pancreatic studies as a book. Thus in 1664, de Graaf had his first publication (*Disputatio medica de natura et usu succi pancreatici*, or Thesis on the nature and function of pancreatic juice). No one seems to have repeated this work until Claude Bernard over 150 years later.

De Graaf went to Paris in 1665. Well-known because of his research, he joined the circle of Louis XIV's personal physician. He traveled widely in France, staying long enough at Angers in northwestern France to get an MD from its university, a celebrated seat of learning until the French Revolution. In 1666, his thesis on pancreatic juice was revised, extended, and published in French in Paris shortly after he had returned to the Netherlands to practice medicine. It is clear that it was not the anatomy of the pancreas that was his goal, but rather its function.

De Graaf went back to Paris in 1667 for another year and then returned to Delft, this time for good. Within a year of his return, he published three more treatises bound in a single volume (1668). One was the invention of a syringe which was surprisingly modern in design. Second was his invention of a device enabling a person to self-administer an enema, which is not as simple as it might seem as rubber tubing did not exist. Third was his first foray into reproductive science. This led to a monograph

A Biographical History of Endocrinology, First Edition. D. Lynn Loriaux.

This work is a co-publication between the Endocrine Society and John Wiley & Sons, Ltd.

on the testis (*De virorum organis generationi inservientibus*, or On the generative organs of men). This small monograph reflected the first part of his work on reproductive organs which he probably began about 1665. It may not have been as original as his other work since at least one other anatomist had studied the testis about 10 years before. De Graaf probably did not know about the previous work.

De Graaf made important contributions to the anatomy of the testis and penile function. At the time it was thought that the testis was glandular and contained only soft amorphous tissue without defined structure or membranous tissues. De Graaf's dissection showed that the testis was largely composed of fine tubules that he called "vessels" and, when teased out, were long and thin or "threadlike." He showed that some of these tiny tubes led to larger "efferent vessels" and thence to the epididymis. This connected with the vas deferens, the whole being the path of the semen to the penis. By tying off the vas deferens he showed that the semen, in fact, came from the testis. Spermatozoa had yet to be discovered and there was no microscopy of the testis to show its fine structure. De Graaf also studied erectile dysfunction. He showed that injection of water (using his syringe) into the arteries leading to an animal's penis caused an erection. He concluded that the main mechanism of erection was vascular rather than neural or muscular [3].

During the seventeenth century, communication among scientists was done by reading each other's books. In 1660, a new intermediary arose: London's fledgling Royal Society. The Royal Society at the time was fairly poor (many members did not pay their dues) but it was dedicated to frequent meetings (weekly or bi-weekly) to demonstrate and discuss new scientific data. The prime goal was to do, analyze, and discuss research. The stated goal was the "promotion of natural knowledge." It was a working scientific group. The members frequently demonstrated experiments to each other as confirmation or refutation of a scientific claim. The members also made a conscious commitment to foster communication among fellow scientists in Europe. Henry Oldenburg was the Society's Secretary for most of the 1660s and 1670s and responsible for turning the Society into an international clearing house for the science of the day. Investigators from all over Europe sent their work to Oldenburg, either as letters or books, usually written in Latin. He would then write of the work to other scientists in Europe. He would help get the work presented at meetings of the Society and, sooner or later, published in the *Philosophical Transactions*. The early issues of the *Transactions* carry work from all over the continent.

Oldenburg convinced many European scientists to write him regularly to report on their own and others' work. For example, Marcello Malpighi, the famous anatomist who later discovered how blood gets from the right heart to the left through the pulmonary capillaries, reported from Bologna on a wide range of investigators. Oldenburg used the erratic postal services and, later, the equivalent of the diplomatic pouch to get the mail through. Even when England was at war he kept up his correspondence with the correspondents' countries. He was once thrown into the Tower for a few weeks on suspicion of spying. His letters and the *Transactions* became a principal means of scientific exchange in Europe.

De Graaf sent his book on the testis to the Royal Society, hoping for a good critique. Oldenburg wrote Malpighi who replied that he strongly approved of de Graaf 's results on the tubular nature of the testis. On the other hand, Dr. Timothy Clarke doubted de Graaf's results so the Society repeated de Graaf's experiment to show the tubules. More correspondence among Oldenburg, de Graaf, and Clarke ensued and several of the Society's members repeated the experiment themselves and, again, demonstrated that the human testis had a tubular structure. The discussion then focused on whether or not the testis was completely made of tubules or perhaps only partly made of tubules. Most doubted that there were only tubules and Dr. Clarke said that, even if it were the case, an English scientist had shown tubules 30 years before. The debate continued into 1669. In July 1669, de Graaf sent the Society a dissection of a testis of the edible dormouse pickled in wine that clearly showed multiple tubules. The Society's consensus was that de Graaf was right. That he was not the first to show the tubules was clear, but his was the better presentation, and that a drawing of de Graaf's dormouse preparation should be published. Oldenburg wrote Malpighi of de Graaf's thesis and his gift of the dormouse testis; Malpighi agreed in a 1670 letter to Oldenburg, that the "very accurate Graaf" was right and that, combined with others' work, "there should no longer be any doubt" [4, 5].

De Graaf was not alone in trying to untangle the mysteries of how animals reproduced. In fact, it was a "hot topic" at the time. His Dutch professors and colleagues, Sylvius, van Horne, and Swammerdam, all still in Leiden, and Stensen, now in Florence in the court of the Grand Duke Ferdinand II, were looking into the issue as well. So was Malpighi in Bologna. By then it was more or less settled that birds' eggs, that is, the structure composed of a yolk surrounded by a clear albuminous fluid and an outer membrane plus a shell, were located in an abdominal organ formerly called the female "testis." Girolamo Fabrici in Padua, also called Fabricius ab Aquapendente, named the reproductive organ of the bird the "ovary" because it contained eggs. Fabrici also knew that these ovarian birds' eggs were closely associated with nearby "tubes," or "small trumpets," named after his Paduan teacher Gabriele Falloppio. Fabrici did not think of the bird egg as originating in the ovary. He thought of the ovary and tube as a kind of complicated brood chamber. Nothing was known of oocytes, spermatozoa, or even cells as individual entities. The roles of the male and female in generating the young chick were purely speculative. The "egg" was the entire structure of yolk surrounded by sticky fluid, membrane, and shell. Fabrici concluded that mammals had no eggs in the "female testis." He could see nothing that resembled a bird's egg. So, for the next 50 years, mammals had female "testes" but not "ovaries." The common thought in the 1660s was that the male testicular essence, the fluid semen, mixed in the uterus with the female testicular essence, a hypothetical female semen, and the mixture somehow turned into an "egg" and a fetus, all in the uterus.

By 1667, Malpighi had seen vesicles and yellowish bodies in the cow's testis but did not know what to make of them and did not publish. The Leiden group saw the same structures. Van Horne and Swammerdam, working together in 1666–1667, thought that the vesicles were similar enough to those in the birds' ovaries that they should be considered eggs. Van Horne published a short note in 1668 and used the word "ova" but did not give a complete description. In his 1667 book on muscles

(*Elementorum myologiae specimen*) Stensen also wrote a short note to the same effect and may have been the first to use "ovarium" as applied to mammals. Swammerdam, who not only knew Stensen from Leiden but had stayed with him when both were in Paris, wrote Stensen to say that he and van Horne had the same idea and asked Stensen to delay further public elucidation of the idea of the female testis as an ovary until they were able to publish their already planned book. Stensen agreed to this bold request. The Leiden partners never wrote up their data. Van Horne's death in 1670 ended the project.

Meantime, Stensen met with Malpighi in Bologna in 1669 and, as Malpighi later wrote, discussed their findings in dissections of the fetus and pregnant uterus. Stensen then traveled to Holland and saw de Graaf, to whom he mentioned Malpighi's data. At that time de Graaf was continuing his work on female reproductive organs – which means that de Graaf and the other Leiden investigators were working on the same topic at the same time in the late 1660s. Stensen wrote Malpighi that de Graaf promised to send Malpighi his (de Graaf's) results before he published them. We do not know if this happened. Among Malpighi's wide-ranging work he continued to take notes on the female reproductive organs. For example, in 1671 he confirmed his previous findings that there were vesicles and yellow bodies in the cow's "testis" and decided that the organ is "really the ovary." Falloppio and others had seen these yellow bodies as well, but Malpighi gave them their modern name: corpus luteum, or yellow body. Curiously, the name stuck even though the corpus luteum is actually yellow only in cows [6]. Malpighi still did not publish any of this despite his role as a reporter to the Royal Society.

The year 1672 was not a good year for the Dutch. The Anglo-Dutch War began again, the third war between the two countries in 20 years. The French under Louis XIV also began a war with the Netherlands that same year. The French invaded the country, but the Dutch opened their dikes to prevent the French from occupying the land. It was in this year of Dutch travail that de Graaf published his little masterpiece on the female generative organs (*De mulierum organis generationi inservientibus tractatus novus*, or A new treatise on the female reproductive organs) [7]. The book is small (about 4 inches by 6 inches), as were many at the time, and would easily fit in one's pocket. In it, de Graaf summarized his work of the previous few years. He discussed the entire female reproductive system, but the two chapters of most interest are those that show the female "testes" are really ovaries. In chapter XII, "On the testes of females, or ovaries," he pointed out that the female "testes" have in them small vesicles full of liquid ("Always found in the testicles are vesicles full of fluid"). By analogy, he thought the fluid in the vesicle corresponded to the albuminous fluid in the bird egg. He confirmed the analogy by showing that heating the vesicles brought about the same changes as occur in heating a hen's egg; both then had the same color, consistency, and flavor. His dissection of a human ovary is one of the earliest. He presumed that the vesicle, or egg, contained something necessary for fetal development. He listed a number of wellknown anatomists who described these vesicles and gave specific credit to his former professor, van Horne, for calling them ova. The difference between him and his predecessors was the quality and comprehensiveness of description. He wanted to show that they occurred in as many species as possible and, with Stensen's help, found them in all mammals studied. That search enabled him to claim that "eggs are found all animals." The organ therefore had to be called the ovary. He observed as well that some of these eggs push up the surface of the ovary "as if threatening to make a quick exit."

De Graaf then went on to describe another type of ovarian body (a "globule") that was not permanent and only appeared from time to time. He gave a good detailed description of what we now call the corpus luteum. De Graaf probably did not know of Malpighi's name for these "globules." De Graaf thought that the corpus luteum appeared only after coitus in all animals. He made this mistake because his principal experimental animal was the rabbit, in which the corpus luteum only appears after coitus. Many regard de Graaf as the discoverer of the corpus luteum because he was the first to publish his description in detail and to relate it to the egg. It was his idea that the glandular material that made up the corpus luteum formed directly from the tissue surrounding the egg, and that the growth of the follicle–corpus luteum pushed the vesicular egg out into the fallopian tube. He thought that the entire fluid-filled vesicle was "shelled out" of the ovary to make its way into the tube as an egg. In fact, the follicle was what was left behind as it formed into the more solid glandular "globule" or corpus luteum.

De Graaf's ovarian studies were detailed and derived from many observations. His observations, however, gave no support to the hypothesis that the "eggs" actually left the ovary and gave rise in some way to embryos in the uterus. De Graaf now focused on understanding reproduction in rabbits. It is an experimental tour de force. He was lucky in his choice of rabbits because his aim was to look for "eggs" in the tubes and uterus at specific times after coitus. As it happens, ovulation in rabbits occurs about 10 hours after coitus. Had de Graaf chosen, for example, the dog, his observations would have been much more difficult to make. He used over 100 rabbits to make his series of observations. In essence, he made what amounted to a slow-motion movie of the stages of rabbit fetal development.

He examined the ovaries, tubes, and uteri of rabbits from 30 minutes to 29 days after coitus. To his delight, he found "ova" in the tubes and uterus, which confirmed his idea that the eggs were released from the ovary and passed through the tubes on their way to the uterus, developing as they went. He was puzzled by the facts that he found no ova for about 3 days and, when he did, the ones he found were only about one tenth the size of the ones presumably released by the ovary. He postulated that some of the fluid in the egg was lost in transit. We now know that the egg or ovum is microscopic compared with de Graaf's "egg," which was the Graafian follicle. What he had seen were blastocysts in the tubes and uterus, which take about 3 days to become big enough to be seen with the naked eye. He assumed that they were the same structures released by the ovary. Without a microscope he could do no better. Though this was an error, in retrospect, it did describe the process of something moving from the ovaries through the tubes into the uterus and becoming a fetus. His observation of a tubal "egg" was original and was supported by his noting cases of tubal pregnancy in women. He was able to match the number of ovarian "globules" (corpora lutea) with the number of developing "ova" (blastocysts), which supported his hypothesis.

He concluded that "all men and animals originate in an egg; not from an egg formed in the uterus by semen, as Aristotle says, or by a seminal essence, as Harvey says, but from an egg that existed before coitus in the female testis." Though the details of his findings were not entirely accurate in light of modern knowledge, he had the process right. He had shifted the view of the female contribution to the fetus from simply offering the uterus as an incubator to providing something substantial and essential from the ovary.

It is clear that de Graaf's egg, the entire fluid-filled follicle, was reasonably named as it was a direct analogy to the entire bird's egg. Our modern use of "ovum" or "egg" to mean the much smaller gamete makes discussion of de Graaf's work confusing. This modern use of "egg" or "ovum" began in the nineteenth century when Karl von Baer was studying fetal development in dogs. In 1827, while tracing backward from larger embryos to smaller ones, he looked at the ovary to see exactly what it was there that led to the embryo. The problem had been considered by many over the years but was considered "insoluble." He looked closely at the follicle with a microscope and saw that each one had in it a small "yellowish-white point." He removed one with the point of a knife, looked at it again in the microscope, and saw what we call the oocyte ("eggcell"). The idea that tissues were made up of cells had not yet been invented and was unknown to both de Graaf and von Baer. Thus, von Baer could not have called it an oocyte ("egg-cell"). He did call it the "ovule" or "little egg." He specifically noted it to be within the "vesicula Graafiana." Later biologists referred to von Baer's discovery as the egg or ovum, hence the modern confusion in reading de Graaf.

De Graaf's name was first attached to his ovarian vesicle in 1765 almost 100 years later. Albrecht von Haller called them "ova Graafiana" or "vesiculae Graafianae." They were called Graafian vesicles into the mid-nineteenth century. The term "Graafian follicle" came into use in 1842 to avoid confusion with the then new term, germinal vesicle.

Texts of the 1990s usually show a picture of the "Graafian follicle," which now refers only to the follicle and its contents when there is a fully developed antrum. In women, in whom there is only one ovulation at a time, the term "Graafian follicle" is often dropped in favor of "dominant follicle." In the broader view of biology, "Graafian" seems better as it applies to all mammals, multi-ovulatory or not.

Despite the political tension between the Dutch and the English in 1672, de Graaf's new book quickly reached Oldenburg and the Royal Society. Oldenburg wrote Malpighi on April 24 that year and asked him what he thought. Malpighi replied in letters on June 7 and August 2 that he had not yet received the book because of the wars in Holland, but that he agreed with de Graaf that eggs do in fact come from the female "testis." Once again, the European network was evaluating de Graaf's work and he actively sought their evaluation. De Graaf's reception in Leiden was not so pleasant. Within weeks of the publication of his book, Swammerdam published a pamphlet that bitterly attacked de Graaf and essentially accused him of plagiarism. As noted above, it is clear that Swammerdam and van Horne in Leiden and de Graaf in Delft were working on the same thing at the same time and probably each knew something of the other's work. Nevertheless, de Graaf was working independently and, most importantly, finished what he started and published his results. By 1672, when de Graaf published, van Horne had died and Swammerdam, who had held off Stensen from publishing still had written nothing. De Graaf countered Swammerdam's complaint with a pamphlet of his own and pointed out that Swammerdam himself had encouraged de Graaf to publish in a letter written in 1670, 2 years before.

Both Swammerdam and de Graaf agreed to look for an impartial decision from the Royal Society. Three Fellows of the Society were appointed to arbitrate and, after due consideration, came to a non-committal conclusion. They sent their nondecision to Holland in 1673 but by then the tragic part of the story had happened: de Graaf had died at the age of 32 years, perhaps of the plague. A modern comparison of what was published by de Graaf, van Horne, and Swammerdam concluded that only de Graaf had seen beyond structure to assess function and had tested function experimentally. De Graaf's work was also more thorough and better illustrated. It seems right to remember de Graaf as the innovator.

But no innovator's ideas are accepted at once even when their apparent importance is emphasized by a dispute over priority. There was still great uncertainty in 1672 about the role of the semen, and sperm were still unknown. De Graaf himself thought that, whatever the semen did, it did it to the ova in the ovary.

A few months before he died in 1673, de Graaf wrote to the Royal Society, again defending himself against Swammerdam. He added a postscript about a colleague in Delft who, though in business as a draper and untrained in science, was making the best microscopes de Graaf had seen. The draper, Antonie van Leeuwenhoek, had made his first microscope in 1671 and, by 1673, his best microscope magnified 270 times. That he made his first one in 1671 when de Graaf was in the last stages of writing his book probably explains why de Graaf had no microscopic data. (Incidentally, "Leeuwenhoek" was his adopted name: it means "Lion's Corner" after his father's corner house near the Lion's Gate in Delft; his actual surname was Thoniszoon [8]).

Though van Leeuwenhoek kept notes, he published nothing. de Graaf saw that the high quality of van Leeuwenhoek's work would never be known without being published. He wrote Oldenburg that "a certain most ingenious person here, named van Leeuwenhoeck (sic), has devised microscopes which far surpass those we have hitherto seen." De Graaf attached a letter from van Leeuwenhoek, containing some of van Leeuwenhoek's work and written in Dutch, to his own letter. The Society had the letter translated and published it in the Society's *Philosophical Transactions*. It became van Leeuwenhoek's first publication and was the first of 308 letters he wrote to the Society over his long lifetime (he lived for 50 more years); he never did write a book as was the custom of the time.

Van Leeuwenhoek worked continuously and kept sending the Society new discoveries. In 1674, he showed that microorganisms were alive and wrote the Society about this in 1676. His main discovery, for our purposes, was his finding in 1677 of animalculi or "little animals" in the semen; they may have first been seen by a student, Johann Hamen, in 1674, who obtained the sample from a patient with a urethral discharge. As usual, van Leeuwenhoek's letter to the Royal Society in November, 1677, did not get published until 2 years later (Observationes de natis e semine genitali animalculis. *Philos Trans Roy Soc* 1679; 12: 1040). Although the savants were happy enough to engage in priority disputes, no one then seemed in a terrific rush to get into print. Van Leeuwenhoek became an "animalculist," or one who thought that the embryo was formed from one of these little animals, or spermatozoa. In van Leeuwenhoek's mind, de Graaf's egg, if it did anything, provided no more than nourishment to the embryo. Research on the topic languished over the next 100 years although theoretical disputes between the animalculists and the ovists, those who maintained the primacy of the egg, continued [9].

De Graaf's ideas on the egg as the precursor to the fetus fell into some disfavor, in part because of the efforts of his Delftian colleague. Another reason was that anyone with a microscope could see the little animals but only someone with great skill and patience could repeat de Graaf's work. Evidence to support the animalculists was easy to obtain. But in 1778, over 100 years after de Graaf's death, William Cruikshank, an assistant to William Hunter in London, thought it was time to repeat de Graaf's studies on fetal development in rabbits. Hunter gave Cruikshank all the rabbits he wanted, Cruikshank did everything that de Graaf did and confirmed de Graaf completely. True to their nature, it was not until 20 years later, in 1797, that the Royal Society published Cruikshank's data [6].

De Graaf's story does make a few points. Science at its basic level has not changed much in 300 years. Most of us still insist on peer review, at least for others, and try to seek it for ourselves lest we look foolish. We are familiar with priority disputes, however unpleasant they are in the nature of science and human personalities. Sometimes our cherished proofs take longer than seems reasonable for our friends to accept. Eventually, if we are right, they do, but not always.

References

1. Catchpole HR: Regnier de Graaf. 1641–1673. *Bull Hist Med* 1940; 8: 1261.
2. Hunter M: *The Royal Society and its Fellows. 1660–1700.* Oxford: British Society for the History of Science, 1994.
3. Setchell BP: The contributions of Regnier de Graaf to reproductive biology. *Eur J Obstet Gynecol Reprod Biol* 1974; 4: 1.
4. Adelmann HB: *Marcello Malpighi and the evolution of embryology.* Ithaca, NY: Cornell University Press, 1966, pp. 329–30, 355–9, 723–6, 780–1.
5. Adelmann HB (Ed.): *The Correspondence of Marcello Malpighi.* Ithaca, NY: Cornell University Press, 1975, pp. 483, 615, 623.
6. Corner GW: The discovery of the mammalian ovum. In *Lectures on the History of Medicine. 1926–1932,* edited by LB Wilson. Philadelphia, PA: W.B. Saunders, 1933, p. 401.
7. de Graaf R: *De Mulierum Organis Generationi lnservientibus Tractatus Novus: Demonstrans tam Homines et Animalia Caetera Omnia, Quae Vivipara Dicuntur, Haud Minus Quam Ovipara ab Ovo Originem Ducere.* Leiden: Hack, 1672 (copy at the Countway Medical Library, Boston, Massachusetts).
8. Dobell C: *Antony van Leeuwenhoek and his "Little Animals."* New York: Dover, 1960.
9. Castellani C: Spermatozoan biology from Leeuwenhoek to Spallanzani. *J Hist Biol* 1973; 6: 37.

This chapter has been reproduced from Loriaux, D. Lynn: Reinier de Graaf (1641–1673). *The Endocrinologist* 2008; 18(1): 1–2.

CHAPTER 18

Antonie van Leeuwenhoek (1632–1723)

The First of the Great Microscopists

Antonie van Leeuwenhoek did not invent the microscope, but he was the first great microscopist. His success can be attributed to his commitment to the exclusive use of small (1–2 mm) spherical glass lenses of enormous magnification power, 200–400×, depending upon the diameter. The clarity and sharpness of his images were far superior to those of his competitors who were using compound microscopes (two lenses) that suffered from marked chromatic and focus distortion.

Van Leeuwenhoek was born in Delft, Netherlands, in 1632. This was a time when the Dutch were world leaders in commerce, art, and science. The van Leeuwenhoek family was financially middle class. His father made a good living with a small basket-making business supplemented by income from a small brewery. When he was 7 years old, his father died. His mother quickly remarried, and Antonie did not get along with his stepfather. He was sent to a boarding school in Warmond. Apparently this did not go well either, and he was sent to live with an uncle in Benthuizen. Two years later, when he was 16 years old, he was apprenticed as a bookkeeper to a Scottish cloth merchant in Amsterdam. He returned to Delft when he was 23 and opened his own draper's shop.

To augment his income, he applied for, and won the job of Chamberlain to the Sheriff of Delft. In this capacity, he managed the day-to-day functioning of the Sheriff's office. The appointment turned out to be a sinecure for life, paying him 800 guilders a year, which continued until his death at 90 years of age. The security provided by this job allowed him to marry a clergyman's daughter in 1666 and start a family. The financial security of the post also allowed him free time to pursue his avocation, lens making.

In his linen business, the quality of various cloths was, in part, related to the "tightness" of the weave, threads per millimeter. The higher the thread count, the more valuable the cloth. Most drapers used a magnifying glass to count threads, but it was wholly inadequate for the finest linens and silks. He needed an optical aid that could be used with the best cloths. He began to experiment with spherical glass lenses. These lenses were extremely powerful.

A Biographical History of Endocrinology, First Edition. D. Lynn Loriaux.

This work is a co-publication between the Endocrine Society and John Wiley & Sons, Ltd.

The magnification power was related to the diameter of the sphere.

$$M = 340 / d,$$

where M is the magnification and d is the diameter of the sphere in millimeters. His first lenses were about 1/8 inch in diameter, 3 millimeters, 100×. This was a huge improvement for cloth grading. Leeuwenhoek became almost obsessed with making smaller lenses of previously unachievable power, 300–400×. It was said that the Leeuwenhoek lenses equaled or surpassed in quality those made by the best lens makers of the time, and that he had a secret technique for grinding and polishing these little lenses. If this was so, he never revealed his process.

Looking back over the glass-making industry, it is likely that we can now understand how he did it. The key was making tiny glass spheres perfectly spherical and without inclusions. The speculation is that he used the "glass filament" approach to the problem. He would start with 2- or 3-mm-thick glass rods of the highest quality optical glass he could find. Using an alcohol lamp and a blow pipe, he would heat the middle of a 12- to 16-inch rod to the point of "sagging," and then quickly pull the ends apart, leaving them attached only by a glass filament the thickness of a human hair. He would break off the filament at one end, leaving a long filament of glass attached to a 5- or 6-inch piece of unaltered glass rod, the handle. Holding the filament by the "handle," he would bring the end of the filament close enough to the flame to melt it into a small glass sphere, the size of which could be controlled by the amount of filament melted and the rate of melting. Surface tension did the rest, ensuring a near perfect sphere, probably more perfect than could be made with grinding of any kind using graded abrasives. To sort the lenses, he needed a perfectly flat surface. For this, he used a pane of "float glass," a glass plate made by pouring molten glass over a pool of mercury or molten tin. The resultant glass plate, cooled and solidified, was almost perfectly flat. He would select only the spheres that rolled straight down the inclined glass plane. Of these, he would discard the spheres that had inclusions or scattered transilluminated light. The result was almost perfect spheres, without ever having to grind or polish at all.

Van Leeuwenhoek made 419 lenses, of which 217 were incorporated into simple microscopes. The microscope looked like a small ping-pong paddle, the lens contained in the paddle portion of the instrument, the handle being composed of a screw that could raise or lower a block of brass that held the sample under study and had a thumb-screw that could move the block toward or away from the paddle surface to allow an entire specimen to be studied, edge to edge and top to bottom. The light source was usually the sun.

Using this simple optical instrument, van Leeuwenhoek made drawings of what he saw that are truly spectacular. His first discovery was an amazing array of protozoa swimming in pond water. He called these organisms his "wee beasties."

> The motion of most of them was swift, and so various, upward, downward, and roundabout, that I admit that I could not but wonder about it. I judge that some of these little creatures were about a thousand times smaller than the smallest one that I have hitherto seen. Some of these are so exceedingly small that millions of millions might be contained in a single drop of water [1].

Van Leeuwenhoek's work came to the attention of Regnier de Graaf in 1668. De Graaf was studying reproductive biology in a number of animals, and he believed that van Leeuwenhoek's microscope would be an invaluable aid in these studies. He knew of Robert Hooke's studies in England using a compound microscope, and believed that van Leeuwenhoek's microscope was superior. He arranged a meeting with Henry Oldenburg, the Secretary of the Royal Society of London for Improving Natural Knowledge (aka The Royal Society). Robert Hooke was asked to verify van Leeuwenhoek's findings, which he did. Along the way, Hooke discovered the cellular nature of cork, leading to the concept that all living things are composed of cells.

De Graaf died suddenly in 1673 at 32 years of age. His death closely followed the death of a child and a growing controversy over some of his scientific findings. Years later, van Leeuwenhoek said that his death could be attributed to an accumulation of "choleric substances" (i.e., melancholia). His introduction of van Leeuwenhoek to Oldenburg, however, led to the publication of all of van Leeuwenhoek's findings as "letters" in the *Transactions* of the Royal Society. There are more than 200 such letters.

It these letters, van Leeuwenhoek describes *Spirogyra* and the flagellated protozoa in pond water, erythrocytes, leukocytes, spermatozoa, urate crystals in gout, the life cycle of the flea, *Giardia*, venous and lymphatic capillaries, volvox, and vorticella, among many more things.

In a letter to the Society in 1723, van Leeuwenhoek writes [2]:

> Not long ago after January finished, I was seized by a violent movement around that large and vital organ we call the diaphragm, so much indeed that those standing around were not a little alarmed. When the movement eased off, searching for a name for this illness, the doctor, who was there, answered it to be a palpitation of the heart. I think the doctor was in fact wrong. For although while the movement was happening I several times felt the arterial pulse with my hand. I did not feel any acceleration. Starting up again every now and then, the violent movement lasted about three days, during which time my stomach and intestine ceased to function. I thought I was at death's door.
>
> I am of the opinion an obstruction was stuck in my diaphragms, not smaller than an imperial penny.

Van Leeuwenhoek had several such attacks. Most believe that it was the cause of his death, others disagree. After van Leeuwenhoek's death, the Minister of his church wrote: "The notion possessed our good old man that he lay a-dying of a distemper of his diaphragm, though in fact 'twas of his lungs" [2].

The constellation of findings that he suffered from is now known to be diaphragmatic flutter. The condition is generally referred to as "Leeuwenhoek's syndrome". Van Leeuwenhoek died in 1723, 90 years of age, a famous man and a transformative scientist. It is not certain that he ever went to school.

References

1. Gillen AL: *The Genesis of Germs: Diseases and the Common Plagues*. Green Forest, AR: Master Books, 2007, p. 51.
2. Rankin JA: Von Leeuwenhoek's disease. *Am J Respir Crit Care Med* 2011; 83: 1434.

CHAPTER 19
John Hunter
(1728–1793)
Embryology of the Hind

John Hunter was the last of 10 children born to John and Agnes Hunter. He was born on February 14, 1728, at Long Calderwood, a farm estate near Glasgow, Scotland. Seven of his siblings died as children or young adults. Infectious disease extracted this savage toll from the Hunter family. The three survivors were John, William, 10 years John's senior, and Dorothea, an older sister. As a boy, Hunter was described as rebellious and lacking in self-control. This was attributed by most to an overindulgent mother, a situation not difficult to understand in the context of his being the last of 10, with seven before him lost at tender ages.

Hunter did poorly in academics, but he was not dull. "When I was a boy, I wanted to know all about the clouds and the grasses, and why leaves changed color in the autumn; I watched the ants, bees, birds, tadpoles and caddisworms; I pestered people with questions about what nobody knew or cared anything about" [1]. He lived with his mother at Long Calderwood until he was 17, at which time he moved to Glasgow to live with his sister and her husband, George Buchanan. George was a cabinetmaker, and John worked with him, finally qualifying as a wheelwright. He found little joy in this work, however, and when his brother William invited him to London in 1748, the offer was eagerly accepted.

William Hunter was a physician specializing in obstetrics. He is described as refined, courtly, and of a sagacious disposition. He spent 5 years at Glasgow University and then apprenticed himself to William Smellie (1697–1763), whose book, *Midwifery*, was the first to describe the techniques of forceps delivery and to define an "abnormal" pelvis on the basis of actual anatomical measurements. Smellie was famous for his obstetrics course, which was given in his home using manikins developed around actual human pelves of different proportions. The cost was three guineas.

The success of this course inspired William Hunter to devise a course of private lectures on human anatomy, operative surgery, and bandaging, a course that evolved into the famous anatomical theater and museum in Great Windmill Street, London, where all of the great anatomists and surgeons of the day trained. As the enterprise

A Biographical History of Endocrinology, First Edition. D. Lynn Loriaux.

This work is a co-publication between the Endocrine Society and John Wiley & Sons, Ltd.

grew, William became the most respected of the London obstetricians. Wealth followed his fame. His basic values, however, remained unaltered. "He never married; he had no country house; he looks, in his portraits a fastidious, fine gentleman, but he worked till he dropped and he lectured when he was dying" [1]. William's greatest legacy is his 1774 *Atlas of the Pregnant Uterus*, illustrated by Riensdigk at Hunter's personal expense. It described, for the first time, the independent fetal and maternal placental circulations, important fundamentals of modern placentology.

John Hunter came into this rarified environment at the age of 20 years. William put him to work as an anatomical assistant. It was one of those happy synergistic combinations that nature sometimes permits. Hunter found himself. The work captured his restless intellect and, by the end of his first year, he was teaching human anatomy unassisted. As his skills grew, he began to accompany William Cheseldon on his rounds. Cheseldon was considered the leading London surgeon of his day. In that pre-anesthetic time, speed was everything, and Cheseldon was the fastest of the lot. He could do a standard lithotomy in 54 seconds. Cheseldon had a stroke in 1752, and Hunter's medical education was given over to Percival Pott (Pott's fracture, Pott's disease). Thus, Hunter's medical foundation came, in aggregate, from three of the greatest physicians of the age. This auspicious beginning was turned to advantage.

In 1760, after 12 years of almost daily human dissection, Hunter suspected that he had contracted "consumption," and he joined the army to seek a posting to a warmer and more salubrious climate. After six months of rehabilitation, he was sent to Portugal and Spain, and he saw action in the Belle Isle expedition of 1761. This conflict provided his experience with gunshot wounds and laid the foundation for the last of his four masterpieces, the *Treatise on the Blood, Inflammation, and Gunshot Wounds*, which was published posthumously in 1795.

Returning to London in 1763, his life work began in earnest, a work so broad in compass that it is difficult to catalog in a simple way. There emerged, in retrospect, six themes: his work with venereal disease (the "Hunterian" chancre) [1], the development of vascular surgery [2], his study of the natural history of human dentition [3], organ transplantation [4], his famous museum [5], and the work on gunshot wounds [6].

That John Hunter inoculated himself with syphilis is disputed by some, but seems certain to me. He describes, in his own handwriting, the experiment designed to separate the natural history of gonorrhea from that of syphilis. "But as I have produced myself a chancre by matter from a gonorrhea that point is now settled" [3].

Hunter scarified his glans and prepuce with a lancet dipped in the urethral secretions of a man suffering from gonorrhea. He soon developed a right inguinal bubo and then a classic syphilitic chancre, followed by the rash of secondary syphilis. Hunter treated the chancre with calomel and rubbed mercurial ointment into his right leg in an attempt to attenuate, but not cure, the disease. After several years of this approach, he began the traditional 3-year mercury "cure" (one night with Venus, three years with Mercury!).

This unfortunate experiment was confounded by the erroneous conclusion made by Hunter that gonorrhea and syphilis were one. On the other hand, with its apparent success at the time, the experimental approach almost certainly influenced Edward Jenner, a pupil and confidant of Hunter, to try the same with cow pox, modified only by the use of a child, James Phipps, a healthy 8-year-old boy, as the subject of the experiment rather than Jenner himself.

John Hunter was fascinated by comparative anatomy and kept a small farm populated with exotic animals for the purpose. In a study of antler growth in deer, he ligated one carotid artery and found that the antler on that side became cool and ceased to grow. One week later, however, the antler warmed, and growth resumed. A dissection revealed the carotid ligature to be intact and the carotid circulation restored through a newly developed collateral circulation. On the basis of this observation, Hunter performed his first operation for popliteal aneurysm. The man, a 45-year-old coachman, had complete resolution of the aneurysm, only to die of a febrile illness 1 year later. Hunter's postmortem examination of the man revealed the aneurysm to be thrombosed and the limb well perfused with blood. This operation marks the beginning of the discipline of vascular surgery.

Hunter's experiments with transplantation have the greatest relevance to endocrinology. In 400 B.C.E. Aristotle had shown that qualities of "maleness," such as coloring and song in certain birds, could be ablated by castration [7]. Hunter showed that these qualities could be restored or produced *de novo* in female birds by testis transplantation. He thus demonstrated that the testis is the source of the "male factor." Hunter sums this up in a succinct statement that is difficult to improve upon, even with all that has gone on since:

> Let us take a testicle from a cock and put in into the belly of a gander. If it were possible that the ducts could unite so as to carry the seed that was secreted in the testicle to the female, the produce would be the same as if a cock had trod the goose, so that the powers of the testicle would remain in the same as if they had never been transplanted, and would continue to secrete the same kind of semen. The inclinations would not be towards the goose; for, although the testicles are the cause of the inclination, yet they do not direct these inclinations: the inclinations become an operation of the mind, after the mind is once stimulated by the testicle [4].

This work and its conceptual derivatives all antedated, and were known, to Arnold Adolph Berthold, whose experiments with testicular transplantation led him to be remembered as the "Father of Endocrinology."

The pathological and anatomical material that Hunter collected during his tour of military service formed the nidus of his extensive collection, which evolved into the Hunterian Museum. During the next 30 years of his life, the collection grew to 13 687 items, a collection rich in comparative and pathological anatomy. At his death, Hunter stipulated that the collection be kept intact and bequeathed entire to the Company of Surgeons (analogous to the American College of Surgeons). In 1811, a new building was built to house the collection, and it increased rapidly in size to more than 63 000 specimens at the time of World War II. On the night of May 10, 1941, however, the museum was hit by several incendiary bombs, and the greater part of the collection was destroyed. About 3500 of Hunter's specimens were salvaged, including the famous skeleton of Charles Byrne, the Irish giant, and the collection is housed to this day at the Royal College of Surgeons [6].

When Hunter was convinced that his luetic condition was adequately treated, he courted and married Anne Home, daughter of a surgical colleague. She is described as beautiful, gracious, and talented. She wrote and published verse, one poem of which was set to music by Haydn ("My Mother Bids Me Bind My Hair") [8]. They had four children in the first 5 years of their marriage.

In the spring of 1772, an anonymous 51-year-old physician read William Heberden's account of angina pectoris and recognized in it his own symptoms. Writing to Heberden, the physician said, "If it please God to take me away suddenly ... an examination of my body will show the cause of it." He died three weeks later, and an autopsy performed by Hunter was unrevealing. However, in three subsequent postmortem examinations of patients with angina, three were found to have ventricular aneurysms and one an apical scar. In addition, Hunter noted that "when I cut into the right ventricle I found the coronary artery, as it goes between the aurical and ventricle, ossified" [9].

During the next year, Hunter had an attack of severe epigastric pain, accompanied by pallor, which lasted 45 minutes. It was his first angina attack, perhaps more than angina alone. The symptoms progressed slowly, and, by 1789, Hunter was continuously plagued by nocturnal pain and exertional discomfort. The end came at a meeting of hospital staff in 1793. At that meeting, Hunter exhorted his colleagues to give more attention to the students and, on being contradicted, flew into a rage, left the room, and collapsed into the arms of a friend, dead. His postmortem examination revealed extensive coronary arterial disease. His wife Anne and the four children were left penniless.

John Hunter was the towering figure of eighteenth-century medicine. He was the founder of experimental and surgical pathology and a pathfinder in physiology and experimental morphology. His contributions to endocrinology largely fill the void between Aristotle and Berthold. The concept that maleness could be tethered to a gland was confirmed by him, and that finding defined the course for the endocrinologic torrent to follow. It is difficult to find any facet of modern medicine not touched by the intellect of this man. It is fitting that he was fascinated by giants. As the children say, it takes one to know one.

References

1. Sigerist HE: *Great Doctors: A Biographical History of Medicine* (2nd edn.). London: George Allen, 1935, p. 224.
2. Garrison FH: *History of Medicine*. Philadelphia, PA: Saunders, 1922, p. 346.
3. Lasky II: John Hunter, the Shakespeare of medicine. *Surg Gynecol Obstet* 1983; 156: 511–18.
4. Forbes TP: Testis transplantation performed by John Hunter. *Endocrinology* 1949; 41: 329–31.
5. Hunter J: *Essays and Observations on Natural History, Anatomy, etc.* Vols. 1–2, edited by Richard Owen. London, 1861.

6. Gray C: The remarkable surgical collection of John Hunter. *Can Med Assoc J* 1983; 128: 1225–8.
7. Aristotle: *Historia animalium*, Book 9, Vol. 4.
8. Cade S: The lasting dynamism of John Hunter: Hunterian oration. *Ann R Coll Surg Engl* 1963; 33: 5–19.
9. Proudfit WL: John Hunter: On heart disease. *Br Heart J* 1986; 56: 109–14.

This chapter has been reproduced from Loriaux, D. Lynn: Historical Note: John Hunter (1728–1793). *The Endocrinologist* 1996; 6(4): 274–6.

CHAPTER 20
Caleb Hillier Parry
(1755–1822)
Thyrotoxicosis

At the end of the eighteenth century some physicians, armed with little other than an understanding of anatomy and outward manifestations of disease, began to describe disorders that are recognizable as conditions we deal with today. Caleb Hillier Parry was one of these individuals. He is credited with one of the earliest descriptions of the form of hyperthyroidism usually termed Graves' disease. His published description preceded that of Robert J. Graves by 10 years.

The Parry family, originally Welsh, moved to Cirencester, Gloucestershire, England, where Parry was born in 1755. His father was a non-Conformist minister who appears to have dissipated his literary expertise in anonymous contributions on political, metaphysical, and satirical subjects. These were later published by his grandson as the *Memoir of the Reverend Joshua Parry*.

Caleb was the eldest of three sons and seven daughters. He grew up in Cirencester where Edward Jenner, later famous for vaccination against smallpox, was a fellow schoolboy and, as it happens, a lifelong friend and associate.

In 1773, Parry travelled to Edinburgh, one of the most popular medical centers of Europe, to take up the study of medicine under the famous William Cullen. Two years later, he transferred to London where he lived with Sir Thomas Denman, the physician-accoucheur to the Middlesex Hospital. He then returned to Edinburgh to complete his course, graduating in 1778 with a dissertation on rabies.

Young Parry's popularity with his fellow students in Edinburgh was reflected in his election as President of the Medical Society, a student organization for which he was instrumental in obtaining a Royal Charter. He was given to delivering speeches full of rhetoric and flowery phrases, typical of the day.

In 1778, Parry married the beautiful daughter of John Rigby of Manchester. After spending some time on the Continent for their honeymoon, visiting Holland, Flanders, and France, they settled down in Bath in 1779. Here Parry remained for the rest of his life, hardly going away even for a day.

A Biographical History of Endocrinology, First Edition. D. Lynn Loriaux.

This work is a co-publication between the Endocrine Society and John Wiley & Sons, Ltd.

For the pacesetters of Parry's day, the city of Bath was the place to go. Its natural attractions were mineral hot springs that gushed "health-giving" water at the rate of half a million gallons per day. It also lured the rich and the aspiring with its open gambling and busy rounds of social events. In this tolerant atmosphere, people of all backgrounds mingled in the temporary suspension of England's rigid pecking order. Bath had been established by the Emperor Claudius about 45 C.E. It was always a place of interest and experienced a great revival in the eighteenth century under an adventurer and gambler named Richard Nash, or later "Beau" Nash, who became the Master of Ceremonies at Bath and gained the title of "The King of Bath." He created a round of social rituals considered compulsory for persons of importance. The express purpose of a stay in Bath was "to take the waters." Fully clothed men and women waded into the steaming mineral-rich water, which rises to the surface at a temperature of over 100°F (38°C), in any one of the city's baths. The cleansing waters could barely penetrate the layers of clothes, but the bathers in any case were not keen on getting washed. Sufferers from such ailments as rheumatism, paralysis, and skin disease also plunged into the same baths.

Daniel Defoe, author of *Robinson Crusoe*, earlier described one of the fashionable baths as follows: "The place being but narrow, they converse freely, make vows and sometimes love." One titled lady said of the resort "Nowhere so much scandal, nowhere so little sin." Horace Walpole remarked that it did him 10 times as much good to leave the city as to enter it.

Because many ostensibly came to Bath for health purposes, Bath also became an important medical center. Parry joined several hospitals in Bath including the Puerperal Charity Hospital and the Casualty Hospital. He was elected Governor of the Casualty Hospital in 1782 and was also physician to the Bath General Hospital, founded in 1742, later renamed the Royal Mineral Water Hospital. Parry's reputation grew quickly and his prosperity grew with it. Once, during an epidemic in Bath, Parry was walking home with a friend. His companion remarked that his waistcoat pockets (large in the fashion of the day) seemed very full, possibly of gold guineas. To this Parry replied "I believe there are 99 and I will make it a round sum [100] before I get home."

Parry had three homes in the Bath district, most notably in the Circus of Bath, where he was a neighbor of Thomas Gainsborough and William Pitt, Prime Minister at the time. The Circus still boasts quite a number of the medical profession, and could also be called the Harley Street of Bath. Parry subsequently moved to Summerfield Park, a farm, where he experimented in horticulture, sheep breeding, and the production of wool.

Parry had a large share in the recognition of angina pectoris, first described by William Heberden [1]. Parry gave an essay on angina pectoris to the small medical society in Gloucestershire and came to the conclusion that disease of the coronary arteries was the cause of angina. John Hunter, the famous anatomist, became a patient of Parry's with his complaint of angina. Parry, however, was unable to be frank about the cause of the angina with Hunter, who had not accepted the idea of the connection to the coronary arteries. Parry later wrote:

> this time my valued friend, Mr. John Hunter, began to have symptoms of angina pectoris too strongly marked upon him, and this circumstance prevented any publication of my ideas on the subject as it must have brought an unpleasant conference between Mr. Hunter and me. I mentioned both to Mr. Clive and Mr. Home (who were anatomists) my notions of the matter at one of Mr. Hunter's Sunday night meetings, but they did not think much of these ideas. When, however, Mr. Hunter died, Mr. Home very candidly wrote to me after the dissection to tell me that I was right [2].

Parry was an inveterate notekeeper and retained the descriptions of the patients that he observed [2]. A description of eight cases of exophthalmic goiter entitled: "Enlargement of the thyroid gland in connection with enlargement and palpitation of the heart" appeared in Parry's "unpublished" works in 1825 (i.e., it was posthumously published by his son, C.H. Parry) [3]. Nothing of significance was omitted from the symptoms and clinical findings, and there is no doubt whatever that these were true cases of "Parry's disease" (as it was termed in Osler's textbooks) or, as we commonly refer to it today, Graves' disease. Although his first case was observed in 1786, he did not publish any reference to the condition until 1815 and his notes on these eight cases did not become public until 1825 [2]. In the meantime, cases were described by Flajani in 1802 and by Demours and Scarpa in 1821; others were later published by Graves in 1835, Basedow in 1840, and Stokes in 1854. Parry's descriptions, however, were the most complete and insightful and he was the first to note the connection between the cardiac manifestations and the thyroid [3,4]. Unfortunately, this recognition came too late to change common usage. The eponym became "Graves' disease" in the English-speaking world and "Basedow's disease" on the European continent.

Parry's second case associated stress with the illness. It was a 21-year-old woman who

> was thrown out of a wheelchair in coming fast downhill, 28th April, last and very much frightened, though not much hurt. From this time she has been subject to palpitations of the heart and various nervous affections. About a fortnight after this period, she began to observe a swelling of the thyroid gland which has since varied at different times so as to be once or twice nearly gone. It is now swelled on both sides but more especially the right, without pain and soreness on pressure. The pulsations of the carotid are very strong and full on both sides. Her head was much relieved by bloodletting, and the swelling of the thyroid gland was evidently diminished. On 25th she was ordered to take thrice a day a teaspoon of a mixture of tincture of digitalis 30 drops, serum of squills an ounce and a half [3].

This was the first instance in which stress seemed to be such an obvious factor in precipitating the disease, a relationship that continues to intrigue us.

Parry was the first to conjecture on the cause of the disorder:

> One can scarcely avoid suspecting that the thyroid gland of which no use whatever has been hitherto hinted at by physiologists, is intended to serve as a diverticulum to avert from the brain a part of the blood, which, urged with too great force by various causes, might disorder or destroy the function of that important organ. This notion, however, I offer as a conjecture which future observations may either establish or annul.

Parry's contribution to our understanding of thyroid disease reflected only one of his many and varied interests. He wrote a dissertation on rabies, a dissertation on tetanus, and began a comprehensive work entitled *Elements of Pathology and Therapeutics*, of which he completed only the first volume. His most original investigation, based on animal experiments, appeared in 1816: "An experimental enquiry into the nature, causes, and varieties of the arterial pulse etc." [4–6]. He was also interested in a wide variety of non-medical topics. He published seven papers in the *Farmer's Journal* and gave 11 papers at the Bath and West of England Society of Agriculture, Arts, Manufacturers, and Commerce. He raised merino sheep and many of his publications were on wool and animal husbandry, including a book entitled *Facts and Observations tending to shew the Practicability and Advantage of Producing in the British Isles Clothing Wool equal to that of Spain* and an essay on "The nature, produce, origin and extension of the Merion breed of sheep," published in the *Transactions of the Board of Agriculture* and for which he received a prize. He was instrumental in showing that rather better wool could be obtained in Britain than in Spain. For this work he was elected a Fellow of the Royal Society in 1800.

His philosophy of clinical enquiry is summarized in his introduction to a discussion on angina:

> but when I consider that truth is the sole foundation of moral and religious virtue and therefore of happiness, my regard for personal delicacy is lost in the more general and greater obligation of public utility. In reality it is of little importance who is the discoverer of truths, however valuable. For mankind, it suffices that the truth is actually known and the good obtained.

In 1816 Parry was stricken with right hemiplegia and aphasia. During the remaining 6 years of this crippled life, he occupied his time by taking entire control of his farm and garden and by reading. Although his speech was almost unintelligible, he collected anecdotes and miscellaneous information of interest and with his daughter's assistance, made several volumes.

One of his last efforts was an essay on the character of Hamlet, which he dictated to his daughter. Parry died in his home on March 9th, 1822. He was buried under the floor of Bath Abbey Church where the monument, translated from Latin, reads:

> Here is the burial place of Caleb Hillier Parry, Doctor of Medicine, Fellow of the Royal Society, an upright man, a faithful steward of God and an astute physician. During the 40 years in this city, he thoroughly discharged his calling in which he excelled as well by his genius and bearing, as by his study of many fields of learning. He matured fruitfully, both by his knowledge and by his brilliant investigations of nature. Lest esteem for so great a nature fall short in any way, his friend and colleagues in the same vocation have erected this marble tablet. He lived for 66 years and died on March 9th, in the year of Our Saviour, 1822 [7, 8].

Parry had four sons, one of whom died in infancy and another at the age of 21 years. The eldest was Dr. Charles Henry Parry, to whom we are indebted for the publication of Parry's notes, including the description of hyperthyroidism as documented by his father. The youngest son, Sir William Edward Parry, was the well-known Arctic explorer.

One of Parry's quotations might serve to close this account: "The most dangerous state incidental to the human mind is a calm acquiescence in the accuracy and extent of its own attainments" [9].

References

1. Parry CH: *An inquiry into the symptoms and causes of the syncope anginosa, etc.* Bath: Cruttwell, 1799, 8 volumes.
2. Parry CH: *Elements of Pathology and Therapeutics, being the outlines of a work.* Bath: Cruttwell, 1815.
3. Parry CH: *Collections from the unpublished medical writings of the late Caleb Hillier Parry,* Vols. 1 and 2. Underwoods: London, 1825.
4. Anonymous: Caleb Hillier Parry. In *Dictionary of National Biography,* 1885–1900, Vol. 43. Oxford: Oxford University Press, 1921–22, pp. 371–2.
5. Rolleston H: Caleb Hillier Parry. *Ann Med History* 1925; 7: 205–14.
6. Anderson HB: Caleb Hillier Parry and something of his contemporaries. *Can Med Assoc J* 1926; 16: 1531–4.
7. Anonymous: Parry of Bath. *Med J Record* 1932; 135: 350–1.
8. Anonymous: Caleb Hillier Parry. *Med Classics* 1940; 5: 1–20.
9. Lewis T: Caleb Hillier Parry, M.D., F. R. S. [1755–1822]. A great Welsh physician and scientist. *Proc Cardiff Med Soc* 1941; 70–89.

This chapter has been reproduced from Sawin, Clark T: Caleb Hillier Parry 1755–1822. *The Endocrinologist* 1994; 4(3): 157–9.

CHAPTER 21

Thomas Addison (1795–1860) Adrenal Insufficiency

Thomas Addison was one of the first to recognize an association between a diseased endocrine organ and a defined clinical syndrome. For this, he is generally regarded as the "father" of clinical endocrinology. He was baptized October 11, 1795 in Long Benton village, 4 miles to the northeast of NewcastleUpon-Tyne, England. His father, Joseph Addison, was a village grocer. There is some confusion about the exact date of Thomas Addison's birth. His tombstone states that he died at 65 years of age, but a wall memorial placed by his widow in Lanercost Priory Church states that he was 68. Equally little is known of his childhood and youth. Only the places of his education are known with certainty. He was first sent to a school managed by John Rutter in Killingsworth, the same school to which George Stevenson later sent his son, Robert Louis. This was followed by the Newcastle Royal Grammar School, which had an excellent reputation for giving its pupils a sound classical education. Addison learned enough Latin to permit him to take his medical school notes in that language. He matriculated at the University of Edinburgh School of Medicine in October 1812.

Addison was granted the MD degree on August 1, 1815. His thesis was on the topic of syphilis. What he did for the next 2 years is not recorded, but subsequent events suggest that he went to the Continent to observe the practice of medicine in the great clinics of Europe. On December 13, 1817, he paid 22 pounds to be designated a perpetual physician's pupil in Guy's Hospital in London.

Clinical teaching was almost unknown in the London medical community of 1817. The only hospital schools of medicine were those attached to large institutions such as the united hospital of Guy's and St. Thomas, close together in Southwark, and St. Bartholomew's and the London Hospital. What Addison did as a perpetual pupil in Guy's Hospital is not precisely known. He must have made a good impression, however, for soon thereafter he was appointed house surgeon at the Lock Hospital for venereal disease. The "Lock Hospitals" were so named because their patients were "locked" out of the city as a consequence of their illness. Addison became an expert in

A Biographical History of Endocrinology, First Edition. D. Lynn Loriaux.

This work is a co-publication between the Endocrine Society and John Wiley & Sons, Ltd.

sexually transmitted disorders during his tenure there. He was licensed by the College of Physicians on December 22, 1819, allowing him to practice as a physician in London.

His next appointment was as physician in the General Dispensary. He worked there for 8 years. He studied skin disease under Dr. Bateman, the foremost dermatologist of his time. Addison developed a reputation as an expert in this branch of medicine. A permanent record of his dermatologic expertise resides in the Guy's Hospital museum in the form of wax models of skin eruptions. Addison was elected assistant physician to Guy's Hospital on January 18, 1824. He took the place of Richard Bright, who had been made physician to the hospital. In 1827, Addison was appointed lecturer in Materia Medica. In this post, his extraordinary skills as a teacher were first revealed. His reputation spread quickly among the students of the London hospitals, and large numbers began to attend his lectures. This led to an appointment as joint lecturer in medicine with Dr. Richard Bright.

In 1839 Bright and Addison published the first volume of *Elements of Practical Medicine*. It seems to have been written primarily by Addison. Among other things, it contained the first accurate description of appendicitis. The second volume never appeared.

Addison concentrated many of his investigations on diseases of the lung. He published five papers on the topic. Before Addison, it was believed that pneumonia was the result of an exudate into the interstitium of the lung. Addison questioned the existence of a true interstitial space in the lung. He revealed through diligent postmortem examinations of patients dying of pneumonia that the disease was associated with an inflammatory exudate in the alveoli. The accepted pathophysiology was wrong.

Addison was also interested in anemia. On March 15, 1849, at a meeting of the South London Medical Society, Addison read a paper on "A remarkable form of anemia" that was later published in *The Medical Gazette* on March 23, 1849. This paper details his first investigations into pernicious, or Addison's, anemia. It was in the course of these investigations that Addison discovered a form of anemia associated with disease of the adrenal glands. The results of these investigations were published in 1855 in a beautiful quarto volume entitled *Disease of the Supra-Renal Capsules*. In this book, Addison describes the clinical picture of pernicious anemia and then describes 11 anemic patients who displayed a remarkable darkening of the skin. In this group, disease of the adrenal glands was uniformly present. He termed the condition, "melasma suprarenale." His first patient was seen in 1829, the last in 1854. Postmortem examinations were described in 10. Most had tuberculosis of the adrenal glands. Two probably had immunemediated adrenal destruction. Case number 4, for example, had small atrophied adrenal glands that, together, weighed 49 grains. Case number 11 had marked vitiligo. No postmortem examination was done. Thus, in this small book, Thomas Addison described two diseases: pernicious anemia and primary adrenal insufficiency. He recognized the two most common types of primary adrenal insufficiency, which we know now to be tuberculous and autoimmune. The clinical description of adrenal insufficiency by Thomas Addison represents the first clear association of a clinical syndrome with an anatomically disordered endocrine gland; it is the benchmark for clinical endocrinology.

Thomas Addison was associated with Guy's Hospital for 40 years. Many regard him as the outstanding personality on the hospital staff of his time. He was at Guy's Hospital at the time of its great flowering; the time of Richard Bright, Thomas Hodgkin, and Sir Astley Cooper. Addison is remembered for his novel descriptions of diseases, his lucid and powerful lectures, and for requiring that clinical clerks write reports about their cases, now a standard of western medical education. Addison was elected President of the Royal Medical and Chirurgical Society in 1849 and held that office for 2 years. It was the single honor paid him in life.

Addison was plagued throughout life with episodes of depression. These became more intense with age. During the winter of 1859, he became incapacitated, presumably from melancholy, and was forced to retire from his hospital duties. He went to Brighton for the sea air. There, isolated from work and family, the death of a close friend and colleague cast him into a despair from which he would not recover. He ended his life on June 29, 1860 by leaping from a second story window onto a stone courtyard.

Thomas Addison believed that the practice of medicine was the noblest of pursuits. His contributions to medicine and to medical education reflect an abiding dedication to that belief. Society owes him a great deal. Clinical endocrinology owes him its beginning.

Sources

Addison T: *On the Constitutional and Local Effects of Disease of the Suprarenal Capsules.* London: Highly, 1855.

Cameron HC: *Mr. Guy's Hospital.* Glasgow: Robert Maclehose, The University Press, 1954.

Munk W: *The Roll of the Royal College of Physicians of London,* Vol. III, 1801 to 1825. London: Royal College of Physicians of London, 1878.

This chapter has been reproduced from Loriaux, D. Lynn: Thomas Addison. *The Endocrinologist* 1991; 1(1): 3–4.

CHAPTER 22
Robert James Graves (1796–1853)
Thyrotoxicosis

The eponym "Graves' disease" is now used to distinguish the most common form of hyperthyroidism, the autoimmune, from the others. Robert James Graves was born in Dublin, the seventh of 10 children. His father and his mother's father were both professors of divinity at Trinity College, Dublin. Robert was well educated. He obtained a BA before going on to his MB (bachelor of medicine) in 1818. He then traveled in Europe for 3 years, including London, Germany, and Denmark. He did this for medical training as well as other trips for his own version of a "grand tour."

Three anecdotes tell something of the young physician. For a while he traveled with the well-known English artist, J.M.W. Turner. They journeyed together through middle and southern Europe, but Graves did not know the name or fame of his companion until they reached Rome, where his main complaint was fleas and bedbugs. They had gotten along so well that they had simply never told each other their names. Another time, he was arrested in Austria as a spy in large part because he spoke German so well that the Austrians could not believe he was Irish. He spent 10 days in prison before he established his bona fides. Finally, having embarked from Genoa to Sicily on a brig of questionable fitness, a storm threatened to sink the ship. The captain and crew were about to launch the only lifeboat and leave the two passenger to their fate. Graves, though ill, rose from bed, stove in the lifeboat with an axe, repaired the leaky pumps with leather cut from his own boots, and helped get the ship to safety. Talented, well-met, and bold when necessary, he returned to Dublin in 1820 to begin his career.

His connections did not hurt, but his talents carried him to the peak of his profession. He made his mark as a lecturer, clinician, and writer. An excellent speaker, for many years he gave lectures at the Meath Hospital and other Dublin institutions on disorders of internal medicine. The lectures are composed of seemingly random topics because etiologies were then thought to be much different. Still, he had his critics. The Dublin Medical Press in 1839 thought he suffered from "chronic medico-literary diarrhea." His clinical practice grew rapidly and he became an expert in febrile illnesses before the era of bacteriology. He suggested that his epitaph be "he fed fevers" but the

A Biographical History of Endocrinology, First Edition. D. Lynn Loriaux.

This work is a co-publication between the Endocrine Society and John Wiley & Sons, Ltd.

suggestion never made it to his tombstone. He was one of the first to offer the bedside teaching of clinical medicine to clinical clerks treated as colleagues with clinical responsibility. While he claimed to have taken the idea from Germany, he brought it to fruition in the English-speaking world. It remains the main form of clinical teaching in the United States to this day.

In 1843 he published his classic textbook of medicine, *A System of Clinical Medicine.* It sold out in short order and spread his name through Europe [1]. That same year, 1843–1844, the high regard of his colleagues elected him president of the Royal College of Physicians of Ireland. He was elected a Fellow of the Royal Society in 1849 [2].

This high regard and reputation did not shield him from the sorrows and difficulties of life. He was widowed twice, and eventually estranged from his third wife. Almost certainly he suffered a major depression when in his forties. This, in turn, was probably a factor in resigning his professorship in 1841 at age 45. Later he resigned from the staff of the Meath Hospital on which he had served for more than 20 years. He died in 1853, probably of hepatic carcinoma, after a fairly lengthy illness at age 57 years.

In his series of lectures at the Meath Hospital in the 1834–1835 session he noted three patients who seemed to be similar: each of the three women had "violent and longcontinued palpitations" along with the "same peculiarity" – enlargement of the thyroid gland. After the lecture his younger, and later equally famous, colleague, William Stokes mentioned a fourth patient who also had exophthalmos. Thus, of the first four cases, at least one had prominent eyes [3]. The journal was obscure and the title of the report did not help. It was called Lecture XII of the Clinical Lectures. The only clue to Graves' disease was the fourth of nine topics listed in the heading: "Newly observed Affection of the Thyroid Gland in Females – its connection with Palpitation with Fits of Hysteria." Few outside England or Ireland knew of either the journal or Graves' report, and several decades later it had been lost from sight even there [4].

Certainly Graves was not the first to publish such a report. Some combination of these symptoms was known in tenth-century Byzantium and in early nineteenth-century Italy and America. Recognition of the combination as a distinct entity, however, probably did not occur until Caleb Parry found it in his practice. Parry did not publish, however, and his writings first appeared in book form in 1825, 3 years after he died.

On the European continent, the disorder we call Graves' disease was called Basedow's disease. Carl Basedow was a physician in Merseberg, near Leipzig, almost an exact contemporary with Graves [5]. In 1840 he, too, reported four cases of the syndrome with a major emphasis on the exophthalmos. That the patients had goiter and palpitations is only apparent on reading the text. As the entity became more widely recognized in Europe through sporadic case reports, it received the eponym of Basedow's disease. Most likely this was not because of continental provincialism or German possessiveness: Basedow was simply thought to have been first. In 1856, for example, Jean-Martin Charcot read an analysis of a case with a thorough review of the literature to the Parisian Society of Biology. Charcot knew of Graves' description but only through Graves' well-known book of 1843, not from the 1835 report. Thus, he gave priority to Basedow and his 1840 report, and agreed with the eponym Basedow's disease.

But the doyen of Parisian medicine, Armand Trousseau, did not agree [6]. Trousseau had long been an admirer of Graves, largely because of his 1843 and 1848 textbooks and because of what Graves had accomplished with clinical teaching. Trousseau clearly knew that Graves' report antedated Basedow's and announced to the assemblage that: "Il nous faudrait substituer au nom de Basedow celui de Graves ... serait dit MALADIE DE GRAYES" ("We must substitute Graves' name for Basedow's ... and call it GRAVES' DISEASE"). Those in the United Kingdom and United States, for the most part, agreed and still call it Graves' disease. Trousseau's colleagues may or may not have thought he was right, but none seem to have openly disagreed. They just ignored him. So in France, as in the rest of Europe, the eponym is still usually Basedow's disease.

The priority dispute aside, it seems clear that Graves' other accomplishments led Trousseau to look upon Graves as worthy. At the time, in the nineteenth century, an eponym was of clear practical use. No one knew the underlying cause. Graves thought it a cardiac disorder; Basedow thought it a "scrofulous dysplasia." Charcot and Trousseau thought it was a neurologic disease [7]. The idea that the thyroid was involved in a major way did not arise until the late nineteenth century. The concept that the thyroid gland was overactive (i.e., that there was hyperthyroidism) did not take hold until the early twentieth century. The existence of an eponym allowed physicians to speak a common language while in dispute over the underlying cause.

Graves knew nothing of hyperthyroidism, of thyroid hormone, or of autoimmunity. What he described did reflect the disorder's clinical presentation: goiter and tachycardia with occasional exophthalmos. He did not distinguish among types of hyperthyroidism, as we do. And so we have kept the eponym for those with a presumed autoimmune origin of hyperthyroidism while we struggle to find out why it occurs and seek at the same time successful therapy. The eponym retains utility and Graves' memory lives.

References

1. Graves RJ: *A System of Clinical Medicine*. Dublin: Fannin and Co., 1843.
2. Taylor S. *Robert Graves. The Golden Years of Irish Medicine*. London: Royal Society of Medicine Services Limited, 1989.
3. Graves RJ: Clinical lectures. *Lond Med Surg J* 1835; 7: 513.
4. Kelly EC: *Medical Classics* 1940; 5: 22.
5. Sattler H: *Basedow's Disease*, translated by GW and JF Marchand. New York: Grune and Stratton, 1952.
6. Bariéty M: Éloge de Armand Trousseau (14 octobre 1801–23 juin 1867). *Bull Acad Natl Med* 1967; 151: 627.
7. Charcot JM: Mémoire sur une affection caraceterisée par des palpitations du coeur et des artères, la tuméfaction de la glande thyroide et une double exophthalmie. *Comptes Rendus Soc Biol* 1857; 3(2 me ser.): 43.

This chapter has been reproduced from Sawin, Clark T: Historical Note: Robert James Graves 1796–1853. *The Endocrinologist* 1994; 4(5): 324–5.

CHAPTER 23

Armand Trousseau (1801–1867)

Diabetes Insipidus

Diabetes is an ancient disorder. It simply means the frequent passing of large amounts of dilute urine. It has been recognized by physicians for over a millennium. The word comes from the Greek word for "siphon" or a "flowing through." One of the earliest descriptions in English is in 1649, when Nicholas Culpeper, an English herbalist who practiced medicine not quite respectably, wrote of "the Diabetes, or continual pissing." Others of the time called it "pot dropsy," a delightful term not recently seen. For most of recorded medicine, the word stood alone, unmodified by "mellitus." There was no need for a modifier because diabetes was characterized not only by a great deal of urine but by the fact that the urine tasted sweet. A much rarer kind of diabetes was first described in the eighteenth century. In this new type of diabetes, the urine did not taste sweet. So, diabetes with the sweet urine was called "mellitus" and diabetes without the sweet taste was called "insipidus" or "tasteless."

The "insipidus" was probably first used by Scottish physician William Cullen who, in 1769, thought some patients with diabetes needed to be separated from others because he could not tell whether or not there was sugar in the urine. He thought all diabetes was due to a kind of nervous disorder. He also thought that the liver and kidney contributed to the excess flow of urine. Though he used the words, there was little in his work on the clinical description of what we would now call diabetes insipidus.

The eighteenth century was the age of the classification of nature, viz., the Linnaean system of naming plants and animals. Many tried to do the same thing in a systematic way with all diseases. Johann Frank was a brilliant peripatetic who came from the German Palatinate, on the edge of the Alsace-Lorraine. He had acquired both a PhD (in France) and an MD (at Heidelberg) and had made the first of his 11 lifetime career moves. In 1794, he was in Lombardy as Director General of Medicine, and was stimulated by the nosologic urge to classify diabetes. Frank thought there were three types: mellitus (the sweetness had by then been attributed to an actual sugar), insipidus (no sugar detectable), and decipiens (deceptive) (urinary sugar without polyuria). Frank is generally thought to be the first accurate describer of what we now call

A Biographical History of Endocrinology, First Edition. D. Lynn Loriaux.

diabetes insipidus. However, his description was not in a medical journal, but in the fifth volume of his magnum opus, *De Curandis Hominem Morbis Epitiome*. Nowadays, or even in the nineteenth century, only a few would have read his work and related it to an actual patient. Nevertheless, the disease was recognized more clearly as a specific entity, and occasional case reports appeared over the next half century after Frank's description.

One of the difficulties in making the specific diagnosis of diabetes insipidus is that one always would have been trying to prove a negative, the absence of sugar in the urine. To show that there was no sugar in the urine required an assay that was believable, yet most assays in the early nineteenth century were not simple, sensitive, or easily quantitated. For example, in 1825, assays of blood from patients with clear-cut diabetes mellitus failed to show any glucose at all (by then the sugar in diabetic urine had been shown to be similar to grape or raisin sugar). Until the mid-eighteenth century, the main glucose assays used fermentation or polarimeter techniques, which improved things somewhat, but for most physicians the taste-test was the standard.

By the 1850s, a copper reduction method for urinary sugar made possible a rough quantitation of the amount of sugar in the diabetic's urine and, conversely, made it possible to say with certainty that there was no sugar in a polyuric urine sample. For instance, Apollinaire Bouchardat, a Parisian physician, had become expert at chemical and polarimetric measurements of urinary glucose. Then, the famous French physiologist Claude Bernard confounded matters in 1855 when he claimed that there was only a slight difference in urine sugar between diabetes mellitus and diabetes insipidus. Both were due to lesions of the brain stem, the only difference being that the former was due to a higher lesion. As we now know, these attributions are not right, but they influenced others, at least in France, for some time.

Armand Trousseau is known to most physicians because his name is the eponym for tetanic contraction of the forearm after arterial occlusion in patients with hypocalcemia. Best known in later life as a teacher and mentor, he originally established himself in the fiercely competitive arena of Parisian medicine in the 1830s with his work on yellow fever (which he himself contracted), on laryngeal tuberculosis, and on tracheotomy for children with croup or diphtheria. After 1840, he focused his publishing on textbooks. His major works on therapeutics and clinical medicine were popular in France and elsewhere. He had served in the National Assembly in 1848 but quit politics in disgust. In 1855 he received one of France's highest medical honors: election to the Imperial Academy of Medicine, subject, of course, to the approval of the Emperor. Trousseau was responsible for the eponyms for both Addison's disease and Graves' disease (although the latter did not catch on in his own country). He was an excellent and active teacher and insisted that students spend a good deal of time in the hospital observing patients. By the 1860s, it is fair to say that he was regarded as the doyen of French medicine.

After Trousseau became famous, he wrote a textbook on clinical medicine. It was titled *Clinique Medicale de L'Hotel-Dieu de Paris.* In essence, Trousseau presented to his eager listeners, and then readers, his analyses of the cases that were in the wards of the Hotel-Dieu. Trousseau's initial edition came out in 1861–1862. It was a great success. The second French edition was published only 3 years later and was translated into English in five volumes over the years 1868–1872.

In Volume 2 of Trousseau's first edition, he presented in his 62nd lecture a peculiar case of "polydipsia," the then-current word for diabetes insipidus (it became the 65th lecture in the English translation). The man had been in the hospital under observation for some months and shown to the audience during Trousseau's lecture. His fluid intake and urine output were enormous: 32 liters per day (the intake was mainly a tisane, a kind of medicinal herb tea). Bouchardat, the hospital pharmacist, tried but failed to find the slightest trace of glucose in the patient's urine.

Trousseau's treatment was to give the patient a large amount of valerian, which, taken over the several months the patient was in the hospital, seemed to Trousseau to be of benefit. Valerian, as an extract or tincture derived from one of several plants of the genus, was an ancient medicine. It was used through the Middle Ages into modern times as a stimulant or antispasmodic, yet it also was used as a soothing agent. The rationale seems to have been that when there was nervousness or "hysteria," what one needed was stimulant for the nervous exhaustion or a calming influence for the highly strung state itself. Trousseau was quite familiar with valerian and its use. He wrote a short section on the drug in his text on therapeutics published in 1836–1839. He apparently used valerian for his patient's problem because he thought that the "polydipsia" was a nervous affliction and felt the treatment needed to be something of a soothing nature. In any case, the therapy either had some beneficial effect or the disorder got better by itself. Of interest is the fact that this therapy persisted well into the twentieth century. Valerian was still recommended in the 8th edition of William Osler's famous text *The Principles and Practice of Medicine*, published in 1919.

Trousseau really did not know what caused this unusual disease but managed to devise what was, for him, a reasonable therapy. The therapy may not even have been original with Trousseau, but he certainly made it widely known. Trousseau's merit was in his incisive description and in his ability to teach his ideas to others. The idea that the disorder was, in fact, due to a lesion of the central nervous system came later.

Sources

Bariety M: Eloge de Armoand Trousseau. *Bull Acad Natl Med* 1967; 151: 627.

Bloomfield AI: Diabetes insipidus. In *A Bibliography of Internal Medicine. Selected Diseases*. Chicago, IL: University of Chicago Press, 1960, p. 130.

Bouchardat A: Du Diabete Sucreo ou glucosurie. Son traitment hygienique. *Mem Acad Natl Med* 1852; 16: 69.

This chapter has been reproduced from Sawin, Clark T: Armand Trousseau and diabetes insipidus. *The Endocrinologist* 1998; 8(3): 139–42.

CHAPTER 24
Arnold Adolph Berthold (1803–1861)
Transplantation of Testes

On February 8, 1849, Arnold Adolph Berthold spoke at a meeting of the Royal Scientific Society in Göttingen [1]. He told the audience about an unusual experiment. He had removed the testes from six young male chickens. In two, he did nothing further. Those chickens served as "controls." In another two he put one testis back into its own abdominal cavity without any attempt at connecting them with blood vessels. Over the next several months, both young castrated chickens with the transplanted testes grew into normal roosters. Their combs and wattles grew, they crowed, they fought, and they ran after the hens just as any normal rooster would. The implanted testes had become revascularized and did whatever testes do to keep roosters from behaving like capons. The two controls remained capons; they did not grow combs or wattles, crowed poorly, and were not at all interested in the hens. The difference was striking and clear. The autotransplant of an entire organ was a success.

Berthold did almost the same experiment with the remaining two animals but with a critical difference. In each of these two, he again implanted one testis into the abdominal cavity but implanted it into the other animal, a "homotransplant," in contrast to an "autotransplant." The result was quite clear. These testes "took" as well. They developed a good blood supply, actually contained actively motile spermatozoa, and caused the birds to grow combs and wattles, to crow, and to chase hens.

If done today, Berthold's experiment would be featured in medical and lay journals, would most likely appear on television and arouse intense interest in immunologists and ethicists. It would lead to speculation about organ transplants for many ailments.

Berthold was born on February 26, 1803, near Munster (in what is now Germany) to a hardworking master carpenter. The boy was the second youngest of six [2]. The family was not wealthy, but his father's hard work kept them out of debt despite the trials of the Napoleonic Wars, which swept over northwest Germany during Berthold's childhood. His early education was poor when he entered the "gymnasium." While there, however, he studied a classical curriculum including Latin and Greek and loved

A Biographical History of Endocrinology, First Edition. D. Lynn Loriaux.

This work is a co-publication between the Endocrine Society and John Wiley & Sons, Ltd.

it. He was most attracted to natural history. He decided to study medicine, and set out on August 1, 1819 for the University of Göttingen.

The University of Göttingen was technically the Georg-August-Universität because it was founded in Hanover by the Elector George Augustus 85 years before. Hanover was an independent German-speaking kingdom. Its ruler was called an Elector because he could vote for the Holy Roman Emperor. By 1819, the Elector also held the title of king since Napoleon's abdication in 1814. The Kings of Hanover in Berthold's student years were also the rulers of Great Britain, George III and George IV, because between 1714 and 1837, the rulers of the two kingdoms were one and the same. When Victoria became queen in 1837 it was against the law for a woman to rule Hanover, so Ernest Augustus (1771–1851), her uncle and the fifth of George III's eight sons, became King of Hanover.

Hanover remained independent during Berthold's lifetime. It was invaded by Prussia in 1866 because the "then" King refused to declare neutrality in a Prussian dispute with Austria. After a brief war, Hanover became a Prussian province.

At Göttingen, Berthold was a well-read and hardworking student. The university had an excellent scientific faculty that included Karl Gauss of the Gaussian distribution and Johann Blumenbach, Göttingen's outstanding physician. Berthold got his medical degree on September 10, 1823 at age 20. His career as a student was interrupted only by scarlet fever. He avoided military service when called earlier in 1823 because of his nearsightedness. The young physician stayed on at Göttingen for almost a year and then visited a number of German clinics and universities. He met J.L. Schonlein and other physicians but retained a great interest in natural science. Finally, probably in 1825, he "settled" in Berlin to practice medicine. He also began to experiment on the effects of mercury and coal gas on the human body. He seems to have "unsettled" himself later that same year and traveled again to several other German scientific centers as well as to Paris, where he attended lectures by G. Cuvier, E. Geoffroy Saint-Hilaire, and A.M.C. Dumeril, some of the nineteenth century's best-known biologists. By the fall of 1825, he had dropped the idea of medical practice, written a paper on the parrot's thyroid gland and come back to Göttingen as lecturer (Privatdozent) in medicine. The 22-year-old physician-physiologist stayed at the university for the rest of his life. He became extraordinary professor of medicine in 1835 and ordinary professor (full professor) the next year at age 33. In 1840 he was also named director of the zoological division of the museum. Perhaps it was in this capacity that he was able to do his experiments on chickens.

Berthold published on a wide variety of topics, such as the length of pregnancy, myopia (his own problem), the formation of hair, and male hermaphroditism. A side venture into toxicology with Robert Bunsen led to an antidote for arsenic poisoning [3]. Berthold's forte was the teaching of physiology. In 1829 he published the first edition of his textbook on the physiology of man and animals. The text went through several editions and seems to have been widely used.

By the end of the 1820s, Berthold, not yet 30 years old, had settled into the steady, quiet life of a nineteenth-century German professor. He was bright, well regarded, and he had developed an excellent reputation. Blumenbach was nominally in charge but was in his seventies. Berthold, along with the well-known surgeon C.J.M. Langenbeck, assumed the medical faculty's leadership in teaching anatomy and physiology [4].

The politics of the mid 1800s were unstable. There was revolution in France and a new king in 1830. The Industrial Revolution swelled the ranks of workers who could not vote but were demanding the franchise. Hanover was not immune to the revolutionary sentiment. The turmoil of 1830 led to a new constitution in 1833 that helped bring the people of Hanover and England together under a common king. But when Ernest Augustus became King of Hanover in 1837, he abrogated the new constitution. The politically active faculty members protested. For their pains, seven faculty, known as the "Göttingen seven," were expelled from the university – including the brothers Grimm, known now for their fairy tales and not for their philology. As far as we know, the medical and science faculty (except for the physicist W.E. Weber) either did not protest or did not care for the new, more liberal constitution in the first place. Berthold, Langenbeck, Gauss, and the others seemed unaffected by all this.

Eventually, Blumenbach died at age 88. He was replaced by Rudolf Wagner, another physician who, like Berthold, was mainly an anatomist and physiologist [4]. Wagner edited a "dictionary" of physiology and pathologic physiology that ran to four volumes. Berthold contributed a 20-page section on sexual physiology, as it was then known, in the first volume in 1842.

Berthold was a good mentor as well as teacher. He encouraged the physiologist Carl Bergmann to study both the production and regulation of body heat in different animals. Bergmann invented the words "poikilotherm" and "homeotherm" [4]. Conceptually, he was responsible for "Bergmann's Rule" (1845). Based on observational data in birds, the rule states that, in a group of related animals, larger species or larger animals within a single species will live in the cooler parts of the available range. Bergmann postulated that this was because larger animals lose less heat per volume per unit time. In the 1840s, Bergmann saw this simply as an example of sensible physiologic adaptation by the organism. There was no concept of survival advantage because Darwin had not yet published his new idea. Nevertheless, the idea of the maintenance of body temperature by changes in the rate of heat generation and loss in the face of heat or cold in the organism's environment was a definite part of Göttingen's mode of physiologic thought. Berthold's support was key to Bergmann's work, and Berthold probably directed him to essential sources of information. Certainly Berthold was familiar with the general concept of physiologic regulation.

With Wagner, physiology at Göttingen got a boost. It is important to note that "physiology" at that time was not the highly experimental science, often with isolated organs, tissues, and cells, that we now equate with the term. It was quite different and based on functional anatomy. The focus was mechanistic ("how does it work?"), as is ours, but not as strictly reductionist as our modern physiology. We assume that we could predict the total organism if only we knew enough about its parts. To the modern mind, it is a bit of a shock to realize that there was another way of doing physiology. Berthold and his colleagues aimed to understand the organism as a whole and its harmonious integration, an idea that is now slowly making its way back 150 years later. Although they were aiming to understand the mechanics, the Göttingen physiologists (in contrast to modern physiology) felt that the organism itself had a uniqueness or "purpose." Could that not be analyzed into its parts? The tools to apply to this task, the understanding of mechanisms within a harmonious whole, were comparative anatomy, the microscope, and a limited amount of vivisection. Even when chemical and physical approaches, such as the measurement of glucose or the observation of muscle contraction on a kymograph, were developed elsewhere in Germany and in France, the Göttingen style found little place for them. Intellectually, they did not fit well. Of course the chemical and experimental school was the wave of the future. Göttingen did not seize this opportunity, and its physiologic preeminence waned.

Such was the intellectual climate of the life sciences in 1840s Göttingen. When the wave of revolution came through Europe in 1848 the university was quiet and so was its faculty, at least politically. For Berthold, it was the year he did his rooster experiment, beginning on August 2 [1].

It is not easy to understand why Berthold did the experiment. As far as we know he had not tried it before. Perhaps he tried it a number of times, unsuccessfully, and simply did not talk about it until it worked. Quite likely his earlier studies, such as those on hermaphroditism, led him to consider how the testes contributed to the harmonious whole. Jorgensen's monograph [5] is the best treatment of this issue. After reviewing many of Berthold's writings and the three editions of his textbook of physiology, the last completed in 1848, Jorgensen felt that Berthold started the experiment to test further potential sites of transplantation and to assess the effect of transplantation on the transplanted tissue itself. Apparently Berthold did not begin with the idea of studying the effect of the transplant on the rest of the organism, in this case, the male chicken. The "sympathies," that is, the set of mechanisms responsible for maintaining harmony among the body's parts and which were thought to be largely neural (hence, our "sympathetic" nervous system), were the issue. Berthold realized from his study that nerves could not be the only means of having a "sympathetic" response and the maintenance of harmony. He realized that the circulating blood could be another sympathetic mediator.

It is doubtful that Berthold's conception of what the testis did, translated sometimes as "secretion," matches ours. A common theory of organ function at the time was that blood itself was a functioning tissue and not simply a passive transporter of things to the body's organs [6]. Some organs transformed the blood so that it might act in different ways on organs elsewhere in the body. Berthold does not say so but, in keeping with the physiologic thought of the time, his likely aims were to assess the body's overall effect on the newly located testis and to figure out how the testis, devoid of nerves, transformed the blood as evidenced by changes elsewhere in the body (e.g., the cock's comb and wattles). He never actually drew a conclusion that can be clearly interpreted as showing that he had an endocrine concept in mind [5,7]. Berthold, in fact, operated well within the framework of Göttingen physiology.

Berthold was not the first to succeed with a testis transplant. John Hunter did almost exactly the same experiment 80 years before [5,8]. John, the irascible younger brother of the more urbane William Hunter, was the most famous surgeon of the eighteenth century, in large part because he strove to put surgery on a scientific basis (both brothers had a high reputation; both were elected to the Royal Society in 1767). No one knows exactly when he did his testicular transplant studies because he never published them. We do know that it was some time before 1771. Hunter did both testicular autotransplants and transplants of rooster testes into a hen's abdomen (a visitor in 1771 noted that he saw many hens with testicular grafts). Hunter himself wrote, in 1794, that he had done transplants to "the abdomen of a hen, and they had sometimes taken root there, but not frequently, and then had never come to perfection." Some of Hunter's specimens still exist today in the Hunterian Museum of the Royal College of Surgeons in London [5]. The testes in the hen's abdomen are clearly vascularized and histologically intact. Hunter's work is definitely not a myth and can be seen by any visitor.

It is thought that Berthold knew about Hunter's chickens. The version of Berthold's work usually quoted [1] was in a widely read journal but was skimpy in the extreme. There is no real introduction or discussion, no mention of Hunter, and it reads like an extended abstract. However, in that same year, 1849, Berthold published almost the same article in the local medical journal [9] and clearly noted Hunter as an influence. This makes better sense because few ideas spring to mind totally without precedent.

If Berthold and his work were solidly placed in at least part of the mainstream of nineteenth-century physiology, one would expect his work to be emulated and expanded, if not by him then by others. However, Berthold's study had practically no effect at all. His own colleague, Wagner, repeated the experiment and it was not a success [5]. Berthold did some work but never published it and clearly did not pursue the problem with any vigor. We do not know why. Perhaps he also was unable to confirm his own work. Perhaps the Göttingen approach to physiology had been rapidly displaced [4]. Carl Ludwig, now considered the principal "father" of modern physiology, was making great strides. Wagner's failure to repeat Berthold's success may have been a major factor in Berthold's failure to influence others and may have been seen by others as an indication that Berthold was simply wrong. Whatever the reason, and despite the clear success of both Hunter and Berthold, no one reported on this phenomenon again until after Charles-Edouard Brown-Séquard's claim of rejuvenation from testicular extract in 1889.

What then of the claims of modern writers that Berthold's "observations ... established a new science" [7], that he did "the first experiment in endocrinology" [10], or that his work was "the foundation of modern endocrinology" [11]? Certainly Berthold and his work are not mythical, but such comments can only be read as efforts to make them legendary and to make them stand in retrospect for more than they were at the time. It is perfectly understandable for endocrinologists to seek older sources of our discipline (which is in reality only about 100 years old) and to find Berthold a kind of hero struggling alone to lead the way down a new and glorious path. The actual story is more interesting and human.

Berthold can be seen as a "forerunner without immediate succession" [12] and his work as a "premature discovery" [13]. Of course, judging whether something is premature can only be done in retrospect; one may find that the apparent prematurity was actually due to active resistance by the scientific community to a scientific discovery [14, 15]. Why Berthold's experiment did not take root in his own time is not fully explained, but certainly it is an example of how science is more than just the collection of data with "true" knowledge then becoming apparent for anyone who can see. Science is also the social phenomenon of acceptance by others that the data are, in fact, "real" and hence, credible.

References

1. Berthold AA: Transplantation der Hoden. *Arch Anat Physiol Wissenschaft Med* 1849; 42–6.
2. Rush HP: A biographical sketch of Arnold Adolf Berthold. An early experimenter with ductless glands. *Ann Med Hist* (new series) 1929; 1: 208–14.
3. Klein M: Berthold, Arnold Adolphe. *Dictionary Scientific Biography* 1970; 2: 72–3.
4. Coleman W: Bergmann's rule: animal heat as a biological phenomenon. *Stud Hist Biol* 1979; 3: 67–88.
5. Jorgensen CB: *John Hunter, A.A. Berthold, and the Origins of Endocrinology*. Odense, Denmark: Odense University Press, 1971.
6. Holmes FL: La signification du concept demilieu interieur. In *La Nécessité de Claude Bernard*, edited by J Michel. Paris, Méridiens Klincksieck, 1991, pp. 53–64.
7. Forbes TR: A.A. Berthold and the first endocrine experiment: some speculation as to its origin. *Bull Hist Med* 1949; 23: 263–7.
8. Forbes TR: Testis transplantations performed by John Hunter. *Endocrinology* 1947; 41: 329–31.
9. Berthold AA: Über die Transplantation der Hoden. Nachrichten GA Univ Konig! *Gesellsch Wissenensch Göttingen* 1849; 1–6 (Feb 19).
10. Setchell BP: *Male Reproduction*. New York: Van Nostrand Reinhold, 1984.
11. Quiring DP: The transplantation of testes [by] Arnold Adolph Berthold. *Bull Hist Med* 1944; 16: 399–401.
12. Klein M: Sur l'article de Berthold: transplantation des testicules (1849). *Arch Anat Histol Embryol* 1968; 51: 380–6.
13. Stent G: Prematurity and uniqueness in scientific discovery. *Sci Am* 1972; 227(Dec): 84–93.
14. Barber B: Resistance by scientists to scientific discovery. *Science* 1961; 134: 596–602.
15. Aronson N: The discovery or resistance. Historical accounts and scientific careers. *Isis* 1986; 77: 630–46.

This chapter has been reproduced from Sawin, Clark T: Arnold Adolph Berthold and the transplantation of testes. *The Endocrinologist* 1996; 6(3): 164–8.

CHAPTER 25

Claude Bernard (1813–1878)

The Discovery of Homeostasis and Internal Secretion

"One gene, one enzyme." "For every action there is an equal and opposite reaction." "The origin of species through natural selection." Accurate or not, these are some of the generalizations around which we structure whole bodies of thought, hypotheses, and scientific enquiry. There is one for endocrinology: the "milieu interieur." The concept was developed by Claude Bernard before the notion of endocrine secretion existed. It evolved over a 20-year period beginning with its first enunciation in 1857 [1], its full exposition in 1865 [2], and its final formulation in 1878: "All the vital mechanisms, varied as they are, have only one object, that of preserving constant the conditions of life in the internal environment" [3]. J.B.S. Haldane thought that "No more pregnant sentence was ever framed by a physiologist" [4]. The concept was distilled into a single word by Walter B. Cannon: "homeostasis" [5].

Claude Bernard was born at 7 o'clock in the morning of July 12, 1813, in the little village of St. Julien-en-Beaujolais, southeast France. A detailed exposition of his life can be found in two old but excellent biographies [6, 7]. He was the eldest of two children; a sister was born several years later. His father was a vintner and, after a reversal of fortune, a village schoolmaster. Claude's education began at 8 years of age with instruction in Latin under the tutelage of Father Bourgaud. The abbes Garets and Desarbes of Chateney recommended him to the priests at the Jesuit College of Villefranche, and he was enrolled there as a student. Bernard was characterized as solitary and "dreamy" – an ordinary student. A fragmentary comment from one of his teachers indicates that Bernard considered reading a waste of time. At 18, because his family could no longer afford the cost of his education, he was apprenticed to a pharmacist in Lyon.

The young Bernard was allowed one free night each month. This he spent in the Theater des Celestins. The productions were comedies, operettas, and vaudeville. The despair of his life in the pharmacy and the relief offered by these evenings inspired him to write a vaudeville of his own, *La Rose du Rhone*. This met with some success and

A Biographical History of Endocrinology, First Edition. D. Lynn Loriaux.

This work is a co-publication between the Endocrine Society and John Wiley & Sons, Ltd.

earned him 100 francs. Thus encouraged, Bernard decided to pursue a literary career and forsake a life of "folding up little squares of paper." In the following year, he wrote *Arthur de Bretagne*, a drama depicting the struggle between Arthur and his uncle, King John, who had usurped the throne of England. Friends of Bernard arranged for the manuscript to be read by Saint-Marc Girardin, professor of literature at the Sorbonne. Girardin said, firmly, "You have done some pharmacy; study medicine. You have not the temperament of a dramatist."

Thus, in the autumn of 1834, at the age of 21, he entered medical school in Paris. Generally a lackluster student, he excelled in anatomic dissection. While an intern at the Hôtel-Dieu, this skill was recognized by Francois Magendie, the leading physiologist of the day, and he took Bernard as his preparateur at the College de France. Thus began a career and a lifelong collaboration that, more than any other single influence, established the validity of physiology as a scientific discipline. In the years that followed, Bernard made major contributions to our understanding of the autonomic nervous system, the function of the pancreas in digestion, and the mechanism of action of certain toxins and drugs.

Perhaps most important was his explicit demonstration of the phenomenon of internal secretion. The studies began with the unexpected finding of sugar in the blood of an animal that had been fasted for several days. "We had a theory here," Bernard later recalled, "which assumed that the vegetable kingdom alone had the power of creating the individual compounds which the animal kingdom is supposed to destroy" [8]. According to this hypothesis, sugar should be found only in the blood of "fed" animals. To better understand the presence of sugar in the blood of starved animals, Bernard began a systematic study of the glucose content in excised rabbit livers. He made duplicate determinations on each specimen, usually several hours after death. One evening, the first measurement was made in the immediate postmortem period and the second was delayed until the following day. The first value was lower than expected; the second was higher. From this observation, Bernard theorized that the liver could make glucose and that it could do so after being removed from the body. This was confirmed when he showed that an isolated perfused liver could produce sugar for several hours after death, the glucose concentration in the hepatic venous effluent being greater than in the portal venous infusate. These findings led to the discovery of glycogen and to the principle of "internal secretion," the fundamental tenet of endocrinology.

Proportionate to the success and joy of his professional life was a painful and, some might say, failed personal life. Bernard married Marie Francoise Martin when he was 32 and she was 26. She was the daughter of a prosperous Paris physician. Fanny, as she was known, was considered by most to be intellectually narrow and bigoted. She had a dowry of 60 000 francs that supported Bernard's scientific career and relieved him of the need to practice medicine. They had four children. The first was a boy who died at three months. Two daughters followed, Jeane Henriette and Marie Louise Alphonsine. Both survived Bernard by many years. The fourth child, a son, lived 14 months. His death was a grievous blow to Bernard.

Fanny developed a horror of vivisection and became a leader in the French antivivisectionist movement. "She led crusades against her husband and cultivated a passionate affection for his victims" [8]. Bernard's daughters were ultimately converted to the cause and, as a result, Bernard became unwillingly and painfully estranged from his wife and children. A permanent separation was arranged in 1870. In the settlement, it is noted that Bernard wished to retain only two things: his books and the playthings of his deceased son.

The vacuum left in the wake of the dissolution of this family was filled with work and an apparently platonic relationship with Marie Raffalovich. Five hundred letters written to Raffalovich between 1869 and 1877 survive. They detail a busy life of experiments, lectures, and an endless stream of meetings generated by his leading role in the French community of scientists. Bernard was chronically ill during these years. He complained of continuous "colds" and sciatica. On New Year's Day of 1878, he became ill on his round of "calls." This evolved into "abdominal rheumatism" and confinement to bed. On Friday morning, February 10, he said he felt cold. A traveling blanket was placed over his feet and legs. "This time it will serve me for the voyage from which there is no return, the voyage of eternity." He died shortly after. He is buried in the Pére Lachaise Cemetery, Paris, in a grave with his two infant sons.

Some years after Bernard's death, his friend Georges Barral succeeded in publishing *Arthur de Bretagne*. It seems that Saint-Marc Girardin was right about the play [9]. His forthright critique and prescient "career counseling" served society well. It is yet another example of the humanities in support of science.

References

1. Bernard C: *Lecons sur les Proprietes Physiologiques et les Alterations Pathologiques des Liquides de l'Organisme*, Vol. 1. Paris: Ballière, 1859, p. 43.
2. Bernard C: *Introduction a la Etrude de la Medicine Experimentale*. Paris: Ballière, 1865, pp. 107–12.
3. Bernard C: *Lecons sur le Phenomenes de la Vie Communs aux Animaux et aux Vegetaux*, Vol. 1. Paris: Baillière, 1878–1879, pp. 121–2.
4. Haldrine JBS: *The Philosophical Basis of Biology*. London: Hodder and Stoughton, 1931.
5. Cannon WB: Organization for physiological homeostasis. *Physiol Rev* 1929; 9: 399–431.
6. Foster M: *Claude Bernard*. London: Fisher and Unwin, 1899.
7. Olmsted JMD: *Claude Bernard. Physiologist*. New York and London: Harper and Brothers, 1938.
8. Bendiner E: Claude Bernard theater's loss was physiology's gain. *Hosp Pract* 1979; 14: 130–9.
9. Olmsted JMD: Claude Bernard as a dramatist. *Ann Hist* 1935; 7: 253–60.

This chapter has been reproduced from Loriaux, D. Lynn: Claude Bernard 1813–1878. *The Endocrinologist* 1991; 1(6): 362–4.

CHAPTER 26
Adolphe Chatin
(1813–1901)
Iodine in the Prevention of Goiter

On March 25, 1850, Gaspard Adolphe Chatin, then 36 years old and a well-established pharmacy educator, medical botanist, and physician, spoke at the weekly meeting of the French Académie des Sciences in Paris. He told the assembly of his new findings that iodine is in fact found in certain freshwater plants and that these plants or their ashes could be used to prevent goiter [1]. He also thought this could be a good treatment for scrofula or tuberculosis.

At that time, brief presentations to the Académie, such as Chatin's, were often printed in another Parisian journal in expanded form. In Chatin's longer version [2] he gave data on the iodine content of 89 different freshwater plants that concentrated iodine from the surrounding fresh water, just as did most iodine-containing sea plants. He also thought that, in addition to preventing goiter, these plants could be used to treat it. Then he wrote that "Perhaps one could establish that (goiter) might be due to [a] ... cause such as the more or less complete absence of iodine in the water" (author's translation). This is the first clear suggestion that iodine deficiency might cause goiter, which is not at all the same thing as using iodine to treat goiter, a therapy then known for 30 years, and not quite the same as proposing iodine as a preventative of goiter.

Chatin was not a member of the Académie, which had an elite, limited membership. One was considered for election only if a member died and, in contrast to the American Academy of Sciences, only if one were reasonably likely to attend the weekly meetings. However, open discussion was the rule. Non-members such as Chatin attended and spoke; the members, in fact, wanted to keep up. When something seemingly significant arose and there was controversy, a few expert members formed a committee (or "commission") to investigate. Sometimes the committee would go beyond simply reviewing the data and repeating the experiment.

After Chatin's presentation, the response over the next several months was what now seems like science's universal response: some thought he must be wrong while others said he was right but they had done it first. This sort of response suggests that Chatin was on to something important.

A Biographical History of Endocrinology, First Edition. D. Lynn Loriaux.

This work is a co-publication between the Endocrine Society and John Wiley & Sons, Ltd.

Adolphe Chatin is hardly known among thyroidologists. He was born on November 13, 1813, in a small village in the mountainous department of Isère in southeastern France. Although he spent his professional career in Paris, the higher rate of goiter in his home department may have sensitized him to the problem. He was apprenticed at 17 to a local pharmacist who rapidly recognized Chatin's high intelligence and sent him on to Paris at 20 years of age to another pharmacist for further training. The Parisian pharmacist, M. Briant, was also struck by Chatin's aptitude and hard work. He saw that the young Chatin would not be content to spend his life in a pharmacist's shop and strongly advised him to pursue a *"purement scientifique"* parallel career. To enable Chatin to do this, Briant took him into his home and supported him through his education. Briant's efforts were well-rewarded. Between 1832 and 1835 Chatin passed two baccalaureate examinations (in arts and in sciences), received a licentiate in sciences, and won a position as an intern in pharmacy in the Parisian hospitals (this was a much higher and more competitive position than are current U.S. internships).

Within a few more years, he won first prize among the interns (1838), and was awarded a DSc (1839), finished his pharmacy training including a thesis and six gold medals in the process (1840), was named chief pharmacist at the Beaujon Hospital (1841), and was appointed agrégé (approximately equal to associate professor) at the Parisian Ecole de Pharmacie (1841). This was a remarkable achievement for the 28-year-old Chatin only 8 years after arriving in Paris.

At the School of Pharmacy he immediately helped revise the curriculum, taught courses officially assigned to other professors too ill to teach, and reorganized the botanical garden. At the time, medical botany was a mainstay of the practice of medicine. As one of Chatin's goals was to make pharmacy a more scientific discipline, he rapidly began to study and publish papers on toxicology and taxonomic botany. Another of his goals was to establish pharmacy as a discipline independent of medicine, a goal which he ultimately achieved. It took a good deal longer than he anticipated. Almost incidentally, in the midst of all this activity, he married in 1843. He now had an income, his MD, DSc, and was writing a thesis on toxicology. Apparently, because he was so good at this job, the school also asked him to teach comparative anatomy, anthropology, and general zoology.

In 1848, two chairs (professorships) of botany at the School of Pharmacy were vacant. The ambitious Chatin, now 35 years old, wanted to be appointed to one of them as he had already been doing most of the work for both professors for 7 years. However, there was a move to reorganize the school and abolish these two chairs (note that all decisions on higher education in France are centralized and need to be approved by the Minister of Public Instruction). Chatin saw his career going down a track he did not like, so he took direct action. He went with his wife in a carriage one evening to the home of the Minister of Health, Hippolyte Carnot, to try to convince him to keep the two chairs active. Carnot agreed but all was not smooth sailing. The chairs were in fact merged into one and, when the school's faculty was asked for nominations. Jean-Baptiste Payer's name was first, Chatin was second. Fortunately, the Académie des Sciences had the power to review faculty nominations at the School of Pharmacy, and they reversed the order of faculty's nominations and put Chatin's name first. And so he was appointed professor.

That year, 1848, was stressful on another front. It was a year of political turmoil throughout Europe. France, especially Paris, was no exception. There were pitched battles in the streets of Paris. Chatin fought as a sub lieutenant in the National Guard. The danger was clear as his sergeant, standing next to him, was killed.

By the 1840s, iodine, discovered only 35 years before, had become widely used as a drug and was widely known to be a poison. Jean-Francois Coindet's use of iodine to treat goiter in the goitrous city of Geneva in 1820 was a bold use of a chemical element to treat a disease. It was, however, based on the prior use of seaweed and sea sponge, then known to contain iodine, for the same purpose. Coindet's success fell into disfavor the next year (1821) as many goitrous Genevans overdosed on iodine and suffered from a peculiar illness we now recognize as iodine-induced hyperthyroidism. Nevertheless, iodine remained on the list of agents used to treat goiter. Analogous thinking led to iodine's use to treat any mass in the neck, including scrofula and, by extension any or illness associated with tissue swelling. These uses were Lugol's claim to fame and his solution is still used today. It was used to sterilize skin wounds as a staple of American home remedies.

In 1831, iodine was proposed as an effective goiter preventative by Jean-Baptiste Boussingault as a result of his years in what is now Colombia, South America. He noticed that goiter was prevalent in some mountainous villages and not in others, and that the crude salt used by those without goiter had iodine in it [3]. He suggested that salt be iodized by the government as a public health measure. Nothing came of it.

In 1848, Jules Grange actually did water analyses in the mountains of Isère, Chatin's home district, and claimed that goiter resulted from too much magnesium in the water. The next year, Grange thought that the effect of this deleterious element could be prevented by iodized salt [4] and said so to the Académie des Sciences. The prevailing dictum of pathology was that a disease such as goiter had to be caused by a noxious stimulus – "*un principal délétère.*" The idea of a deficiency causing a disease was a heretical idea.

Such was the context of Chatin's presentation in 1850. France had recovered from the strife of 1848 and was rapidly drifting toward the more conservative Second Empire under Napoleon III. Chatin was now a professor. His research in toxicology led him to study arsenic, copper, and iron in plants and organic material. Perhaps he was plagued by Grange's work or perhaps he wanted to see if he could detect iodine in freshwater plants with a sensitive method for measuring iodine. Whatever the direct stimulus, he clearly thought he had solved the problems of both the cause and the prevention of goiter.

The committee appointed to report on his work actually did so and with speed. A.A.B. Bussy, a senior botanist in the Académie des Sciences, told the group less than a month after Chatin's paper that Chatin's work was sound but needed better quantitation. At a later meeting, Bussy noted that he personally confirmed Chatin's data. Chatin responded in kind in August 1850 with new data. He now confidently stated that "too little iodine in the drinking water ... seems to be the principal cause of goiter." Chatin's focus then became iodine in the environment. He studied air, soil, food, and water from all over France. The data in general confirmed his thesis that low iodine was associated with goiter (*"il y a coincidence générale entre l'abondance de l'iode ... et l'absence complete du goiter et du cretinsime"*) [5].

It was clear. Iodine deficiency caused goiter and iodine should be given to prevent goiter and cretinism. More data came in from other workers. Grange himself agreed with most of Chatin's findings, but he found some areas of France where he detected no iodine in the water and the people had no goiter. Others agreed with Grange.

Chatin improved his assay for iodine. He did more studies, and rebutted his critics. Curiously, he never studied individual patients and never tried to correlate urinary iodine with the presence or absence of goiter (although he did find iodine in the Parisian sewers!) [6]. The Académie des Sciences weighed in on October 11, 1852 [7]. They agreed with most of Chatin's data but thought he needed more. They disagreed with his assertion that low iodine caused goiter. They urged him to study individual patients with goiter.

Why Chatin did not then study goitrous persons is a mystery. The closest he came was a report of two villages on the Rhone called Fully and Saillon [8]. People living in Fully had goiter and cretinism and those in Saillon did not. Saillon's water had much more iodine. This was apparently not sufficient to sway the Académie.

Chatin published 11 papers on iodine in the 1850s. No further committee reports appeared during the 1850s and any enthusiasm for Chatin's idea had faded. At the end of the decade, from 1858 to 1860, a controversy broke out in Paris over the apparent toxicity of tiny amounts of iodine. It culminated in a lengthy discussion in the Paris Academy of Medicine that ran from February 28 to April 9, 1860. Some thought it might even be dangerous to breathe the air at the seaside. Chatin's ideas were effectively dead.

Discussions on goiter continued to engage French investigators, always looking for the active or positive action of a noxious agent. A complete review in 1867 by St. Lager [9] concluded that Chatin's data were contradicted by many others, that something in the water actively caused goiter, and that the best preventatives would be better living conditions, better hygiene, and the draining of swamps. Years later in 1876, Chatin fired his last salvo: investigators simply must learn how to measure iodine accurately [10].

Toward the end of the century, one of France's best chemists, Armand Gautier, repeated many of Chatin's iodine measurements and essentially concluded that Chatin was right [11]. But this had no effect on the prophylaxis of goiter. The idea lay dormant until 1918–1920 when Marine and Kimball in the United States repeated Grange's studies and showed that iodine prevented goiter in schoolgirls in Akron, Ohio. It was still a few more years before iodine deficiency and goiter were clearly connected.

Chatin was intelligent, scientifically ambitious, and well-placed. He worked in a context of reasonable prior knowledge of iodine and produced data of high quality. In his case, these did not matter. There was enough difference of opinion over the data, which resonated with physicians' fear of iodine toxicity, to kill the thesis of "iodine deficiency" as a cause of goiter. There were more than 70 years between Chatin's first proposal and the general consensus that he was right.

Chatin himself, despite the failure of his efforts in the 1850s to convince others, went on with his career. He remained as professor at the School of Pharmacy until retirement in 1886. In his last 13 years he was Director of the entire school. He finally succeeded in achieving some independence for pharmacy from the oversight of the faculty of medicine. He was elected to both the Académie de Médicine and the Académie des Sciences and became the latter's president after he had retired from the school. He published over 200 papers, many after retirement, and became France's botanical expert on truffles. He died at age 87 years, in his home country, a well-honored and well-respected man.

References

1. Chatin A: Existence de l'iode dans les plantes d'eau douce. Consequences de ce fait pour la geognosie, la physiologie vegetale, la therapeutique et peut-etre pour l'industrie. *CR Acad Sci* 1850; 30: 352–4.
2. Chatin, A: Existence de l'iode dans les plantes d'eau douce. Consequences de ce fait pour la geognosie, la physiologie vegetale, la therapeutique et peut-etre pour l'industrie. *J Pharmacie Chim* 1850; 17: 418–30.
3. Boussingault JB: Recherches sur la cause pui produit le goiter dans les Cordilieres de la Nouvelle-Granada. *Annales Chim Phys* 1831; 48: 41–69.
4. Grange J: Recherches sur les causes du poitre et du cretinisme. *Annales Chim Phys* 1849; 26: 129–37.
5. Chatin A: Recherches de l'iode dans l'air, les eaux, le sol et les produits alimentaires des Alpes de la France et du Piedmont. *CR Acad Sci* 1852; 34: 51–4.
6. Chatin A: Recherche comparative de l'iode et de quelques autres matieres dans les eaux (et les egouts) qui alimentent Paris, Londres et Turin. *CR Acad Sci* 1852; 35: 46–9.
7. Bussy AAB: Rapport sur les travaux de M. Chatin, relatifs a la recherché de l'iode et sur differentes Notes ou Memoires presents sur le meme sujet, par MM Marchand, Niepce, Meyrac. *CR Acad Sci* 1852; 35: 505–17.
8. Chatin A: Un fait dans le question du goiter et du cretinisme. *CR Acad Sci* 1853; 36: 652-
9. St. Lager J: *Etudes sur les Causes du Cretinisme et du Goitre Endemique*. Paris: Balière et fils, 1867.
10. Chatin A: Des causes d'insucces dans la recherché de minims quantites d'iode. *CR Acad Sci* 1876; 82: 128–32.
11. Gautier A: L'iode existe t-il dans l'air? *CR Acad Sci* 1899; 128: 643–9.

Sources

Bonnier G: Adolphe Chatin. *Rev Gen Bot* 1901; 13: 97–108.

Bornet E: Notice sur AD Chatin. *Bull Soc Bot France* 1901; 48: 26–38.

Guignard L: Notice sur M. Adolphe Chatin. *J Pharmacie Chimie* 1901; 13: 151–60.

Perrot E: Biographie M. le docteur Adolphe Chatin. *Bull Sci Pharmacol* 1901; 4: 23–32.

This chapter has been reproduced from Sawin, Clark T: Adolphe Catin (1813–1901): Iodine in the prevention of goiter. *The Endocrinologist* 1995; 5(3): 165–8.

CHAPTER 27
Sir James Paget
(1814–1899)
Osteitis Deformans

On November 14, 1876, James Paget spoke to the assembled Royal Medical and Chirurgical Society (RMCS) of London at its four-story home at 53 Berners Street. Although the Society's membership was several hundred, about 35 usually came to the biweekly meetings. The main attraction of the Society was its huge medical library; it was one of the largest in the United Kingdom and the Society was always looking for more space. Paget, by then Sir James, was 62 years old. He was in the second year of his Presidency of the Society and was widely known as one of England's preeminent surgeons. His topic that evening was an unusual disorder that he described as a "chronic inflammation of the bones" or "osteitis deformans" [1].

Paget's description of this rare disease has become a classic. Paget had followed a single patient for 20 years until the patient died from osteosarcoma. In his presentation that November, Paget described the evolution of the disease over that 20-year period. The patient, a country gentleman from the North of England, first noticed aching in his thighs and legs in 1854 when he was 40 years old. When Paget first saw him in 1856, there was some distortion of the left tibia with apparent thickening of the periosteum and a lesser degree of similar changes in the left femur. Paget thought that this represented some sort of ill-defined inflammation and prescribed potassium iodide which did not help (iodide was then in common use for any chronic inflammatory condition, e.g., syphilis or tuberculosis). Three years later the tibia was larger and bowed; the left femur and right side of the skull had grown as well. The patient did not suffer much discomfort and continued his usual activities.

Paget rarely saw him over the next 17 years but learned from others that the disease had progressed inexorably. The patient's height shrank from 73 to 69 inches and his chest and pelvis became distorted. By 1872 he began to lose his hearing and had a variety of diffuse aches and pains. In late 1875 the patient had photographs taken: these are the pictures redrafted into the sketches that illustrated Paget's published paper in 1877.

In January, 1876, the patient developed pain in the left elbow and forearm which rapidly became worse. When Paget saw him in February there was a clear-cut swelling

A Biographical History of Endocrinology, First Edition. D. Lynn Loriaux.

This work is a co-publication between the Endocrine Society and John Wiley & Sons, Ltd.

of the upper radius: "it seemed certain that a firm medullary or osteoid cancerous growth was forming. The patient developed a pleural effusion and failed quickly: he died on March 24th." Paget did the autopsy himself and obtained the specimens of skull and femur that most endocrinologists have seen reproduced in texts and advertisements (a colleague, Henry Butlin, prepared the histologic sections).

There was certainly no rush on Paget's part to publish the clinical description although it could have been written any time during the 20 years of follow-up. Some likely reasons for his hesitancy are that he did not know whether the disorder was unique, or what to call it. Another likely reason is that one of Paget's claims to fame was his thoroughness in pathologic description. Once the patient died and had been autopsied, Paget had a complete story to tell: the slow development of the clinical disorder over many years combined with a full autopsy including histologic sections (such sections were then uncommon in published descriptions of disease). Finally, he had already made his reputation and had no need to enhance it. He could afford to wait until the story was there to tell.

Although Paget had seen three similar patients over the years before 1876, only one was his personal patient and he saw this man, a master of hounds, in the 1860s only for the purpose of surgically removing a cancerous arm. The patient survived only a few days. None of these three had an autopsy. The only previously autopsied patient was one described by his younger London colleague, Samuel Wilks. This patient had been cared for by William Gull (who later described what we now call hypothyroidism). Wilks called the disease "spongy hypertrophy of the bones" [2]. Wilks' description was not only convincing, but also thoroughly acknowledged by Paget. Both Wilks and Gull were members of the RMC Society, but it is unclear if they were present at Paget's lecture in 1876, or whether Wilks' case was even discussed. Even at Paget's presentation in 1876, neither he nor Wilks were sure they had seen a new disease.

Paget had found three other possible cases in the European medical literature but the descriptions were fuzzy and perhaps only one had the same disease he described. Paget made no claim of priority. He called the disorder "osteitis deformans" because it seemed to be inflammatory, but he readily admitted that "a better name may be given when more is known of it."

How was it that Paget, a well-known surgeon, came to speak in November, 1876, about a patient who had no surgery? Few medical practitioners were knighted – why was Paget? He was, in fact, a successful surgeon but he was a physiologist and pathologist as well. These other disciplines were actually the prime sources of his early reputation, which was well established before he engaged in full-time surgical practice.

Paget came from Great Yarmouth, a seaport in Norfolk on the North Sea about 100 miles northeast of London and about the furthest east one can go on land in Great Britain. His father, Samuel was a prosperous brewer and ship owner of the town and fathered 16 other children. George, James' older brother by 5 years, had been well-educated at private school and then gone off to Caius College in Cambridge in 1827. By the time James was old enough to go to secondary school, the family finances had suffered. James was forced to attend a local school and there was no chance of attending the University. He recalled that his school was "not of a very high order." By this, he meant that he did not go beyond reading Horace, Virgil, Homer, and Xenophon in the original.

The young James was attracted by the sparkling uniforms worn by sailors when in town and he decided on a Navy career when he was 16 years old. This almost came to pass, but his mother finally convinced his father that she would be most distressed if her James wound up at sea. The arrangements were canceled and James was apprenticed to the family's physician for the next 4 years upon a payment, by his father, of $100. James was to be a medical practitioner. His duties were varied but were essential to learning the tasks of any family physician of the time. He recalled long, hard days attending patients who "usually were bled until they fainted," at the end of which, there were "leeches to be put in their boxes." But all was not work. James and another brother, Charles, learned a good deal of the botany (James) and entomology (Charles) of the area which led to their first published paper in 1834 [3].

When his apprenticeship was over, James could have stayed locally and practiced. No further training or licensing was needed. But he chose to go to London. No doubt influenced by George who, by 1834, had been awarded a medical fellowship at Caius College. He trained in medicine at St. Bartholomew's Hospital in London and received his MB degree from Cambridge. James could not follow his brother to the University nor could he follow his own desire of surgical training. Both required money that simply was not there. He did follow his brother to Bart's to "begin my hospital work" in 1834. By his own admission, he "was not a diligent attendant at their lectures" but was nevertheless a spectacular student.

In the early 1800s, there was no fixed curriculum at a hospital-based medical school in England. Students may or may not have had experience, such as Paget's apprenticeship. They could attend lectures as they wished. Clinical work was not prescribed. In fact, clinical experience went only to those who actively sought the opportunity and paid the fees. The only requirements were to register, spend a certain amount of time, and, if one wanted to practice in London, pass a test.

Paget arrived, determined to learn all he could. During his first year he did attend some lectures but, more importantly for him, read and dissected at every opportunity. He had already learned French on his own while an apprentice. In addition, at Bart's, he learned enough German, Dutch, and Italian to read the important European medical scientific texts of the time. In his first year, 1834–1835, he noticed little "specks" in the muscles of some cadavers. These were known to be common enough but Paget pursued the matter with the microscope. The school did not have one, but he was in touch with a botanist at the British Museum called Robert Brown (whose name is the origin of the term "Brownian motion") and got permission to use his microscope. This was how Paget found the small worm in the muscle we call *Trichinella spiralis*, the cause of trichinosis. Paget's student discovery is not usually attributed to him because his teacher sent some of the same tissue to Richard Owen, then a senior scientist in London, who diagnosed a parasitic worm and published the discovery.

The year Paget arrived at Bart's, the school began a series of prize examinations. The prize was usually a book. Towards the end of his first year, in early 1835, Paget seemed to have won every prize the school offered, in medicine, surgery, chemistry, and botany. It was fortunate that he had an extensive apprenticeship because in his second, clinical year at Bart's, there was "very little active practical teaching in the wards." He would do as many autopsies as he could. Again, he swept the range of prizes: anatomy and physiology, clinical medicine, and medical jurisprudence. At the end of his second year, he qualified to take the oral examination of the Royal College of Surgeons. If he passed he was allowed to practice in London. No medical degree was needed. He passed, early in 1836. He was now a member of the College. There were no Fellowships, so he could not have been FRCS.

Paget was 22 years old in 1836. To begin a practice was hard and Paget had no regular independent income. Nevertheless, consciously or otherwise, and in part driven by quiet ambition, he made a firm decision to stay in London and take his chances. He did, in fact, begin to practice. For years, however, it brought in little income (usually less than 15 pounds per summer). Moreover, he had become so attached to Bart's that, for practical purposes, he never left. To support himself he tutored a few students. Still, this brought in little income. Again, following in his brother George's footsteps, Paget went to Paris for three months in early 1837 to learn something of French medicine. He heard lectures by some of the famous French physicians and scientists: Magendie, Broussais, Andral, and Louis, but he developed a low opinion of French medical students: "Students here are the most ruttingly ill-looking set of fellows he had ever seen." He thought American students in Paris were the worst.

Paget returned to London and eked out a living that year by medical writing. Here, too, there was little income but it was much more valuable for his future. He met some of the senior physicians and editors of London. He was, for example, sub-editor of the *London Medical Gazette* for 5 years. He reported on the London scene, and wrote and translated the European medical literature. Few could do this as well as he. He wrote annual reports on progress in anatomy and physiology as well as a number of reviews and short biographies. He recalled two merits of this period: "I learned more than ever the necessity of verifying every reference and learned the value of dates and raisins for averting hunger." He managed to get by while waiting for something better.

In 1837, Paget was appointed Curator of the Museum at St. Bartholomew's Hospital. The work required long hours and he was responsible for preparing bodies for dissection and for all the material needed to illustrate other lectures. The job paid only 100 pounds per year, but he finally had an appointment at his medical school. It taught him about the management of pathology specimens and was a clear step in the right direction, even though it almost completely shut him off from practice. Two years later he got another assignment from the school. He was appointed as an unpaid demonstrator of morbid anatomy. Here the only task was to perform medical autopsies, but he also taught students during these autopsies. He taught so well that, although not permitted to give formal lectures, the students insisted, and so began his lecturing career. Part of his ultimate reputation stems from this time; he became renowned as a superb lecturer. Even though the position had no pay, it clearly paid off.

Paget still sought a career in surgery, but had no surgical appointment and one did not seem in the offing. In 1841, he was offered the appointment of demonstrator in anatomy, a much more formal appointment than the one in morbid anatomy and one which was known as a stepping stone to a surgical appointment. But medical school politics intervened as so often is the case. He was not qualified, men said, because he had not served on the surgical wards, and what of the others who had been waiting for years? The offer was withdrawn. Paget suffered a "bitter disappointment." Ever resourceful, however, he expanded his surgical experience when he was appointed surgeon to the Finsbury dispensary.

The next year, Paget's career took a decided turn for the better. His teaching ability, his curatorship of Bart's pathologic museum, and his writing connections led to an offer to write the *Pathological Catalogue of the College of Surgeons Museum*. This was a monumental task. John Hunter's original collection from the seventeenth century, the Hunterian Museum, was the basis of the museum collection and had never been carefully arranged in a systematic way or catalogued so that one could learn from it. Further, the collection had expanded during the 40 years since Hunter's death so that there were more than 3000 specimens to be described and organized. Paget felt that, with time, there had to be case histories for the learner. He took on the further task of writing these. Others, including the same Richard Owen who published on trichina a few years before, envied Paget this assignment, but it was not withdrawn and Paget moved ahead. His approach was that "nothing was to be told but what could be then and there seen." His work style was simply to add anything new he took on to whatever he was already doing. One wonders where he found the time, but find it he did. The resulting *Catalogue* came out in five volumes from 1846 to 1849 and was considered a remarkable achievement [4]. By the time the last volume was published, Paget's reputation had risen far. He was seen as the master of surgical pathology and as the "English Virchow."

In that same year, 1842, the school finally decided to split the single lectureship in anatomy and physiology into two. Now one need not compete for the anatomy position in the face of the surgeons but one could seek the physiology appointment separately which, at the time, included "general anatomy," synonymous with "microscopic anatomy." Paget competed for the position and succeeded. He was named Lecturer in General Anatomy and Physiology in 1843. This appointment was probably his most important. Paget told his brother Frank, who was in London when the news came, that Frank and the rest of the family should "make much of it; my fortune is made!" Paget's lectures in physiology took place five days a week during the course; as before in pathology, they were quite popular with the students. One student, William Kirkes, later used them as the basis for a textbook of physiology. In the first edition of this text (1848) Kirkes notes that "I cannot sufficiently express my obligations to Mr. Paget, from whom I have received the most liberal aid in every stage of the work." The text continued well into the twentieth century.

Paget's reputation in physiology lasted throughout the nineteenth century despite the fact the he did no experimentation. He was elected an Honorary Member of the Physiological Society in 1882, 6 years after its founding.

Paget was soon immersed in the curriculum of the school at Bart's. He was named Warden of the school's newly established college. In practice, this meant that he was housemaster to a select group of medical students in a new dormitory-like arrangement (the "College"), advisor to them as well as to many other students, and finance officer for the school. Paget was not only teaching but administering. Later in 1843, he was elected as one of the first 300 Fellows of the Royal College of Surgeons, no doubt a result of his work on their catalogue.

As Warden, he settled into the college where he lived for the next 8 years. His personal finances improved and he finally married in 1844. He was responsible for seeing that the students in fact paid attention to the reason they were there: to study medicine. He found some to be good students but there were others that were "always wanting guidance and encouragement, (and were) seldom improved by it." He worked on his lectures with great care; all were thoroughly prepared. For any important lecture he would prepare "every word long before, and learned, if I could, every word by heart." Despite his intelligence and the knowledge that his talks were well-received, he "could conceal my nervousness but it always weighed on me."

His long-desired appointment to the surgical staff came through in 1847 after intensive political canvassing. The usual objections that he had not been trained on Bart's surgical wards did not prevail. He was now assistant surgeon to the hospital. His position was more firmly established than ever. That year, he was chosen as professor of anatomy and surgery (this meant that he had to give an occasional lecture at the College but had no other duties, and he was not expected to move from Bart's. The lectures he gave for this annual professorship were, again, so well-received that he was re-elected to the professorship for six consecutive years. He made the microscope the centerpiece, particularly in the diagnosis of tumors, which was a great advance at the time. These lectures resulted in a book, *Lectures on Surgical Pathology*, that stood as a standard text for more than two decades.

By 1851, Paget decided that he needed more income to support his expanding family. He had six children. He also needed money to help pay off debts incurred by his father's business failure years before but which were still outstanding. His fame had spread. Owen now thought of Paget so highly that he said that Paget could either be the best physiologist in Europe or the best surgeon in London. He was 37 years old. Paget resigned his position as Warden at Bart's and went into full-time surgical practice in London. Within a few years, he had one of the most lucrative practices in England. His forte was not skillful surgery, although he was quite competent and was greatly aided by the new anesthesia, but rather in thoughtful diagnosis and gentle operation. He continued the frenetic pace of his earlier years. For the 20 years after 1851 he worked 12–16 hours a day and traveled 5000–8000 miles a year within the United Kingdom to see patients. It was during this time that he first saw the patient he presented to the RMCS in 1876.

His fame spread to England's upper class. He saw his first royal patient in 1858 and promptly bought a portrait of Queen Victoria with the fee. That year he was named Surgeon Extraordinary to the Queen (the usage does not mean he was better than ordinary but rather that he might be called in if the "ordinary" or usual surgeon needed help). He was so busy that in 1859 he resigned as Lecturer in Physiology, in part because he no longer needed the income but mainly because he was not able to do for the students what he thought he should. In 1861, the hospital promoted him from Assistant Surgeon to Surgeon and the Prince of Wales appointed him his Surgeon-in-Ordinary. In this last capacity he sometimes accompanied the Prince to the continent. The royal practice expanded. One day in 1865, he noted that "I have to see a Baron, a Viscount, a Countess, and a Marquis!!!" He collected honorary degrees from Oxford and Bonn (1868) and was elected President of the Clinical Society of London (1869), the same Society before which Gull and Ord would soon describe that curious disease, myxedema. The 1850s and 1860s were enormously successful decades for Paget.

Paget's older brother George, to whom he had always looked for advice, also did well as an academic physician. He was named Physician to Addenbrooke's Hospital, the major hospital in Cambridge, and held the position for 45 years. He held his Caius fellowship until 1851 when he married and had to resign it. He was instrumental in revitalizing the Cambridge Medical School, which, until his arrival graduated few students. He began, for the first time in the United Kingdom, the clinical examination of patients as part of the MB examination. The 1860s were a good decade for him as well; he was president of the British Medical Association in 1864 and, like his younger brother, fostered the development of physiology in the medical school. He was also elected a Fellow of the Royal Society in 1873. One wonders how extensive the contacts were between the two brothers as their reputation spread through British medicine. We do know that James relied heavily on George whenever he needed to make a major decision.

James Paget, now aged 57 years, suffered a grievous infection, probably septicemia, in 1871 after doing an autopsy. While he was ill, he had advice from many other physicians. He later recalled that a fellow surgeon, Sir William Lawrence, had said that "he had not known anyone recover on whose case more than seven had consulted." Paget did recover, but as a result of his illness cut back on his work and resigned his position as Surgeon to St. Bartholomew's Hospital, although he remained as Consultant. His reputation and royal connections led to a baronetcy the same year (hence Sir James Paget). Although his medical responsibilities decreased, he seemed to work as hard as before, staying up until 1 to 2 a.m. The Royal College of Surgeons elected him their president in 1875 – and so did the Royal Medical and Surgical Society to whom he presented his patient with osteitis deformans the following year.

Recognition continued although Paget stopped operating in 1878 when he was 64 years old after consulting once again with his brother George, who was now Cambridge's regius professor of physics. By then, James Paget was the serjeant-surgeon to the Queen (that is, the chief surgical consultant). He thought that the peak of his career, however, came in 1881 when he was chosen as president of the Seventh International Medical Congress. More than 3000 came to London and heard him give the opening address; William Osler, who heard Paget speak, thought that Paget's speech was the highlight of the meeting. Paget later became an honorary member of the Massachusetts Medical Society, but that seems to have been one of his few American connections. He continued to work and think. In a lecture on cancer to the Royal College of Surgeons in 1887, now aged 73, he said that "I believe that microparasites, or substances produced by them, will someday be found in essential relation with cancer." Was this prescience or just a lucky guess?

For our story, however, the key year in Paget's later life was 1882. That year, on June 13th, he spoke again on osteitis deformans to the Royal Medical and Surgical Society. He had been looking for more of these patients ever since he spoke on the topic in 1876. Between 1878 and 1882 he had personally seen seven more cases, three of whom were women. None had a complete autopsy, but the clinical findings were so characteristic that he felt it was time to "justify the giving of a distinctive name and a definite general description of the disease" [5]. His uncertainty of 6 years before as to whether he had described a unique entity had gone. In 1882 he made up his mind. There were now enough cases to crystallize the condition as a distinct nosologic disorder. His 1876 paper is often used to denote Paget's "discovery" of the disease, but it was his later paper in 1882, even though it did not have the dramatic illustrations of the older paper, that finally convinced him he had something new.

In his 1882 presentation, Paget did not refer to any previous paper on the topic, including Wilks', except to note that an 1873 German paper had used the same term, "osteitis deformans," to describe what Paget thought was an entirely different disorder. He seemed to want to focus on cases he had seen himself before deciding that he had described a discrete disease.

Paget himself, of course, never referred to the disease as "Paget's disease" as this would have been wholly inappropriate. The eponym arose when Jonathan Hutchinson (of "Hutchinson's teeth"), another famous London surgeon 14 years Paget's junior and Paget's former pupil, referred to Paget's descriptions as "models for us all." Hutchinson wrote that "Osteitis Deformans, a malady which, were it not that the brow of its discoverer wears already so many laurels, we might be tempted to propose should be known as Paget's disease" [6].

The eponym is with us still, in large part because we remain ignorant of the disease's cause and so have difficulty calling it by another name. But the eponym serves us well: it calls to mind the efforts of a brilliant practitioner and scientist who advanced knowledge within the framework of what was then possible. As both physicians and scientists, we are no different. Science 150 years ago was, as it is now, not only the doing of experiments in the laboratory but, more broadly, the practice of an inquisitive mind seeking to unravel nature's codes. Were it not for the eponym, Paget would likely be lost to view. And we would have lost another small piece of our own heritage.

Paget died on December 30, 1899, at the age of 85 years, 2 days after receiving Holy Communion from his son, Francis, then the Bishop of Oxford. Though frail and ill, his mind was clear to the end. He was buried in Westminster Abbey. His other son, Stephen, followed in his father's steps and became Surgeon to St. Bartholomew's Hospital but retired from the profession when he was 42 years old to become a successful biographer and essayist (one biography was of his father and another was of Victor Horsley). The family tradition of public service continued well into the twentieth century. One of Paget's grandsons was an archbishop in Africa and the other a prominent general in the Second World War.

References

1. Paget J: On a form of chronic inflammation of the bones (osteitis deformans). *Med-Chir Trans* 1877; 60: 37.
2. Wilks S: Case of osteoporosis, or spongy hypertrophy of the bones (calvaria, clavicle, os femoris and rib, exhibited at the Society). *Trans Pathol Soc Lond* 1869; 20: 273.
3. Paget CJ, Paget J: *Sketch of the Natural History of Yarmouth and its Neighborhood*. Yarmouth: Skill, 1834.
4. *Pathological Catalogue of the College of Surgeons Museum* (5 Vols.). London: Royal College of Surgeons, 1846 (Vol. 1), 1847 (Vol. 2), 1848 (Vol. 3), 1849 (Vols. 4 and 5).
5. Paget J: Additional cases of osteitis deformans. *Med-Chir Trans* 1882; 65: 225.
6. Hutchinson J: The Bradshawe Lecture on Museums: In their relations to medical education and the progress of knowledge. *Br Med J* 1888; 2: 1257.

Sources

The principal source is Paget's own partial autobiography and his letters, all of which were compiled and edited by his son, Stephen. There also is good information in more recent short papers on Paget as well as in standard sources such as the *Dictionary of National Biography* and the *Encyclopedia Britannica* (11th edn., 1910–11). Paget's 1876 and 1882 papers have been reprinted twice, though not in facsimile (*Selected Essays and Monographs*, London: New Sydenham Society, 1901; 1: 5); readers may find these easier to access than the original journal. Those used here include:

Goldstein HB: Sir James Paget. *Am J Dermatopathol* 1980; 3: 27.

Lefanu WR: *British Periodicals of Medicine. A Chronological List*. Baltimore, MD: Johns Hopkins Press, 1938.

Moore N, Paget S: *The Royal Medical and Chirurgical Society of London. Centenary, 1805–1905*. Aberdeen: Aberdeen University Press, 1905.

Paget S: *Memoirs and Letters of Sir James Paget*, edited by Stephen Paget, one of his sons (2nd edn.). London: Longmans, Green. 1901.

Proger LW: Sir James Paget and the Museum of Pathology. *Ann R Coll Surg Engl* 1964; 34: 59.

Reed K, Grage TB: The Paget tradition revisited. *Am J Surg* 1982; 144: 498.

Rolleston HD: *The Cambridge Medical School. A Biographical History*. Cambridge: Cambridge University Press, 1932.

Shenoy BV, Sheithauer BW: Sir James Paget, F.R.S. *Mayo Clin Proc* 1983; 58: 51.

Shenoy BV, Sheithauer BW: Paget's perspectives in pathology. *Mayo Clin Proc* 1988; 63: 184.

This chapter has been reproduced from Sawin, Clark T: Sir James Paget and osteitis deformans. *The Endocrinologist* 1997; 7(4): 205–10.

CHAPTER 28
Sir William Gull
(1816–1890)
Adult Cretinism and "Jack the Ripper"

On Friday, October 24, 1873, Sir William Withey Gull spoke to the Clinical Society of London about two syndromes, adult cretinism and anorexia nervosa. The first is the one of most interest to endocrinologists as it is the disorder later called "myxedema," which we now know as hypothyroidism. Gull's description of hypothyroidism in the Society's *Transactions* in 1874 [1] was the first report of this disease. Although Gull thought that the "cretinoid state" was a disorder of the nervous system, it can be said that he crystalized the clinical picture of the disorder which led to the first successful endocrine therapy, the treatment of myxedema with thyroid extract.

William Gull was one of England's best-known physicians in 1873. Still, his eminence was not predictable as a circumstance of birth or privilege. Born in Colchester, he was the son of a bargeman, the youngest of eight children. Shortly after he was born, the family moved to Thorpe-le-Soken in Essex. His father died of cholera when Gull was 10 years old, leaving his mother with limited means to raise the large family. She managed and William was able to attend local schools. His mother seems to have moved to the village of Beaumont in 1832 to live on property owned by Guy's Hospital. As an "earnest Churchwoman" she regularly attended church and observed the eating of fish on Friday.

In 1834, Gull left home to attend Mr. Abbott's school, where he became a kind of student-teacher. For example, he began to teach himself Greek and, although not particularly proficient, was asked by Mr. Abbott to teach it to the younger boys on the theory that he would learn more as he taught. After 2 years at the school, at about age 19 years, Gull decided that he wanted to go to sea. His mother disapproved and convinced William to come to Beaumont and study further with Beaumont's rector, Mr. Browell. William came and studied. After about a year, the desire to get to the sea faded and he decided that he wanted to do medicine, although at the time there was no way that he could do so: finances would not permit. The next step in Gull's career is a bit cloudy but is hinged on the fact that Mr. Browell was the nephew of Benjamin Harrison Jr. who had been, for some years, the powerful treasurer of Guy's Hospital.

A Biographical History of Endocrinology, First Edition. D. Lynn Loriaux.

This work is a co-publication between the Endocrine Society and John Wiley & Sons, Ltd.

Though nominally subservient to the hospital's governors, the treasurer was, in fact, the person who ran the hospital. One version of the story tells that Harrison came to visit his nephew and was taken by, or was told of, William's intelligence, and so offered William a position at Guy's. Another story is that Mr. Browell sent William to London with an introduction to Harrison to help find something for him. Whatever the details, William went to London in September, 1837, at the age of 20 years, to live at Guy's under Harrison's protection and sponsorship.

At Guy's, Gull was not immediately a medical student. Things were not that simple. The special arrangement gave him the privileges of apprenticeship but he seems not to have been an actual apprentice. He was expected to provide for himself which, as a student, would have been almost impossible. Harrison provided rooms and about $50 per year. Gull's initial work was to copy Guy's museum catalog, which had earlier been drawn up by Thomas Hodgkin. During his first year Gull attended lectures and learned more of the classical languages. After that year, Gull formally matriculated at the new University of London as a medical student. As the university was an examining body and did not hold classes, he also needed to enroll in a school. Once again his sponsor provided. Harrison arranged free entry to Guy's Hospital School of Medicine and for Gull to be a "perpetual student" or "perpetual pupil." His finances assured, Gull proceeded to win most the prizes offered. He received his MB in 1841 with honors in physiology, comparative anatomy, medicine, and surgery. He also qualified, as was then common, by becoming a member of the Royal College of Surgeons (MRCS) on passing its qualifying examination. Gull's intelligence was now known and he was admired for his retentive memory, his attention to detail, his thoroughness, and his breadth of clinical expertise.

Gull did not leave immediately to go into practice as most then did. He elected to stay at the hospital where he continued to live – or at least to live nearby – for most of the decade after graduating, even though he had no official position. It was a "trying period." But Harrison's hand was felt again. In 1842 Harrison arranged for the new graduate to teach materia medica. In return, Gull got the use of a house and $100 per year. He also assisted the full-time hospital apothecary, which meant that he would visit patients in the hospital and attend to urgent cases. In 1843 Gull also became lecturer in natural philosophy. He taught physics to the medical students, tutored medical students for modest sums, and, when the hospital governors were forced to name a Medical Superintendent for the patients with mental illness housed in the "lunatic wards," Gull got the job. One of his first moves was to clean these wards and decrease the use of restraints, then thought by many to be effective treatment. By 1851, he was able to abolish restraints entirely against the wishes of many others. This experience had a notable effect on his view of mental and psychosomatic illness. He concluded that "moral therapy," what we would call psychotherapy now, was preferred over medical treatment. At the same time he developed a major interest in neurologic disease.

Gull began a small practice about 1843. Once he saw a patient, that person tended to stay with him. This satisfaction seemed to come from Gull's attitude, and he was confident as well as knowledgeable. He had "a strong sympathy with suffering in every form" and felt that "the young, the aged, or the sick ... must always be helped." For him, "no detail in the comfort or well-being of the patient was too minute for his attention." Although he was not always correct in his diagnosis, he seemed to radiate assuredness. An anxious hypochondriac was once encouraged by Gull's telling him that, "he was a healthy man out of health," and wondered why no one had told him this before. Others said that, "he treated men, not diseases."

During most of the 1840s Gull learned more and more in his constant attendance at the hospital. He developed into an excellent lecturer. The students liked him because he not only gave them what they thought they needed but did so in a firm and confident manner. Gull was a hard worker as well. One of his mottoes was, "work is an essential condition of life." Ward rounds on Sunday morning were usual. But he was not one who could get by with little sleep: he slept a full 8 hours each night and, when fatigued, "he could sleep anywhere and at any time."

Another of Gull's characteristics was an intolerance for most of the prescriptions then used to treat illness. His later reputation as a therapeutic nihilist is unjustified, however, as he did use those few drugs he thought would actually benefit a patient – digitalis, opium, etc. "I do not say that no drugs are useful; but that there is not enough discrimination in their use." Moreover, "in cases of cardiac dropsy his belief in, 'Addison's pill,' of digitalis, squills, and mercury was unbounded." Nevertheless, he was also intolerant: he "never tired of exposing the absurdity of much of the traditional polypharmacy." This attitude did not endear him to many of his colleagues. He was sometimes criticized when he refused to write a prescription he thought was not needed. Occasionally, his attitude got in the way of dealing with patients who expected their medicine. Once, a patient at Guy's recovered from typhoid fever under Gull's expectant treatment. When Gull congratulated him on his successful outcome, the patient replied, "Yes, and no thanks to you either."

Gull's later effort to show that rheumatic fever can be successfully treated with a placebo backfired. He tried to show that a mint–water placebo could result in a successful outcome. He published his cases as examples [2]. Readers then took the placebo to be an active treatment and looked on mint–water as a cure! Gull was certainly against the tenor of the times, but while he did not hesitate to comment on others' overuse of drugs, he may have been a bit unfair to the large number of practicing apothecaries who were not then paid for their medical advice but only for the drugs they would dispense. No doubt this was at the root of Gull's life-long antipathy to the licensing of apothecaries to practice medicine.

Gull continued with his education and went on to write a thesis for his MD on "paralysis," a reflection of his continuing interest in neurologic disease. His 1846 thesis won the gold medal. That same year other work came his way, probably guided there by Harrison. Gull was appointed to another lectureship, this time in physiology and comparative anatomy, subjects in which he had won honors as a student. He held this lectureship for the next 10 years, giving it up only when he joined a Guy's colleague, George Rees, in practice and the patient load went beyond his capacity. The work included teaching pathology as well as physiology. Gull believed that "diseases are but perverted life processes" and "the pathologist follows the steps of the physiologist, and often the work is but one." Again, he was a successful lecturer with a reputation that went beyond his school. The next year, 1847, he was elected Fullerian Professor of Physiology at the Royal Institution for a 3-year term and became a friend of Michael Faraday, the contemporary Fullerian Professor of Chemistry. Gull also paid attention to the medical school's curriculum and helped institute graded clinical responsibilities for students in place of the random choices of the students themselves.

Gull progressed rapidly. In 1848 he was elected a Fellow of the Royal College of Physicians (FRCP), one of the peaks of a London elite physician's career. The next year he gave the traditional Gulstonian Lectures, for which he again chose nervous diseases as the topic. He became an official resident physician at Guy's in 1848, a position that seems to have been created specifically for him. It may have been Harrison's final bit of help for Gull as Harrison retired from his treasurer's position that year. A later commentator noted that Gull was so "favored by Mr. Harrison as to excite not a little jealousy." But 1848 was a year of sorrow as well. His fiancée had died and he was depressed. A colleague invited Gull to his wedding and Gull almost failed to attend. It is as well he did because at that wedding he met his colleague's sister, Susan, and married her later that year.

In the late 1840s, Gull's practice was expanding and he was becoming known in London as well as at Guy's. He was elected a Fellow of the Royal Medical and Chirurgical Society as well as FRCP, but he still had no established position at the hospital where he had been for over a decade. In 1851 his wait came to an end. He was appointed to the position of assistant physician. Even now the hand of Harrison may have been present although Harrison had been retired for 3 years. The positions of assistant physician and physician had by then become fixed; no one was appointed until a previous appointee retired, which was mandatory at age 60 years, or died. But that year the governors seem to have decided that they needed four rather than three assistant physicians and so Gull was appointed. The 34-year-old Gull now had status and was a true colleague of Thomas Addison (1793–1860). His position was firm for years to come. Now he hoped for a promotion to physician.

Gull published seven papers by 1851, mainly clinical reports, as were almost all of his 92 lifetime publications, including his only paper with Addison on xanthelasma [3]. During the 1850s Gull seems to have lived the life of the successful practitioner and teacher. His practice became quite lucrative as the "carriage trade" gravitated to him. He wrote on the successful treatment of tapeworm, on steatorrhea in cases of mesenteric adenitis, on several skin diseases including leprosy, and co-authored a major report on cholera with William Bayley for the College of Physicians. He elucidated a number of causes of paraplegia such as spinal cord tumor, venereal disease, and obstruction of the abdominal aorta. He began to give lectures on medicine when he was appointed to the medicine lectureship in 1856. Finally, on the death of Henry Hughes after only 4 years as a physician, Gull succeeded to a physicianship at Guy's. He was more established among the elite physicians of London than ever.

One sign of his persistence and ambition was his pursuit of an autopsy on a young man he had seen with darkening of the skin, weakness, and lethargy. The patient left the hospital and died at home. Gull wanted the adrenal glands to confirm his suspicion that the patient had the disease described by Addison. He went to the boy's home but the father refused permission. Gull, though polite, stubbornly refused to leave the house. Finally, he went up to view the body in the presence of a family observer. There he removed the adrenal glands anyway, put them in a bottle he carried, and cautioned the observer not to upset the father by speaking of what he had done. The glands became part of the collection of the pathological museum at Guy's.

The 1860s brought more of the same. Gull's practice flourished. He continued to describe disease in his thorough and inquiring manner with continued attention to diseases of the nervous system. He was the first to describe syringomyelia in 1862 [4] and one of the first to use the eponym "Addison's disease" [5] the year after Addison killed himself while depressed. He got into a scientific argument with Charles-Edouard Brown-Séquard over whether or not there was an obligatory lesion of the spinal cord in patients with bladder paralysis. Brown-Séquard was then in London practicing neurology and was a fellow Gulstonian lecturer. Gull is said by his contemporaries to have "won" but in retrospect probably did not. Despite Gull's outspoken nature and his tendency to irritate others with his intolerance of what he called "bumbledom," he became a leader in his profession. He was the first medical graduate to serve in the Senate of the University of London in 1856. He was one of the founders of the Clinical Society of London, which was later to publish the endocrinologically famous report on myxedema. By 1868 his practice had apparently become so large that he resigned his coveted physicianship at Guy's well before the mandatory age of 60 years. Three years later, the hospital appointed him as consulting physician, a position without obligation to the hospital or the school.

Perhaps the highest professional honors came at the end of the 1860s. In 1868 he received an honorary degree from Oxford and the next year was elected a Fellow of the Royal Society. His contributions to his discipline, largely clinical, were seen as high science and worthy of his belonging to the scientific as well as the medical elite.

Gull came to public prominence in 1871 when he was one of those in attendance to the then Prince of Wales (the future King Edward VII). In November, the 30-year-old, pleasure-loving Prince had become seriously ill with typhoid fever at Sandringham, the 7000 acre estate in Norfolk he bought in 1861. The disease was more worrisome than usual for the British because he was the heir apparent to the throne and everyone remembered that typhoid had killed Prince Albert, the Prince's father, 10 years before. Most members of the royal family had court-appointed physicians and surgeons. Such appointments were considered a clear honor as well as a call to duty. In 1863 the Prince had appointed two physicians-in-ordinary (for obscure reasons a higher title than physician-extraordinary): William Jenner, an expert on infectious disease who had been among the first to distinguish typhus from typhoid, and Edward Steveking. By 1871, Steveking had, for unclear reasons, temporarily fallen from favor so when it was evident that the Prince was indeed seriously ill, Jenner was called to Sandringham from London but Steveking was not. Jenner may have then called for Gull to come, or perhaps the local doctor who saw the Prince when he first became ill, Oscar Clayton, may have asked for both Gull and Jenner. In any event, both came to attend the Prince along with the Queen's appointed surgeon, Sir James Paget, a personal friend of the Prince. The situation was so critical that Queen Victoria came as well. Gull remained with the Prince for most of December and personally cared for him, doing what would now be done by a skilled nurse: "He seemed to combine the duties of physician, dresser, dispenser, valet, nurse ... passing at times twelve or fourteen hours at that bedside." The Prince recovered and Gull got much of the credit although, of course, there was no specific therapy for typhoid. Gull later remarked that the Prince "was as well treated as if he had been a patient in Guy's Hospital." Gull became nationally famous for his care of the Prince and was knighted within the month.

On a Friday evening in October, 1873, Gull lectured on his two syndromes to the Clinical Society. Gull was a founder of the Society and had just completed a 2-year term as its President. His prominence had led to his attendance at the autopsy of the French emperor, Napoleon III, earlier in the year in London where the emperor had fled after his defeat in the French-Prussian war. Now Gull came to the Society's meeting as a famous but ordinary member. He gave his presentation on anorexia nervosa first and then spoke on the cretinoid state in women. Most refer to Gull's five cases but, in fact, he spoke of only two. The first was postmenopausal and noted that she was progressively more "languid" over time and described "her much like the full moon at rising." She spoke "as if the tongue were too large for the mouth." The other patient was premenopausal and had "too profuse" menses.

Gull gave credit to his brilliant younger colleague at Guy's, Charles Hilton Fagge, then the morning assistant physician, for describing sporadic cretinism in children 2 years earlier [6]. Fagge had written that Gull himself had taught him about cretinism when he was a student and agreed that many of the sporadic cretins had "a wasting of the thyroid body" (the functions of the thyroid gland were not then known). He further speculated that this "wasting" might "possibly be the cause of the other changes which make up that morbid state." Gull in his talk considered that the disorder might be due to heart or kidney disease. Strangely, he did not mention the thyroid body except to note that it was not enlarged in his patients. He concluded that "I am unable to give any explanation of the cause," although he was later inclined to a neurological origin.

Gull's presentation could hardly have been the first time that such patients had been seen by physicians, yet no one reported anything like this in adults before. Byrom Bramwell, a prominent Edinburgh physician, later said that his father had mentioned cases like this to him in 1869 but had never published. Certainly Gull had been primed by his knowledge of childhood cretinism but he was thinking more widely than others and saw in his adult patients what others did not.

The adult disease was named "myxedema" a few years later by William Ord [7], another physician at Guy's. He, too, thought it a nervous disease and theorized that the mucinous infiltrate, myxedema, impeded the flow of nervous impulses to the brain, which in turn led to the clinical findings. Ord later chaired the Committee of the Clinical Society to look into the cause of this peculiar and incurable disease. Gull was appointed but seems not to have served. That is another story.

Gull's other presentation on that October evening was on anorexia nervosa [8]. It actually led to a good deal more discussion than on adult cretinism [9]. Gull is usually credited by English speakers with defining that syndrome as well. As with adult cretinism, he had followed his patients some time before presenting them to the Society. He noted that he had mentioned this syndrome, almost in passing, in a major speech on another topic 5 years before, but was now giving much more detail, including some comments on its outcome. The discussion makes it apparent that many members of the Society had also seen such cases; they had simply not bothered to write them up. Perhaps this is the reason for the more extensive discussion on anorexia; they had not seen anyone with myxedema and so had nothing to discuss.

Gull probably had a reason for quoting himself in this case: it was a matter of publishing priority. Earlier in 1873, Ernest Lasègue, who was a Parisian psychiatrist, a member of the French Academy of Medicine, and the editor of the *Archives Générales de Médecine*, had written on the same topic [10]. Further, his paper had been translated into English and published in a London medical journal about a month before Gull's talk. Gull mentioned that he had written his speech and only then was told by Dr. Webb of Lasègue's reports. It appears that both Gull and Lasègue reported on the disease independently [11] but that Lasègue was in print first with a substantive description. There was no real priority dispute although Lasègue's later comments were somewhat barbed [12].

A thread that runs through Gull's work is his attention to the mental state of the patient and the benefit that calming it can bring to the patient's condition, whether the disorder is the mind, as in the case of the "healthy man," or clearly of the body, as in the case of the British heir apparent. He did seem to seek a neuroanatomical explanation for these many neurological malfunctions as seen in his interaction with Brown-Séquard, but accepted that one might not be found as in adult cretinism or anorexia nervosa.

Gull's career proceeded apace. His personality did not change. He remained honest and outspoken and tolerated fools not at all. His "love of argument was great" and "his humor was generally critical and sometimes sarcastic." While he maintained that he did not hesitate to say "I do not know," his expressed views "not infrequently provoked antagonism and gave offence when none was intended" and "on two or three occasions incurred some degree of professional censure." Some likened him to the first Napoleon. Still, he was in fact careful not to speak so bluntly to a patient or to anyone junior to him; he was simply no politician and saw no reason to be one [13].

Nevertheless, this acerbic character and his skill at speaking made him a strong advocate. He was openly in favor of experimental medicine, although he did none himself. Even the public knew this. The magazine *Vanity Fair* caricatured him as the "Physiological Physic" in 1875, the year of the turmoil over animal experimentation in the United Kingdom that led to the Cruelty to Animals Act of 1876.

Another episode arose over the role of nurses in the hospital. It embroiled Gull in the public press and led to uproar from the audience when he was given an honorary degree at Cambridge in the 1880s. Gull refused to allow the Vice-Chancellor to stop the din and "stood calmly until it had subsided." The case was that of Pleasance Louisa Ingle, a nurse at Guy's Hospital who was accused of manslaughter because, while walking a sick patient, the patient died. The patient's physician, Frederick Pavy, had an international reputation for his work on diabetes mellitus. But in this case his patient had undiagnosed tuberculous meningitis and Pavy encouraged the patient to walk in an attempt to relieve her muscular weakness. The nurse took the recommendation to heart and vigorously walked the patient, during which the patient died. At her trial, Pavy testified that the nurse had caused the patient's death. Gull felt the patient would have died anyway, that the nurse was in no way at fault, and that her prosecution was unjust. The nurse was nevertheless convicted. The public was on Pavy's side, hence the uproar at Cambridge. Gull once again said what he thought in the face of opprobrium.

In October, 1887, when Gull was 70 years old, he suffered a stroke while vacationing in Scotland. He knew what had happened, and though aphasic and with right-sided weakness, he was able to walk to his house. Recovery was good but he felt he should no longer practice and retired. It was during the year after his first stroke that the Whitechapel murders occurred (August–November, 1888). The murderer of the five prostitutes has never been identified though theories are many. The killer was named by the press as "Jack the Ripper" because the women were all killed by knife and mutilated. Eighty-eight years later, in 1976, a journalist's theory that Gull was Jack the Ripper was a sensation of sort [14]. The book was made into a television "documentary" with Gull's name prominent in the scrolled end-notes. The theory's background was that Gull was carrying out the wishes of "royalty" who were eager for a cover-up. The basis of the theory was that only a physician with knowledge of anatomy and surgical skill could have done the murders. Gull was the only physician who lived near enough and was present in the area and was a physician. That Gull had had a stroke was of no moment. Sensational though it was, the theory's rebuttal and counter conclusion a decade later by a professional policeman and crime writer seem more reasonable. No one knows who Jack was [15].

In 1890, after several seizures and further strokes, Gull died in London, aged 73 years, on Wednesday, January 29. He did not quite make it to the time of effective thyroid therapy, successfully applied by George Murray the next year. Friends, including James Paget, accompanied the coffin by train from Liverpool Street Station to his boyhood village of Thorpe-le-Soken, where he was buried in the churchyard on the following Monday. He died a wealthy man. His estate was $344 000, equivalent to more than US$28 million today. While this fortune was "unprecedented in the history of medicine," his colleagues felt that "few men have practiced a lucrative profession with less eagerness to grasp at its pecuniary rewards." His own view was clear: "If I am anything, I am a clinical physician."

References

1. Gull WW: On a cretinoid state supervening in adult life in women. *Trans Clin Soc London* 1874; 7: 180.
2. Gull WW: Cases of rhematic fever treated for the most part by mint water. *Guy's Hosp Rep* 1865; 11: 392.

3. Addison T, Gull WW: On a certain affection of the skin. Vitligoldea-a: plana; b. tuberosa. *Guy's Hosp Rep* 1851; 7: 265.
4. Gull WW: A case of progressive atrophy of the muscles of the hands. Enlargement of the ventricle of the cord in cervical region with atrophy of the grey matter (hydromyclus). *Guy's Hosp Rep* 1862; 8: 244.
5. Gull WW: A case of Addison's disease. *Med Times Gaz* 1861; 2: 57
6. Fagge CH: On sporadic cretinism, occurring in England. *Med-Chir Trans* 1871; 54: 155.
7. Ord WM: On myxedema. *Med-Chir Trans* 1878; 61: 57.
8. Gull WW: Anorexia nervosa (apepsia hysterca, anorexia hysterica). *Trans Clin Soc* Lond 1874; 7: 22.
9. Hewitt P: Clinical Society of London. *BMJ* 1873; 1: 385.
10. League EC: De Tanorexie Hysterique. *Arch Gen Med* 1873; 1: 385.
11. Vandereycken W, van Deth R: Who was the first to describe anorexia nervosa Gull or Lasègue? *Psychol Med* 1989; 19: 837–45.
12. Silverman JA: Lasègue's editorial riposte to Gull's contributions on anorexia nervosa. *Psychol Med* 1992; 22: 307.
13. Hunter RA, Greenberg HP: Sir William Gull and psychiatry. *Guy's Hosp Rep* 1956; 105: 361.
14. Knight S: *Jack the Ripper: the Final Solution*. New York: David Mckay, 1976.
15. Rumbelow D: *Jack the Ripper. The Complete Casebook*. Chicago, IL: Contemporary Books, 1988.

Sources

Acland TD (Ed.): *A Collection of the Published Writings of William Withey Gull, Bart, M.D. F.R.S. Medical Papers*. London: New Sydenham Society, 1894, p. 17.

Acland TD (Ed.): *A Collection of the Published Writings of William Withey Gull. Bart, M.D., F.R.S. Memoir and Addresses*. London: The New Sydenham Society, 1896.

Anonymous: Sir William Gull. *BMJ* 1890; 1: 256.

Anonymous: In memorian Sir William Gull. *Guy's Hosp Rep* 1890; 47: xxv.

Cameron HC: *Mr. Guy's Hospital, 1726–1848*. London: Longmans, Green and Co., 1954.

French RD: *Antivivisection and Medical Science in Victorian Society*. Princeton: Princeton University Press, 1975.

Wilks S, Bettany GT: *A Biographical History of Guy's Hospital*. London: Ward, Lock Bowden & Co., 1892, pp. 261–74.

This chapter has been reproduced from Sawin, Clark T: Sir William Gull, adult cretinism, and "Jack the Ripper." *The Endocrinologist* 1997; 7(5): 279–84.

CHAPTER 29

Charles-Edouard Brown-Séquard (1817–1894)

Glandular Extract Therapy

Charles-Edouard Brown-Séquard is best known to most medical students and physicians for the eponymic neurological syndrome in which damage to the spinal cord on one side results in a loss of position and vibration sensation on the other side. Most of Brown-Séquard's life work focused on the nervous system, both clinically and physiologically, and was consistent with the main current of regulatory thought in the nineteenth century, which maintained that the nervous system was the principal controller of the body's functions. He was also an innovator in what we now call endocrinology.

The year after Thomas Addison's description in 1855 of damaged adrenal glands associated with hyperpigmentation and death, Brown-Séquard showed that bilateral adrenalectomy in animals always led to death. It did so specifically because of the absence of the adrenal glands and not because of infection, hemorrhage, or local injury. Death was caused by, and not just associated with, absence of these glands. His findings were controversial since others had removed the adrenal glands without causing death. The idea that this was a fruitful phenomenon worth pursuing did not catch on and Brown-Séquard dropped the idea.

His initial work was done under uncomfortable conditions. His father, an Irish-American sea captain, died before Edouard was born on the island of Mauritius, then a British possession in the Indian Ocean. He was raised by his mother in what were called "modest circumstances." He moved to Paris in 1938 and hoped for a career in letters but, as with Claude Bernard, his hopes were dashed by a Parisian critic. Shifting to medicine, he took his MD degree in 1846 at the relatively late age of 29 years. His thesis was on the physiology of the spinal cord. He was poor and lacked research funds but had the compulsion to experiment and answer physiologic questions. He eked out a living in the years immediately following his MD. He said he worked "very hard, taking no exercise and living in a vitiated atmosphere. [He] slept very little, and usually passed eighteen or nineteen hours a day writing, reading or experimenting. [His] diet was miserable."

In 1851, the empire in France was restored and Brown-Séquard, being a known Republican, felt it better to leave. Thus he began a peripatetic life. Until he finally

A Biographical History of Endocrinology, First Edition. D. Lynn Loriaux.

This work is a co-publication between the Endocrine Society and John Wiley & Sons, Ltd.

obtained a Parisian professorship on Claude Bernard's death in 1878, Brown-Séquard traveled almost constantly to England and America and back, crossing the Atlantic more than 60 times during these years in the days before steamships and airplanes. Two of his three wives (all died before he did) were U.S. citizens and the third was English. At one time, he was on the senior staff of London's National Hospital for Diseases of the Nervous System including Paralysis and Epilepsy, the famous "Queen Square Hospital." He was professor of the physiology and pathology of the nervous system at Boston's Harvard Medical School, the first person to hold that position. He was also a member of the U.S. National Academy of Sciences and of the British Royal Society, largely on the basis of his neurological work. Nevertheless, it is clear that his constant desire was to find a place in Paris. His spoken English was not good, and neither America nor England was, at the time, fertile ground for experimental physiology. He continued to make a living wherever he was by the practice of medicine, financing his research largely out of his personal income.

Brown-Séquard returned about every 10 years to endocrinology. While his adrenal work led to no further experiments, he claimed in 1869 in Paris that the adrenal glands, the kidneys, and the sexual glands, "give to the blood, by an internal secretion, principles which are of great importance if not necessary" (written in 1893). Whether these claims were backed by unpublished experiments is not clear. In 1875 he was back in Boston visiting his friend, Louis Agassiz, the Harvard paleontologist and zoologist who had emigrated from Switzerland, at the Agassiz's summer cottage in Nahant. Here, he first tried testicular grafts from guinea-pigs to elderly dogs in an attempt to rejuvenate the dogs. There are no published data (despite his otherwise enormous bibliography), but he felt that he had "confirmed the correctness of the view [he] had advanced."

Another decade passed and Brown-Séquard, now age 72 years, was firmly ensconced in his professorship of medicine at the College de France. He announced to the membership of the Société de Biologie on June 15, 1889, that he had injected himself with watery extracts of dog and guinea-pig testes and had "regained at least all the strength I had a number of years ago." He could work longer, his own strength was better (measured with an instrument, the dynamometer), and his urinary stream went further. He was no charlatan; he clearly noted that others should repeat the study and that the results could have depended on "mon idiosyncrasie personelle." His lofty position gained much respect for these unusual findings. Further, he provided carefully prepared extracts for others to use free of charge and at his own expense; he did not profit.

Nevertheless, the scientific climate of the time did not insist on experimental controls. Some became enthusiastic and tried extract of testes and other tissues, which we know contain little if any biologic activity, in a wide variety of diseases with apparent success. Physicians, including the internationally famous William Osler, claimed benefits, for example, from adrenal extracts. Others castigated Brown-Séquard and denounced his therapy. The public as well as the medical profession clamored for his "elixir of life." By August 1889, the New York Times reported that testicular extracts were being used at Bellevue Hospital, while others noted that "it was repugnant to true science to parade crude and untried theories before the public." So the controversy had spread to America within two months. Within another month *The Times* had reported a death from this therapy.

Brown-Séquard remained convinced of the efficacy of his treatment until the day he died in 1894. He had strong support for his ideas in the United States. Both clinicians and physiologists agreed that there was something to his work. Still, his extracts as he prepared them were, in retrospect, not effective.

Henry P. Bowditch (1840–1911), the eminent Harvard physiologist of the late nineteenth century, knew Brown-Séquard well. He wrote that Brown-Séquard's work on the "elixir of life," was "received with so much incredulity by most physicians that it gave an important stimulus to the study of the internal secretions of glands." One of Brown-Séquard's "strongest claims to remembrance rests upon the stimulus to research which flowed from his activity." While Brown-Séquard's specific facts were wrong, his general idea that glands secreted what we now call hormones was right. This concept led to the successful therapy with thyroid extract of an incurable disease, myxedema, by George R. Murray (1865–1939) only 3 years after Brown-Séquard's announcement to the Société de Biologie.

Sources

Brown-Séquard CE: Des effects produits chez l'homme par des injections sous-cultanees d'un liquid retire des testicules frais de cobaye et de chien. *CR Soc Biol* 1889; 41: 415–19.

Brown-Séquard CE: On a new therapeutic method consisting in the use of organic liquids extracted from the glands and other organs. *Br Med J* 1893; 1: 1145–7, 1212–14.

Bowditch HP: Memoir of Charles Edouard Brown-Séquard 1817–1894. *Biog Mem Natl Acad Sci* 1902; 4: 93–7.

Grmek MD: Brown-Séquard, Charles Edouard. *Dict Sci Biog* 1970; 2: 524–6.

Jefferson M: Brown-Séquard: a biographical assay. *Lancet* 1952; 1: 760–1.

Olmsted JMD: *Charles-Edouard Brown-Séquard. A Nineteenth Century Neurologist and Endocrinologist.* Baltimore, MD: Johns Hopkins University Press, 1946.

Ott I: Dr. Brown-Séquard. *Med Bull* 1896; 18: 361–6.

Stockwell GA: Historical, critical, and scientific aspects of Brown-Séquard's discovery – the so-called "elixir." *Ther Gaz* 1889; 13: 812–14, 14: 14–19.

Tyler HR, Tyler KL: Charles Edouard Brown-Séquard: professor of physiology and pathology of the nervous system at Harvard Medical School. *Neurology* 1984, 34: 1231–6.

Wilson, JD: Charles-Edouard Brown-Séquard and the centennial of endocrinology. *J Clin Endocrinol Metab* 1990; 71: 1403–9.

This chapter has been reproduced from Sawin, Clark T: Charles-Edouard Brown-Séquard (1817–1894). *The Endocrinologist* 1991; 1(2): 73–4.

CHAPTER 30

Franz Leydig

(1821–1908)

Testosterone Secreting Cells

Franz Leydig was born in Rothenburg ob der Tauber in 1821 [1]. His father was a clerk in a salt shop (*Salzamtsdiener*). Like so many great biologists, Leydig was fascinated by the natural world at a very early age. Taxonomic classification and a rudimentary microscope fueled his appreciation of the complexity of the world of insects, birds, and small mammals. He went to Latin school where he had the advantage of being the only student in the class. As a result, school was transformed into one long tutorial with a committed teacher interested in natural history. He went to the Unirversity of Munich in 1840, studying philosophy and zoology, which he found "disappointing." Thus, he set his mind on the study of medicine, and moved to the University of Wurzburg in 1942.

Because of his academic facility and his need for money, he began assisting in the anatomy and physiology courses. When the University decided to develop a Microscopy Institute, Leydig was invited to guide its implementation. A laboratory was built around a modern microscope and an incubator in which to culture organisms of interest. This became his scientific home for many years. Leydig earned a "lectureship" in 1849, largely on the basis of his work on the relationship between Cowper's glands and the prostate. Shortly thereafter, he submitted a manuscript on his histological studies of the male reproductive system in a number of laboratory animals. The article included the first histological description of the "Leydig cells" [2]:

> Near the end of the article is a 12-page summary of findings for the various organs, including a page on the testis, with a 13-line summary about the Leydig cells ... "From the comparative histology of the testis it is clear that, in addition to seminiferous tubules, blood vessels, and nerves, one finds an additional constant component in the mammalian testis, a cell-like mass that when present follows the course of blood vessels between the seminiferous tubules but, when more developed, becomes a mass in which the seminiferous tubules are imbedded. Its main constituents are small granules of fatty appearance, which are unaltered by acetic acid and sodium hydroxide treatment, i.e., colorless, or yellowish, and encompass clear, bubble-like nuclei. Its semi fluid ground substance may condense into a cell membrane, and at least in some mammals, the entire granular mass is surrounded by a sharp outline. Also, at times, the entire structural aggregate is of such an appearance that one can speak of it as a complete cell" [3].

A Biographical History of Endocrinology, First Edition. D. Lynn Loriaux.

This work is a co-publication between the Endocrine Society and John Wiley & Sons, Ltd.

In 1857, Leydig published his textbook *Lehrbuch der Histologie des Menschen und der Theire* (*Textbook of Human and Animal Histology*), which was the first such work on comparative histology. Leydig moved to the University of Tübingen in that year as professor of zoology and comparative anatomy, and then moved again in 1875 to the University of Bonn as professor of anatomy. At Bonn he continued his histological studies and taught students. He was remembered by his students as an inspiring teacher. In the Germanic tradition, he taught anatomy at the blackboard with colored chalk. He would draw figures of symmetrical structures, such as the brain, simultaneously with right and left hand [4]. Leydig retired when he was 66 years of age and returned to Wurzburg and Rothenburg ob der Tauber, where he died at the age of 87.

As histological techniques of preservation, staining, and sectioning improved, descriptions of the Leydig cells advanced apace. Friedrich Reinke, in 1896, was the first to observe crystals in human Leydig cells in tissue from a 25-year-old executed criminal. He looked for these structures in 10 other specimens, and found them in all but a 15-year-old boy and a 65-year-old man [1]. The endocrine nature of the Leydig cell was deduced in 1903 by Pol Bouin and Paul Ancel. They correctly concluded that the cells are endocrine, synthesizing and secreting some substance that is essential for the maintenance of "maleness" [5]. Thus they closed the loop proposed by Aristotle in his *Historia Animalium*, Book 9, Volume 4, in which he demonstrated that castration of the rooster causes regression of male characteristics, and in songbirds the loss of the song. Aristotle also showed that "transplanted" testes can restore these qualities. Nothing is new under the sun.

References

1. Ober UB, Sciagara C: Leydig, Sertoli, and Reinke: three anatomists who were on the ball. *Pathol Annu* 1981; 16: 1–13.
2. Leydig F: Zur der Männlichen Geschlechtsorgane und Analdrüsen der Sängethiere. *Z Wiss Zool* 1850; 2: 1–57.
3. Christensen AK: A history of Leydig cell research. In *The Leydig Cell in Health and Disease*, edited by AH Payne and MP Hardy. Totowa, NJ: Humana Press, 2007, p. 6.
4. Nussbaum M: Franz von Leydig. *Anat Anz* 1908; 32: 503–6.
5. Bouin P, Ancel P: Recherches sur des Cellules interstitielles du testicule des mammiferess. *Arch Zool Exp Gen Ser A* 1903; 1: 473–523.

This chapter has been reproduced from Loriaux, D. Lynn: Franz Leydig (1821–1908). *The Endocrinologist* 2007; 17(6): 297–8.

CHAPTER 31
Adolf Kussmaul
(1822–1902)
Ketoacidosis

Adolf Kussmaul was born February 22, 1822, in Graben, Germany. His father and grandfather were both physicians. The young Kussmaul often accompanied his father on his rounds, and even occasionally into the autopsy suite. He began his medical studies in Heidelberg at the age of 18. He graduated in 1845 and went to Vienna to continue his studies.

Kussmaul was a military surgeon between 1848 and 1849, and then entered private practice in Kandern, Switzerland, in 1850–1853. He married Luise Amanda Wolf in 1850 and they had five children: Helene, Luise, Eduard, Hedwig, and Ida. Two died young: Eduard drowned in the Rhone River and Ida died from tetanus.

Kussmaul left private practice because of poor health and moved to Würzburg to be in the same institution with Rudolf Virchow. He became a doctor of medicine there in 1855.

He returned to Heidelberg in 1857 as professor of medicine, and moved again in 1859, accepting the chair of internal medicine in Erlangen. He moved to the same position at Freiburg in 1863, and again to Strassburg in 1876. He lived in Strassburg for the remainder of his life.

Kussmaul worked across the breadth of internal medicine as it was in the nineteenth century. He made important discoveries in psychology, neurology, pathology, and pathophysiology. This can be seen from his list of eponyms: Kussmaul breathing, Kussmaul's sign, Kussmaul disease (polyarteritis nodosa), Kussmaul coma (diabetic ketoacidosis), and Kussmaul's aphasia (selective mutism). He was the first to describe "word blindness" (dyslexia), polyarteritis nodosa, progressive bulbar paralysis, and mesenteric embolism, and was the first to perform gastric lavage, thoracentesis, esophagoscopy, and gastroscopy.

Wilhelm Petters demonstrated the presence of acetone in the urine of diabetic patients in 1857, and Karl Gerhardt demonstrated acetoacetic acid in the urine of diabetic patients with acetonemia. Kussmaul proved that diabetic coma was caused by ketoacidosis, and it was in these patients that he first described Kussmaul's respiration.

A Biographical History of Endocrinology, First Edition. D. Lynn Loriaux.

He called it *diese grosse athmung* ("this great breathing"). He described dyspnea, indicative of air hunger, even when the patient was in diabetic coma. The breaths are rhythmic, deep, often sighing, not particularly fast, but faster than would be expected for a patient at rest.

Kussmaul was first to describe pulsus paradoxus, the disappearance of the peripheral pulse with inspiration in patients with constrictive pericarditis. In this same disease, he described Kussmaul's sign, the increase in the height of the jugular venous pulse with inspiration. The pathophysiology of these two signs is still not perfectly understood.

Kussmaul made a careful study of a famous sword swallower and, by noting the position in which the sword swallower held his head, realized that it would be possible to introduce an inflexible tube through the esophagus and into the stomach. Kussmaul thus developed the first endoscope. He also developed the first ophthalmoscope. His book on aphasia remains a classic to this day.

Adolf Kussmaul was one of the most creative minds in the history of medicine. He was the most prolific translational investigator of the nineteenth century. He died of a myocardial infarction on the morning of May 28, 1902.

Sources

Gerhardt J: Diabète sucré und acetone. *Wein Presse Med* 1865; 6: 672.

Kussmaul A: Zur Lehre vom diabète sucré. *Dtsch Arch Klin Med* 1874; 14: 1–46; 55: 81–94.

Petters W: Untersuchungen über die Honigharnruhr. *Vierteljahrschr Prakt Heilk* 1857; 55: 81–94.

This chapter has been reproduced from Loriaux, D. Lynn: Adolf Kussmaul: 1822–1902. *The Endocrinologist* 2010; 20(3): 95.

CHAPTER 32

Jean-Martin Charcot (1825–1893)

Exophthalmic Goiter

In May 1856, Jean-Martin Charcot, a young Parisian physician, presented the first thorough description of a peculiar entity termed "exophthalmic goiter" or "exophthalmic cachexia" to his colleagues at a meeting of the Société de Biologie. This odd disease had been well-described in the United Kingdom and in Germany, but not in France where it was known mainly to specialists in eye diseases.

Charcot later became nationally and internationally famous for his work on neurologic diseases. For many, he practically invented the specialty of neurology at a time when there were few specialists of any sort. He also became known and, to some, infamous for his studies on hysteria, a disease that is now, strictly speaking, no longer a disease according to *Diagnostic and Statistical Manual of Mental Disorders* criteria, although it has clear remnants in recognized entities such as "conversion disorder." However, all of that came long after his permanent appointment to the Salpêtrière Hospital in Paris in 1862, and his gradually increasing focus on neurologic disorders in the patients who came there.

Charcot did not come to medicine easily. Parisian by birth, his family was not wealthy but was able to send him to the local school mainly attended by lower middle class boys. There was probably a choice to be made between his becoming an artist or entering medical school, though the former seems not to have been pursued with any great fervor. In any case, in 1843 at age 17, he went to the Paris Medical School after he had finished high school. At the time, students had a relatively loose curriculum. They could attend lectures or not and, in fact, were expected to learn mainly on the wards of the hospitals. Graduation as a physician could take a varied length of time, often up to 8 or 9 years, and depended on passage of several examinations as well as the completion of a thesis. Charcot was successful in his first year examination and so was able to proceed.

Charcot seems to have decided on an academic career. In Paris at the time, such a choice was by no means an easy one. There were two parallel paths, a hospital path and one based on faculty of the medical school. A medical academician had to master

A Biographical History of Endocrinology, First Edition. D. Lynn Loriaux.

This work is a co-publication between the Endocrine Society and John Wiley & Sons, Ltd.

both paths to succeed. To do this, he (there were no women) had to be intelligent and make a good impression on his superiors. But more than this, he had to publish and cultivate highly placed sponsors to plead his case with the doyens of the profession. In the hospital pathway, many students acted as externs after completing 2 years of school and passing a not too rigorous examination. However, for there to be any hope of later promotion in the academic world, the student had to compete for the elite and limited post of "interne." The interne post was far from what we now call internship, a one-year clinical appointment at the end of medical school. Each of 4 years was spent at a different Parisian hospital under the tutelage of a different clinical professor. Only a few were chosen, and almost all who later became professors in the medical school had earlier been internes.

Charcot first competed for the externship in 1845 and spent the 2 years 1846–1848 attending to patients in various hospitals, changing dressings and performing common treatments such as bleeding. He tried for the *internat*, or internship, in 1847 but failed. For his hospital experience that year he took a temporary internship at the St. Louis Hospital under J.G.A. Lugol, the proponent of iodine solutions for the treatment of tuberculosis. The next year, in December 1848, he was one of only 19 students in the Parisian student body to achieve the desired position of interne des hôpitaux. During the next 4 years, 1849–1853, he rotated among four hospitals. In 1850, for example, he spent the year at the Charité Hospital with Pierre Rayer, who was later physician to the emperor, Napoleon III. In 1851, Charcot was at the Pitie Hospital with Pierre Piorry, and the last of his four internship years was spent at the Salpêtriére Hospital. Both professors at the Salpêtriére became mentors and were influential in his later career (the hospital, incidentally, was an arsenal in prior centuries and was so named because saltpeter had been stored there).

Charcot finally graduated from medical school in 1853, 9 years after he began. His thesis was not the routine review of the literature proffered by most students. Rather, Charcot based his thesis on direct observation of 41 patients with gout or rheumatoid arthritis whom he had seen the previous year in the Salpêtriére Hospital. Piorry presided over Charcot's thesis presentation.

Two years before his graduation in 1851, Charcot widened his professional circle further by joining the new liberal Société de Biologie, which had been founded in 1848 to give young investigators a forum for experimental and scientific data and to connect clinical and laboratory work. It met frequently and heard from such eminent figures of experimental medicine as Claude Bernard with little of the stuffiness of the usual academic society. The young mixed with the old, and it was the data that counted, not the prestige of the person. In fact, the young Charcot co-authored a paper with Bernard. The Société remained an important place for Charcot as well as for French biologic science for the rest of the century.

Charcot's prestigious internship was over in 1853. He then sought and received an appointment on the first step of the academic ladder, a 2-year appointment as chef de clinique, roughly the equivalent of an assistant professor. These appointments were prized and were under the complete control of the responsible clinical professor. Nevertheless, though necessary for further advancement and with little obligated work, there was little honor or financial reward attached. Worse, it narrowed the kinds of patients Charcot could see. The saving grace was that it was under the supervision of his former professor, Piorry, now at the Charité Hospital. That there were not many fixed obligations was also a boon because another of Charcot's mentors, Rayer, referred a wealthy patient, Benoit Fould, to Charcot. Fould, with Charcot as his physician, went on a tour of Italy for his health. The results for Charcot were education in Italian art, a substantial sum with which he was able to begin a private practice, and lifelong friendship with a wealthy and politically connected family.

Following his 2-year stint as chef de clinique, Charcot now needed a hospital appointment of his own while making further plans on what to do about the academic path. He was chosen as a médecin du Bureau central, or médecin des hôpitaux. Although it sounds important today, the work was mainly outpatient triage (i.e., quickly evaluating hundreds of applicants for admission to one of the Paris hospitals and sending them on to the correct institution). There was almost no connection to the patients in the hospital and Charcot was now basically cut off from his work. The idea was that promising young physicians who might want to stay on the hospital path had to serve in these outpatient positions until there was an opening as a chief of a hospital service (médecin de l'hôpital). Further, to boost one's chances at rising up the hospital path and to be able to teach students sent to the hospital, one needed to rise on the academic path as well. The hospital path was mainly a waiting game. One simply had to wait for an opening and have enough clout to obtain it. The academic path probably was based more on merit, but the path was perilous and still required powerful sponsors.

Charcot continued his clinical work as best he could and wrote extensively. His next competition, in 1857, was in the academic path for the aggregation (an agrégé is the rough equivalent of associate professor). One undergoes a stiff series of oral examinations, and submits and defends a thesis. Charcot failed in 1857. He was able to teach but only outside the official curriculum. His teaching included topics such as gout, rheumatoid arthritis, fevers, neuroses, poisons, and parasitic diseases. He tried again for the aggregation in 1860 and succeeded in becoming one of only six physicians who became agrégé stagiaire that year. It required Rayer's personal intercession to achieve this. Two years later, he became agrégé en exercise, which permitted him to teach in an official capacity whenever a full professor was absent, and provided a small, inadequate salary. In 1862, still agrégé (as he was to remain until 1872, when he became professor), he finally got an appointment as a médecin de l'hôpital at the Salpêtrière Hospital. He stayed for the rest of his career.

Charcot's major theme on beginning at the Salpêtrière was chronic disease. The patients, in fact, directed him. His job was to care for the service in the hospital that had women over the age of 60 who had chronic illnesses. He began with his colleagues to diagnose and classify these patients and, by 1866, was able to give a series of lectures on diseases of old age. These lectures, done before his major interest in neurology developed, began to change the reputation of the Salpêtrière from a hospital on the margins to one that was attractive to students. They also brought recognition to Charcot as a leader in gerontology. Overall, his focus remained on chronic illness for most of the 1860s, with publications on topics such as diabetic gangrene and syphilitic or neuropathic arthropathy, Charcot's joint.

Toward the end of the 1860s, Charcot began his emphasis on nervous diseases which brought him his lasting fame. During his career, he focused not only on hysteria, with a degree of skepticism from some of his colleagues, but also described multiple sclerosis, amyotrophic lateral sclerosis, and named Parkinson's disease. His lectures were ever more regular. In particular, his Tuesday Lectures, given from 1887 to 1889 were world famous and were a true innovation for their time because Charcot did not give formal lectures as did most of his fellow professors. Instead, he spoke about patients presented to him in person whom he may not have seen before and thus ran the risk of being in error. He preferred that mode because it more nearly mimicked the true clinical situation.

When Charcot presented a paper on exophthalmic goiter to the Société de Biologie in 1856, no one knew about hormones and there was no such thing as endocrinology. He had finished his 2 years with Piorry as chef de clinique and was working in his outpatient triage job. He recognized that there had not been a complete description of exophthalmic goiter in France and wanted to bring it to the attention of the scientists in the Société as a complex syndrome rather than as a peculiar form of eye disease. He had already developed a reputation for thorough reviews of the extant literature, and his talk on this occasion was no exception. His review included the cases described not only by Parry, Graves, Stokes, and Basedow, but also the older probable case described by Flajani.

Charcot's patient, Caroline C., was a 24-year-old woman whom he had seen in February 1855 while on Piorry's service at the Charité Hospital. She had palpitations of the heart, goiter, and bilateral exophthalmos. Charcot noted that she eventually underwent a spontaneous remission, although he realized that the disease could recur. He did not like the available terminology, exophthalmic cachexia, because not all patients had all three findings. Still, there was no better term, so he used it. Charcot did not accept any of the proposed explanations of the disorder, and strongly felt, in the face of overt criticism from his mentor, Piorry, that the findings did in fact represent a specific syndrome and not a random association of signs. Charcot thought that the pathophysiologic explanations offered were faulty, and that the disorder was "une affection du système nerveux." His reasoning was that the most prominent symptoms were the palpitations and the tremor which Charcot seems to have been the first to note. He attributed the goiter and exophthalmos to excessive blood flow to these parts. This interpretation was reflected in the type sizes used in his published paper: "palpitations" is in 18-point type and "exophthalmos" is in 8-point type.

In agreement with those Europeans who said that the disorder, which we now call hyperthyroidism, was too diffuse and nonspecific in its etiology to be named on the basis of its cause, Charcot felt that an eponym was called for. He decided that "Basedow's disease" was a good one because Basedow had first described it reasonably fully. The difficulty was that even he, in his thorough search of the literature, had missed Graves' first report in 1835 and missed the opportunity to recognize Graves. Another of Charcot's teachers, Armand Trousseau, changed this in the 1860s and insisted that the disease be called "Graves' disease." Although Trousseau's idea took hold in English-speaking parts of the world, it largely remained "Basedow's disease" in Europe.

Charcot's description appeared in the popular medical press in 1856 and then, the next year, in the Société's *Memoires*. It never appeared in English, which is perhaps why it is not as well-known as it might be.

Charcot became a full professor on the academic path in 1872. He was named a professor of pathological anatomy. Other honors came. He was elected to the French Academy of Medicine in 1872 and then to the Academy of Sciences. In 1882 he also was elected to a professorial chair in nervous diseases created for him. Full of honors and wealthy to boot, Charcot kept working, although slowed a bit by angina pectoris, until he died of pulmonary edema while on vacation in 1893 at age 67.

Neurologists and gerontologists remember Charcot as a founder of their fields. For most endocrinologists Charcot is, if anything, a French-sounding name attached to an unusual problem that occurs in the foot of a diabetic patient. It is well to recall that he was one of the first to realize the unity of the autoimmune disease we now call Graves' or Basedow's disease and had the concept that it was somehow a systemic disorder.

Sources

Beeson BB: Jean-Martin Charcot. A summary of his life and works. *Ann Med Hist* 1928; 10: 126.
Bonduelle M: Portrait de Jean-Martin Charcot. *Bull Acad Natl Med* 1993; 177: 865.
Charcot JM: Mémoire sur une affection caracterisée par des palpitations du Coeur et des arteres, la tumefaction de la glande thyroid et une double exophthalmie. *Comptes-Rendus des Séances et Mémoires de la Société de Biologie* 1857; 3(2nd ser.): 43.
Goetz CG: Visual art in the neurologic career of Jean-Martin Charcot. *Arch Neurol* 1991; 48: 421.
Goetz CG, Bouduelle M, Gelfand T: *Charcot. Constructing Neurology*. New York: Oxford University Press, 1995.
Micale MS: Charcot. An essay review. *J Hist Med Allied Sci* 1996; 51: 358.
Sawin CT: Therories of causation of Graves' disease. A historical perspective. *Endocrinol Metab Clin North Am* 1998; 27: 63.

This chapter has been reproduced from Sawin, Clark T: Jean-Martin Charcot (1825–1893) and exophthalmic goiter. *The Endocrinologist* 1999; 9(2): 153.

CHAPTER 33

Jean Baptiste Boussingault (1802–1887)

Iodine and the Goiter

Jean Baptiste Boussingault, whose full name was Jean Baptiste Joseph Dieudonné Boussingault, was a well-known nineteenth-century French scientist. He was elected to the French Académie des sciences at the young age of 37 years and was regarded well enough in the twentieth century to be included in the *Dictionary of Scientific Biography (DSB)* [1]. His inclusion in the *DSB*, however, notes only work in agricultural chemistry and does not mention iodine at all. In fact, his reputation, as outlined in the *DSB* as well as in the 1910 "Scholar's" 11th edition of the *Encyclopedia Britannica* [2], derived only from his pioneering studies of chemistry and physiology as they relate to agriculture. These sources ignore his early studies on goiter. He was probably the first to suggest that goiter could be prevented by the prophylactic use of iodine.

Boussingault was born in Paris. His father, Charles, was the proprietor of a tobacco shop. His mother, Elizabeth, grew up in Wetzlar, Germany near Giessen. His family was poor and lived in a poor area of the city. He was not a good student. He had no education in the sciences, and he quit the lycée the year before he was to graduate. This eliminated any chance he had of attending a university. This was not a promising start for a future academician. The one thing he had that could lead to an advanced education was a year he spent helping clean the laboratory of Louis Thénard, a well-known chemist at the Collége de France. When Thénard found out that the young Boussingault was working in his laboratory, he fired him. Years later, Thénard remarked, "if only I could have foreseen."

The teenage Boussingault seems to have been brighter than his record at the lycée would suggest. The spark was probably science. Boussingault read chemistry and physics on his own.

His mother bought him Thénard's four-volume treatise on chemistry (*Traité de chimie élémentaire, théorique et pratique*), and he attended free lectures that were open to the public on a wide range of scientific topics: chemistry, botany, crystallography, and geology. He later recalled that "after all I was only 14 to 16 years of age and there was

A Biographical History of Endocrinology, First Edition. D. Lynn Loriaux.

This work is a co-publication between the Endocrine Society and John Wiley & Sons, Ltd.

no time to digest all that I had learned." The times were difficult for his family as well. These were the years of Napoleon's two defeats and the Prussian occupation of Paris. His mother's ability to speak German helped mitigate the situation for the family.

At 16 years of age, Boussingault thought of joining the French navy, but promotion in the officer corps depended on connections that he did not have. A new school of mines had just opened at Saint-Etienne, near Lyon. There were laboratories, a library, and geologic specimens. So, in 1818, having convinced a friend to join him, the two walked from Paris to Saint-Etienne to begin the 2-year course. Toward the end of his second year, Boussingault was awarded the position of student-demonstrator. This gave him access to the laboratory for his own study. He had his first publication, at 19 years of age, on the presence of silicon in steel and platinum.

In 1820, Boussingault took a position at a lignite mine in Alsace and then, in 1822, received an appointment to the National School of Mines in Bogotá, Colombia. Boussingault was to be a professor for a term of 4 years at a salary four times greater than his salary in Alsace. In addition, Boussingault received a commission as a lieutenant-colonel in Bolivar's army which he was to hold until he left South America 10 years later.

The 20-year-old Boussingault left for South America as a member of the scientific expedition organized by Alexander von Humboldt. The main emphasis of the expedition was geology, geography, mining, and surveying. Included was the physician-naturalist François Roulin. The political climate in South America was unstable and the French government, now under the monarchy again, was decidedly unfriendly to the revolutionaries in South America. Boussingault and Roulin took their own ship to Colombia and Venezuela via Belgium and England. Roulin went directly to Bogotá and Boussingault disembarked in Venezuela and proceeded overland to Bogotá to make geologic and climatologic observations along the way. He traveled with a group of Bolivar's soldiers: capture by the Spanish army could be fatal.

Once in Venezuela, Boussingault was struck by the many women with goiters. He noted that even the dogs had goiters (this finding is reminiscent of David Marine's first visit to Cleveland almost 100 years later where he noted goiter in both women and dogs in the streets of the city). When he finally arrived in Bogotá in May 1823, Boussingault found goiter there as well. He also saw that some families avoided goiter by "drinking water from a particular source." He hypothesized that some water had a noxious substance in it that caused goiter. He thought that drinking rain water, therefore, would prevent goiter. He also noted the presence of many cretins who were seen by the local population as special people and were accorded a protected status. One of the cretins stabbed him, fortunately not seriously.

Although Boussingault taught at the school of mines between 1823 and 1824, he did not start right away. He was just assigned to survey mining sites, particularly for gold and other precious metals (platinum, incidentally, was thought to be a nuisance because it interfered with the extraction of gold and was generally thrown away once separated).

It is not known whether or not Boussingault knew of the work of the Swiss physician Jean François Coindet. Coindet showed that endemic goiter could be treated with iodine. Boussingault connected the absence of goiter in the cordilleran mines with the possibility that the mine water and the salt made from it might contain iodine. He used his expertise with mineral assays to see whether the salt preparations had iodine. He used the standard assay at the time which depended on the ability of iodine to turn a starch solution blue. His results were clear. The salt from the mines did not have detectable iodine, but the oily material present after the salt crystallized did contain iodine [3]. He went beyond Coindet's conclusion that iodine was a treatment for goiter to conclude that iodine in the drinking water, or in iodized salt, could prevent goiter from forming in the first place. Boussingault's conclusion was not novel because the local inhabitants had been using this salt and the oil to prevent goiter for at least 100 years. His conclusion that the prevention of goiter was related to iodine, however, was original.

Boussingault finished his term as professor in 1826–1827 but did not renew it. He signed on to work for the Colombian Mining Company which had, as its main interest, the finding and working of former Incan gold mines. He spent most of his time doing what he did while a professor: inspecting mines, traveling, and making a series of scientific observations. Before returning to France in 1832 he attempted to climb seven of the highest Andean mountains. One of these, Chimborazo, was considered, at that time, to be the highest mountain in the world. He did not reach Chimborazo's peak, although he might have reached the highest altitude of any European climber to that date.

In 1832, after 10 years in South America, Boussingault went home to France. Roulin had returned to Paris in 1828. In 1835, Roulin developed the "Minutes of the Académie des sciences" into the *Comptes Rendus*, which remains to this day the record of the Académie's weekly proceedings. Boussingault authored 33 papers in South America. Included were papers on geology, chemistry, medicine, and climatology.

Two of these papers, one published in 1831 and the other in 1833, describe his remaining work on iodine in South America. In these two papers [4, 5] he discussed more details about iodine as a preventive for goiter. In the first, he notes that "the reason why goiter does not occur in Antioquia is because all the inhabitants of this province take iodine every day with the salt that they consume." He also thought that "goiter would certainly disappear from the Cordilleras if the authorities would establish in each town a depot of iodine-containing salt. In New Granada this question was very important because goiter not only disfigured people but exerted a deadly effect on their intellectual faculties." He pursued the topic in his paper of 1833 in which he distinguished between the use of iodine itself, which could lead to "very serious accidents," and the "iodized salt, used as seasoning on food, which is always followed by happy results." Curiously, he never made the connection that iodine deficiency caused goiter and cretinism. That iodine prevented these disorders did not mean, in his time, that iodine intake was deficient, however obvious it might seem to us. The concept that a dietary deficiency could cause a disease did not exist. Boussingault's best idea, by his own reckoning, was that goiter was caused by drinking water that did not have enough air in it.

His recommendations about the use of iodized salt were not followed in Colombia. Generations passed before a more aggressive approach in the twentieth century met with some success in eliminating goiter and cretinism.

When Boussingault returned to France in 1832, he wanted a connection to the French center of science in Paris. He obtained a professorship in chemistry at Lyon but stayed there only a short time. In 1835, after visiting old friends in Alsace, he married Adèle LeBel, the daughter of the proprietor of the Bechelbronn farm. He first met Adèle when she was 6 years old when he was working in the lignite mine in Alsace. The marriage gave Boussingault access to the farm and a laboratory to study chemical and physical problems related to farming. He spent the rest of his career in this field. He is thought to have established the first agricultural experiment station. He showed that plants grow best with a mixture of nitrogen and phosphate fertilizers. He originated modern metabolic balance studies. Many of these studies were published in book form and translated later into English [6].

He was appointed to the faculty at the Sorbonne in 1837. Two years later he was elected to the Académie des sciences in the field of rural economy. The following year he became one of the editors of the *Annales de Chimie et de Physique*, the journal in which he had published most of his South American work. Finally, in 1845, he received a Parisian professorship as the professor of agriculture at the Conservatoire des Arts et Métiers. This was not an appointment of the highest status, but it was high enough. It enabled Boussingault to spend considerable time in Paris. He kept his professorship until the end of his life, but lost the Bechelbronn farm during the Franco-Prussian War of 1870. He moved to Saint-Etienne, where he had trained 50 years before, to work with an old colleague at a steel mill. For a few years he returned to the metallurgy that had started his career.

In 1851, after he had been elected to the Académie des sciences, he was appointed to one of the Académie's committees to evaluate a report by Jules Grange. Grange had eliminated most of the proposed causes of goiter with an application of geographic medicine, and concluded that goiter had something to do with a change in the character of the soil and that goiter was basically caused by too much magnesium in the diet. The committee's response was to adopt Grange's hypothesis and encourage him to continue his studies. Boussingault's committee thought that the best way to prevent goiter would be to change the drinking water. If this were not practical, then people should be given slightly iodinated salt. There was still no disagreement, 20 years after Boussingault's return to France, that magnesium could cause goiter. Boussingault now mentions that, in 1835, 3 years after he had left the South American government of New Granada, iodized salt was distributed to the population in goitrous areas and that "this trial was followed by an incontestable success." To our knowledge, the success was never written up, published, or emulated. The committee made no comment on the lack of follow-up but encouraged Grange to pursue these trials [7].

Science and the advancement of knowledge are quirky beasts indeed. Even when knowledge is gained, it is open to interpretations that are colored by the fixed ideas of the time and the lessons supposedly learned might need to be learned again.

References

1. Aulie RP: Boussingault, Jean Baptiste Joseph Dieudonné. *Dictionary of Scientific Biography* 1970; 2: 356.
2. *Encyclopedia Britannica* (11th edn.) 1910; 4: 334.
3. Boussingault JB: Sur l'existence de l'iode dans l'eau d'une saline de la province d'Antioquia. *Ann Chim Phys* 1825; 30: 91.
4. Boussingault JB: Recherches sur la cause qui produit le goıtre dans les cordilières de la Nouvelle-Grenade. *Ann Chim Phys* 1831; 48: 41.
5. Boussingault JB: Mémoire sur les salines iodifères des Andes. *Ann Chim Phys* 833; 54: 163.
6. Boussingault JB: *Rural Economy in Its Relations With Chemistry, Physics, and Meteorology: or, An Application of the Principles of Chemistry and Physiology to the Details of Practical Farming* (2nd edn.). London: H. Ballière, 1845.
7. Dumas JB, Boussingault JB, de Beaumont LE: Rapport sur les recherches de M. le Dr. Grange, relatives aux causes du crétinisme et du goıtre, et aux moyens d'en préserver les populations. *CR hebd Seanc Acad Sci* 1851; 32: 611.

This chapter has been reproduced from Sawin, Clark T: Historical Note: Jean Baptiste Boussingault (1802–1887) and the discovery (almost) of iodine prophylaxis of goiter. *The Endocrinologist* 2003; 13(4): 305–8.

CHAPTER 34

Bernhard Naunyn (1839–1925)

Dietary Treatment of Diabetes

Bernhard Naunyn is one of the giants in the history of medical science. He worked successfully in many clinical areas including the pathophysiology of gallstone disease, hepatogenic icterus, aphasia, the clinical course of mitral insufficiency, the mechanisms of fever, the relationship between blood flow and CSF pressure, epilepsy, syphilis, and the clinical categorization of transudates and exudates. He is best remembered, however, as the guiding force in developing the first clear understanding of the pathophysiology of diabetes mellitus type 1, and in developing the first successful treatments for it.

Among the many books written by Naunyn is this gem: *Erinnerungen, Gedanken, and Meinungen* (Memories, Thoughts, and Convictions) [1]. It is an autobiography of sorts, and gives us a first-hand view of his work and his time. We can follow Naunyn's life in his own words. He was born in Berlin on Sunday, September 2, 1839:

> I understand I was often ill in my early years and it was said that I had the "onset of water on the brain." Thus, it was only at the age of 4 that I learnt to speak distinctly; I was one of those children whose initial vocabulary happens to be particularly rich in self-created words of completely puzzling etymology [2, p. 12].
>
> Both my father and my mother were of old East-Prussian descent. This name appears as early as 1360 when a Noynyn, who had property near Bartenstein, sold a field to the city of Bartenstein [2, p. 14].
>
> My mother was a quiet woman who seemed quite shy; she had a very kind heart and immense goodwill. Her self-assuredness and total unpretentiousness enabled her to rise splendidly to any occasion, but she preferred to remain in the background; she had a strong streak of middle class pride. The relationship between my parents was exemplary. An austere outlook on life enveloped us: firm middle class morality [2, p. 19].
>
> My father, since he had worked his way up by his own efforts, being somewhat pedantic and very serious, and having a tendency to moral hypochondria, made great demands on us and made our school days very difficult. He was stern but not harsh, at least not with me as the second son. He never hit me. It must be pointed out about father that he was not really a stimulating influence on his sons. He was skilled in everything, had good refined tastes, but had

A Biographical History of Endocrinology, First Edition. D. Lynn Loriaux.

This work is a co-publication between the Endocrine Society and John Wiley & Sons, Ltd.

himself as a child lacked a stimulating influence. Above all, he was the admonishing teacher and far too much our reproving conscience for him to have been able to give direction to our lives. In spite of all this, my memory of my parental home is not a very happy one. This still weighs on me [2, p. 18].

My father called me sullen. According to modern psychiatry, I was a cyclothyme, one of those who are periodically weighed down by attacks of depression. Perhaps these depressive notions have gained the upper hand and muddled my memories [2, p. 21].

Naunyn's early education was typically European; rigorous, steeped in the classics, languages, and literature. He decided to become a doctor.

It was a good thing that my decision to become a doctor held firm; I knew that I had to study medicine. My father let me do so, but unhappily. He had decided that I was to become a government official, but I stayed with medicine. I cannot explain how I arrived at this decision. It was partly due to the notion that a doctor's job was an independent one as well as one dedicated to the good of his fellow men; the great esteem that our family doctor had received from us also played no small role [2, p. 38].

Naunyn's medical studies were tedious, he even thought of switching to forestry, but things fell into place with his first clinical rotation.

The very first hour under Frerichs appealed to me. He introduced a young man who suffered from gastrorrhagia, a simple case of peptic ulcer (*Ulcus simplex*). What Frerichs then explained about gastrorrhagia due to various causes was excellent: the manner in which he demonstrated the case, the vividness of his presentation, his clear, concise diction, the serious and austere solemnity of his delivery, his objectivity and his refusal to allow it to be distracted by secondary considerations impressed me so much that I became an enthusiast. I feel today that it is from the time of this first class with Frerichs that I began to see my goal. Soon thereafter, I realized that my life belonged to internal medicine, and I have never since been unfaithful to my banner, not once even in my thoughts [2, p. 53].

Thus, the power of an effective teacher early in one's educational experience.

To cement his commitment, he became interested in the ontology of echinococcal infections, and began his first scientific studies.

I truly had very little time, for I had occupied myself with the echinococcus since the beginning of the seventh semester. The early morning found me at the microscope, before I went on duty at the clinic, and when I came back in the afternoon, I sat at the microscope again, preferring to sit there well into the night, I had early learned microscopy even by lamp light. I found the cilia on the inner surface of the echinococcal membrane – which no mortal eye seems to have seen since [I saw it] with my small Schiekschen microscope by dim lamp light [2, p. 54].

Following medical school was a 6-year period of apprenticeship. He was most fortunate in his mentor, the great Frerichs whose patient presentation had led Naunyn to internal medicine in the first instance.

The apprenticeship with Frerichs led to Naunyn's first academic appointment, Dorpat, in Russia, followed by appointments in Bern, Konigsberg, and Strassburg over a period of 35 years. In these years, Naunyn contributed in a substantive way to disease entities that stretch across the breadth of internal medicine, from neurology to endocrinology, and a professional association with some of the greatest academics of the nineteenth century – Müller, Quincke, Trendelenburg, Romberg, Cohnheim, Billroth, Kussmaul, Recklinghausen, Hoppe-Seyler, Ludwig, Madelung, Traube, Virchow, and so on.

Naunyn's greatest contribution, however, was the intellectual driving force for the emerging understanding of the pathophysiology of juvenile diabetes mellitus. Naunyn's early work focused on the origin of glucose in the disease. He demonstrated that glucose could be derived from protein (gluconeogenesis) and that control of plasma glucose levels in diabetic children required dietary limitations on both carbohydrates and protein.

He pushed the diets of diabetic children to the point of "near starvation" to control glycosuria and hyperglycemia. This concept was the foundation for F.M. Allen's studies of dietary therapy for diabetes, and led to the more famous "Joslin diet" which was shown by Elliott Joslin to extend life in diabetic children.

Naunyn's student, Dieter Hallervorden (of the Hallervorden–Spatz syndrome) recognized that urinary ammonia excretion was elevated in severe diabetes. He reasoned that it was associated with increased acid excretion, and Stadelmann soon recovered large amounts of a volatile acid from diabetic urine, crotonic acid, that Minkowski showed to be derived from hydroxybutyric acid: diabetic keto-acidosis [3]. This was the same Minkowski who, with Von Meering, produced diabetes mellitus in dogs by pancreatectomy, the experiment that led directly to the triumph of Banting and Best who isolated insulin for the first time and paved the way for the first truly life-saving treatment of this disease.

Naunyn codified all of this in two books, *Die Diatische Behandlung des Diabetes Mellitus*, describing the dietary treatment of diabetes in 1889, and the now classic text, *Der Diabetes*, in 1898 [4]. These books brought focus to the field and propelled a generation of translational research.

One final note: while Naunyn was Rector of Konigsberg University in the 1880s, the statutes of a new student body were brought to him for approval. The statute explicitly denied membership to Jews. He refused to approve. The issue was taken "up" to the University Senate where the statutes were approved in spite of Naunyn's objection. Some things never change, but the event does tell us something important about the man.

References

1. Naunyn B: *Erinnerungen, Gedanken, and Meinungen*. Munich: J.S. Bergmann, 1925.
2. Naunyn B: *Memories, Thoughts, and Convictions*, edited by DL Cowen. Canton, MA: Watson Publishing, 1994.
3. Woodyatt RT: Bernhard Naunyn. *Diabetes* 1952; 1: 240–1.
4. Naunyn B: *Der Diabetes Mellitus*. Vienna: Alfred Holler, 1906.

This chapter has been reproduced from Loriaux, D. Lynn: Bernhard Naunyn (1839–1925). *The Endocrinologist* 2006; 16(5): 239–40.

CHAPTER 35
Enrico Sertoli (1842–1910)
Gametes and the Testes

Sertoli was born June 6, 1842 in the small town of Sondrio, north of Milan on the Swiss border. He studied medicine at the University of Pavia, graduating in 1865. After graduation he studied with Ernst Wilhelm von Brücke in Vienna, and with Felix Hoppe-Seyler in Tübingen. From 1870 until 1907, Sertoli was at the Royal School of Veterinary Medicine in Milan as professor of anatomy and physiology. He purchased his first microscope in 1862 and began his research under the direction of Professor Eusebio Oehl.

Sertoli began his studies with human testis specimens preserved in ammonia and mercuric chloride. His studies included microdissections of individual seminiferous tubules, thin sections of testis, and frayed sections of tubules. As was the custom, he drew what he saw in the microscopic field. He described the cell that carries his name as a cell with many branches with "blobs" at the ends. About this time, Sertoli became aware of the stain extracted from logwood (*Haematoxylum campechianum*) collected in Central America. Waldeyer was the first to propose that this dye could be used to stain histological sections. Sertoli used the stain in his first descriptions of the Sertoli cell. He drew the cell as a multinucleated syncytium. He concluded that the cells were protecting or embracing the germ cells.

> IV. Finally, some special cells, which I saw in moderate number in the preparations and which, to my knowledge, have not previously been observed and described by anyone. They appear in the form of irregularly cylindrical or conical cells, with indistinct margins, provided with a nucleus always containing a nucleolus. Their contents comprise fine droplets of fat in a substance that is reasonably transparent because it is homogenous. These cells almost always have quite transparent extensions, in the interior of which fine droplets of fat can frequently be seen. They have an irregularly shaped body from which often protrude one or more extensions, and two extremities of which the upper is usually large and bounded by well-marked margin that sometimes appears double . Lower down the cell often is contracted somewhat, formed like a sort of collar. The other luminal extremity becomes narrower and forms an extension which often ends abruptly in a rounded tip with delicate outlines. Often the tip is torn and it is not possible to determine how it ends normally. I have observed that other cells bifurcate and send out secondary extensions [1].

A Biographical History of Endocrinology, First Edition. D. Lynn Loriaux.

This work is a co-publication between the Endocrine Society and John Wiley & Sons, Ltd.

In the last figure of Sertoli's manuscript he showed germ cells and spermatozoa associated with the Sertoli cell. He concluded that the Sertoli cells were the "mother," or the sustentacular cells of the seminiferous tubule.

This was his first paper [2]. Subsequent papers described the germ cells, spermatogonia, spermatids, spermatozoa, the spermatogenic wave, and the cytoplasmic bridge between Sertoli cells. He showed that Sertoli cells do not divide. His work led directly to the discovery of the blood–testis barrier, and the endocrine nature of the Sertoli cell, including the elaboration and secretion of inhibin and activin.

Sertoli retired in 1907.

> He returned to his hometown of Sondrio, due to an illness, and there he lived until his death on January 28, 1910. Sertoli never married and devoted his adult life to teaching and his research [3].

References

1. Setchell BP: Male reproduction. In *Benchmark Papers in Human Physiology Series*, edited by LL Langley. New York: Van Nostrand Reinhold, 1984, pp. 10–20.
2. Sertoli E: Dell' esistenza do particolari cellue ramificate vie canalicoli seminifers del testicolo uinano. *Morgagni* 1865; 7: 31–40.
3. Hess RA, Franca L: History of the Sertoli cell discovery. In *Sertoli Cell Biology*, edited by MK Skinner and MD Griswald. San Diego, CA: Elsevier Academic Press, 2005, p. 10.

This chapter has been reproduced from Loriaux, D. Lynn: Enrico Sertoli: 1842–1910. *The Endocrinologist* 2009; 19(6): 249.

CHAPTER 36
William Osler
(1849–1919)
Treatment of Addison's Disease

William Osler, the eighth of nine children of Featherstone Lake Osler and Ellen Free Picton Osler, was born on the Canadian frontier in Bond Head Parsonage, Tecumseh, Upper Canada. The place is near Lake Simcoe, between Lakes Ontario and Huron. Featherstone Osler came from a Cornwall family steeped in the traditions of the sea. He began a promising career in the Royal Navy, but abandoned it to be with his father in his declining years. He studied for holy orders and, with ordination, took his new bride to the Canadian wilderness. Service, kindness, faith, and works were his watchwords. The tradition would be handed down in full measure to his children.

William was a bright and willful child. In grammar school he led a group of boys in bad behavior and, finally, was expelled because of it. He was sent to a boarding school in Barrie, and became the leader of "Barrie's Bad Boys." He was moved to a stricter environment at Weston's School, where liberal "caning" by an austere headmaster was to be expected. When the head matron emptied a bucket of kitchen waste over one of his friends, Osler devised a revenge that led to a short stay in jail. He concocted a mixture of molasses, pepper, and mustard, and put it on the stove beneath the floor grate of the head matron's room. The smoke was stifling. When she tried to close the opening over the stove, the boys pulled the rags away and fanned the conflagration on. The woman was finally rescued by the headmaster. She filed charges of battery and the young Osler and his companions were jailed for 3 days [1].

This seems to have been the extremity of Osler's youthful indiscretion. When we read of him thereafter, he is a model student. It was about this time that Osler came under the spell of Father Johnson and Dr. Bovell. These two faculty men, one a theologian and the other a biologist, shared a passionate interest in natural history. Their view of the world, based upon objective scientific study leavened with humanism and theologic philosophy, found fertile ground in Osler. It was Bovell who introduced Osler to the world of books and, under his tutelage, Osler made his first purchase: the *Globe Shakespeare*. His second was the 1862 edition of Sir Thomas Browne's *Religio Medici*. That book became his *compagnon de voyage* and was buried with him 52 years later.

A Biographical History of Endocrinology, First Edition. D. Lynn Loriaux.

This work is a co-publication between the Endocrine Society and John Wiley & Sons, Ltd.

Osler intended to follow his father into the ministry. He went to Trinity College in Toronto and applied himself to this goal. After the first few days of the second year, however, he decided upon medicine. Dr. Bovell was delighted and enrolled him in the medical school in Toronto. Of this turning point, Osler says,

> In my school days I was more bent upon mischief than upon books. I say it with regret now but as soon as I got interested in Medicine I had only a single idea and I do believe that if I have had any measure of success at all, it has been solely because of doing the day's work that was before me just as faithfully and honestly and energetically as I could [2, Vol. 1, p. 81].

Dr. Bovell came to believe that it would be in Osler's best interest to transfer to the "better" medical school in Montreal. When Bovell mysteriously moved to the West Indies in 1870, Osler was freed of his last "medical" connections with Toronto and he left for McGill Medical School. He took with him a philosophical structure, a love of books, and a sense of direction that would energize and sustain him for the rest of his life.

McGill provided Osler's next mentor in the person of Robert Palmer Howard. Dr. Howard guided the formative years of Osler's professional development. Osler was not a gold medalist at McGill, but the faculty awarded him a special prize for his thesis "greatly distinguished for original research." Dr. Howard advised a period of study in Europe, and the winter of 1872 found Osler working in the physiology laboratory of John Burdon-Sanderson at the University College Hospital, London. This is the same Burdon-Sanderson that Osler would follow as Regius Professor of Medicine 34 years later. Osler's most important scientific contribution was made in that year. He had developed an expertise on the morphology of the formed elements of blood as a result of his interest in blood-borne parasites. This paved the way for his discovery of the platelets, previously described only in fixed preparations, never before seen in circulating blood. Burdon-Sanderson presented Osler's findings to the Royal Society and Osler presented them to the Royal Microscopical Society. An academic appointment at McGill was thus secured and he returned as lecturer in 1874. Rising rapidly through the ranks, he was appointed Physician to Montreal General Hospital in 1878.

S. Weir Mitchell was instrumental in moving Osler to Philadelphia in 1884. Osler stayed at the University of Pennsylvania for 4 years as professor of clinical medicine before moving to Baltimore and the Johns Hopkins Hospital. Johns Hopkins, on his death, left seven million dollars for a university and for a hospital to relieve suffering. Daniel Coit Gilman, brought from California, was installed as President of the university and John Shaw Billings was appointed medical advisor to the hospital. The university opened its doors in 1876, but the hospital was long delayed. Gilman developed the staff along department lines, each department with a chief. Welch was named head of Pathology in 1883; Osler as chief of the Medical Department in 1888.

Osler proceeded to create what Welch called "the first medical clinic in any English speaking country worthy of the name." The clinic was built along Teutonic lines, a system that had placed German medicine foremost in the world. Osler said that, "If I have done anything to promote the growth of clinical medicine, it has been in this direction, in the formation of a large clinic with well-organized series of assistants and house physicians and with proper laboratories in which to work at the intricate problems that confront us in internal medicine." To the German method he added the English system of clinical clerkships and thereby created the American system as we know it today. The nascent staff of the Johns Hopkins Hospital were young. Osler was the oldest at 40. Welch was 39, Halsted 37, and Kelly 31. They created a system of medical education that, for the first time in America, permitted medical students to have formal clinic rotations and "postdoctoral" resident physicians the opportunity for ongoing clinical training, analogous in concept to that provided for post-doctoral fellows in the preclinical sciences.

Although the hospital was functioning efficiently, it would be 5 more years before the medical school officially opened its doors. This relieved Osler of the greater part of his teaching burden and, in this hiatus, he wrote one of the great textbooks of internal medicine.

> On several occasions in Philadelphia I was asked by Lee Brothers to prepare a work on Diagnoses and half promised one. Indeed, I had prepared a couple of chapters but continually procrastinated on the plea that up to the fortieth year a man was fit for better things than textbooks. Time went on and as I crossed this date I began to feel that the energy and persistence necessary for the task were lacking. In September 1890 I returned from a four months trip to Europe, shook myself, and towards the end of the month began a work on practice. I had nearly finished the chapter on Typhoid Fever when Dr. Granger, Messrs. Appleton's agent, came from New York to ask me to prepare a text-book on Medicine. We haggled for a few weeks about terms and finally, selling my brains to the devil, I signed the contract. My intention had been to publish the book myself and have Lippincott or Blakiston (both of whom offered) handle the book, but the bait of a guaranteed circulation of 10,000 copies in two years and $1500 on the date of publication was too glittering and I was hooked. October, November, December were not very satisfactory months and January first 1891, saw the Infectious Diseases scarcely completed. I then got well into harness. Three mornings of each week I stayed at home and dictated from 8 A.M. to 1 P.M. On the alternate days I dictated after the morning Hospital visit, beginning about 11:30 A.M. The spare hours of the afternoon were devoted to reference work. Early in May I gave up the house at 209 West Monument Street and went to my rooms at the Hospital. The routine there was: 8 A.M. to 1 P.M. dictation. 2 P.M. visits to the private patients and special cases in the wards, after which revision, etc. After 5 P.M. I saw my outside cases; dinner at the club about 6:30. Loafed until 9:30; bed at 10:00. Up at 7 A.M. I had arranged to send manuscripts by the first of July and on that date I forwarded five sections but the publishers did not begin to print until the middle of August. The first two weeks of August I spent in Toronto and then, with the same routine, I practically finished the manuscript by about October the 15th. During the summer the entire manuscript was carefully revised for the press by Mr. Powell of the English Department at the University. The last three months of 1891 were devoted to proof reading. In January I made out the Index, and in the entire work nothing so wearied me as the verifying of every reference. Without the help of Lafleur and Thayer, who took the ward work off my hands, I never could have finished in so short a time. My other assistants also rendered much aid in looking up references and special points. During the writing of the work I lost only one afternoon through transient indisposition and never a night's rest. Between September 1890 and January 1892, I gained nearly eight pounds in weight [2, Vol. 1, p. 339–45, 3].

Thus, in 16 months of diligent application, the medical text of its age was written. Over 23 500 copies were sold in the first edition, giving Osler unexpected lifelong financial security. The constant revisions for new editions proved a burden, and Thomas McCrae became a co-editor with the eighth edition. With Osler's death in 1919, McCrae assumed full control of the ninth through the twelfth editions. The mantle passed then to Henry Christian at Harvard. He maintained the single author tradition and carried the book through the sixteenth and final edition. It was a run of 55 years; publication ceased in 1947. As Osler observed, "even great textbooks die like their authors."

Following the death of Osler's close friend Samuel Gross in 1888, Osler married his widow, the former Grace Revere Linzee of Boston, on Saturday, May 7, 1892. Harvey Cushing said that with this marriage, Osler's phenomenal luck reached its apogee. A son, Revere, was born December 28, 1895.

Osler became the Regius Professor of Medicine at Oxford in 1905. The First World War brought the death of his son, Revere, on a battlefield in France. Osler was haunted by the fact that Revere was initially rejected from military service because of bad eyesight. Only his father's intercession with "the authorities" allowed him to get into uniform and across the channel to France and an artillery emplacement.

> A grieving Osler was stricken with influenza in the great pandemic. A pneumonia followed by empyema proved fatal. Near the end of his illness, too weak to read to himself, family and friends took turns reading selections from his favorite books, from Walter Pater's "Marius"; the Peach Blossom and Wine chapter in Gaston de Latour; from Andrew Lang; from his beloved Plato; Matthew Arnold's "On Translating Homer"; Sir Thomas Browne, of course; and from Bridge's anthology, "The Spirit of Man", the things which Revere particularly liked. One night he asked for something from the "Jungle Books", and after Malloch had read "The King's Ankus" and had sat quietly in the darkened room thinking his listener was asleep, came a whispered voice saying: "He was a fine boy" [2, Vol. 2, p. 684].

The end came quietly following a hemorrhage from a thoracentesis wound at 4:30 in the afternoon of December 29, 1919.

What has all of this to do with endocrinology? Osler was one of the first to treat Addison's disease with glycerin extract of pig adrenal gland, sometimes successfully, and sometimes not [4, 5]. The point, however, is a larger one. American medicine is created in Osler's image. Hippocrates said, "I will honor as my father the man who teaches me the Art." We owe that to Osler. He is remembered as the foremost clinician of his day and the architect of the American system of medical education. More importantly, he is remembered as the complete physician, saintly in his generosity and compassion. The following anecdote reveals all.

> He visited our little Janet twice every day from the middle of October until her death a month later, and these visits she looked forward to with a pathetic eagerness and joy. There would be a little tap low down on the door which would be pushed open and a crouching figure playing goblin would come in, and in a high pitched voice would ask if the fairy godmother was at home and could he have a bit of tea. Instantly the sick room was turned into a fairyland, and in a fairy language he would talk about the flowers, the birds, and the dolls who sat at the foot of the bed who were always greeted with "Well, all ye loves!" In the course of this he would manage to find out all he needed to know about the little patient.

The most exquisite moment came one cold, raw November morning when the end was near, and he mysteriously brought out from his inside pocket a beautiful red rose carefully wrapped in paper, and told how he had watched the last rose of summer growing in his garden and how the rose had called out to him as he passed by, that she wished to go along with him to see his little lassie. That evening we all had a fairy tea party at a tiny tea table by the bed. Sir William talking to the rose, his little lassie, and her mother in the most exquisite way; and presently he slipped out of the room just as mysteriously as he had entered it, all crouched down on his heels; and the little girl understood that neither the fairies nor people could always have the color of a red rose in their cheeks, or stay as long as they wanted in one place, but that they nevertheless would be very happy in another home and must not let the people they left behind, particularly their parents, feel badly about it; and the little girl understood and was not unhappy [6].

References

1. Burrow, G: The trial and tribulation of Egerton Yorick Davis. *West J Med* 1991: 80–2.
2. Cushing, H: *Sir William Osler*. Oxford: Clarendon Press, 1926.
3. Bliss, M: *A Life in Medicine: William Osler*. Oxford: Oxford University Press, 1999, p. 183.
4. Osler, W: On six cases of Addison's disease, with the report of a case greatly benefitted by the use of suprarenal extract. *Int Med Magazine* 1896; 5: 3.
5. Osler, W: Case of Addison's disease–death during treatment with the suprarenal extract. *Johns Hopkins Bull* 1896; 7: 208–9.
6. Reid, Edith Gittings: *The Great Physician: A Short Life of Sir William Osler*. New York: Oxford University Press, 1931.

This chapter has been reproduced from Loriaux, DL: William Osler (1849–1919) and the treatment of Addison's disease. *The Endocrinologist* 2004; 14(2): 51–3.

CHAPTER 37

Emil Fischer

(1852–1919)

The Stereochemical Nature of Sugars

Emil Fischer made pioneering insights into the stereochemistry of the simple sugars, using the analogy of a lock-and-key fit between an enzyme and its substrate. He discovered that proteins are polypeptides. He characterized and synthesized caffeine and theobromine, and made landmark contributions regarding purines. He was awarded the Nobel Prize in Chemistry in 1902, and his work influences every endocrinologist to this day.

Hermann Emil Fischer was born near Cologne, Germany on October 9, 1852 [1]. His father ran a prosperous lumber business, and it was Emil's good fortune throughout his life to have substantial financial resources as a result of that family enterprise. He loved physics, but a mentor at the University of Bonn, Adolf von Baeyer, who had worked with August Kekulé of the benzene ring, advised Fischer to study chemistry. Von Baeyer won the Nobel Prize in Chemistry in 1905, three years after Fischer.

After receiving his PhD in 1874, Fischer became an assistant instructor at Strasbourg University, where he worked out the structure of phenylhydrazine, the first hydrazine base. This discovery would influence his later work because phenylhydrazine became the first useful tool for analyzing sugars. Von Baeyer was invited to move to the University of Munich in 1875, and Fischer followed him there. Fischer rose to the rank of associate professor of analytical chemistry in 1879, and was appointed professor of chemistry in 1881 at the University of Erlangen.

He was approached in 1883 to take the position of scientific director at a private firm, Badische Anilin-und Soda-Fabrik, BASF. Although Fischer was tempted, he loved academic research, and the family money gave him the freedom to turn down the offer.

In 1887, Fischer experienced a bout of severe gastritis and took a one-year leave of absence before moving to the University of Würzburg. After four productive years as professor of chemistry there, he made his final academic move to the University of Berlin in 1892. There he succeeded A.W. Hoffmann as the Chair of Chemistry, and he retained that Chair until his death in 1919.

Jean-Baptiste Biot demonstrated, in 1815, that some chemicals in solution rotated the plane of a polarized light. Louis Pasteur [2], pursuing his first important experiments

---

A Biographical History of Endocrinology, First Edition. D. Lynn Loriaux.

in the late 1840s, noted that the tiny crystals of tartaric acid in French wine came in two varieties. Using a magnifying glass, Pasteur observed that the two crystal types appeared to be mirror images of each other. He used tweezers to separate the two types and found that, when dissolved in an aqueous solution, one type of crystal rotated polarized light to the right and the other to the left. Years later, Fischer mentioned Pasteur's experiments in his Nobel Prize lecture [3].

Jacobus H. van 't Hoff and J.A. Le Bel independently developed the concept of the asymmetric carbon atom in the early 1870s [4]. Although his doctoral thesis in 1874 dealt with cyanoacetic and malonic acid, van 't Hoff's early fame actually derived from a small pamphlet that he published a few months before entitled "Voorstel tot Uitbreiding der Tegenwoordige in de Scheikunde gebruikte Structuurformules in de Ruimte" (Proposal for the development of 3-dimensional chemical structural formulae). Consisting of 12 pages of text and 1 page of diagrams, the paper showed that the asymmetric carbon atom could explain the occurrence of isomers of compounds despite their identical chemical formulae. Van 't Hoff also explained how such stereochemistry could be related to optical activity. The first publication about the asymmetric carbon atom occurred just as Fischer was finishing his doctorate. The assignment as a D- or L-sugar began based on whether the plane of polarized light was rotated to the right or left (dextrorotatory or levorotatory). Today, optical isomers of monosaccharides are assigned as either D- or L- based on their absolute configurations as relative to D-glyceraldehyde, as proposed by Rosanoff, an American chemist, in 1906 [5].

The structural formula for an aldohexose (such as glucose) contains four asymmetric carbon atoms, each marked by an asterisk. Thus, there are 16 possible stereoisomers having this general formula; eight pairs of enantiomers, as we would say today. This is the family of aldohexoses. All 16 compounds have been created by synthesis or isolated from nature, and include the very common compounds glucose, mannose, and galactose, each with a D- and an L- form.

The way that Fischer worked out the correct configurations of the aldohexoses demanded years of trial and error, ingenuity, and logic. While working at the University of Munich in the early 1880s, Fischer found that phenylhydrazine converted sugars into osazones whose crystals had characteristic forms that could be identified. Fischer found that two distinct monosaccharides, D-glucose and D-mannose, yielded the same osazone. Because osazone formation destroyed asymmetry about carbon 2 without changing the configuration of the rest of the molecule, it followed logically that D-glucose and D-mannose were identical except that they had configurations around carbon 2 that were mirror images. Today we call D-glucose and D-mannose epimers. Fischer knew that D-glucose, the most important monosaccharide, was an aldohexose, and in 1888 he set out to learn which of the 16 possible configurations of $C_6H_{12}O_6$ was the correct formula for naturally occurring glucose.

Fischer published his formula in 1891 while at the University of Würzburg, and this triumph was primarily responsible for his award of the Nobel Prize in Chemistry in 1902 [6]. During his Nobel Lecture, delivered on December 12, 1902, he showed the 16 formulae of the aldohexoses, of which only 12 had actually been synthesized or isolated from nature.

During the early twentieth century, Fischer turned his attention to identifying the individual amino acids and was the discoverer of proline. He coined the term "peptide bond." He synthesized short peptides. He studied enzymes and fats. In 1902, at the meeting of the Society of German Scientists and Physicians in Karlsbad, Fischer followed the eminent chemist Franz Hofmeister on the program. Hofmeister presented a plenary lecture about the possible structure of proteins, and Fischer spoke about the isolation of amino acids from protein hydrolysates and suggested that proteins were made from amino acids linked together. Thus was born the Fischer–Hofmeister theory of protein structure.

A brilliant and patient man, Fischer is said to have had a keen memory but was not a great speaker. In 1888, he married Agnes Gerlach, who was the daughter of the anatomy professor at Erlangen. Although she died in the seventh year of their marriage, they had three sons. One son was killed in the First World War, and another took his own life at age 25 while distraught over compulsory military service. A third son, Hermann Otto Laurenz Fischer, eventually became a professor of biochemistry at the University of California at Berkeley. Shortly after the First World War, his health failed, possibly as a result of chronic exposure to chemical solvents. Amid the shambles of postwar Germany, these problems overwhelmed him and it is believed that he took his own life in 1919 [7].

Shortly after Fischer's death, the German Chemical Society established the Emil Fischer Memorial Medal, viewed as a prestigious scientific award. The field of carbohydrate chemistry moved onward. In the 1890s, Fischer himself provided evidence that glucose actually was a cyclic structure, and Tollens, Tanret, and many others contributed to this concept. In 1909, C.S. Hudson of the U.S. Public Health Service made proposals about nomenclature that were widely accepted, and the enantiomer of alpha-D-[+]-glucose became alpha-L-[−]-glucose. He discovered the structure and the way to measure the compound in biological fluids. This was one of the major hurdles along the way to understanding the disease of diabetes mellitus.

References

1. Adolf von Baeyer–Biography (official web site of the Nobel Foundation). June 23, 2003.
2. Geison GL. *The Private Science of Louis Pasteur*. Princeton, NJ: Princeton University Press, 1995.
3. Emil Fischer–Nobel Lecture (official web site of the Nobel Foundation). April 7, 2004.
4. Jacobus H. van 't Hoff–Biography (official web site of the Nobel Foundation). April 15, 2004.
5. Morrison RT, Boyd RN (Eds.): *Organic Chemistry* (2nd edn.). Boston, MA: Allyn and Bacon, 1969.
6. McBride JM: Emil Fischer: On the configuration of grape sugar and its isomers. *Berichte d d chem Gesellsch* 1891; 24: 1836.
7. Reynolds R, Tanford C. Enzyme action. Emil Hermann Fischer 1852–1919. In *The Science Book*, edited by P Tallack. London: Weidenfeld & Nicolson, 2003, pp. 218–19.

This chapter has been reproduced from Magner, James A: Emil Fischer (1852–1919): The stereochemical nature of sugars. *The Endocrinologist* 2004; 14(5): 239–44.

CHAPTER 38

William Stewart Halsted (1852–1922)

Surgery of the Thyroid Gland

William Stewart Halsted was arguably the best known surgeon in the United States in the first decades of the twentieth century. Yet, in today's medical environment, he would likely have been dismissed from his professorship at the Johns Hopkins Medical School and Hospital, labeled as an "impaired physician." He was addicted to cocaine, a problem which lasted most of his professional life, and to morphine, which he was given initially in an attempt to cure him of the cocaine addiction. Halsted was one of several surgeons who worked out the details of thyroidectomy to make the procedure, then associated with what today would be considered completely unacceptable mortality and complication rates, a safe operation.

Halsted was born in New York City, the son of a wealthy dry goods merchant. He was educated at the Phillips Andover Academy in Massachusetts, a private boarding school, and then at Yale College where his main distinction was football. He was captain of the team. He later claimed that he never took a book out of the College's library. In contrast, he did well in medical school, New York's College of Physicians and Surgeons, then a proprietary school only loosely associated with Columbia University. After graduation in 1877, he interned at Bellevue Hospital and became quite interested in surgery as an area of medical practice.

There were then no formal training programs in surgery or, for that matter, any limitations on which physicians could perform surgery. In fact, his surgical training was essentially a set of short apprenticeships, some in New York and some in Europe where he spent 2 years, largely in Vienna. On his return to New York, he taught anatomy at his medical school and was on the staff of Bellevue and Roosevelt Hospitals. At Bellevue, he got to know a young pathologist, William H. Welch, who also had graduated from both Yale College and P&S and had further training in Europe, and who later became the first professor appointed to the Johns Hopkins Medical School. Halsted lived well in New York and put on "frequent dinner parties and musicales" at the house he shared with another bachelor surgeon, no doubt supported by his family's income, some of which seems to have come from his father's embezzlement of company funds [1].

A Biographical History of Endocrinology, First Edition. D. Lynn Loriaux.

This work is a co-publication between the Endocrine Society and John Wiley & Sons, Ltd.

Note that at this time the importance of the concept of a clean surgical field to minimize infection was not universally accepted as necessary. Bacteriology was still an infant discipline. Welch became one of its leaders. Halsted and Welch became fast friends, which was truly fortunate for Halsted a few years later. Within a few years of his arrival back in New York, Halsted established himself as a competent and busy surgeon as well as an excellent teacher.

In 1884, Carl Koller of Vienna noted that cocaine rendered the cornea and conjunctiva insensitive to pain (i.e., it was a local anesthetic for mucosal surfaces). Until then, cocaine mixed into wine had been widely used as a popular tonic for the treatment of alcoholism and morphine addiction. Halsted and his colleagues thought that if cocaine anesthetized mucosa, it must act on the pain-sensitive nerves in these membranes. If so, then cocaine might also anesthetize pain-bearing nerves anywhere in the body. Halsted and his associates proceeded to prove that this was so and, in essence, founded the fields of local and spinal anesthesia. The profession did not then realize the addictive potential of the drug (although Sigmund Freud said that addiction did occur but only in those already addicted to morphine). The result was that Halsted and several of his colleagues, whose experiments in local anesthesia were often done on themselves, became addicted to the drug.

Halsted continued his surgical practice for a while, but his attendance at meetings "dropped precipitously." In an attempt to cure his habit, he admitted himself to the Butler Sanitarium in Providence, Rhode Island, but the cure did not succeed. It was probably at this time that he was given morphine to counteract the craving for cocaine. As a result, he ended up addicted to both cocaine and morphine. Another result of the cocaine addiction was that he was unable to compete for the Chair of Surgery at P&S in 1886. With his teaching and practice now failing, although still well off financially, his cover was suffering in New York. Welch, now professor of pathology at Johns Hopkins, asked Halsted to join him in Baltimore. For a year or two, Halsted worked in the surgical laboratory only doing surgical research. He saw no patients. Another trial at curing his addiction at the Butler institution in 1887 fared no better, although he was thought to have been cured of his addiction to morphine, which in time was found to be untrue.

Several observers commented on the different personality he presented in Baltimore compared with how he had appeared in New York. In Baltimore, he was more reserved and distant and more sarcastic in his dealings with colleagues and subordinates. He often failed to complete administrative matters he was responsible for as chief surgeon and professor at the Johns Hopkins Hospital and Medical School. Harvey Cushing, who received his surgical training under Halsted, noted that despite his close contact with Halsted over approximately 15 years, he was invited to Halsted's home only five times. This stood in contrast to Cushing's frequent visits to the home of William Osler, the well-known professor of medicine at the Hopkins institutions [2].

In spite of his medical problems and attitude change, or, perhaps because of his efforts to deal with his addictions, noted in retrospect by colleagues such as William Osler, Halsted achieved a great deal. One example is the use of rubber gloves during surgical procedures. In Halsted's time, surgical operators did not wear gloves or face masks, although they did wear cloth caps. The standard story is that Halsted's chief operating room nurse, Caroline Hampton, whom Halsted later married, complained in the winter of 1889–1890 that the solution used to wash the hands before surgery caused serious irritation of her hands and made it difficult to do her work. Halsted responded by contacting the Goodyear Rubber Company and asked them to make some rubber gloves, which they did. The innovation seems to have been effective, because we hear no more of irritated hands. However, Halsted was certainly in no rush to publish his innovation. Prompted by his colleagues to do so, he finally did write up the experience with rubber gloves more than 20 years later [3].

Clearly, the initial intent was to decrease hand irritation and not to decrease surgical infections. Nevertheless, one of Halsted's residents, Joseph C. Bloodgood was able to show that surgical gloves were associated with a marked diminution in postoperative infection after herniorrhaphy at the Johns Hopkins Hospital. Bloodgood wrote a long paper on his recollections of Halsted's contributions to surgery and of what life was like as Halsted's assistant [4]. The use of gloves did not catch on immediately, even at Johns Hopkins, where it took the better part of a decade for all surgery to be performed with gloved hands. Elsewhere, many surgeons resisted the practice, stating that they could not feel structures and lesions as well with gloves on compared with gloves off. However, with time, the benefit of lower infection rates became clear, and after the first decade of the twentieth century, most surgery was done wearing gloves.

It turns out that the gloved hand in surgery was not an original idea with Halsted. The idea had even been patented in the United States several decades earlier. There was also a modest priority dispute among the Johns Hopkins family. Another Johns Hopkins surgeon, Hunter Robb, claimed priority. He wrote up and published his version many years before Halsted got around to it. Most likely, Robb simply wrote down under his own name what Halsted was already doing. Whatever the case might be, it is certain that Halsted had the idea and acted on it. Whether original or not, the use of surgical gloves was not previously known to him, and Halsted did ensure that gloves were eventually used by all those operating on his service.

Halsted's other achievement during this time was his work with the professor of anatomy, Franklin P. Mall, on intestinal anastomosis. They were the first to show that the suture line had to include the intestinal submucosa for it to hold [5]. This paper was the only one of Halsted's 169 publications that was included in the 1993 celebratory volume of facsimile reprints of fundamental research done at the Johns Hopkins institutions over the previous 100 years [6]. Done correctly, this technique eliminated later bowel leakage and the consequent peritonitis.

Surgery on the bowel was hazardous indeed. Halsted's work on this problem was done in dogs. The results, however, may not have had clear application to man [4]. Halsted's perfectionism in hemostasis was also reflected in his personal habits. He was "always extraordinarily careful of his attire" and a fussy dresser almost to the extreme. He had his shoes and shirts made in Paris. His suits were made in London, and he sent his shirts to Paris for laundering. He wore a silk hat when most others had stopped wearing them. Wrinkles in a tablecloth were ironed out on the spot, on the table. He chose his own coffee beans individually and prepared his coffee almost ritualistically.

When Halsted went to Baltimore to join Welch in 1886, he did not have a hospital or a medical school appointment. Given his medical history, one can understand the Trustees' reluctance to offer appointments despite Welch's sterling recommendations as to Halsted's skill based, of course, on Welch's knowledge of Halsted from their common time in New York. By 1889, however, Welch succeeded in convincing the Trustees that Halsted should be appointed to the Johns Hopkins Hospital. Halsted's initial appointment was not as the Chief of Surgery at the Hospital, it was as Surgeon-in-Chief to the Dispensary and as Acting Surgeon to the Hospital, the latter for only 1 year. Halsted did well in his surgical work. Osler noted that "Halsted is doing remarkable work in surgery" and recommended Halsted's appointment to the hospital itself and not just the dispensary [7]. The Trustees agreed; Halsted was appointed to the medical school faculty as associate professor of surgery in 1889, the year that the hospital opened. The next spring, in March 1890, Halsted was made a full professor of surgery, a post he held until he died in 1922. He was also named Surgeon-in-Chief to the Hospital at the same time as the appointment to his professorship.

Halsted's other accomplishments were several. He perfected the now seemingly routine operation of inguinal herniorrhaphy [8]. Before he perfected this procedure, accurate and precise repair of inguinal hernia was not thought to be possible without recurrence. He offered a "radical" procedure (i.e., one that was aimed at curing the condition) [9]. Admittedly, unknown to Halsted, the Italian surgeon Edoardo Bassini had done the same thing 2 years before, but Halsted remains an innovator in any case. Both Bassini and Halsted went on to improve their herniorrhaphy procedures so that they were no longer quite so similar technical operations [10]. Halsted also devised what came to be known as the radical mastectomy procedure, done in an attempt to cure breast cancer. Many of his patients, based on what we would call historical controls, did survive longer than expected and so were "cured" [11]. He had a 40% 3-year survival rate in patients who often had advanced disease when first seen.

The characteristics of the operative procedures that distinguished Halsted from most other surgeons of his time were fourfold. First, he maintained careful attention to hemostasis using large numbers of small clamps. If there was a good deal of bleeding in a procedure, Halsted would give the blood lost back to the patient, if it was easily collectible and not clotted. Shock after surgery as a result of blood loss was common then and was routinely treated only with stimulants. Halsted's patients rarely lost significant amounts of blood so he rarely used stimulants which would, in retrospect, not have helped much in any case. Second was the gentle handling of all tissues. Third was the use of the finest sutures available (he was an advocate of fine silk here), and fourth was the avoidance of any unnecessary tension in approximating the tissues cut through during surgery.

Halsted's main influence on the practice of surgery in the United States was probably none of these technical achievements, but rather the institution of his surgical training program at Johns Hopkins. As exemplified by his own career, there was no standard way to become a surgeon in that era. In essence, one had to be an apprentice to one or more well-known surgeons. Halsted's exposure to the European clinics of his time was responsible for his devising a training program that, by diffusion through its graduates, influenced American surgery for decades, and to some extent still does. Halsted consciously copied the German–Austrian model of a major professor who has a senior assistant. At Johns Hopkins this was the resident, who might stay on for a number of years until finding a position at Johns Hopkins or elsewhere in the United States. Halsted did not intend to train surgeons for practice, but rather to train teachers of surgery who would then train practitioners. The program was intentionally "harshly competitive and exceedingly selective" [12]. It was the classic "pyramidal system" in which few became "the resident." It took 6 years on Halsted's surgical service before one could be "the resident." The resident was paid $40 a month, whereas the three assistant residents were paid only in kind: room, board, and laundry. All trainees were truly residents in that they lived in the hospital. "The resident" is now usually termed the "chief resident" in most institutions. At Johns Hopkins, "the resident," after a few years, would be as competent in most areas as was the professor. Many went on directly to professorships at other medical institutions. Others went into the several surgical subspecialties.

One of Halsted's greatest accomplishments was in the improvement of thyroid surgery, particularly that of thyroidectomy for hyperthyroidism or, as it was then called, exophthalmic goiter. There was a high mortality associated with this procedure, mainly as a result of blood loss and sepsis. Some said that the operation should simply not be done because the consequences were too severe. Halsted's first contact with thyroid research came during part of his European sojourn in 1879–1880 when he was working in Vienna with Anton Wölfler who was then the first assistant to the famous Viennese surgeon Theodor Billroth. For unclear reasons, Halsted was working with Wölfler on the histology of the salmon thyroid, although no publication resulted from this work. In late 1887, he began to study the dog thyroid gland at Welch's suggestion. Welch had an interest in the thyroid for some time but never wrote up any of his work for publication. Halsted's interest in the thyroid gland is beautifully encompassed in his lengthy monograph on goiter and its treatment [13]. Halsted never saw a thyroid operation when he was in New York, nor did he see one in Vienna. Much of this monograph is given over to an extensive review of prior thyroid operations and their outcomes.

His experiments with dogs involved assessment of the effects of partial thyroid removal on the remainder of the dog's thyroid. The remnant became hyperplastic, which is not a surprise to us today but was inexplicable then. These changes were recognized as similar to those seen in the thyroid glands of patients with Graves' disease, yet the dogs showed no sign of thyroid overactivity which was quite mysterious to Halsted and others. Halsted began this work in 1887 and had these results within a year but did not publish them until years later in 1896 [14]. It seems reasonably clear that Halsted did these experiments to determine how better to treat Graves' disease. One of his questions was exactly how much of the normal thyroid gland a dog needed to live. The parallel question in hyperthyroid patients was how much of the gland should be removed at surgery. Halsted was quite aware of the dangers that thyroid surgery might provoke. The worst were tetany or, if the gland were completely removed, myxedema. He also knew that the tetany was the result of interference with the parathyroid glands, either by their inadvertent removal or, more likely in his opinion, interdiction of their blood supply. This complication he defined better with the help of a medical student, Herbert McLean Evans, who later became one of the most prominent endocrinologists in the United States [15].

Halsted learned much of the technique of thyroidectomy for Graves' disease from his European mentor, Theodor Kocher [16], whom he visited many times and who was probably the world's foremost thyroid surgeon in the late nineteenth and early twentieth centuries. Halsted knew that Kocher was the one of the first to realize that total removal of the thyroid gland led to myxedema. Myxedema, was, of course, what we now call hypothyroidism and, until 1891, was an untreatable and incurable disease. Halsted later wrote "Many times during the last 20 years I have stood by the side of Professor Kocher at the operating table" [13]. Halsted probably helped Kocher in the understanding of the parathyroid glands. The two men last met in the spring of 1914 a few months before World War I began. By then, Halsted had performed 650 operations in 500 patients with Graves' disease. Most of these were unilateral lobectomies with "an approximate cure in possibly 60%" and a mortality of less than 2% [17].

Halsted never did understand why the dog's thyroid remnants became hyperplastic. Although the finding was confirmed by others, Halsted himself was not able to confirm his own results when he repeated the studies many years later in 1913. He thought perhaps the earlier results were the result of local lack of cleanliness or infection. The puzzle remains today as to why his later studies did not confirm his earlier ones. Halsted was regarded as one of the great surgeons of his time both in the United States and in Europe because of his research and skill, an outcome all the more remarkable in light of his addictions. He died in 1922 from complications of surgery on his biliary tract.

References

1. Rutkow IM: William Halsted, his family, and "queer business methods." *Arch Surg* 1996; 131: 123.
2. Rutkow IM: The unpublished letters of Wil-liam Halsted and Harvey Cushing. *Surg Gynecol Obstet* 1988; 166: 370.
3. Geelhoed GW. The pre-Halstedian and post-Halstedian history of the surgical rubber glove. *Surg Gynecol Obstet* 1988; 167: 350.
4. Bloodgood JC: Halsted thirty-six years ago. (William Stewart Halsted, Professor of Surgery, Johns Hopkins University and Chief Surgeon, Johns Hopkins Hospital, 1889–1922). *Am J Surg* 1931; 14: 89.
5. Halsted WS: Circular suture of the intestine–an experimental study. *Am J Med Sci* 1887; 94: 436.
6. Harvey AM, Cameron JL, Lane MD, et al.: *A Century of Biomedical Science at Johns Hopkins*, Vol. I. Baltimore, MD: Johns Hopkins University School of Medicine, 1993.
7. Nunn DB: William Stewart Halsted. Transitional years. *Surgery* 1997; 121: 343.
8. Halsted WS: The radical cure of hernia. *Johns Hopkins Hosp Bull* 1889; 1: 12.
9. Brieger GH: From conservative to radical surgery in late nineteenth-century America. In *Medical Theory, Surgical Practice*, edited by C Lawrence. London, New York: Routledge. 1992.
10. Halsted WS: The cure of the more difficult as well as the simpler inguinal ruptures. *Johns Hopkins Hosp Bull* 1903; 14: 208.

11. Halsted WS: The results of operations for the cure of cancer of the breast performed at the Johns Hopkins Hospital from June, 1889 to January, 1894. *Johns Hopkins Hosp Rep* 1894–5; 4: 297.
12. McClure RD, Szilagyi DE: Halsted–teacher of surgeons. *Am J Surg* 1951; 82: 122.
13. Halsted WS: The operative story of goitre. The author's operation. *Johns Hopkins Hosp Rep* 1920; 19: 71 (reprinted in Surgical Papers by William Stewart Halsted in Two Volumes). Baltimore, MD: The Johns Hopkins Press, 1924.
14. Halsted WS: An experimental study of the thyroid gland of dogs, with especial consideration of hypertrophy of this gland. *Johns Hopkins Hosp Rep* 1896; 1: 372.
15. Halsted WS: Preservation of the parathyroids during thyroidectomy. *Trans Am Surg Assn* 1907; 25: 60.
16. Harwick RD: Our legacy of thyroid surgery. *Am J Surg* 1988; 156: 230.
17. Becker WF. Pioneers in thyroid surgery. *Ann Surg* 1977; 185: 493.

This chapter has been reproduced from Sawin, Clark T: William Stewart Halstead (1852–1922): Thyroid surgeon. *The Endocrinologist* 2004; 14(1): 1–4.

CHAPTER 39

Charles Eucharist de Medicis Sajous (1852–1929)

The First President of the Endocrine Society

On June 4, 1917, Charles E. de M. Sajous, MD, then 65 years old, was elected the first president of the Association for the Study of Internal Secretions (ASIS), which is now the Endocrine Society, a thriving organization of more than 13 000 physicians and scientists. A few years later he was also the first in the United States to be named to a professorship specifically in endocrinology at the University of Pennsylvania. Some call him the "father" of American endocrinology [1].

Sajous thought that epinephrine was the key to all life processes, that the intermediate lobe of the pituitary was a sense organ for toxins in the body, and that the thyroid gland was a repository of white cells which, on release to the blood stream, carried an organic form of iodine to the body's tissues where it maintained tissue oxygenation. Sajous' successor thought this a sad tale because, even in Sajous' own time, his ideas were not widely accepted. Sajous never published any experimental data and spent his entire career as a medical editor and writer while maintaining a clinical practice in downtown Philadelphia.

Sajous was born on board an American ship on the way to France. He received his early education in France, but grew up in Mexico and California. Coming east to Philadelphia on horseback, he graduated from Jefferson Medical College in Philadelphia in 1878. He may have studied with the famous Brown-Séquard in the late 1870s, but it is not clear where this might have been. The peripatetic Brown-Séquard, although considered French, spent much of the 1870s in the United States. After graduation, Sajous practiced in Philadelphia and developed a thriving practice in otolaryngology, authoring a text on the subject in 1885. He was a well-established practitioner [2].

Mr. F.A. Davis, owner of the publishing company in Philadelphia which had published Sajous' book on diseases of the nose and throat, thought Sajous might be interested in editing a massive annual medical encyclopedia, the *Annual of the Universal Medical Sciences*. Sajous was indeed interested, and the first set of five volumes appeared in 1888. At five volumes per year, Sajous relentlessly and tirelessly wrote letters, reviewed published papers, recruited more than 70 associate editors, many

A Biographical History of Endocrinology, First Edition. D. Lynn Loriaux.

This work is a co-publication between the Endocrine Society and John Wiley & Sons, Ltd.

well-known academics, to write articles, and put the whole thing into a shape suitable for American practitioners. Over 100 000 sets of these five volumes were sold over the next 9 years and provided an excellent income for Sajous.

In fact, he closed his practice in 1891 and returned to France to learn endocrinology. Sajous stayed in Europe for 7 years, returning to Philadelphia in 1897 only because he had been named Dean of the Medico-Chirurgical College and its Professor of Laryngology. The College was later absorbed by the University of Pennsylvania. Where Sajous worked during his time in Paris is unknown. There are no known endocrine publications by him while he was away. Finances were not a problem. He continued to edit the *Annual* while in Paris and got weekly paychecks and royalty payments even though the publisher was in financial difficulty for much of the 1890s. The "panic" of 1896 lowered physicians' incomes enough, however, to cause the *Annual* to cease publication that year. This stopped neither Sajous nor the Davis Co. The venture was converted into a purely clinical encyclopedia for general practitioners called the *Analytic Cyclopedia of Practical Medicine*. It went through 10 editions from 1898 to 1927 and sold over 70 000 sets, providing yet more royalties to Sajous [3].

While in Paris, he seems to have adopted a strain of French theoretical medicine that now seems inconsistent with sound medical thought. He believed that a thorough study of others' work from many sources can be combined to generate a grand theory that explains all biology and disease. His life as an encyclopedist in the 1880s and 1890s and his fascination with both clinical and experimental endocrinology, combined with this theoretical approach, led to a massive two-volume work, *The Internal Secretions and the Principles of Medicine*, again published by the Davis Co. The first volume of 800 pages appeared in 1903. The book had a reasonable tone in many of its parts, carefully reviewing the extant endocrine literature. When critical data did not exist, however, he makes "reasonable" assumptions in order to complete his theoretical explanations instead of simply saying that more data are needed. The focus of Volume 1 was on normal endocrine function. The focus of Volume 2 was on pathophysiologic theory. Volume 2 appeared 4 years later. It seems to imply that almost all illness is endocrine in nature and all patients might benefit from endocrine therapy, often injections of epinephrine. Volume 1, which was the first comprehensive treatise on the internal secretions, received mixed reviews. Some admired it as "a great uplifting to the science of medicine," but others thought that "fact and fancy are inextricably woven." No matter. Thousands of copies were sold and the book went through 10 editions, the last being published in 1922. Sajous became nationally known as an endocrinologist [4].

He continued his practice in Philadelphia, sometimes diagnosing and prescribing endocrine treatment by mail. Editing, however, still paid the bills. To meet a publication deadline he might take off for a month or two. He added to his work in 1911 with the editorship of the *New York Medical Journal*. But at this point there was no evidence of any desire to form a national organization.

Enter Henry R. Harrower. Harrower was an enthusiast, a promoter, and an entrepreneur. Born in England in 1883, he seems to have grown up in Chicago and attended the nearby American Missionary Medical School, graduating in 1907. He did no missionary work but went into practice in Kankakee and then Chicago, Illinois. His entrepreneurship got him into trouble, early on, with the American Medical Association (AMA), then, as now, headquartered in Chicago. He advertised a urinalysis program to the public, wrote in a "fifth-rate" journal, and solicited subscriptions, and defended what was considered a "quack device." Enamored of endocrinology, by 1912 or 1913 he returned to England for a year or two, and was loosely associated with an American manufacturer of oral glandular preparations. There, he wrote a book, *Practical Hormone Therapy*, in 1914. It had a laudatory foreword by the Austrian pioneer in endocrine disease, Artur Biedl. The young hyperactive physician went back to New York in 1914 and then to Glendale in southern California the following year. There he practiced clinical endocrinology. He manufactured his own glandular products. None of this endeared him to the AMA, which, fortunately for us, kept a file on him.

Harrower had corresponded with Sajous in 1914 about his book. In early 1916, Harrower began a letter-writing campaign to wellknown practitioners, including Sajous, to organize an "internal secretions round-table" at the upcoming AMA meeting in Detroit in June 1916. He generated a good deal of resentment, probably because of his "blind" letters and general "pushiness." What Harrower really wanted was to organize a national group, and he drafted a proposal for Sajous' approval, saying that Sajous ought to be its president. In April 1916, Sajous politely tried to fend him off by saying that he (Sajous) had already thought of it and decided that such a group would not work. Sajous also wrote to the AMA saying he did "not favor the formation of such a society." Sajous' aim was to establish local "endocrine clubs."

Harrower, however, was not put off. Sajous' colleagues felt it was too late to turn him aside and suggested that they "cooperate and get the right sort... interested." Harrower appointed himself "secretary pro-temp" of the incipient group. Sajous was annoyed, of course, but agreed to put a notice into the *New York Medical Journal* about a possible meeting in Detroit for those interested. The meeting did take place as Harrower wanted. About 60 interested physicians attended and were asked to join the ASIS. More cautious senior physicians put together a Committee on Organization with George M. Hoxie of Kansas City, Missouri, as Chairman, and Harrower as Secretary. By the end of the meeting, Harrower claimed over 200 members. He continued to arouse suspicions by his methods of canvassing for more members but wasted no time in getting at his other goal, a journal. He found paying advertisers and put together the *Bulletin of the Association for the Study of Internal Secretions* in short order, working with Hoxie's approval.

But there was still no "official" ASIS. It was only an organizing committee, the best-known member being Lewellys F. Barker of Baltimore, former professor of medicine at Johns Hopkins. He had contributed to the new journal. In January 1917, The AMA learned of the nationally respected Barker's presence on the committee and saw Harrower's name on the same letterhead. Dr. Simmons of the AMA wrote Barker about Harrower's past and created consternation in Barker's mind. Barker attempted to stop publication of the *Bulletin*, but Harrower had already printed, and it was sent to the members (those who had signed up in June 1916 and afterward) of the still ill-defined association in February 1917. It was now named *Endocrinology: The Bulletin of the Association for the Study of Internal Secretions* and remains *Endocrinology* to this day.

The organizing meeting finally took place at the AMA meeting in June 1917, and the ASIS was brought into existence. There was no more talk of not needing a national association, nor did Sajous decline to hold office. By then, two issues of the *Bulletin* had appeared with articles by well-known scientists such as Swale Vincent and Edward Kendall as well as by Harrower and several clinicians. Several case reports were presented at the meeting in June and the officers were elected, included Sajous as President and Harrower, now age 34, as Secretary for the year 1917–1918. Harvey Cushing was a Vice-President and Barker a member of the Council, the actual governing body of which the President was only a member. At the same meeting, Roy Hoskins, Walter Cannon's first doctoral student, was named editor of *Endocrinology*, with Harrower now as only business or editorial manager, an overt sign of the group's unhappiness with Harrower.

Harrower continued his efforts in his capacity as Secretary during the rest of 1917 and early 1918. In the meantime, the Association was formally incorporated in Delaware in January 1918 by the East Coast members of the Council. It is not clear what then happened. At the first official Council meeting only two months later, in March 1918, held in Barker's Baltimore home, Harrower's resignation as editorial manager of the Association was accepted. He was sent a letter of thanks. His role as Secretary was ignored. Sajous, as President, eagerly recruited new members, noting to a friend that Harrower was "out of it." At the next annual meeting in June 1918, the first after incorporation, Harrower was not re-nominated as Secretary, although another southern Californian was. Sajous completed his term as President. The 65-year-old clinician gave a long presidential address to the now official and incorporated Association. He again propounded his theory of adrenal control of respiration and thought that the physiologist ought to do more to help the clinicians.

Sajous remained on the Council for some years, but others, even other Council members, thought little of his ideas. He was so affable and kind-spoken, however, that his ideas never got in the way of his personal relationships. His affability may have helped get him the appointment as professor of endocrinology at the University of Pennsylvania, but probably more important was the absorption of part of the Medico-Chirurgical College by the University. His idea of local endocrine clubs did not die; it was resurrected by the Endocrine Society's Council in 1991. He died at age 76 of cardiac and renal failure.

Harrower continued to be a consultant in endocrinology in Glendale and built a manufacturing plant for oral glandular preparations sold nationwide (they were similar to those sold today in some health-food stores). He had a last shot at the Association in 1920 when he asked them for $150 as partial reimbursement for his expense in setting up the original meeting in Detroit in 1916. On Barker's motion he got no money, but did get a letter suggesting that he should "take pleasure in knowing that he was instrumental in bringing about the organization of so thriving an institution, and that this ... should be ... sufficient compensation." He died in Glendale in 1935.

Harrower was clearly the driving force in organizing the Association and in getting Sajous to be its President. Harrower rightly judged Sajous as attractive to general physicians – as most members then were – and by his energy which made it difficult for the others not to form the Association. The journal he began–again by forcing it before there was full discussion–has, with its successors, been the linchpin of the Endocrine Society. In retrospect, the glandular products he advocated were almost certainly without biologic activity (except for those containing thyroid gland derivatives). They were no different from others approved by the AMA, such as antithyroidin, a sheep serum preparation for the treatment of hyperthyroidism. He was eased out as quickly as possible because of his failure to comply with the then-current norms. It was expected that physicians could own, make, sell, and advertise medical products. Times have changed [5].

References

1. Knobil E: Presidential address: the Endocrine Society. *Endocrinology* 1971; 101: 1647–51.
2. Sajous papers, College of Physicians of Philadelphia.
3. Anders JM: Memoir of Charles Eucharist de Medicis Sajous, M.D., Sc.D., LL.D. *Trans Stud Coll Phys Phila* 1930; 52: Lxv–Lxx.
4. Robinson V: Charles Eucharist de Medicis Sajous. *Med Life* 1925; 32: 3–21.
5. Hafner AW: *Guide to the AMA Historical Health Fraud and Alternative Medicine Collection*. File no. 3–42, Harrower, Henry R. Chicago: AMA, 1992.

This chapter has been reproduced from Sawin, Clark T: Charles Eucharist de Medicis Sajous (1852–1929). *The Endocrinologist* 1993; 3(2): 83–6.

CHAPTER 40
Pierre Marie (1853–1940)
Acromegaly

Pierre Marie was born into a wealthy Parisian family in 1853. After boarding school at Vauves, he went to law school at the bidding of his father. He was not happy there, however, and was successful in convincing his father that a career in medicine would be equally satisfactory. He did well in medical school and, in 1878, as an intern, he began his association with the great Jean-Martin Charcot at the Salpêtrière and Bicêtre hospitals. Charcot was quick to recognize Marie's aptitude, and soon appointed him chief of Charcot's laboratory and clinic. Marie chose Basedow's disease as the topic of his doctoral thesis, and was perhaps the first to point out the value of the fine tremor in the outstretched hand as a specific diagnostic sign of the disease. Based largely on the quality of this dissertation, Marie was awarded the MD degree in 1883.

It was at this same time that Marie's interest in acromegaly began. The literature of the time contained two excellent descriptions of the disease, by Vicenzo Brigidi in 1877, and Fritsche and Klebs in 1884. Both reports contained detailed clinical descriptions of the disease and, in both cases, enlargement of the pituitary body was noted.

Marie had accumulated two cases of his own which he reported in 1886, "Sur deux cas d'acromégalie. Hypertrophie singulière non congénitale des extrémités supérieures, inférieúres et céphalique" [1]. Marie, in a stroke of genius, assigned the problem of acromegaly to his new fellow, Jose Dantas da Souza-Leite. Souza-Leite combed the literature for unidentified cases and began collecting cases of his own. It became the subject of his doctoral dissertation. When published, it consisted of a thorough review of the literature, 38 cases, and 10 new ones.

Marie's first report and Souza-Leite's thesis were translated into English by Proctor Hutchinson and published together by the New Sydenham Society in 1891. The title of the new combined work was *Essays on Acromegaly* [2]. The publication attracted considerable attention, especially Souza-Leite's comments on the associated pituitary pathology: "The most specific of these lesions which may be considered as essential, since it has not been found absent, is the considerable increase in size of the pituitary

A Biographical History of Endocrinology, First Edition. D. Lynn Loriaux.

This work is a co-publication between the Endocrine Society and John Wiley & Sons, Ltd.

body. The gland is changed into a hypertrophical mass of which the size varies from that of a pigeon's egg or even an apple."

Thus, Marie and Souza-Leite did for the pituitary gland what Addison had done for the adrenal gland: related a specific glandular abnormality to a specific clinical syndrome. It is generally agreed that the publication of the English translation of Marie and Souza-Leite's work marks the beginning of clinical endocrinology and of the endocrinology of the pituitary gland and its disorders.

Marie, however, was first and foremost a neurologist, not an endocrinologist. His career advanced along the neurological path, not the endocrinologic path. He was appointed professor agrégé to the Paris faculty of medicine in 1889 based, in large part, on a series of lectures on spinal cord disease. In 1897, Marie created the legendary Neurological Service at the Hospice Bícêtre. It became the world's leading center for the study of neurological disease. It was there that Marie described Charcot–Marie–Tooth muscular dystrophy, pulmonary hypertrophic osteoarthropathy, hereditary cerebellar ataxia, cleidocranial dysostosis, and rhizomelic spondylosis, all for the first time.

Marie's private life was a quiet one. He shunned acclaim and public appearances. He and his wife liked art and opera. Marie also liked fencing and golf. They had two children, André, who became a physician, and Juliette. Juliette died of appendicitis as a child. André, after becoming a physician, worked as a scientist at the Pasteur Institute. As a result of an experiment gone awry, he died of botulism. And then, Marie's wife of many years died of erysipelas. These repetitive shocks were too much, and Marie became a recluse in his last years. He died at home at the age of 86.

References

1. Marie, Pierre. Sur deux cas d'acromégalie. Hypertrophie singulière non congénitale des extrémiteś supérieures, inférieúres et céphalique. *Rev Med* 1886; 6: 297–333.
2. Marie P, de Souza-Leite JD: *Essays on Acromegaly*. London. New Sydenham Society, 1891.

This chapter has been reproduced from Loriaux, D. Lynn: Pierre Marie (1853–1940). *The Endocrinologist* 2007; 17(5): 243.

CHAPTER 41
Victor Horsley
(1857–1916)
Treating Myxedema with Thyroid Extract

Victor Horsley was one of the first neurosurgeons and is remembered by some as a co-inventor of the Horsley–Clarke stereotactic apparatus for brain studies. Endocrinologists, however, should know that he was the first to produce experimental hypothyroidism, then called myxedema, by removing the thyroid gland from several mammals, including sheep and monkeys. In so doing, he showed that the thyroid gland had an essential function, not previously defined, and produced one of the first animal models of a human disease.

Horsley was "of good birth," meaning that his family was well off and well connected. He was named after Queen Victoria at her request. As a boy, he wanted to become a cavalry officer. His father demurred, saying that he could not afford it. When his father suggested medicine instead, the boy agreed, provided he could be a surgeon. And so it was.

After medical training at University College Hospital (UCH) Medical School, Horsley became the surgical registrar (or resident) at UCH, a very competitive position. At the same time he was appointed assistant professor of pathology at the school. He began a private practice, not then against the rules. He also began some experimental work on cerebral localization with Edward Schafer, one of his professors at University College London (UCL). This was the start of several years' work on brain function, defined by electrical stimulation of the brain of anesthetized animals, for which he became famous.

By 1884, now 27 years of age, Horsley was appointed Professor Superintendent of the Brown Animal Sanatory Institution, probably through the influence of another professor, John S. Burdon-Sanderson. This was an unusual London Institution, separately endowed and loosely connected to the University of London. Its main aim was the care of sick animals. It was also, however, one of the few places in London where animal experiments could be done, largely because of the restrictions of the Cruelty to Animals Act of 1876. Horsley began other work on localization with Charles Beevor while continuing the work with Schafer.

A Biographical History of Endocrinology, First Edition. D. Lynn Loriaux.

This work is a co-publication between the Endocrine Society and John Wiley & Sons, Ltd.

At about the same time of his appointment to the Brown Institution in the fall of 1884, he began his work on the thyroid gland. The suspicion was that three illnesses – spontaneous myxedema, cretinism, and the peculiar Swiss syndrome that occurred after total thyroidectomy – might all be due to the lack of the thyroid gland. This caused the Clinical Society of London to appoint a committee to look into the matter in December in 1883. No experiments were done, however, until Horsley was asked to join the committee in 1884. Little work was done at UCL. Almost all of it was done at the Brown Institution, mainly because he could work with larger animals.

His approach to thyroidectomy was simply to take it out. No vessels were tied off; they were "torn out of the gland" and bleeding stopped with "light pressure of carbolized wool." There was almost no knowledge about the parathyroid glands, and so the muscular fibrillations and tetany were attributed to the loss of thyroid tissue. There was no measurement of basal metabolic rate or of serum thyroxine. Observations of the animals for their similarity to human disease had to be his end-points. Animals that died within a few days, particularly cats and dogs, were thought to have "acute myxedema," which we now know was parathyroid deficiency. Probably because of his surgical skill and attention to antisepsis, some animals lived longer. Monkeys were the best example and, not least, were the experimental animals most similar to humans. By several weeks after thyroidectomy, "the change from the well-known vivacious condition of the healthy monkey is very obvious, ... this one is ... quite characteristic [and is] ... in the advanced condition of imbecility following the operation." He also found that these animals were anemic, lost their hair, and had a low body temperature. After death, the monkeys had "swollen, jelly-like" subcutaneous tissues.

Previous surgeons had thought the symptoms after thyroidectomy were due to the local effects of surgery, either in humans or in dogs. Horsley, on the other hand, clearly believed that the thyroid gland had a specific, although ill-defined, function: "in using the expression 'loss of the thyroid body,' I mean loss of its functional activity' and, personally, I believe, in those cases of well-marked myxedema where a thyroid body is found, whether anatomically altered or not, that it is not acting normally."

Horsley's straightforward experimental approach thus confirmed the Clinical Society's suspicion. His work was a crucial part of the final committee report, not completed until 1888, which defined the role of the thyroid gland in these apparently disparate conditions. The report, now a classic in endocrinology, concluded that "myxedema, as observed in adults, is practically the same disease as that named sporadic cretinism when affecting children; that myxedema and endemic cretinism .... While these ... depend on, or ... [are] associated with, destruction or loss of the function of the thyroid gland, the ultimate cause of such destruction or loss is at present not evident." Despite this remarkable advance in pathophysiologic understanding, no treatment was offered or even suggested. But Horsley had made his mark.

The still young surgeon was made a Fellow of the Royal Society in 1886 because of his neural and thyroid work. He went on to define neurosurgery as a specialty in Great Britain. He removed for example, a tumor near the spinal cord for the first time successfully in 1887.

Although a successful scientist and surgeon, Horsley was of fixed opinions. He was against smoking and alcohol from his student days to the end of his life. He was for women's suffrage, a national health service, and democratic reform of the medical profession. Such "black-or-white" opinions were not popular. He ran for Parliament but was never elected. His overt intolerance for the views of others did not help. William Osler, the internist's internist and one of Horsley's close friends, asked later: "what demon drove a man of this type into the muddy pool of politics?"

In academic life he was equally rigid. After becoming professor of pathology in the 1890s, he fired a bacteriologist who spent much time teaching because he "evinced no interest in the research going on in or outside the laboratory." That teacher was later a leader in his field. He also was estranged for some years from his mentor, Schafer, because of a difference of opinion over an academic appointment. Charles S. Sherrington, a contemporary and future winner of the Nobel Prize for his work in neurophysiology, actually suppressed some of his research findings until after Horsley's death to avoid a clash.

When World War I broke out, Horsley was internationally famous. At age 57, he insisted on active duty, which was grudgingly given. Sent to France in 1915, he was shortly transferred to Egypt, where he spent most of the last year of his life. There was not much to do in Egypt (the Army was probably intentionally keeping him out of harm's way), so he went on to India in 1916, stayed less than a month, and then went to Mesopotamia, now Iraq. Although he did little surgery there, he continued in his typical hyperactive way to try to solve obvious and serious logistical problems. Probably because he persisted in walking about in the midday sun, he developed heat stroke and died in July 1916.

References

Horsley V: The Brown lectures on pathology. *Br Med J* 1885; 1: 111–15, 211–13.

Merrington WR: *University College Hospital and its Medical School: A History*. London: Heinemann, 1976.

Osler W: In memoriam. Sir Victor Horsley. *Br J Surg* 1916–1917; 4: 327–31.

Page S: *Sir Victor Horsley. A Study of His Life and Work*. New York: Harcourt, Brace and Howe, 1920.

Power D'A (Ed.): *Plarr's Lives of the Fellows of the Royal College of Surgeons of England*, Vol. 1. Bristol: John Wright and Sons, 1930.

Tepperman J: Horsley and Clarke: a biographical medallion. *Perspect Biol Med* 1970; 13: 295–308.

Wilson G: The Brown Animal Sanatory Institution. *J Hyg* 1979; 82: 155–76. 337–52, 501–21; 1979; 82: 171–97.

This chapter has been reproduced from Sawin, Clark T: Victor Horsley (1857–1916). *The Endocrinologist* 1991; 1(3): 207–8.

CHAPTER 42

Archibald Edward Garrod (1857–1936)

Orchronosis and Human Genetics

Archibald Edward Garrod was born in London on November 26, 1857. He was the youngest of four sons born to Alfred Baring Garrod and his wife Elisabeth. The Garrod family was one of exceptional intellectual accomplishment. Alfred Garrod was a pioneer in contemporary scientific medicine. He was the first to differentiate gout from other rheumatic diseases by showing that uric acid was elevated in the serum and tissues of gouty patients, and he published a now "classic" textbook in 1859 in which he coined the term "rheumatoid arthritis."

> Although unwilling to add to the number of names, I cannot help expressing a desire that a name might not be found for this disease (Rheumatic Gout), not implying any necessary relation between it and either gout or rheumatism. Perhaps Rheumatoid Arthritis would answer the object, by which term I should wish to imply an inflammatory affection of the joints, not unlike rheumatism in some of its characters but differing materially from it [1].

For these contributions, Alfred Garrod is widely regarded as the "Father of Modern Rheumatology" [2]. His eldest son, Alfred Henry, 11 years older than Archibald, became one of the leading zoologists of his day. At the time of his death from tuberculosis at age 33, he had published 75 papers, held two professorships, was the Prosector of the London Zoo, and a Fellow of the Royal Society. He is remembered mainly for the definitive anatomical classification of the passerine birds. Herbert, 8 years older than Archibald, had a distinguished career in humanities. Nurtured and challenged by this environment, Archibald's professional achievements would change the face of modern biology and medicine.

Archibald attended preparatory school at Harrow, and entered Marlborough at 15. He was an average student with a flair for the sciences. He was admitted to Oxford as a commoner at Christ Church in 1875. He flourished there and, in his last year, was awarded the Johnson Memorial Prize for an essay entitled "The Nebulae – A Fragment of Astronomical History." He left Oxford with a First in the natural sciences, and decided to follow his father into the medical profession. He entered Saint Bartholomew's

A Biographical History of Endocrinology, First Edition. D. Lynn Loriaux.

Hospital in 1880, "qualifying" in 1884. He spent the next year in the Algemeines Krankenhaus in Vienna where he was introduced to the laryngoscope. Returning to England, he wrote his first book on the clinical applications of this instrument [3]. He became a member of the Royal College of Physicians in 1885, and was elected a Fellow in 1891. In 1886, Garrod married Elisabeth Smith, eldest daughter of Sir Thomas Smith, a prominent surgeon to St. Bartholomew's Hospital. They had four children–three sons and a daughter. He was appointed assistant physician to the West London Hospital in 1888, and joined the staff of the Hospital of Sick Children at Great Ormond Street in 1889.

Garrod's interest in disorders associated with "pigmented" urine began at this time. His first paper on the subject appeared in 1892 [4]. Of particular importance was his introduction to the disease of alkaptonuria in 1897. The disease had been first described by Bodeker in 1859 [5], and black pigment in the urine identified as homogentisic acid by Wolkow and Baumann in 1891 [6]. Like most diseases at that time, it was thought to be caused by an infectious agent. In the case of alkaptonuria, an intestinal bacteria that altered the metabolism of tyrosine was suspected. Garrod searched diligently for this organism and, failing to find it, concluded that the disorder was more likely explained by "metabolic error" [7]. In an extensive study of the families of patients with alkaptonuria [8], Garrod could find no single instance of direct transmission of the disorder from parent to child. He concluded that it was unlikely to be an example of simple hereditary transmission:

> Lifelong Alkaptonuria is sometimes met within several members of a family, but although brothers and sisters are apt to share this peculiarity, I know of no instance in which it has been transmitted from one generation to another. When it occurs in families, some members are apt to escape, and a child born between two alkaptonuric members may pass normal urine [8].

About this time, Garrod conceived of a way to "prove" that alkaptonuria was congenital and not infectious in origin.

> Garrod knew that the mother of one of his alkaptonuric patients was pregnant with her fifth child. When the baby was born on May 1, 1901, Garrod instructed the nurse to examine the diapers carefully for any trace of darkening or staining. Fifteen hours after birth, there were stains. By the morning of the second day, the diapers were slightly stained, and by 10:30 AM, on March 3, just fifty two hours after birth, the infant's diapers had changed color and were deeply stained [9].

In the same article [10], Garrod recognized an increased consanguinity in the parents of children with alkaptonuria:

> However, although brothers and sisters share this peculiarity, there is, as yet, no known instance of its transmission from one generation to another.... On the other hand, I am able to bring forward evidence which seems to point, in no uncertain manner, to a very special liability of alkaptonuria to occur in the children of first cousins.

The work of Gregor Mendel on the laws of dominant and recessive inheritance had just been rediscovered after being "lost" for more than 40 years. William Bateson, a leading botanist of the time, translated Mendel's work into English in the now classic *Mendel's Principles of Heredity* [11]. Learning of Garrod's work, Bateson referred to it in a report to the "Evolution Committee" in 1901 [12]:

> In illustration of such a phenomenon (the persistence of hidden recessives) we may perhaps venture to refer to the extraordinarily interesting evidence lately collected by Garrod regarding the rare condition known as "alkaptonuria". In such persons, the substance, alkapton, forms a regular constituent of the urine, giving it a deep brown color which becomes black on exposure.
>
> The condition is extremely rare, and though met with in several members of the same families, has only once been known to be transmitted from parent to offspring. Recently, however, Garrod has noticed that no fewer than five families containing alkaptonuric members, more than a quarter of the recorded cases, are offspring's of the unions of first cousins.
>
> ... we note that the mating of first cousins gives exactly the conditions most likely to enable a rare and usually recessive character to show itself.

Garrod and Bateson began a correspondence in late 1901 or early 1902 [9]. Out of this emerged the framework for the examination of human disease in terms of Mendelian genetic principles. Of equal importance is that, in the context of this correspondence, Garrod conceptualized the linkage between the biochemical constitution and the phenotype of a given individual:

> I have for some time been collecting information as to specific and individual differences of metabolism, which seems to me to be a little explored but promising field in relation to natural selection, and I believe that no two individuals are exactly alike chemically any more than structurally. I fancy that monstrosities or rather malformations, vestigial remnants and individual differences all have their chemical analogues [9].

Thus, in the 5 years between 1897 and 1902, Garrod had disproved the infectious theory of the etiology of alkaptonuria, shown that it was a congenital disorder, clarified the concept of autosomal recessive inheritance in humans, demonstrated the importance of consanguinity in diseases of this nature, and formulated the idea of biochemical identity and the consequences of metabolic error. In the next few years, Garrod applied these principles to albinism, cystinuria, and pentosuria. The work was codified in "The Croonian Lectures on Inborn Errors of Metabolism", delivered before the Royal College of Physicians of London in June 1908. The lectures were published as a single volume, *Inborn Errors of Metabolism*, one year later [13]. As often the case with insights that require more than a little revision of prevailing dogma, the world was unprepared for change and the work received little attention or comment.

Garrod was impressed by the Flexner reports of 1910 and 1911:

> If it be true that the scientific spirit is not in evidence in the places in which the training of the future members of our profession is carried out, this must be reckoned a grave defect in our British system of education [14].

He developed plans for academic reform that were interrupted by the First World War. He was stationed in Malta as a consultant physician and remained there for the duration of the war. His military career was distinguished, and King George V appointed him a Knight Commander of St. Michael and St. George. Garrod's personal sacrifice to the war, however, was immense: all three of his sons lost their lives. The first two, Alfred Noel and Thomas A., were killed in action. The third, Basil Rahere, died in occupied Germany in the influenza pandemic that devastated Europe in the immediate post-war period.

On his return to London, Garrod was asked to be the head of the first Medical Professional Unit in London at the St. Bartholomew's Hospital. He was in this position less than 1 year when called upon to succeed William Osler as Regius Professor of Medicine at Oxford. He took this position, retiring from it at age 70. He died on March 28, 1936, 80 years of age, from myocardial infarction.

More than any other person, Garrod set the stage for modern human genetics and the "one gene, one enzyme" concept. His contributions were encapsulated best by George Beadle in his Nobel Lecture of December 11, 1858:

> In this long, roundabout way, first in Drosophila and then Neurospora, we had rediscovered what Garrod had seen so clearly so many years before. By now we knew of his work and were aware that we had added little if anything new in principle [15].

References

1. Garrod AE: *The Nature and Treatment of Gout and Rheumatic Gout*. London: Walton and Maberly, 1859.
2. *Journal of the American Medical Association*, Cover Story: Sir Alfred Baring Garrod, FRS, Primer on the Rheumatic Diseases. *JAMA*, Suppl No. 5, 1973.
3. Garrod AE: *An Introduction to the Use of the Laryngoscope*. London, 1886.
4. Garrod AE: On the presence of urohematoporphyrin in the urine in chorea and articular rheumatism. *Lancet* 1892; i: 793.
5. Bodeker H: Mittheilungen aus dem chemischen Laboratorium des Physiologischen Institutes zu Gottingen. *Zeit F Rationelle Med* 1859; 7: 130.
6. Wolkow M, Baumann E: Ueber das Wesen der Alkaptonurie. *Zeit F Physiol Chemie* 1891; 15: 228.
7. Hopkins FG: Archibald Edward Garrod. *Obituary Notices of the Royal Society* 1938; 2: 225–8.
8. Garrod AE: A contribution to the study of alkaptonuria. *Medico-Chir Trans* 1899; 82: 369.
9. Bearn AG, Miller ED: Archibald Garrod and the development of the concept of inborn errors of metabolism. *Bull History Med* 1979; 53: 315.
10. Garrod AE: About alkaptonuria. *Lancet* 1901; 2: 1484–6.
11. Bateson W: *Mendel's Principles of Heredity*. Cambridge, 1902.
12. Bateson W: *Report of the Evolution Committee of the Royal Society (London) December 17, 1901*. London, 1901, p. 133.
13. Garrod AE: *Inborn Errors of Metabolism*. Cambridge, 1909.
14. Bearn AG: Inborn Errors of Metabolism. 1. Archibald Garrod and the Birth of an Idea. 2. Present Concepts and Future Directions. Lettsoonian Lectures, February 9 and 23, 1976.
15. Beadle GW: Genes and the chemical reactions in Neurospora. Nobel Lecture. December 11, 1958, *Nobel Lectures in Medicine or Physiology 1942–62*. Amsterdam, London, New York: Elsevier, 1964, p. 59.

This chapter has been reproduced from Loriaux, D. Lynn: Archibald Edward Garrod (1857–1936). *The Endocrinologist* 1992; 2(5): 284–6.

CHAPTER 43

John J. Abel

(1857–1938)

Isolation of Hormones

On January 13, 1893, William Osler, the well-known physician who was then the professor of medicine at Johns Hopkins University School of Medicine, wrote to John J. Abel, the 35-year-old professor of materia medica and therapeutics at the University of Michigan's medical school, to ask: "On what terms could you be dislocated?"

Osler's faculty had, the day before, decided that it needed a professor of pharmacology and authorized him to approach Abel. At that time, although it had appointed several professors and its affiliated hospital had been open for several years, the Hopkins medical school had no Department of Pharmacology and, in fact, had no students. The planned opening of the school had been delayed because of a shortage of money; its endowment income had suffered from the recession of the mid 1890s. The school sought the needed money from a group of wealthy Baltimore women who agreed to provide it on condition that women be admitted on an equal basis with men. The trustees and faculty took some time to agree and thus delayed the opening of the school.

Osler approached Abel because the school was finally going to open in the fall of 1893. Abel had been at Michigan for less than 2 years and the Michigan position was his first job. He had been hoping for, and had trained for years, to assume a research-oriented academic position in which he could apply chemistry to the problems of human disease (a chancy idea at the time as there were then few full-time chemistry or biochemistry faculty in American medical schools and no full-time pharmacologists except Abel himself). There was, however, some further delay in the financing from the women's group so Abel did not receive a definite offer from Johns Hopkins until March 2, 1893. He accepted 5 days later with the proviso that his actual title be professor of pharmacology and not professor of materia medica. He thus became the first such professor in the United States.

The distinction made all the difference to him and to the discipline to which he would make immense contributions. His aim was to establish pharmacology as an independent investigative discipline, based on the chemistry of drugs and of the body,

---

A Biographical History of Endocrinology, First Edition. D. Lynn Loriaux.

This work is a co-publication between the Endocrine Society and John Wiley & Sons, Ltd.

which would be parallel to, but separate from, physiology, and to distinguish it clearly from materia medica, then taught by rote lectures with little fundamental understanding of the theory and practice of prescribing drugs.

Coincidently, Abel came to Baltimore at the same time that hormones, not then named as such, came to the medical and public eye as potent regulators of body function. The main thread that runs through his career, though by no means the only one, is the isolation of the active principles of endocrine glands. He saw this as essential to establish the reality and credibility of these substances and necessary to determine ultimately their structure and synthesis. Overall, in this specific venue, he had only modest success. He determined no hormonal structure, defined no hormone's action and, in fact, successfully isolated only one hormone in his lifetime, insulin. This isolation was itself surrounded by controversy. Nevertheless, he clearly focused attention on the need to define the endocrine substances being given to patients and, because of his premier position and the commitment of his new school to "scientific" medicine, became a leader and mentor to others who in turn spread the pharmacologic word through North America.

Abel was born, the oldest of eight children, to German immigrants in Cleveland, Ohio, on May 19, 1857. He was named after his maternal grandfather, John Jacob Becker. He was an excellent student in high school and went on to the University of Michigan in 1876. He left the University for financial reasons after only 3 years, during which he took only a few science courses. He worked for 3 years as a principal, and then superintendent of schools in La Porte, Indiana, a modest-sized town about halfway between South Bend and Gary. While in La Porte, for unclear reasons, he decided on medicine as a career with a leaning toward research rather than practice. There, he also met his future wife.

In the late nineteenth century and often well into the twentieth century, one did not need an undergraduate degree to go to medical school. Abel debated whether to get direct training in research, to go directly to medical school, or to return to college. He chose the last and graduated from the University of Michigan in 1883 with the PhB degree, Bachelor of Philosophy. He married that summer and spent the next year (1883–1884) at Johns Hopkins University as a graduate student with Henry Martin, the British-trained physiologist. He then planned to spend 2 years in Europe with Carl Ludwig, the world-famous physiologist, before returning to the United States to study for a PhD. This planned 2 years in Europe stretched out to 7 years, perhaps the longest incubation of any American scientist of his time. Finances were tight; he managed on loans from his father and, later, on money sent by his wife who returned to the United States in 1889 to work as a nutritionist in Boston, Massachusetts. Abel felt he needed clinical as well as laboratory experience and his wife agreed. After his 2 years with Ludwig, he went to Strassburg, then in Germany as a result of the 1870 Franco-Prussian war, to learn physiological chemistry with Felix Hoppe-Seyler. Once there, however, he switched to the pharmacologic laboratory of Oswald Schmiedeberg, mainly because the laboratory was better equipped and the professor more accessible. This serendipitous switch was his first real exposure to the new discipline of pharmacology.

Because he believed it would be hard to find a purely academic position in the United States and that he would likely have to practice part-time medicine, he got his MD, rather than PhD, from Strassburg in 1888. That year was not a good one for the young couple. A search for a position in the United States yielded nothing, and their 3-year-old daughter died of poliomyelitis. A clinical year in Vienna followed, and then Abel moved to Berne, Switzerland, to do biochemical work. By the end of his European experience he had studied not only with Ludwig, Hoppe-Seyler, and Schmiedeberg but also with the internist Adolf Kussmaul, the pathologist Friedrich von Recklinghausen, the neurologist Wilhelm Erb, the metabolic physician Bernhard Naunyn, the neurologist and therapeutist Hermann Nothnagel, the biochemist and pharmacologist Edmund Drechsel, and the medical chemist Marceli Nencki. It is a striking array.

In early 1890 Abel got an offer from the University of Michigan's medical dean (who had taught him in his fourth year of college) to teach physiological chemistry. The details and salary were vague so Abel deferred the offer until the next year. Then, because of local politics, Michigan's dean wrote again in July 1890 that he could offer Abel the chair of materia medica and therapeutics. Abel accepted it at a salary of US$2000, probably thinking of it as a stepping-stone to better jobs in biochemistry. He arrived in Ann Arbor in 1891 to find no laboratory equipment, no on-going research, and no demonstrations of drug effects in the medical students' curriculum. He had to start from scratch.

He went back to Europe the next summer, 1892, for more study and brought back laboratory equipment in November. By then he had started his research again, finished one project, reorganized the medical pharmacology course with actual animal demonstrations for the class, and begun an advanced laboratory course for a select few students. Thus he stood when Osler wrote him two months later.

In 1893, aged 35 years, Abel had published only six research papers, including his MD thesis, all but one in German and in German journals. This was, in part, because there were no American journals for biochemistry or pharmacology, in part because he was in German-speaking lands when the work was done, and in part because Abel was emotionally attached to German science. This publication record, skimpy though it would be for us today, was in fact not seen by the Johns Hopkins medical faculty as something negative. They knew Abel, or at least his reputation, from his post-graduate year in Baltimore, his previous letters inquiring as to positions, and chance meetings with him in Europe. He was alone in the United States in the quality and extent of his training. He fit the model that the Johns Hopkins medical school had adopted: an adaptation for all students of the German "learn-by-doing" approach based on the assumption that training in basic science would lead to better physicians.

Abel did not, in fact, teach pharmacology that first year in Baltimore (1893–1894). Pharmacology was planned as a second-year class. Instead, he was asked to teach physiological chemistry to the 75 first-year students, which he did as the school had no one else to teach it. Although Abel delegated the biochemistry course to others after only 1 year, the school had no separate biochemistry department for 15 years. Although minor, this episode shows the ambivalence of the most "modern" medical faculty to newly arising areas in the "basic" sciences and is an example of how blurred were disciplinary lines at the time. Abel is in fact seen by some as one of the founders of American biochemistry, although he agreed to take on its teaching only as a stopgap "to give us time to look about."

Abel was not a strong lecturer nor was he eager to lecture. He thought teaching medical student a most important activity, but often found himself otherwise occupied when the time came to do it. His fame arose from his laboratory, its lunchtime conversations, and its reputation. He stayed at the Johns Hopkins School of Medicine for the rest of his career and, in 1932 at age 75 years (39 years after he began), he was the last of the original faculty to retire.

The 1890s were the beginning of the active age of internal secretions, later named "hormones" by Vesey, Hardy, and Starling in 1904. Because these glandular extracts were almost immediately and widely used for a range of reasons soon after Brown-Séquard's rejuvenative claims beginning in 1889, and because Murray demonstrated specific benefit of thyroid extract in a defined thyroid illness, myxedema, in 1891, there was intense interest in the nature of the active principles of these glandular extracts. Within a year of Abel's arrival at Johns Hopkins, he was attempting to find the essence of thyroid extract. Progress was painfully slow. When the German chemist Eugen Baumann discovered iodine in the thyroid gland in 1895 and made a thyroid preparation called iodothyrin, Abel ceased work on the thyroid without publishing anything and shifted to another gland, the adrenal, even though Baumann's preparation was fairly crude and was not itself the thyroid's active principle.

The adrenal, or suprarenal gland, had just been shown by George Oliver and Edward Schafer in England (1894–1895) to have a powerful effect on blood pressure. Many thought that a cure for Addison's disease was in the offing (at the time, no one made the necessary distinction between the adrenal cortex and medulla, which took another 20 years to be fully realized). Abel and his colleagues attacked the problem with vigor. By 1897 he reached seeming success. They made crystals–a major criterion of uniformity and purity–of sheep adrenal extracts and named the substance "epinephrine" (from the Greek *epinephros*, "on top of the kidney"). Success, though seemingly hard-won, was not at hand. It turned out that what was isolated was a monobenzoyl derivative of the actual adrenal material, a fact realized in 1901 by others who got both the isolation and molecular weight more or less right. Abel was forthright about his failure to take the last one or two steps but bitterly disappointed. Nevertheless, he came as close to isolating the first chemically identified hormone as it is possible to come without actually doing so, and certainly laid down 95% of the path taken by others.

Although Abel continued to write about the adrenal until 1905 (a total of 15 papers) and lost his right eye in a laboratory explosion while trying to improve his preparation in 1900, he shifted again, away from glands, to study mushroom poisons (1906), laxatives (1909), and cardiac function and tetany in frogs (1910). His experience with the adrenal allowed him to find epinephrine in a tropical toad's parotid gland (1911), an example of "the prepared mind." His curiosity about whether free amino acids existed in blood led to the "vividiffusion" apparatus (1913–1914), a precursor of the modern hemodialysis machine. His technique was too primitive to work for long in animals or to work at all in humans, but it did manage to keep dogs with severe renal failure alive for a few days longer. In 1912 he was honored, probably for his adrenal work, by election to the National Academy of Sciences.

It is hard, however, to turn away from what one thinks is truly important. Abel came back to hormones. He made a pass (read: "worked intensively for months") at the duodenal hormone secretin, probably in 1913–1914, but nothing was published. In 1915, after Kendall had isolated his crystals of thyroxin, Abel went back again and again to the thyroid gland. He tried an enzymatic isolation technique, gentler than Kendall's, for isolating the gland's hormone and designed a few experiments to try to show that the thyroid gland secreted thyroxin into the thyroid veins, the true mark of a hormone. Nothing came of these attempts, either.

About 1917, he took up the posterior pituitary gland, which by then (albeit in the midst of World War I) was known to have powerful oxytocic and antidiuretic activities. The idea that guided his approach to purification of these activities was that there was only one hormone with two activities. He first thought that this hormone was histamine (1917) but backed away from this idea by 1920. In part because of this persistent unitary belief, he never succeeded in isolating or even highly purifying either hormone, although he worked at it off and on for over 10 years. Vincent du Vigneaud, one of Abel's postdoctoral fellows in 1927–1928, went on to isolate and synthesize mammalian oxytocin and vasopressin and won the Nobel Prize as a result.

The hormone of most interest to all in the 1920s was insulin, after Frederick Banting, Charles Best, J. Bertram Collip, and John J.R. Macleod showed in 1921–1922 that a stable, active pancreatic extract could reliably lower the elevated serum glucose concentration in pancreatomized dog (the four names were listed alphabetically at Macleod's suggestion). This "cure" for juvenile diabetes mellitus brought "scarecrow" looking children back to health and won a Nobel Prize for Banting and Macleod the very next year, 1923. No one knew what insulin actually was in a chemical sense, and the extract was recognizably impure. The discoverers themselves did not think it was a protein.

In 1924, Abel saw an opportunity for his talents. He was by now 67 years old. Many scientists in Europe and North America were trying to find out what insulin was. Abel thought that he did not have the expertise or financial backing to attack the problem. But that year, Arthur Noyes, a chemist at California Institute of Technology and fellow member with Abel in the National Academy and on the editorial board of its *Proceedings*, suggested that Abel come to Pasadena and work on the crystallization of insulin. Supplies and the large amount of crude insulin needed would come from a yearly grant of US$12 000 given to Noyes by a local physician for insulin work. So Abel left for Pasadena in October, 1924, with an associate from Johns Hopkins.

Abel stayed in Pasadena for four months. While there, with his chemical "nose," he made a key observation. He smelled something sulfur-like in one of the biologically active fractions of crude insulin that he was making and found that the biologic activity paralleled the sulfur content. He could now speed up his trials. Instead of doing tedious bioassays to track insulin's activity in the various fractions, he could simply measure the sulfur content, much as Kendall had used iodine to track thyroxine in his thyroid fractions 10 years before. Abel took the project back to Baltimore and on a Saturday afternoon in October (or perhaps November), 1925, achieved a major success. He saw insulin crystals under his microscope. While this success did not change patients' treatment (it was too costly to prepare the crystals and the cruder preparations worked reasonably well), getting crystals of anything was seen as a key to purity, structure, and synthesis. It also promised better therapy.

Abel's work was reported in the *Journal of the American Medical Association*, in the *British Medical Journal*, and in many newspapers as a great achievement. Within two months, the work was in print in the February 1926 issue of the *Proceedings of the National Academy*. Abel easily got support from the Carnegie Foundation (US$10 000) and drug companies (US$6000) for his insulin work. But, as had happened to Kendall in the year after he isolated thyroxine crystals, disaster struck. Beginning in March 1926, Abel could get no crystals. Further, his work was widely criticized in Europe and America because his data also implied that insulin might be a protein (although in 1926 he did not say so). At the time, "everyone knew" that proteins were large, inactive molecules of little or no biologic activity. Although proteins might carry or loosely bind other active molecules, the active substances themselves could not be proteins. Abel did not accept this criticism, but his thesis was hard to defend when he himself could not make the crystals.

In the meantime, James Sumner of Cornell was criticized for the same reason when he wrote that he had crystallized the protein enzyme urease in August 1926. Whether enzymatic or hormonal, biologically active molecules "could not" be proteins. Theory clearly overwhelmed the evidence. But Abel persisted as he always did. Now 69 years old, he was able to make insulin crystals again by January 1927 and never lost the knack again.

This did not, however, answer the criticism that insulin was actually some small molecule absorbed in some way to crystals of something else. There was no simple way to rebut this critique. In a sense, it was like trying to prove that something is not so. After 1927, Abel left the problem to others in his laboratory but watched over it like a mother hen. The approach chosen was to recrystallize the insulin crystals and see if the activity was the same as that of the old ones. Although not a direct disproof of the "adsorption" critique, it was reasonably acceptable to the criticizers because it seemed unlikely, a priori, that a substance would adsorb nonspecifically to a crystal of something else in the same ratio time after time. The laboratory thus aimed for crystallizing to constant specific activity.

The problem with this criterion, itself somewhat "soft," is that it requires a valid standard insulin preparation as a benchmark against which to compare the crystals. By 1929, the British scientists, who generally opposed equating Abel's crystals with insulin, had completed a comparative study of Abel's crystals with others and found that all had about 24 U/mg of biologic activity. Most were now convinced that Abel was right. George Barger, the co-synthesizer of thyroxine with Charles Harington, was convinced simply by the physical beauty of the crystals themselves. Nevertheless, in the absence of a "clean" proof, the controversy died down slowly over the 10 years or so after Abel first got his crystals. The insulin crystals, although they did not directly affect patient care, showed that insulin was a homogeneous substance, permitted the validation of an international insulin standard, and led the way to the determination of insulin's structure. Insulin was, in fact, a protein.

Abel's laboratory was a place of high intellectual stimulation, in large part because Abel facilitated the talk and because those who came almost always had advanced degrees (Abel was opposed to PhD degrees in pharmacology and Johns Hopkins did not grant them until 1969). The quality was not produced by Abel directing his "students" to key problems. These "post-docs" were basically "turned loose… to sink or swim," an educational approach that caused a "great deal of mental anguish." Quality was certainly not evident in the facilities. Abel's laboratory was a third-floor walk-up in a building notably dingy most of his career. There was no elevator and even the dumbwaiter had to be worked by hand. The laboratory was poorly equipped (a single microscope, ancient kymographs) and poorly heated (workers often needed extra clothes in the winter) with no heat at all at night. The talk at the daily lunch-table (an old kitchen table in the laboratory covered with oilcloth) was legendary and it took the place of seminars, attended by visitors from around the world. The cockroaches in the laboratory, no doubt enticed by the leftovers of the Spartan bread and cheese lunches were equally legendary. No one opened the laboratory door without first stepping back to let the roaches run away, nor put on a hat to leave without first shaking it out. Budgets were tiny and one wonders at the comparison with modern laboratories. No one now would consider for a moment working in a laboratory like Abel's. Yet the famous Flexner Report of 1910 called the laboratory facilities "unexcelled." Perhaps those at other schools were even worse.

It was not just with his laboratory that Abel professionalized pharmacology. He began new journals and societies so that like-minded scientist would have places to publish and talk. He stimulated the start of the *Journal of Experimental Medicine* (1896) and was a principal in both the *Journal of Biological Chemistry* (1905) and the *Journal of Pharmacology and Experimental Therapeutics* (1909), which he edited for 23 years until his retirement. He also took the lead in organizing the American Society of Biological Chemists (1906) and the American Society for Pharmacology and Experimental Therapeutics (1908). These organizational stimuli, originating as they did from a locus of high prestige, may have done as much or more for Abel than his laboratory to make him the man who made pharmacology in the United States.

Abel's attraction to endocrinology and his independent, almost stubborn, streak persisted after his retirement. When he was 75 years old, he and his co-workers were set up in a separate Laboratory for Endocrine Research, funded by the Carnegie Foundation (note that the overhead was only 3%!). His colleagues worked on hormones, especially insulin, but he chose, for reasons known only to him, to work on tetanus toxin. He published three papers in his last year of life, and was in his laboratory almost until the day he died, at age 81 years, on May 26, 1938. He left an estate of US$103 000.

No one is perfect in life or in science. Abel was both forgetful and single-minded. Few now recall his influence on the field of endocrinology. But, despite his limited success at his chosen goal, the isolation of hormones, he did succeed with insulin and late in life at that. His broader success was in keeping medicine's eye sharply focused on chemically identifiable hormones and not allowing it to drift back, as it persistently tended to do, into the vagueness of glandular extracts.

Sources

Abel JJ: Chemistry in relation to biology and medicine with especial reference to insulin and other hormones. *Science* 1927; 66: 307–19, 337–46. A personal overview of his hormonal work.

Kohler RE: *From Medical Chemistry to Biochemistry: The Making of a Biomedical Discipline*. Cambridge, Cambridge University Press, 1982, 399 + ix pp. Has a number of entries on Abel.

Lamson PD: John Jacob Abel. A portrait. *Bull Johns Hopkins Hosp* 1941; 68: 119–57. Another personal view with tales of Abel's laboratory.

MacNider, WdeB: Biographical memoir of John Jacob Abel. 1837–1938. *Biogr Mem Natl Acad Sci* 1946; 24: 231–57.

Murnaghan JH, Talalay P: John Jacob Abel and the crystallization of insulin. *Perspect Biol Med* 1967; 10: 334–80. Excellent on the insulin story.

Parascandola J: *The Development of American Pharmacology: John J. Abel and the Shaping of a Discipline*. Baltimore, MD: Johns Hopkins University Press, 1992. 212 + xxvii pp. This is a superb resource and is the main one used for this essay: the only thing better is the Chesney Archives at Johns Hopkins Medical Center and the book is naturally easier to use.

Rosenberg CE: Abel, John Jacob Abel. 1857–1938. *J Pharmacol Exp Ther* 1939; 67: 373–406. A personal view with some material on unpublished work.

This chapter has been reproduced from Sawin, Clark T: John J. Abel (1857–1938) and the isolation of hormones. *The Endocrinologist* 1995; 5(6): 391.

CHAPTER 44
Oskar Minkowski (1858–1931)
Diabetes and the Pancreas

Oskar Minkowski was born in Alexoten, in Tsarist Russia. In 1872, antisemitic ordinances forced the family to leave Russia for Königsberg in Prussia. Oskar went to medical school at the University of Königsberg. His mentor in medical school, Bernhard Naunyn, was invited to become the professor of medicine in Strasbourg, and he took Minkowski with him as a young assistant professor.

It was in Strasbourg that Minkowski met Joseph von Mering and they discussed a commercial preparation of pancreatic enzymes, Lipanin, which von Mering asserted was necessary to break down fatty acids in the gut. Minkowski was skeptical. He proposed that they test the hypothesis by examining fatty acid metabolism in a pancreatectomized dog. Pancreatectomy was widely believed to be an operation that no experimental animal could survive, but Minkowski was sure that he could do the operation successfully. He attempted the operation the same afternoon. The surgery was a technical success and the dog survived the immediate postoperative period. It was in this period that Minkowski observed the abrupt appearance of polyuria, polyphagia, and polydipsia. He correctly deduced that the factor responsible for glucose homeostasis was pancreatic in origin and that pancreatectomy led to diabetes mellitus. This was the first fundamental breakthrough in elucidating the pathophysiology of juvenile diabetes [1] and paved the way for the subsequent extraction of insulin from pancreas.

Two years later, in 1891, Minkowski gave a lecture to the Strasbourg Society of Natural Science and Medicine which was published in the *Berliner Klinische Wochenschrift*. In this lecture, he pointed out again that pancreatectomy caused diabetes in the dog. More importantly, however, he showed that a pancreatic autograft under the skin could prevent the diabetes from appearing [2].

Minkowski next moved to Breslau as chief of the Department of Internal Medicine. His fame spread, and he was soon chairman of the German Association of Internal Medicine. He was known at the time as one of the greatest consultants in internal medicine in all of Europe.

A Biographical History of Endocrinology, First Edition. D. Lynn Loriaux.

This work is a co-publication between the Endocrine Society and John Wiley & Sons, Ltd.

Minkowski married Marie Johanna Siegel in 1894. Their daughter Laure, with her husband and two sons, fled the Nazi regime to Argentina. She died in Buenos Aires in 1983. Minkowski's son, Rudolph, was an astronomer at the Mount Wilson Observatory and has a galaxy named in his honor. Minkowski died in Fürstenberg, Mecklenburg on June 18, 1931. His remains are buried in the cemetery on Heerstrasse in Berlin, protected as a national historical monument.

References

1. von Mering J, Minkowski O: Diabetes mellitus nach pankreasexstirpation [in German]. *Arch Exp Pathol Pharmakol* 1890; 26: 37.
2. Minkowski O: Weitere mittheilungen uber den diabetes mellitus nach exstirpation des pankreas [in German]. *Berliner Klin Wochenschr* 1892; 29: 90–4.

This chapter has been reproduced from Loriaux, D. Lynn: Oskar Minkowski (1858–1931). *The Endocrinologist* 2006; 16(1): 1.

CHAPTER 45

Frederick Gowland Hopkins (1861–1947)

Vitamin(e)s and Biochemistry

In 1912, the *Journal of Physiology*, the United Kingdom's premier journal in this field, published an article entitled, "Feeding experiments illustrating the importance of accessory factors in normal dietaries" [1]. The author, Frederick Gowland Hopkins, was then 51 years old and a reader in chemical physiology at Cambridge University. He was also praelector in biochemistry at the University's Trinity College, a position he had held for just 2 years. Hopkins was by then well established, but his field of biochemistry was not. During that time, biochemistry was seen mainly as a branch of physiology (as was histology). The apparently banal title of his article, however, caught the attention of the world of scientific medicine and it was, in fact, the clearest and most forceful statement to date that what we now call vitamins actually existed.

Ninety years ago, no vitamin had ever been isolated and none had a known chemical structure. The evidence came solely from feeding experiments performed in laboratory animals. These experiments used "purified" diets that were not, in fact, particularly pure nor were they easy to duplicate. The idea of performing controlled experiments was in its infancy and was not always insisted on or seen as necessary. The parallel between feeding experiments and dietary deficiency was new and not universally accepted. After 6 years of work, Hopkins' article brought clarity to the problem. He achieved this through a combination of well-controlled studies in rats, a careful review of previous publications (some of which were unknown to him when he began), recognition of the similarity between dietary diseases in humans and disturbed growth in rats eating artificial diets, and by looking at what constituted a minimally complete diet.

Although Hopkins shared a Nobel Prize in 1929 for this work, it was only a marginal part of his career. His odd lifeline would not have gotten him far today. He had no PhD, which is now an absolute necessity for a university appointment. He was known, by those who recall him at all, as the founding father of British biochemistry based on his discovery of vitamins.

Hopkins grew up in Eastbourne, England, where he was born in 1861. His family was solidly middle class and worked in business. Frederick's parents had married in

A Biographical History of Endocrinology, First Edition. D. Lynn Loriaux.

This work is a co-publication between the Endocrine Society and John Wiley & Sons, Ltd.

London where most of the family lived, but moved soon after their wedding to Eastbourne. His father died when Frederick was an infant. Though there were sufficient funds to support the small family, Hopkins' childhood was a lonely one.

At age 10, he and his mother moved to Enfield, not far from London, to live with his maternal grandmother and an uncle, James Gowland. At first Hopkins did well at school, particularly in chemistry, and seemed on his way to Cambridge. However at the age of 14 he decided that he would rather wander the countryside and the city of London while pretending to his family that he was at school. After some weeks of this, including a summer vacation, the truth came out. He was asked to leave the school by the headmaster. Hopkins recalled that this was the only time he had ever spoken with the headmaster. The university was no longer possible. After three more years in private school, his uncle arranged a position as a clerk in an insurance firm. This lasted only a few months. Frederick then became an apprentice to a chemical analyst. Although interesting at first, the job was tedious and long. Hopkins later thought the only benefit might have been that he was trained to be careful and precise in the laboratory.

When his grandfather died, he left Frederick a modest inheritance. At age 20, Cambridge was again a possibility, but instead he chose to learn chemistry and attended the Royal School of Mines in London. There, he did surprisingly well and became an Associate of the Institute of Chemistry. He was interested in attending medical school, which was then the only real way to get a higher degree in a biomedical science, but money was not available. So, at that point, with his knowledge of chemistry expanded, he went to work for Thomas Stevenson, who was the "Medical Jurist" at Guy's Hospital in London. Stevenson's task was to perform chemical analyses in cases of possible poisoning deaths and to testify in court. As a result, when Hopkins came to work for Stevenson, he was involved in the analyses for several famous murder trials, such as the case of a woman accused of killing her husband by having him swallow chloroform. Hopkins spent 5 years working for Stevenson. He recognized the need for a degree if he were ever to get ahead so he attended the "external program" of the University of London. In that way, he could learn while he kept his job. It meant that he had to do almost all his studying during the 3 hours each day that he traveled on the train to and from work. He got his London BSc in 1887.

With Stevenson's help, Hopkins was admitted to Guy's Hospital Medical School in 1888. He was awarded the first Gull Studentship, named after W.W. Gull, who first described adult myxedema. This award came with some financial support and the obligation to perform some investigation. Hopkins managed to do both. He had a retentive memory and no fear of hard work.

In 1890, he traveled to the Continent to visit the famous clinics. He caught a glimpse of Pasteur himself when he was in Paris. He thought that the Parisian hospitals had "extraordinarily bad nursing arrangements." By the time he finished medical school and qualified to practice, in 1894, he had published eight articles, all on the chemical analysis of some bodily substance. He had invented a new assay for urinary uric acid. His work was recognized well enough that he was elected a member of the Physiological Society in 1892. Clearly, he was more than the usual medical graduate. At 33, he was older than most by several years. He was a highly trained chemical analyst who had begun to study aspects of what we would call biochemistry.

Hopkins was taken on as a demonstrator in practical physiology at Guy's under the guidance of the famous physiologist Ernest Starling. Over the course of the next 4 years, 1894–1898, Hopkins taught physiology and worked in the laboratory. He turned out 12 papers during this time, three of which were co-authored with Archibald E. Garrod and six of which were published in 1898 alone.

At Guy's, perhaps influenced by Starling, Hopkins added to his studies of well-known urinary compounds such as urobilin, and the study of proteins. The dominant theory at the time was that proteins in the body were simply part of an agglomeration "protoplasm," that had no particularly distinct features. Hopkins thought, however, that it was indeed possible to analyze proteins. He was able to crystallize egg albumen, making the point that a particular protein had a constant composition. In doing so, he began the destruction of the prevailing "protoplasmic myth" and was on his way to defining intracellular compounds as definable and measurable. In a sense, this idea was a major founding stone of modern biochemistry. He was now 37 years old and in quite a junior position. More importantly there were no positions in London for a scientist interested in the chemistry of life, biochemistry.

At a meeting of the Physiological Society in 1898 in Cambridge, Michael Foster, the doyen of British physiology, took Hopkins aside for a chat. Foster was internationally famous by that time. He had been a professor of physiology at Cambridge for 28 years and a Fellow of the Royal Society for more than 14 years, but had not been able to build the chemical side of his discipline. He asked Hopkins if he would do just that. Hopkins was paid only £200 per year, an amount somewhat more than the average laborer. His new position did not include a Fellowship at any of Cambridge's colleges, which would have provided free housing and other benefits. The job was not just to work in the laboratory. He had to teach the entire class of medical students what they needed to know in the field of chemical physiology. When he arrived in Cambridge, Hopkins also found that he was responsible for teaching gross anatomy to some students. Whatever the work entailed, this was an opportunity and Hopkins took it.

While carrying out his teaching duties for the next 12 years, Hopkins also achieved much in the laboratory, despite its primitive facilities. He performed all of his analyses and maintained his rats. The floor centrifuge was not attached and wandered around the laboratory when in use.

His first major discovery was an "accident." In the student laboratory one day, Hopkins was supervising an experiment that required an assay for protein. The test was to add sulfuric acid to a solution of an unknown in glacial acetic acid. A violet color showed that there was protein in the unknown. The assay, however, failed to work with the control solution protein. Looking further into it, Hopkins realized that the assay itself was poorly founded. The color reaction was not caused by the acetic acid, but rather by a contaminant of glyoxylic acid. The acetic acid used on the day when the test failed was a purer batch than most.

Hopkins asked why protein reacted with glyoxylic acid. He was able to isolate a crystalline substance that gave a powerful color reaction in this assay. It had been known for some time that trypsin hydrolysates of some proteins gave a red color when bromine water was added. This reaction was called the tryptophane reaction because it made a color appear (*phane* from the Greek "to appear") from the tryptic digest. Because the newly crystallized material also gave a strong tryptophane reaction, Hopkins called it "tryptophane," named after the reaction. The name was later shortened to "tryptophan," as being more in keeping with biochemical convention. Hopkins had isolated a new amino acid that others had been hunting for some time, and he had made another mark in his career. The article, published in 1901, appeared in a physiology journal and not in a biochemical one. There were biochemical journals in Europe, but none in the United Kingdom. Hopkins was elected to the Royal Society in London.

The next year, Hopkins was promoted from lecturer to reader (about the same as associate professor in the United States) There was a modest increase in salary. He pursued the tryptophane problem as an issue in nutrition. Was this amino acid important, and, if so, in what way? Feeding experiments in rats showed that it was important. Rats without tryptophane in their diets died. Tryptophane was an essential amino acid. When he wrote about that diet in 1906, he wrote, "It is suggested that the tryptophane is directly utilized as the normal precursor of some specific 'hormone' essential to the processes of the body." Thus, he linked nutrition and endocrinology only one year after his old colleague, Starling, had first used the word "hormone."

In that same paper in 1906, he raised the hypothesis that there were essential dietary needs other than particular amino acids. He was well aware that there were disorders in humans, such as scurvy and rickets, which were curable by certain foods. He thought that whatever it was in those foods that helped people with these diseases they could be examples of specific essential dietary substances. In retrospect, other European workers had the same idea, but Hopkins did not know of their work. They had either published in Dutch, not a widely read language by non-Dutch scientists, or in German journals in articles with obscure titles. From this point on, Hopkins performed a long series of feeding experiments culminating in the publication of the article, 6 years later, that led to the Nobel Prize.

Emmanuel College at the University gave him the position of science tutor. The new title came with a great deal of teaching. It also came with a Fellowship at Emmanuel.

The work that got Hopkins really interested in intermediary metabolism was somewhat of an accident. There were conflicting data on how lactic acid was handled by muscle. Some thought its production by muscle occurred with any contraction, and others that it was produced only when the muscle became fatigued.

These questions seem minor today, but at the time, the idea that one could quantitatively assess what was going on inside a muscle cell by assaying specific analytes was a novel idea. Hopkins wanted to look at the problem in detail and worked on it from 1905 to 1907 with a colleague, Walter Fletcher. Using contracting muscle of frogs, they found that lactic acid was produced with contraction and that, with rest, the lactic acid disappeared. Without oxygen, the lactic acid kept accumulating. Thus, no special chemistry was needed to study muscle metabolism.

Hopkins' abilities came to the fore in the muscle experiments. Two major contributions were technical. He ground up the muscle before analysis in ice cold alcohol rather than at room temperature, and he made the assay for lactic acid more precise and accurate. The first avoided glycogen breakdown to lactic acid in the process of performing the experiment. The second gave quantitative results that could be trusted. He knew that he had to use controls for every experiment, something not everyone did in those days. Henry Dale, who worked with Hopkins as a student, said, of Hopkins' report on lactic acid, published in 1907: "Few papers in the history of physiology can have had so great an influence." Note that Dale was still referring to Hopkins as a physiologist and not a biochemist. The Biochemical Society was not founded until a few years later in 1911.

While Hopkins' main interests were intermediary metabolism and proselytizing for the recognition of biochemistry as a discrete discipline, he continued his feeding experiments. In 1910, he had a major personal setback. He struck his head on an iron staircase in his laboratory and soon afterward, cardiac symptoms and "months of extreme mental and bodily discomfort" developed. He was unable to work, and he feared that his career might be over. Fortunately, he recovered within the year, a recovery perhaps enhanced by the fact that Trinity College in Cambridge elected him a Fellow and appointed him to a praelectorship in biochemistry. The former assured him a more substantial income and the latter, though technically still only the equivalent of an associate professorship, was the appointment that he prized most, a true appointment in his discipline. The 49-year-old Hopkins finally had a position in which he could devote all of his time to teaching in his chosen field and to the laboratory, and Trinity asked no more of him than that.

For a few more years, his minimalist facilities seemed to be enough. He began his search for "essential" dietary components. There was no particular rush to print. In essence, Hopkins performed carefully designed feeding studies in rats fed diets containing all the protein, fat, and carbohydrate needed for normal growth but in pure form so that little was in them other than these dietary elements. What happened was that the rats grew poorly despite a good appetite and completely adequate intake of calories. Remarkably, whatever it was that was needed for good growth was present in 2–3 mL of milk added to an otherwise constant diet. The growth curves were startling: growth was flat without the milk and perfect with it.

Hopkins had not actually identified any particular "vitamine," as these mysterious factors had been called by Casimir Funk, nor had anyone else. Funk was a Polish immigrant then working at London's Lister Institute. He had obtained his PhD in Bern, and worked on steroid chemistry. He became quite famous for his work on vitamins (the terminal "e" was dropped in 1920). In the United States, he performed a great deal of work for commercial vitamin companies. During 1911 and 1912, Funk visited Hopkins during the Christmas holidays to discuss his "vitamines". The result was that Hopkins supported Funk for one of the prestigious Beit fellowships that would enable Funk to continue his work.

Hopkins' 1912 article pulled together much of the world's literature and removed many objections that others had towards the idea of the existence of these essential, or "vital," dietary factors. The rats did not find the diet monotonous and did not eat less. They consumed the same amount of calories as the rats that ate a normal diet. He also showed that absorption of the food was not a factor in the failure to grow. Even more important, Hopkins made it quite clear that the interpretation of dietary experiments hinged on the use of proper controls. Anyone who has performed these experiments in animals knows the importance of control over the dietary components and of the absolute need to use controls in all studies. His results were measurable and quantitative. This part alone convinced many who were intolerant of results presented without numbers. He was even more explicit in tying together the historical information on diseases such as scurvy and rickets with the concept of dietary needs. By linking all these ideas with his data, Hopkins' article drew widespread attention to the matter.

Hopkins' won the Nobel Prize in 1929, sharing it with Christiaan Eijkman who, in 1890, cured malnourished chickens with an experimental diet. Hopkins' work was not without controversy. Some just did not believe it. Some tried to repeat his studies and failed. Hopkins was lucky. Milk does not contain only one vitamin, nor does it contain all vitamins. To some degree, it was a fluke that his experiments worked as "cleanly" as they did. The failure of others to repeat his studies was probably caused by subtle variables in the composition of the experimental diets and also by the fact that rats are coprophagic and can obtain vitamins made in the gut that are excreted into but not absorbed from the lower intestine.

Hopkins' response to these objections was exemplary. Rather than bicker or argue about possible reasons why others failed to get his results, he took the objections seriously. He went back to his laboratory, and simply repeated his own studies and tried to duplicate those of others. Usually, he got the same result that he got previously. Vitamins were nevertheless considered theoretical substances by some until the 1920s. Hopkins spent most of World War I studying nutrition, writing reports on the dietary needs of people in the United Kingdom, and advising his government on food policy. In 1920 the British Medical Association had a meeting in Cambridge on vitamins. There were many skeptics. One announced that "as far as their composition is concerned, [vitamins] seem to be a figment of the imagination." Some feared the accusation of quackery. Could anyone adopt as real something that had no known chemical composition? The issue was not settled until the chemical structures of these molecules were elucidated.

Hopkins was promoted to a newly created professorship of biochemistry in 1914. He got a new laboratory in 1920. It was an abandoned chapel, but was definitely better than what he had before. Then, with the help of truly significant private donations, the Dunn Institute was created and Hopkins was named to head it as professor in 1921. He was 60 years old, and held this position for 22 years, until 1942. He worked until the day he died. His last paper on glyoxylate was published posthumously in 1948.

Hopkins was a small, slender man who walked to work every day. His colleagues thought his major talent was attention to detail and precision. He made connections that others had missed. His approach to controversy was moderate and not overtly critical. He would simply ask questions that brought light to the issue. Because he had never worked with a true professional chemist, he thought himself "an amateur intellectually." He wrote no book. He presented lectures that were appreciated by all who listened. He thought it better to explain what was not yet known than to dwell completely on what we did know.

Hopkins gathered many honors, including 12 honorary degrees from universities around the world. Both Cambridge and Oxford so honored him, as did Harvard University in the United States at its tricentennial in 1936. He was asked to be, and served as, President of the Royal Society for 5 years from 1930 to 1935. His biochemical legacy is clear. He died on May 16, 1947, at age 85, after several difficult years, including progressive blindness that seemed not to dampen his desire to continue in the laboratory. He managed. As he said of himself, "I know well how much I owe to fortunate circumstances and to happy chance."

Reference

1. Hopkins FG: Feeding experiments illustrating the importance of accessory factors in normal dietaries. *J Physiol* 1912; 44: 425.

Sources

Dale HH: Frederick Gowland Hopkins.1861–1947. *Obituary Notices of Fellows of the Royal Society* 1948; 6: 115.

Fletcher WM, Hopkins FG: Lactic acidin amphibian muscle. *J Physiol* 1907; 35: 247.

Harris LJ: *Vitamins in Theory and Practice.* Cambridge: Cambridge University Press, 1955, Chapter 1.

Harris LJ: The discovery of vitamins. In *The Chemistry of Life,* edited by J Needham. Cambridge: Cambridge University Press, 1971, p. 156.

Harrow B: *Casimir Funk. Pioneer in Vitamins and Hormones.* New York: Dodd Mead, 1955.

Hill AV: *Trails and Trials in Physiology.* Baltimore, MD: Williams and Wilkins, 1966, pp. 2–5.

Hopkins FG, Cole SW: A contribution to the chemistry of proteids, Part I. A preliminary study of a hitherto undescribed product of tryptic digestion. *J Physiol* 1901; 27: 418.

Needham J: Sir Frederick Gowland Hopkins, O.M., F.R.S. (1861–1947). *Notes Records R Soc London* 1962; 17: 117.

Needham J, Baldwin E (Eds.): *Hopkins and Biochemistry 1861–1947.* Cambridge: Heffer and Sons, 1949.

Willcock EG, Hopkins FG: The importance of individual amino-acids in metabolism: Observations on the effect of adding tryptophane to a dietary in which zein is the sole nitrogenous constituent. *J Physiol* 1906; 35: 88.

This chapter has been reproduced from Sawin, Clark T: Frederick Gowland Hopkins (1861–1947), vitamin(e)s, and biochemistry. *The Endocrinologist* 2001; 11(6): 437–42.

CHAPTER 46

George R. Murray
(1865–1939)
Treatment of Hypothyroidism

In 1891, George R. Murray was a young physician, 26 years of age, in Newcastle-upon-Tyne, England, without a hospital or medical school appointment. Then, in July of that year, he reported his successful treatment of a woman with myxedema to the British Medical Association assembled in Bournemouth, England. He told them of a revolutionary new approach, the subcutaneous injection of sheep thyroid extract, and the conspicuously clear-cut improvement in the patient's condition.

Murray had good reason to try this odd therapy of injecting a glycerine–phenol extract from a common farm animal into a patient. His mentor, Victor Horsley, had helped show that it was the lack of the thyroid gland that produced the myxedematous condition. Hypothyroidism was common to patients with cretinism, those who had thyroidectomy, and patients with spontaneous myxedema with an atrophic, fibrotic thyroid gland.

Horsley had investigated the problem of the causation of myxedema through much of the 1880s and had done the first experimental thyroidectomies to show that clinical hypothyroidism follows upon the removal of the thyroid gland. His work was done as part of a multifaceted investigation sponsored by the Clinical Society of London. The results of the investigation, done by a committee whose work took 5 years to complete, became the famous "Myxoedema Report." The actual Report is entitled the "Report of a Committee of the Clinical Society of London, nominated December 14, 1883, to investigate the subject of Myxoedema."

The Committee's findings were presented on Friday, May 25, 1888, to the Society at its last meeting of that academic year. Usually sparsely attended, there was a crowd this year. The interest in myxedema was not only local. This disease, though clinically rare, aroused interest not only because it resembled the ancient disease of cretinism, but also because its understanding might shed light on the role of the thyroid gland, heretofore an organ with no known function.

The Committee's final conclusions stand today:

> a general review of symptoms and pathology leads to the belief that the disease described under the name of myxoedema, as observed in adults, is practically the same disease as that named

A Biographical History of Endocrinology, First Edition. D. Lynn Loriaux.

This work is a co-publication between the Endocrine Society and John Wiley & Sons, Ltd.

> sporadic cretinism when affecting children; that myxoedema is probably identical with cachexia strumipriva; and that very close affinity exists between myxoedema and endemic cretinism.

The Committee also noted that "while these several conditions appear ... to depend on ... destruction or loss of the function of the thyroid gland, the ultimate cause of such destruction or loss is at present not evident."

The Committee's results were rapidly picked up in the United States. Notes, abstracts, or editorials commenting on the Committee's work appeared in medical journals published in New York City, Philadelphia, Cincinnati, and Indianapolis, some within a month of the Committee's final presentation. However, the Committee, despite its modern-sounding and ultimately accurate conclusions, offered nothing substantial in the way of therapy. Specifically, they did not connect thyroid deficiency with any suggestion of thyroid replacement.

Some had tried implantations of thyroid tissue in animals or humans in the 1880s in an attempt to overcome the deleterious effects of the gland's removal. Moritz Schiff, an Italian and Swiss physiologist, tried to prevent death in dogs after thyroidectomy by implanting part of a dog's own thyroid gland into its abdomen. Theodor Kocher, the famous Swiss surgeon, and the only person to win a Nobel Prize for studying the thyroid gland, also tried this in a man after thyroidectomy with little success. Neither had any real understanding of what the gland did and their procedures were really "shots in the dark."

The year after the Myxoedema Report, in 1889, the Parisian physiologist and physician, Charles-Edouard Brown-Séquard, who was then in his 70s, startled the medical world with his announcement that testicular extracts from dogs and guinea-pigs, injected into an older man with failing powers (i.e., himself), brought about a reversal of some of these deficiencies. In a matter of months, this therapy, now called organotherapy, was extended to extracts of other organs for the treatment of many diseases. As it happens, Brown-Séquard never did try thyroid extracts for myxedema and we know now that his organotherapy's effects were largely those of a placebo. Organotherapy, though viewed with suspicion by some, was well-regarded and accepted by many respectable physicians, including practitioners in the United Kingdom and the United States. The therapy spread through the western medical world, and from there to Russia.

After the Myxoedema Report there were further efforts to transplant thyroid glands from sheep and monkeys into patients with hypothyroidism, now with a clearer rationale. Although Horsley himself was a strong advocate of this approach to therapy for hypothyroidism, he seems not to have tried it himself but urged others to do so (perhaps the rarity of the disease or his burgeoning interest in neurosurgery got in the way). In any case, such implants were tried in France, the United Kingdom, and Switzerland with varying success. There were occasional claims of true vascular connections but, overall, the results were sketchy at best. Sometimes there was a transient effect, the disappearance of which was attributed to the disintegration of the implant.

About this time, 1890, Murray advanced Horsley's idea of implantations by suggesting that injection of a thyroid extract could accomplish the same thing. Admittedly, injections would have to be more or less continual as opposed to a single permanent therapy. Horsley was not too supportive, but told Murray that it was worth a try. Murray was ridiculed by his own local medical society in Newcastle but went ahead after his father, a respected local practitioner, referred him a patient with myxedema. In the spring of 1891, he made his crude extract by simply mincing a sheep thyroid gland in glycerine, adding a few drops of phenol (as a disinfectant), letting the mixture sit for a while, and then straining the result through cloth. He injected the pinkish liquid under the patient's skin with a hypodermic syringe. Benefit was apparent in a few weeks. There was a cure for the incurable.

Murray knew that with only a single case he had to be cautious in his claims. However, in the late spring of 1891, Horsley had read of another case treated by sheep thyroid implant. The authors concluded that the rapid onset of the benefit must have been due to resorption of thyroid juice from the implant and not from the generation of true vascular connections. The authors, Antonio-Maria Bettencourt Rodrigues and Jose-Antonio Serrano of Lisbon, had presented their patient almost a year before, in August 1890, at the annual meeting of the French Association for the Advancement of Sciences in Limoges [1]. One can assume an influence of Brown-Séquard in the author's interpretation of their results. Horsley read only the French abstract [2] before Murray had either presented it to an audience or published, and quickly wrote to Murray that he should "publish at once", which he did. Murray was widely and justifiably credited with a major advance in therapy, one that put the success of Brown-Séquard's organotherapy on a much firmer footing.

What Horsley had not done was read Bettencourt and Serrano's complete paper, which was published in early 1891 in the proceedings of the Association's meeting [3]. There, they not only noted that benefit was likely due to absorption of thyroid juice, but also stated that when they returned home to Lisbon, they planned to treat their next patient with this disease with hypodermic injections of glandular juice ("chez une autre malade, atteinte aussi de myxoedeme et actuellement à la 'Maison de sante,' nous proposons d'essayer les injections hypodermiques de *suc* glandularie") [2]. Their presentation in Limoges in the summer of 1890 was only a proposal, but the proposal was exactly the same as Murray's, conceived later that same year (1890) but unknown to him or, apparently, to anyone else in England. Bettencourt and Serrano did, in fact, find a patient after they returned to Lisbon and proposed the therapy. She initially refused to have this strange treatment but, after she became worse a few weeks later, she agreed. Bettencourt reported their results to the Lisbon Society of Medical Sciences on November 15, 1890 "after four or five injections ... experienced notable improvement; the sensation of cold in the dorsal region disappeared, her movements are easier, and she sleeps well. The menstrual periods are now regular, and the areas of alopecia have disappeared" [3].

There was little notice of their report. It was published only as a note in the proceedings of the Society and, as it was in Portuguese, few outside Portugal saw it. Murray's reputation was made for the rest of his life. It is clear that, whatever might be the issue of priority, so dear to competitive scientists, the idea of how one might treat hypothyroidism was "in the air" as a result of the confluence of the Myxoedema Report and Brown-Séquard's therapy. Treatment of hypothyroidism with thyroid extract, bizarre though it may have seemed at the time, was in fact the first successful endocrine therapy and helped establish endocrinology as a discipline.

References

1. Bettencourt A-M, Serrano J-A: Un cas de myxoedème traité par la greffe hypodermique du corps thyroïde d'un mouton. *Semin Med* 1890; 10: 294.
2. Bettencourt-Rodrigues A-M, Serrano J-A: Un cas de myxoedème (cachexie pachydermique) traité par la greffe hypodermique du corps thyroïde d'un mouton. *Comptes Rendus de l'Association Française pour l'Avancement des Sciences* 1891; part 2: 683.
3. Bettencourt-Rodrigues A-M: Communicaçöes scientificas. *J Soc Sci Med Lisboa* 1890; 15: 114.

Sources

Brown-Séquard C-É: Des effets produits chez l'homme par les injections souscutaneés d'un liquide retiré des testicules frais de cobaye et de chien. *C R Soc Biol* 1889; 41: 415.

Merklen P: Sur un cas de myxoedème amelioré par la greffe thyroïdienne. *Bull Mém Soc Méd Hôp Paris* 1890; 7: 859.

Murray GR: Note on the treatment of myxoedema by hypodermic injections of an extract of the thyroid gland of a sheep. *BMJ* 1891; 2: 796.

Ord WM (Chairman): Report of a committee of the Clinical Society of London nominated December 14, 1883, to investigate the subject of myxoedema. *Trans Clin Soc Lond* 1888; 21(Suppl.): 1–215.

Osler, W: The thyroid gland and myxoedema. *Med News* 1885; 46: 381.

This chapter has been reproduced from Sawin, Clark T: The invention of thyroid therapy in the late nineteenth century. *The Endocrinologist* 2001; 11(1): 1–3.

CHAPTER 47

William Bayliss and Ernest Starling (1860–1924) (1866–1927)

Molecular Messengers

At the end of the nineteenth century, the prevailing wisdom was that the pancreas secreted its juice in response to a meal by means of a local neural reflex. Food went from the stomach to the duodenum and small intestine, where it stimulated local nerves to tell the pancreas to secrete the fluid and enzymes needed for the food's digestion. The leader in this work was the wellknown Russian physiologist Ivan Pavlov, who developed the experimental model and techniques to study digestive physiology during the last decades of the nineteenth century. It was for this work that he won one of the early Nobel Prizes (1904). Pavlov and his coworkers were firmly committed to the idea of neural control of the entire digestive process, including pancreatic function.

In England, a pair of younger workers were attacking the same general problem. Ernest H. Starling was a brilliant, ebullient, impatient, and outgoing man of limited financial means who trained as a physician at Guy's Hospital Medical School. There he won every prize in sight and qualified as MB in 1889. He had become enamored of physiology and stayed on at Guy's Hospital to devote himself to experiments rather than to medicine. The pay was low, but it was his life.

By 1899, Starling had published over two dozen papers on the physiology of the heart, the body fluids, and the gut. He had written a short textbook. He had delivered the Arris and Gale lectures to the Royal College of Surgeons on lymph formation (1894), the development of ascites (1896), and on congestive heart failure (1897). He had an excellent reputation and was a forceful advocate for physiology. He was indefatigable in the laboratory although he was personally "rather bored with details of technical method." In 1899 he was elected a Fellow of the Royal Society. He was the outspoken man who rose from a low beginning solely through merit, the prototype of the new scientist, the professional.

The other Londoner, William M. Bayliss, was some years older than Starling, with a very different personality. Bayliss was wealthy by birth and his career began slowly. He was thoroughly learned and probably as brilliant as Starling, though quietly so.

A Biographical History of Endocrinology, First Edition. D. Lynn Loriaux.

This work is a co-publication between the Endocrine Society and John Wiley & Sons, Ltd.

In contrast to Starling, he was cautious, methodical, loved to work with his hands and to "do it himself." He was calm where Starling was ardent; Bayliss had the better critical judgment.

After finishing school, Bayliss tried his father's business for a while but this did not suit him. He then began the study of medicine, entered University College London, won several prizes or scholarships and a BSc degree (1882). He was greatly influenced by two professors, John S. BurdonSanderson and E. Ray Lankester, to think of physiology as a career. He never got to be a physician as he foundered on the anatomy examination, which he failed, and gave up medicine for good. What he did between 1883, when he seems to have left medical school, and 1885 is unclear, but in that year, he followed BurdonSanderson, now professor of physiology, to Oxford. There he enrolled to pursue another undergraduate degree, now in the natural sciences. The 25yearold student was much older than most of his classmates (he was known to them as "father Bayliss" both because of his age and his beard) but made friends with them easily and graduated with firstclass honors in 1888. Then he returned to London to work for BurdonSanderson's replacement at University College, Edward A. Schäfer, as an assistant in physiology. At first, transportation from his home to the laboratory was difficult so he solved the problem for a while by building his own laboratory at home. But London's public transportation system soon expanded so, after a few years, he did most of his work in the University College laboratory. The pair, Bayliss and Starling, exemplified the transition in the late nineteenth century from science as something one did if one could afford it to science as a profession worthy of itself.

Starling's facilities at Guy's were meager and funds for research were almost nil. Shortly after his official appointment to the faculty at Guy's, he sought resources and help from Schäfer's laboratory at University College. Schäfer was helpful and invited Starling to work in his laboratory, where he met Bayliss. The two opposites seemed hit it off from the beginning. They began work on the electrical activity of the mammalian heart and within a few months published their first paper together. Over the next 16 years they were to publish 21 papers.

Although they did not work together after 1906, they remained close friends for life and, in fact, became brothersinlaw after Bayliss married Starling's sister, Gertrude, in 1893. Starling moved permanently to University College in 1899 when Schäfer resigned to become professor of physiology at Edinburgh. Starling's appointment to the professorship at University College put him, the younger man, in charge of Bayliss. This did not seem to matter. Their work together continued, if anything, at a greater rate. Bayliss remained an assistant until 1903 when he became assistant professor. After 1912, he was professor of general physiology, a position created expressly for him in a field he hoped to develop into a discipline independent from medicine.

Their work varied. Starling was the more famous but Bayliss' personality seems to have been oblivious to that. Starling was the demanding and insistent purveyor of his discipline, urging better facilities for experiment and pushing for his own designs in medical education. Bayliss was the more relaxed on these topics and eager to get on with his laboratory work. He was the skilled experimenter. They focused for a while on the heart in the 1890s. They then broadened their view to include studies of arterial and venous flow and the neural control of the heart and of blood flow to various organs. By the end of the 1890s, their studies on the blood supply and innervation of the gut established that food moved through the digestive tract by contraction of the gut from above with relaxation below.

They were puzzled, however, by the relationship of the gut to the pancreas. If food were to be digested in a coordinated manner, there had to be linked neural contraction and relaxation and properly timed release of bile and pancreatic juice; otherwise, digestion would not proceed apace. Because all control seemed neurological, there had to be a neural connection from the gut to the pancreas. Pavlov was convinced that there was such a connection. He thought that when acid reached the duodenum, the low pH stimulated nerves in the wall of the small intestine which, in turn, reflexly stimulated the pancreas. The reflex had to be local because, even though vagal stimulation brought about this secretion, acid still brought about this secretion when the vagi were cut. But what nerves mediated the action? In 1900 and 1901 other workers had repeated Pavlov's experiment and had cut the sympathetic nerves as well as the vagi. Acid still stimulated the pancreas to secrete. Some of these other works concluded that the neural pathway must be from the pyloric wall to scattered ganglia in the nearby pancreatic head. Others, however, were able to show that acid did not have to be put into the duodenum to stimulate the pancreas. It would work just as well if it were put into the jejunum, even when reflux back into the duodenum was prevented. The conclusion had to be that the ganglia involved were in the solar plexus.

Bayliss and Starling already had experience with investigating the local reflexes of the small intestine, including the jejunum. They realized that they might be able to extend their work by looking at the problem of pancreatic secretion. They first wanted to do a control experiment because previous workers had not done it. If the solar plexus nerves were the pathway for local reflex, then it would be best to remove these nerves and see whether the acid still stimulated the pancreas. The earlier discovery that acid put into the jejunum, as well as into the duodenum, stimulated the pancreas was critical for them. Anatomically, one cannot easily free up the duodenum and ensure that all nerves are removed, but one can do this with the jejunum.

So it was, that on January 16, 1902, the two physiologists and a few onlookers isolated a jejunal loop in one female dog and dissected and divided all mesenteric nerves. The loop was "connected to the body of the animal merely by its arteries and veins." First they made sure that the animal's duodenum showed the expected response. It did: acid introduced into the duodenum brought about a brisk secretion of pancreatic juice. They expected that the totally denervated jejunum would not show the same response. They predicted no pancreatic secretion in the complete absence of intestinal nerves. But the opposite happened: acid put into the jejunum elicited the same response as it did when put into the duodenum. They immediately realized that the pathway to the pancreas had to be via the blood. They knew that what went through the blood to stimulate the pancreas was not the acid itself; that had been tried and it failed. The messenger had to be something released from the gut by the acid.

They immediately took the same jejunal loop from the same dog, cut it out, scraped off the intestinal mucosa, ground it up with sand and a little hydrochloric acid, filtered it, and injected the crude extract into a peripheral vein of the dog. There was an immediate, nonspecific fall in blood pressure followed in about 70 seconds by a clear increase in pancreatic secretion. They had shown for the first time that a humoral substance, carried by the blood stream and completely independent of the nervous system, was the mediator of a physiologic action.

Charles J. Martin, a Londoner who was an exact contemporary of Starling and a professor of physiology in Melbourne, was visiting Bayliss and Starling that day in 1902 and was in the room during the experiment. He later wrote in Starling's obituary that when Starling saw the pancreas secrete vigorously after putting acid into the denervated jejunum, he said, "Then it must be a chemical reflex" [1].

The two physiologists moved quickly. They showed in a day or so that a duodenal or jejunal extract, without prior exposure to acid, had no effect, whereas an extract of ileum, which had no effect on pancreatic secretion, did lower the blood pressure. So the hypotensive effect had to be due to a different substance than the one that stimulated the pancreas. The pancreatic effect depended on prior instillation of acid into the gut, which meant that the pancreatic stimulator existed in an inactive form in the gut wall before acid converted it to the active material. Because the active substance (or "body" as they called it) increased pancreatic secretion, they called it secretin and the precursor was then prosecretin.

This was the first use of the prefix "pro"to identify a hormonal precursor. All of this, including the names, was written up in less than a week and sent to the Royal Society. As noted, Starling was a member. The Society received the short twopage paper on January 22, 1902, six days after the experiment and the paper was read the next day. It was in print shortly thereafter.

This classic experiment by Bayliss and Starling, along with the lengthy followup studies they performed during the rest of that year, is sometimes thought to be the origin of modern endocrinology. Bayliss and Starling were, however, not the first to think that organs might make substances that affected other organs via the blood stream, nor were they the first to present experimental support for the idea. Beginning in 1889, Charles-Edouard BrownSéquard had made organ extracts and claimed biologic effects when they were injected. In 1891, George R. Murray did the same with a thyroid extract. This time there was a clear and powerful biologic action. It proved to be a successful treatment for the disease of myxedema. Schäfer himself knew well the effects of glandular extracts. He and George Oliver had shown in the 1890s that the adrenal gland contained a potent pressor agent. The idea that there were biologic effects of the socalled "bloodglands" was a current one in the 1890s. What was different about Bayliss and Starling's remarkable finding was twofold. First, they connected the biologic effect of a tissue extract with parallel evidence that the active substance actually circulated through the blood to give the same biologic effect, and second, they showed such an effect was not limited to the recognized vascular glands.

Secretin took most physiologists by surprise. To them, neural control of the gut was an "established" fact. It seems unlikely, however, that BrownSéquard, Murray or others of similar mind were surprised at all. The idea of internal secretions as a major regulatory system of the body was only beginning to take hold of scientists' minds.

It had simply not filtered through to those whose focus was the heart or the gut. Perhaps the failure of BrownSéquard's work to be confirmed and the excesses of some in calling it a "fountain of youth" kept the cautious away from the concept.

Pavlov learned of Bayliss and Starling's work through an abstract journal and did not believe it. He had two of his colleagues inject various tissue extracts and concluded that any effect on the pancreas was nonspecific. He held on to his neural hypothesis. But when Bayliss and Starling published the complete version of their work later in 1902, Pavlov asked another colleague in the fall of 1902 to repeat the English experiment exactly. Pavlov's student Boris P. Babkin, writing almost 50 years later, remembered that

> the effect of secretin was selfevident. Pavlov and the rest of us watched the experiment in silence. Then, without a word, Pavlov disappeared into his study. He returned half an hour later and said, "Of course, they are right. It is clear that we did not take out an exclusive patent for the discovery of truth" [2].

Bayliss and Starling went on to check a range of other animals and performed further studies from January to March, 1902, when they completed their work. Publication was "delayed by extraneous circumstances". The full 29page description of their studies on secretin appeared in the fall of 1902 in the *Journal of Physiology*. This paper is a classic in both endocrinology and physiology. They wanted to be sure that sercretin was not peculiar to dogs. It was not; they found it in every mammal they studied, including humans. They were also careful to note that they had not excluded a neural effect but had only added a humoral one. They felt, however, that a neural effect was unlikely to play much of a physiologic role. They also showed that secretin, partially purified, stimulated the pancreas. They never attempted to find what we now know as gastrin. In fact, they dropped the project altogether with a remark that "we are unable to continue these experiments" and never again studied the humoral control of digestion.

After 1902, as a result of Bayliss and Starling's work, humoral mediation in biology left the realm of the questionable and became a clear part of the mainstream of physiologic thinking. There still were debates over whether or not a particular phenomenon was humoraly mediated or not. That there was a humoral mechanism, essential to much of physiology, was no longer in doubt.

Neither Bayliss nor Starling pursued humoral internal secretions after 1902. Both advocated recognition of these secretions as an important regulatory system of the body. In their Croonian Lecture to the Royal Society in 1904, entitled "The chemical regulation of the secretory process," they described their work on secretin in detail and suggested that secretin represented but one part of an integrated system of chemical messengers. They wanted, however, a better term for "chemical messenger." They wanted a single word that would convey the idea. After much discussion in the laboratory, one of their colleagues, William B. Hardy, discussed the problem with his classical colleague at Cambridge, W.T. Vesey, who thought that "hormone" would be good. He derived the word from the Greek word όρμή, meaning "to stimulate or arouse." The next year, in June, 1905, Starling gave a different set of Croonian Lectures to the Royal Society of Physicians, reviewing what was known about these chemical messengers and used the new word for the first time in public: "'hormones' ... as we might call them."

Bayliss continued to be the quiet man and spent his time investigating the control of osmotic pressure in the 1900s and studying enzymes and their mode of action in the 1910s. By 1908 he had written an entire treatise on enzymes which was so popular that it went into five editions, the last being published by his son, Leonard, after the senior Bayliss died in 1924. The senior Bayliss spent the better part of 2 years writing and personally illustrating his renowned *Principles of General Physiology*, which reflected his life's work and which went through several editions before he died. He dedicated this "summa" of his career to Starling, his "fellowworker." Though he was personally willing to talk and discuss physiology with anyone, his text assumed high competence on the part of the reader. The text itself was not easy. It included a good deal of biochemistry and physical chemistry. Although his hope for a separate discipline of general physiology never came to pass, the book was so popular that "Bayliss clubs" formed at several American universities specifically to discuss it. The text did not die with Bayliss. Decades later his son, retiring early from his position as reader in physiology at University College, spent several years completely revising his father's text. This fifth edition of 1960 was the last.

Bayliss was elected to the Royal Society in 1903. Other honors included a knighthood in 1922. One might have almost predicted that this modest man was somewhat annoyed that, to be knighted by the King, he had to go to Buckingham Palace and miss a meeting of the Physiological Society. He died in 1924 of a "blood dyscrasia."

Starling was a textbook writer as well, but aimed more at the medical community. He began with his *Essentials of Human Physiology* in 1892, which went through many editions, and came out with a large text, *Principles of Human Physiology*, in 1912. This book was also popular among students. It went to four editions during Starling's lifetime. After his death in 1927, his text went on for several more decades. One of his students, and a successor to his professorship at University College, Charles Lovatt Evans, edited the textbook until 1958.

The two physiologists, Bayliss and Starling, brought respectability to internal secretions in an era when there was confusion and uncertainty. Their discovery was a major one simply in terms of physiological knowledge. It put the discipline of endocrinology on solid footing. Their memory lives on in the Bayliss and Starling Society, which still meets yearly in the United Kingdom.

References

1. Martin CJ: Ernest Henry Starling – 1866–1927. *Proc R Soc Lond B* 1927; 8: 102: xvii.
2. Babkin BP: *Pavlov. A Biography*. Chicago, IL: University of Chicago Press, 1949 [1974].

Sources

Bayliss LE: William Maddock Bayliss, 1960–1924; life and scientific work. *Perspect Biol Med* 1961; 4: 460.

Bayliss WM: *Principles of General Physiology*. London: Longmans, Green and Co., 1915.

Sir William Maddock Bayliss – 1866–1924. *Proc R Soc Lond* 1925; 6: 99: xxvii.
Bayliss WM, Starling EH: On the causation of the socalled "peripheral reflex secretion" of the pancreas. (Preliminary communication). *Proc R Soc Lond* 1902; 69: 352.
Bayliss WM, Starling EH: The mechanism of pancreatic secretion. *J Physiol* 1902; 28: 325.
Bayliss WM, Starling EH: Croonian Lecture. The chemical regulation of the secretory process. *Proc R Soc Lond* 1904; 73: 310.
Chapman CB: Ernest Henry Starling. The clinician's physiologist. *Ann Intern Med* 1962; 57 (Suppl. 2). Includes a complete bibliography.
Chapman CB: Starling, Ernest Henry. *Dictionary of Scientific Biography* 1975; 12: 617.
Colp R Jr: Ernest H. Starling. His contribution to medicine. *J Hist Med Allied Sci* 1952; 7: 280.
Evans CL: *Reminiscences of Bayliss and Starling. First BaylissStarling Memorial Lecture.* Cambridge: Cambridge University Press, 1964.
Evans CL: Bayliss, William Maddock. *Dictionary of Scientific Biography* 1970; 1: 535.
Hill AV: Bayliss and Starling and the happy fellowship of physiologists. The third BaylissStarling memorial lecture. *J Physiol* 1969; 204: 1.
Rolleston HD: *The Endocrine Organs in Health and Disease with an Historical Review.* London: Oxford University Press, 1936, p. 2.
Starling EH: The Croonian Lectures on the chemical correlation of the functions of the body. *Lancet* 1905; 2: 339, 423, 501, 579.
Starling EH: *Principles of Human Physiology*. London: J. & A. Churchill, 1912.
Verney EB: Some aspects of the work of Ernest Henry Starling. *Ann Sci* 1956; 12: 30.
Winton FR: Bayliss, Leonard Ernest. *Dictionary of Scientific Biography* 1970; 1: 533.

This chapter has been reproduced from Sawin, Clark T: William M. Bayliss, Ernest H. Starling, and the discovery of secretin. *The Endocrinologist* 1998; 8(1): 1–5.

CHAPTER 48
Harvey Williams Cushing (1869–1939)
Pituitary Basophilism

Harvey Cushing arose from Puritan stock rich in the medical tradition. Matthew, the first Cushing in America, sailed from Gravesend on the *Diligent* in 1638. He arrived in Boston on the tenth day of August and settled in Hingham, Massachusetts. Harvey Cushing arrived eight generations later. His great grandfather, David, was a physician in Stafford Hill, Vermont, and both his grandfather, Erastus, and father, Henry, were physicians in Cleveland, Ohio. Harvey was the last of 10 children born to Henry Kirke and Betsy Maria Williams Cushing. Educated in the Cleveland public schools, he was a popular student and was elected president of his senior class. He went to Yale, where he was distinguished primarily by athletic prowess. He played shortstop and right field on the varsity nine during his last 3 years. Amos Alonzo Stagg, who pitched on that championship team, recalled "that Harvey was good at batting and in fielding and in running" [1].

Cushing entered Harvard Medical School in 1891. In his second year, he worked as an anesthetist for Maurice Richardson, James Warren, and John Homans, surgeons at the Massachusetts General Hospital. The death of a patient while he was administering anesthesia focused his attention on the haphazard approach to the administration of volatile anesthetics. Cushing and a friend, Amory Codman, developed a system for the continuous recording of temperature, pulse, and respiration on a flow chart throughout an operation. This allowed the anesthetist and surgeon to tell, at a glance, the condition of the patient. Later, Cushing encountered the Riva-Rocci pneumatic blood pressure recording device in Pavia and modified the chart to include blood pressure. This chart is our anesthesia record of today [2]. Thus, as a second-year medical student, Harvey Cushing made an important contribution to modern surgical technique.

This experience set Cushing's career on a "surgical" path from which he never deviated. He was appointed a surgical extern and then intern at the Massachusetts General Hospital upon graduation and, the following year, joined the surgical program at Johns Hopkins Hospital under the legendary William Halsted. After a year as assistant surgical resident, he was appointed to the prestigious surgical resident position in

A Biographical History of Endocrinology, First Edition. D. Lynn Loriaux.

This work is a co-publication between the Endocrine Society and John Wiley & Sons, Ltd.

1897. Halsted was "of indifferent health" stemming from an addiction to cocaine that grew out of studies of its properties as a local anesthetic. As a result, the hospital surgical service was left largely in the hands of the surgical resident. Cushing performed admirably and was appointed an instructor in surgery for the next 2 years.

Following a year abroad in the great clinics of Europe, Cushing returned to Hopkins as a junior staffman in 1901. He was a "latch-keyer," one of the young physicians living in the house at 3 West Franklin Street next door to William Osler. He was given a latch key to the Osler house so that he could come and go as he pleased. He married Katherine Crowell, a childhood friend and fiancée of 2 years, on June 10, 1902. They were married for 37 years and had five children.

Cushing remained at Hopkins until 1912. His great achievement in these years was the experimental delineation of the effects of hypophysectomy in the dog. This led naturally to an interest in patients with disorders of the pituitary gland. Of particular interest is the early formulation of the disorder now referred to as Cushing's syndrome. Five cases of the "pluriglandular syndrome," as Cushing called it, are described, in *The Pituitary Body and its Disorders*, published in 1912 [3]. The best example is case number XLV, a young woman with painful obesity, amenorrhea, and hirsutism. After describing her case, he notes:

> It will thus be seen that we may perchance be on the way toward the recognition of the consequences of hyperadrenalism. Heretofore the only recognizable clinical state associated with primary adrenal disease has been the syndrome of Addison, and the grouping of these cases may possibly add one more to the primary maladies of the ductless glands.

Previous cases of this syndrome had been linked to neoplasms of the adrenal gland. In this case, however, the clinical findings were those of increased intracranial pressure and progressive constriction of the visual fields. Accordingly, an operation was performed in September of 1911. A "wet brain with low grade hydrocephalus" was revealed, but no tumor found.

In 1912, Cushing was recruited to Harvard Medical School as professor of surgery and surgeon-in-chief at the new Peter Bent Brigham Hospital. He worked there for 20 years. During this time, he established the field of neurosurgery in the United States. Landmarks of the period include the refinement and, in some cases, the development, of operations for ablating the Gasserian ganglion in trigeminal neuralgia, transsphenoidal and transfrontal hypophysectomy, and operations for meningioma and acoustic neuroma. He was largely responsible for introducing cautery and bone wax to neurosurgical technique.

With the outbreak of the First World War, Cushing formed the surgical unit that staffed Base Hospital No. 5, the unit that sailed for France on May 11, 1917, and remained there until the end of the War in November, 1918.

Cushing operated intensively during this period, primarily on wounds of the head and spinal cord. In the midst of the conflict he contracted a strange illness characterized by fever, loss of deep tendon reflexes, paresthesia of the palms and soles of the feet, and muscle wasting. It was diagnosed as "trench fever" or "polyneuritis ambulatoria." Remarkably, in the course of this illness it was discovered that both femoral arteries were completely thrombosed. Were it not for documented disease in the larger arteries it would be tempting, in retrospect, to diagnose Buerger's disease: Cushing was an incessant lifelong smoker. In any event, claudication dated from this time. It became so severe in the later years of his career that he would stay in the hospital for days to avoid walking and would be brought to and from the operating room by wheelchair.

It was during the War that Cushing's friendship with William Osler took an unexpected and tragic turn [4]:

> Thursday, 30 August 1917 .... Rather used up, I was preparing to turn in at 10 last night, when came this shocking message: "Sir Wm. Osler's son seriously wounded at 47 C. C. S. Can Major Cushing come immediately?" The C. O. let me have an ambulance, and in a pouring rain we reached Dosinghem in about half an hour. It could have been worse, though there was a bare chance – one traversing through the upper abdomen, another penetrating the chest just above the heart, two others in the thigh, fortunately without fracture. The local C. O. would not let me cable, and I finally insisted on phoning G. H. Q. – got General Macpherson on the wire and persuaded him to send to Oxford via the London War Office: "Revere seriously wounded, not hopelessly: conscious: comfortable."
>
> Crile came over from Remy with Eisenbrey, and after a transfusion, Darrach, assisted by Brewer, opened the abdomen about midnight. There had been bleeding from two holes – in the upper colon and the mesenteric vessels. His condition remained unaltered, and about seven this morning the world lost this fine boy, as it does many others every day.
>
> We saw him buried in the early morning. A soggy Flanders field beside a little oak grove to the rear of the Dosinghem group – an overcast, windy, autumnal day – long rows of simple wooden crosses – the new ditches half full of water being dug by Chinese coolies wearing tin helmets – the boy wrapped in an army blanket and covered by a weather-worn Union Jack, carried on the shoulders by four slipping stretcher bearers. A strange scene – the great-great-grandson of Paul Revere under a British flag, and awaiting him a group of some six or eight American Army medical officers – saddened with the thoughts of his father. Happily it was fairly dry at this end of the trench, and some green branches were thrown in for him to lie on. The Padre recited the usual service. A bugler gave the "Last Post" and we went about our duties. Plot 4, No. 7

Lady Osler wrote a few days later:

> Dearest Harvey, Our one comfort is that you were with him – No one in the world could have done as much and no one been fonder of him – I can only think what an agony it was for you when you saw him come in. You will tell us everything I know, Dear Revere, he was living for his leave – a letter last evening told what we would do – I hope he knew you and could talk to you. It is very hard – and we are getting old. There was a fine life in store for the boy – but it couldn't be. I always expected this to happen – but I never could be ready. Our Love, Grace Osler.

Cushing was to know this pain first-hand when, in 1926, his eldest son William was killed in an automobile accident while an undergraduate at Yale University. Cushing recovered, but William Osler could not. He caught the influenza in the great pandemic and it evolved into chronic empyema, from which he died on the afternoon of December 29, 1919. In his room was found a slip of paper on which he had written these words: "The Harbour almost reached after a splendid voyage with such companions all the way and my boy awaiting me" [5].

Grace Osler asked Harvey Cushing to undertake the "official" biography of her late husband. It required more than 4 years to complete. The two-volume *Life of Sir William Osler* [6], published by Oxford University Press in 1925 and awarded a Pulitzer Prize in 1926, remains a classic of American medical biography. In addition to this work of a lifetime and his demanding surgical schedule, still more was accomplished. During his years at Brigham it is estimated that Cushing wrote 5000–10 000 words each day. In addition to the Osler biography and the voluminous scientific material, there are four books: *Consecratio Medici and other Papers* [7], *From A Surgeon's Journal* [4], *The Medical Career* [8], and *A Bio-bibliography of Andreas Vesalius* [9].

The events surrounding the recognition of "pituitary basophilism" as a clinical entity began with Cushing's preparations for the Lister Lecture in 1930. In the course of his reading, he chanced upon a paper from Prague by Dr. William Raab in which a case was described that resembled in every way a case of "pluriglandular syndrome" under his care. The Raab case was found at autopsy to have a small basophilic adenoma of the pituitary gland [10]. Shortly thereafter, H.M. Teel, a former resident of Cushing's, published a second case of pluriglandular syndrome associated with a basophilic adenoma of the pituitary gland [11]. Cushing, in contrast to his predecessors, recognized that the clinical syndrome was likely to be the result of the basophilic adenoma rather than the cause of it. In the famous monograph of 1932, he presented 12 cases to make the point [12]. Ten of the cases were extracted from the literature; two were his own. These two were case XLV from the 1912 monograph and "case 11," the dentist under his care at the time of the "Raab revelation." Neither had died at the time the 1932 monograph was published and Cushing could not be sure of a basophilic adenoma in either. Three years later, however, case 11 died and, on hearing of this, Cushing persuaded the widow to allow an exhumation autopsy. The long-suspected basophilic adenoma was revealed. Cushing was 63 years old.

Cushing's retirement from the Brigham was not an amicable one. The new chief thought it best that Cushing be insulated from the day-to-day activities of the surgical department, a decision that did not "set well" with Cushing who, at the peak of his professional career, had much yet to give. He accepted a position as professor of neurology at Yale, his alma mater, and left Boston on October 12, 1933. His departure from the institution that he had "put on the map" passed largely unnoticed.

> Harvard University, now separated from this vigorous pioneering spirit, could settle back into a more peaceful way of life without his periodic agitation about medical education, the full time plan, internationalism, and the sanctity of the Common. Yale in its turn regained her most eminent son in medicine, and she also acquired a unique pathological collection and one of the great libraries of our time [1].

Cushing's final years were marked by honor upon honor and by the increasing ravages of arteriosclerosis. On the evening of October 3, 1939, an attack of substernal pain occurred that intensified through the night. Signs of heart block developed the next day. For 2 days his heart beat at a rate of 30 per minute and, on the morning of the 7th, he died.

Harvey Cushing was a marvel. He excelled at all he did. As an educator, a surgeon, a scholar, and a scientist, he was in the front rank. His biography of Osler occupies the pinnacle of achievement. It is given to few men to stand at the "head of the class," even fewer to stand at the head of two. And then there is Harvey Cushing.

References

1. Fulton JF: *Harvey Cushing – A Biography*. Springfield, IL: Charles C. Thomas, 1946.
2. Beecher HK: The first anesthesia records (Codman, Cushing). *Surg Gynecol Obstet* 1940; 71: 689–93.
3. Cushing H: *The Pituitary Body and its Disorders*. Philadelphia, PA: JB Lippincott, 1912.
4. Cushing H: *From a Surgeon's Journal, 1915–1918*. Boston, MA: Little, Brown, and Co., 1936.
5. Reid EG: *The Great Physician: A Short Life of Sir William Osler*. Oxford: Oxford University Press, 1936.
6. Cushing H: *The Life of Sir William Osler*, 2 Vols. Oxford: Oxford University Press, 1925.
7. Cushing H: *Consecratio Medici and Other Papers*. Boston, MA: Little, Brown, and Co., 1928.
8. Cushing H: *The Medical Career and Other Papers*. Boston, MA: Little Brown, and Co., 1940.
9. Cushing H: *A Bio-Bibliography of Andreas Vesalius*. New York: Schuman's, 1943.
10. Raab W: Klinishce und rontgenologische Beritage zur hypophysaren und zerebralen Fettsucht und genital Atrophie (case 2). *Wein Arch F Inn Med* 1924; 7: 443–530.
11. Teel HM: Basophil adenoma of the hypophysis with associate pluriglandular syndrome. *Arch Neurol Psychiatry* 1931; 26: 593–9.
12. Cushing H: The basophil adenomas of the pituitary body and their clinical manifestations (pituitary basophilism). *Bull Johns Hopkins Hosp* 1932; 50: 137–95.

This chapter has been reproduced from Loriaux, D. Lynn: Harvey Williams Cushing (1869–1939). *The Endocrinologist* 1992; 2(1): 2–5.

CHAPTER 49

Leo Loeb and Max Aron

(1869–1959) (1892–1974)

Thyrotropin

In 1929 Leo Loeb, then 60 years of age and the chairman of the Department of Pathology at Washington University School of Medicine in St. Louis, wrote a short paper that described marked hyperplasia of the guinea-pig thyroid gland after the injection of bovine pituitary extract [1]. This paper, along with a similar, short, but completely independent paper by Max Aron of Strasbourg [2], came to be seen by later endocrinologists as the "discovery" of thyrotropin, also called thyroid-stimulating hormone or TSH. George Corner, the well-known endocrinologist active in the 1920s, thought that "actual isolation ... in crude form was accomplished" [3], and Herbert Evans, an equally eminent contemporary, felt that the "discovery" of thyroid-stimulating effects from anterior pituitary substance ... by Loeb and Aron in 1929" [4] provided the first "convincing evidence of the existence of this hormone" [5].

Leo Loeb, born in Mayen, Germany, was the younger brother of the more famous Jacques Loeb. Leo was orphaned at age 6 years and was raised by relatives. After short periods of study at several German universities, he left Germany in 1890 because he disapproved of the rising German militarism. He studied medicine at the University of Zurich and completed his clinical work in Edinburgh and London, returning to Zurich to qualify and practice. Loeb was also interested in research, and went on to do laboratory work for an MD thesis, which he obtained in 1897. That year he left Switzerland for the United States, following his brother. He remained there for the rest of his life.

Although he began a medical practice in Chicago, where his brother was professor of physiology, he gave it up after only 10 months to study wound healing and tissue culture in a rented space in the back of a local drugstore. During the next 12 years, he continued his work where he could get a job: Johns Hopkins School of Medicine, the Marine Biological Laboratory at Woods Hole, McGill University, and the University of Pennsylvania.

Finally he came to St. Louis in 1910 where he stayed until he died in 1959. His initial appointment at St. Louis was as the director of research at the Barnard Skin and Cancer Hospital. In 1915 he was appointed as professor of comparative pathology at Washington University and, in 1924, he assumed the chairmanship of the pathology

A Biographical History of Endocrinology, First Edition. D. Lynn Loriaux.

This work is a co-publication between the Endocrine Society and John Wiley & Sons, Ltd.

department which he held until he retired in 1937. His research continued to focus on cell growth and its control, always seeking the reason why some cells became cancerous. Another major theme was the problem of transplantation and the individuality of the organism. He was not really an endocrinologist. While studying transplantation, one of the cell types that he was able to transplant was a carcinoma of the thyroid gland. This finding led to his studies on the control of thyroid growth.

In the early twentieth century, the control of thyroid growth by TSH was unknown. In fact, the pituitary hormones themselves were unknown. The function of the pituitary gland, if any, was quite mysterious. It was thought that iodine had something to do with the formation of a goiter, but the relationship was far from clear. By the 1920s when Loeb successfully transplanted the thyroid tumor, some progress had been made on the problem of the relationship between the thyroid and pituitary glands. Pituitary removal in amphibians prevented thyroid growth and caused the thyroid gland to shrink. By then, some were beginning to think that there was "something" in the pituitary gland. It was all done in amphibians. What was true for amphibians might not be true for mammals. Only amphibians really undergo metamorphosis, after all, and few thought it reasonable to transfer the idea of a pituitary thyroid stimulator to other classes of animals.

Although amphibian work focused on the possible function of the pituitary gland, suggesting a thyroid stimulant, mammalian work had gone in a somewhat different direction. Crude pituitary extracts, usually of bovine pituitary glands, made rats grow. The conclusion was that there must be a growth factor in the pituitary gland. These extracts also made the thyroid gland grow and stimulated the growth of a host of other tissues as well. At the time, the principal thought was that the pituitary gland had one hormone, leading to "one gland, one hormone." Growth hormone was thought by most to explain all of the pituitary effects on the enlargement of body tissues.

Beginning in 1919, the year after his transplantation of the thyroid tumor, Loeb published a long series of papers on compensatory hypertrophy of the thyroid gland. The following decade was spent in an attempt to understand why this hypertrophy occurred. The original phenomenon of compensatory hypertrophy of the gland had been described by Halsted at Johns Hopkins years before [6]. The phenomenon itself was straightforward. If one removed part of the thyroid gland from, for example, a dog, the remaining thyroid tissue grew larger in "compensation." How this happened had never been satisfactorily explained. In fact, Halsted had actually retracted his own original observation and attributed it to an unsuspected infection.

Loeb hoped that the thyroid gland would serve as a model for cell and tissue growth, and, if he could figure out what controlled the thyroid growth, he might make a real contribution to the understanding of cell growth in general. He pursued the thyroid issue quite vigorously. Twelve of his 96 publications between 1919 and 1928 were about the thyroid gland in one way or another. In the next decade, 36 of 86 papers were thyroid in nature. He called most of his thyroid papers "Studies on compensatory hypertrophy of the thyroid gland." He explored many aspects of thyroid growth in the guinea-pig, an animal he chose because it did not develop goiter spontaneously, but it did develop thyroid hyperplasia as did dogs and humans in the St. Louis of the time [7].

He found no effect of iodine on the thyroid gland, or tethelin, a supposed pituitary growth factor, or thymus tablets, or a meat diet, all given by mouth, but he did find a dramatic effect of thyroid tablets given by mouth. They completely prevented the compensatory hypertrophy. Loeb thought the thyroid tablet had a direct effect on the thyroid gland itself [8].

He went on to try a pituitary preparation. Because a prior publication showed that commercial pituitary tablets, taken orally, had biologic activity, he gave some of these tablets to guinea-pigs. As had happened with the thyroid tablets, these pituitary tablets also inhibited compensatory thyroid growth. Loeb concluded that a pituitary factor inhibited thyroid growth and thought that pituitary preparations might help patients with Graves' disease [9]. He thought he had found a situation in which the pituitary inhibited rather than stimulated growth. In retrospect, he was clearly on the wrong track.

Four years later, in 1928, he repeated his study with the pituitary extract and got the same results. He raised the possibility that the tablets might contain a thyroid-like substance but never tested the possibility. Philip Smith had already shown, in 1921, that the commercial pituitary tablet probably contained thyroid substance. Loeb seems not to have known about Smith's paper and never resolved the issue of whether or not the pituitary preparation he used was contaminated with thyroid material. He concluded that the "action of anterior pituitary substance on the thyroid gland in mammals and in an amphibian may be different in kind" [10]. The pituitary gland was thus an inhibitor of mammalian thyroid growth and a stimulator in amphibians.

Loeb went on to repeat one of the amphibian experiments in his guinea-pigs. He gave bovine pituitary extract by injection rather than pituitary tablets by mouth. Now he observed a clear-cut thyroid hyperplasia: "All the signs of compensatory hypertrophy were thus initiated." This was his "classic" paper wherein he "discovered" TSH [1]. Curiously, he never studied the pituitary tablets again. He held to his previous observation that the pituitary could inhibit the thyroid gland, and concluded that there were two pituitary effects on the mammalian thyroid gland: an inhibitory one and a stimulatory one. He had been chasing the wrong fox for almost 10 years and he got onto the right one almost by chance.

Loeb did not claim that he had isolated a new hormone but only that the guinea-pig thyroid responds to a pituitary injection. He did not suggest a name for the presumed stimulatory substance, and he implied that the pituitary had something specific to do with the thyroid gland.

Aron, like many others at the time, had served in the First World War as a physician. After the War he had gone into research at the University of Strasbourg's Institute of Histology. Like Loeb, his tools were largely histologic. Aron's prime interest was in development of mammalian embryos. In 1929, knowing of the pituitary–thyroid relationship already shown in amphibians, he thought it would be interesting to try the same experiment in a mammal. He practically duplicated Loeb's 1929 experiment. He gave crude extracts of bovine pituitary glands to guinea-pigs by injection and found histologic signs of increased activity ("suractivité fonctionelle") such that the glands resembled "goiter exophthalmique" [2]. He, too, never claimed isolation of a hormone, nor did he then propose a name for the presumed thyroid stimulatory substance. He did, however, offer his finding as indicating specificity for the thyroid gland.

These, then, are the findings that others said constituted the "discovery" of TSH. In fact, they were qualitatively no different from previous data in amphibians, so one could as validly claim that the amphibian workers really had made the discovery, as some did at the time. But to make such claim of a discovery of a specific thyroid stimulator, one would have to show the community of investigators that the substance had broad significance outside the amphibian world. To do this one would have to ignore the prevailing idea that there was a single pituitary hormone and that it was growth hormone, at least in mammals. Even though the actual data provided by Loeb and Aron were essentially the same as the amphibian data, the fact that they studied mammals was important. They may not have been the first to show a stimulatory effect of the pituitary on the thyroid gland, but they did show that the effect was a broad one and that it applied to several different classes of animals.

Another reason for the perception that Aron and Loeb had "discovered" TSH was that, by the end of the 1920s, endocrinologists as a community were beginning to suspect that the idea of a single pituitary hormone might not be sound. So, when the two investigators published in 1929, the endocrine community was better prepared for the concept. The idea of several separate pituitary hormones was beginning to spread, and so the histologic findings of Loeb and Aron could be seen as support for the new idea. It would then be important to look back on their findings as a "discovery" so that there would be a point of origin for the multi-hormone concept.

In 1929 no one had isolated a pituitary hormone in the modern sense of a chemically pure preparation or had even shown that a pituitary preparation contained only one hormone and was free of others. These "discoveries," separating TSH from other pituitary hormones and purifying it to homogeneity, were to come later. Before it could happen, the concept that there was a separate hormone called thyrotropin had to become so widely accepted that it made sense for scientists to put time and energy into the problem.

Loeb and Aron solidified the effects of the pituitary on the thyroid gland. They helped define an entity, a thyroid stimulator from the pituitary gland, only vaguely suspected before. They fostered a way of looking at the pituitary gland that altered previous views. Writing a few years later in 1935, Oscar Riddle, one of the "discoverers" of prolactin, said that "the really decisive evidence for TSH has slowly accumulated" [11].

References

1. Loeb L. Bassett RB: Effect is hormones of the anterior pituitary on thyroid gland in the guinea pig. *Proc Soc Exp Biol Med* 1929; 26: 860.
2. Aron M: Action de la prehypophyse sur le thyroide chez le cobaye. *C R Seances Soc Biol* 1929; 102: 682.
3. Corner GW: Herbert McLean Evans 1882–1971. *Bio Mem Natl Acad Sci* 1974; 45: 169.
4. Evans HM: Present position of our knowledge of anterior pituitary function. *JAMA* 1933; 101: 425.

5. Evans HM: Clinical manifestations of dysfunction of the anterior pituitary. In *Glandular Physiology and Therapy*. Chicago, IL: American Medical Association, 1935, p. 20.
6. Halsted WS: An experimental study of the thyroid gland of dogs, with especial consideration of hypertrophy of this gland. *Johns Hopkins Hosp Rep* 1896; 1: 373.
7. Loeb L: Studies on compensatory hypertrophy of this gland. I: A quantitative analysis of the thyroid gland. *J Med Res* 1919; 40: 199.
8. Loeb L: Studies on compensatory hypertrophy of the thyroid gland. V. The effect of the administration of thyroid, thymus gland and tethelin and of a meat diet on the hypertrophy of the thyroid gland in guinea pigs. *J Med Res* 1920; 4: 77.
9. Loeb L: Studies on compensatory hypertrophy of the thyroid gland. VI. The effect of feeding anterior lobe of the thyroid gland in guinea pig. *J Med Res* 1924; 44: 557.
10. Loeb L: Studies on compensatory hypertrophy of the thyroid gland. VIII. A comparison between the effect of administration of thyroxin, thyroid and anterior pituitary substance on the compensatory hypertrophy of the thyroid gland in the guinea pig. *Am J Pathol* 1929; 5: 71.
11. Riddle O: Contemplating the hormones. *Endocrinology* 1935; 19: 1.

Sources

Goodpasture EW: Leo Loeb. *Biog Mem Natl Acad Sci* 1961; 35: 205.
Loeb L: Autobiographical notes. *Perspect Biol Med* 1958; 2: 1.
Parker F: Loeb L. *Dictionary of Scientific Biography* 1973; 8: 447.
Schafer P: Biographical notes on Dr. Leo Loeb. *Arch Pathol* 1950; 50: 661.

This chapter has been reproduced from Sawin, Clark T: Leo Loeb, Max Aron, and thyrotropin. *The Endocrinologist* 1997; 7(1): 1–4.

CHAPTER 50
W.G. MacCallum
(1874–1944)
Tetany and the Parathyroid Gland

In March 1908, a short paper, barely one page long, appeared in the monthly bulletin of the Johns Hopkins Hospital. In it, William G. MacCallum, then an associate professor of pathology at the Johns Hopkins Medical School, and his chemical colleague, Carl Voegtlin, briefly described some of their findings in dogs that had the parathyroid glands removed [1]. It had been known for more than a decade that this procedure would cause tetany, but no one knew exactly why. The MacCallum–Voegtlin team showed that the operated dogs got better if they were given injections of calcium salts. The dogs had a low level of calcium in the blood.

MacCallum was Canadian and came to Hopkins from the University of Toronto where he was a bright student. He was enamored of the classics and majored in Greek, intending to make its study his life's work. His father, a general practitioner from Ontario, insisted that William take sufficient science courses to qualify for medical school [2]. William did this, then, when he heard that there was a new medical school in Baltimore that had just opened in 1893 and not only required a college degree but also a reading knowledge of French and German and the ability to translate Latin, he thought that would be just the place for him. Because he had taken all of those science courses, he thought he deserved advance standing. He not only applied for admission to the Johns Hopkins Medical School but asked that he be admitted as a second-year student. A physician friend of his family who knew the famous professor of medicine at Hopkins, William Osler, suggested that MacCallum write Osler to ask for the advanced placement. Osler turned him down. Undaunted, MacCallum then wrote to the dean, William H. Welch, who was also the professor of pathology, and asked the same question. MacCallum came to Hopkins as a second-year student that fall.

MacCallum graduated from medical school at 23 years of age at the top of his class of 15. All but one did a rotating internship at the Hopkins hospital. The other joined the faculty directly. MacCallum wanted to go onto Osler's service to do a residency in medicine. Once again, Osler turned him down. MacCallum turned again to Welch, who took him on as the only assistant resident in pathology for the next 2 years

A Biographical History of Endocrinology, First Edition. D. Lynn Loriaux.

This work is a co-publication between the Endocrine Society and John Wiley & Sons, Ltd.

(1898–1900). MacCallum's career in pathology was set for life. After the 2 years were over, Welch appointed MacCallum "resident pathologist," and MacCallum essentially ran the service. Technically, MacCallum's hospital appointment remained "resident" for the next 9 years; apparently, there were no other hospital appointments available. He progressed rapidly in the school's academic hierarchy and became associate professor of pathology in 1902. In large part because he developed an innovative course in pathological physiology, he was appointed to a newly founded professorship in that field in 1908. By this time the 34-year-old had become quite well known. The next year, 1909, MacCallum became a professor in Columbia Medical School's Department of Pathology, and pathologist to the Presbyterian Hospital, where he stayed for most of the next decade. His last academic move came in 1917 when he returned to Baltimore to replace his former chief, Welch, as Hopkins' professor of pathology.

Voegtlin was not a physician, but came to Hopkins as a PhD in 1906. He was originally recruited to the Department of Medicine by Lewellys Barker, who had replaced Osler as professor of medicine in 1905. Barker thought that a Department of Medicine ought to be actively involved in research so he set up three modest laboratories within the department. One was physiological, one was biological (which turned out to be largely infectious diseases and immunology), and the third was chemical. Voegtlin, who was Swiss, came to Hopkins via Freiburg, Manchester, and Madison, Wisconsin. He was appointed as director of the chemical laboratory. He stayed only 2 years in that position before moving to the Department of Pharmacology in 1908. Five years later, he left academia to join the U.S. Government's Hygienic Laboratory, the precursor of the NIH, as a pharmacologist. Eventually, in 1938, he was appointed to head the National Cancer Institute.

MacCallum's interest in the parathyroid glands began about 1902. He worked with William Halsted, Hopkins' professor of surgery, on the pathology of the thyroid and parathyroid glands. Halsted was perfecting his surgical approach to the thyroid and wanted to consistently save the parathyroids that were so easily damaged during that surgery. His goal was to avoid postoperative tetany, which was known to be related to damage of the parathyroid glands. Halsted knew about the fragile blood supply to these tiny glands. He and Herbert McLean Evans, then a medical student and, later, one of America's best-known endocrinologists, carefully defined the parathyroid vascular anatomy [3]. Careful surgery to preserve these vessels averted parathyroid damage. Perhaps the parathyroid glands secreted something that prevented muscle tetany. The prevalent theory was that the substance was an antitoxin that prevented unidentified toxins from acting. Some thought that tetany was caused by a "tetany toxin" that the parathyroid glands either metabolized or neutralized to prevent it from acting. MacCallum and others had tried using parathyroid extracts to treat postoperative tetany. Sometimes there was success, and sometimes not. In 1906, for example, Halsted had a patient who developed tetany. MacCallum gave Halsted his entire supply of bovine parathyroids to give to this patient by mouth. Other patients received parathyroid emulsions subcutaneously with apparent benefit. MacCallum had no evidence, however, as to whether the parathyroid glands made a hormone or a detoxicant.

MacCallum began to investigate the role of calcium in the tetanic phenomenon. There was no precedent for an intermediary between a hormone and the responding tissues. Jacques Loeb, the polymath and founder of general biology, had shown various effects of different salt solutions on muscle twitching and the suppression of twitching by calcium or analogous ions such as magnesium. MacCallum's younger brother, also a Hopkins medical graduate, who died of tuberculosis in 1906, had made similar findings. Further, animals without parathyroids sometimes did not develop tetany if the diet contained a good deal of milk, an obvious source of calcium.

Whatever the precise reason, MacCallum, the pathophysiologist, and Voegtlin, the laboratory chemist, got together and gave several salt solutions to parathyroidectomized dogs to see what would happen. Their own words tell the story: "all violent symptoms produced by parathyroidectomy, muscle twitching, and rigidity ... etc., may be almost instantly cured by the injection of a solution of a calcium salt" [1]. They went on in their complete paper, published the next year, to show that this result was consistent and that parathyroidectomy caused a clear-cut fall in the serum calcium [4]. One would have thought that these data would have settled the issue and would be immediately received as a major advance in endocrinology. They were not.

MacCallum himself advocated the idea that the parathyroid glands prevented tetany by mobilizing calcium, but he was still willing to consider the idea of a toxin. Further, he himself had shown that the effect was not specific to calcium; magnesium also worked but had more side effects. Others, unable to confirm MacCallum's work, chose to regard the calcium effect on blunting tetany as a simple pharmacologic effect, a sedative of sorts. Others had trouble showing that there was a low level of serum calcium after parathyroidectomy. The measurement of serum calcium was not simple. Voegtlin's method seems to have required 50 mL of blood for each assay.

MacCallum's overall work in pathology was highly regarded. He was one of relatively few physicians elected to the National Academy of Sciences (1921). He lived a full life at Hopkins though his last years were difficult. After suffering a debilitating stroke that paralyzed his right side and left him unable to speak, he died, bedridden in February, 1944, at 69 years of age.

References

1. MacCallum WG, Voegtlin C: On the relation of the parathyroid to calcium metabolism and the nature of tetany. *Bull Johns Hopkins Hosp* 1908; 19: 91.
2. Longcope WT: Biographical memoir of William George MacCallum 1874–1944. *Biographical Memoirs*, Vol. 23. National Academy of Sciences, 1914, pp. 337–64.
3. Halsted WS, Evans HM: The parathyroidglandules. Their blood supply, and their preservation in operation upon the thyroid gland. *Ann Surg* 1907; 46: 489.
4. MacCallum WG, Voegtlin C: On the relation of tetany to the parathyroid glands and to calcium metabolism. *J Exp Med* 1909; 11: 118.

Sources

Dolev E: A gland in search of a function: The parathyroid glands and the explanations of tetany 1903–1926. *J Hist Med Allied Sci* 1987; 42: 186.

Harvey AM: *Adventures in Medical Research. A Century of Discovery at Johns Hopkins*. Baltimore, MD: Johns Hopkins University Press, 1976.

Harvey AM, Brieger GH, Abrams SL, McKusick VA: *A Model of Its Kind*. Vol. I. *A Centennial History of Medicine at Johns Hopkins*. Baltimore, MD: Johns Hopkins University Press, 1989.

MacCallum WG: *A Text-book of Pathology*. Philadelphia, PA: W.B. Saunders, 1916.

This chapter has been reproduced from Sawin, Clark T: What causes tetany after removal of the parathyroid glands? MacCallum, Voegtlin, and calcium. *The Endocrinologist* 2003; 13(1): 1–3.

CHAPTER 51

Moses Barron (1883–1974)

Pancreatic Duct Stone

Most endocrinologists are familiar with the story of the discovery of insulin. Frederick Banting was born on a small farm in Alliston, Ontario in 1891. He was the youngest of five children. He was an average student. He went to the University of Toronto in 1912 where he enrolled in medicine. He was an average medical student. His 4-year course was shortened because of the war. Banting spent a year in England, and then was transferred to the "front" as a battalion medical officer. He received the Military Cross for courage under fire but suffered a shrapnel wound in one arm as well. After a long convalescence, he returned to Toronto in 1919. He became a resident in surgery at the Sick Children's Hospital and soon developed an interest in orthopedics. Failing to receive an appointment on the staff of the hospital, Banting set up a practice in London Ontario. He saw his first patient on July 29, nearly a month after opening his practice doors, and his income for the month of July was $4.00. He needed a paying job, so he took one at Western University as an assistant to the professor of physiology. On the night of October 31, 1920, Banting was preparing to give a lecture on carbohydrate metabolism to the physiology students. He had little interest in the subject. He studied what was in the textbooks at the time, and went to bed with the latest issue of *Surgery, Gynecology, and Obstetrics*, where his attention was drawn to an article by Moses Barron on "The relation of the islets of Langerhans to diabetes with special reference to cases of pancreatic lithiasis" [1].

In Banting's 1940 memoir, "The Story of Insulin," he describes the events of that night [2, 3]:

> It was one of those nights when I was disturbed and could not sleep. I thought about the lecture and about the article and I thought about my miseries and how I would like to get out of debt and away from worry.
>
> Finally about two in the morning, after the lecture and the article had been chasing each other through my mind for some time, the idea occurred to me that by the experimental ligation of the duct and the subsequent degeneration of a portion of the pancreas, that one might

A Biographical History of Endocrinology, First Edition. D. Lynn Loriaux.

This work is a co-publication between the Endocrine Society and John Wiley & Sons, Ltd.

> obtain the internal secretion separate from the external secretion. I got up and wrote down the idea and spent most of the night thinking about it.

This is what he wrote in his notebook:

> Diabetes. Ligate pancreatic ducts of dogs. Keep dogs alive till acini degenerate leaving islets. Try to isolate the internal secretion of these to relieve glycosuria.

The rest of the story is one of those "medical miracles" that come along only once in a great while. What was in the Barron paper that could so clearly show Banting the way? And, who was Moses Barron anyway?

Moses Barron was born in Korno, Russia, on November 8, 1883. His family immigrated to the United States when he was 5 years old. They settled on a farm in western Minnesota, but soon moved to Fargo and, finally, St. Paul, Minnesota. He went to Central High School. A good scholar, he qualified for the 6-year pre-medical and medical course at the University of Minnesota at the age of 22 years. He received his MD in 1911 and was the only intern at the newly constructed Elliot Memorial Hospital. In the following year he was appointed as instructor in pathology at the medical school.

Barron joined the Army Medical Reserve Corps and served in Base Hospital 26 at the Hospital Center in Allerey, France. Barron was the director of the laboratory that served all 10 of the hospitals in the Center. He returned to the University of Minnesota in the Department of Pathology in 1919 and, in that year, he performed an autopsy on a 40-year-old man who had died with diabetic ketoacidosis and coma. The postmortem examination revealed a markedly atrophic pancreas. Probing the pancreatic duct revealed an obstruction caused by a chalk white calculus, 5 × 6 × 12 mm in diameter. It completely and firmly occluded the pancreatic duct. The stone was composed of calcium carbonate. Microscopic examination of the pancreas showed numerous islets of Langerhans, many of which were entirely normal. There was no normal acinic tissue found.

Most students of the events surrounding the discovery of insulin attribute Banting's experimental plan to the example of this patient. I think not. The patient, who had many normal islets, died of diabetic ketoacidosis. Banting could not have concluded, in the face of these facts, that the "active principle" could be extracted from these islets. I think that Banting was guided by animal experiments described by Barron in his review of the literature. The following passage, from Barron's 1920 article, was, I believe, the key to Banting's plans:

> Kamimura conducted very extensive experiments for the elucidation of the problem relative to the effect of duct ligation on the islets. His results are based on the study of one hundred rabbits. At the end of the first week after ligation, he found very little change. At the end of the second week, the normal structure was lost – the tissue was scarcely recognizable as pancreas. There was atrophy with beginning sclerosis. The fifth week, very few nests of parenchyma were visible, and the entire organ was replaced by connective-tissue stroma. After 10 weeks, there was contraction of the connective tissue and fat cells began to appear. In about 15 weeks, there was scarcely any parenchyma visible and there was considerable fat replacement. The

> islets, however, remained normal throughout. In contrast to the findings following the extirpation of the gland, examinations of the blood and urine showed neither hyperglycemia nor glycosuria present during any stage of these experiments. He concludes that the ligation of the pancreatic duct leads to a slow, progressive atrophy of parenchyma with replacement by connective tissue, until there is practically no acinic structure left, but the islets remain intact. The animals suffered no digestive disturbances, they ate well and assimilated their food. They reacted normally after injection of adrenalin. The author is, therefore, convinced that the islets control the carbohydrate metabolism, since these animals appeared entirely normal as long as the islets were left intact for the production of the internal secretion; the profound alterations in the glandular portion of the pancreas had not had the slightest effect upon the utilization of sugar [1].

Similar experiments, with similar results, are described for guinea-pigs, cats, and dogs.

Barron's review of the literature contains the design of Banting's experiments. Banting's insight was that the active principle might be better extracted from a duct ligated atrophic pancreas than a normal one. That insight remains his and, indeed, he made the best of it.

Moses Barron remained at the University of Minnesota Medical School for his entire career. He is credited with another important observation – the recognition of the rapid increase in the incidence of carcinoma of the lung which he reported in 1922 [4]. He noted that the postmortem incidence had risen from about 0.05% between 1880 and 1900, to 0.9% in 1919–1921. It was the first warning of the epidemic to come. He attributed the increase to the ravages of the 1917–1918 influenza epidemic. It was up to Alton Ochsner to connect the disease to cigarette smoking.

Barron spent a year in Vienna at the Allgemeines Krankenhaus and returned to Minnesota in private practice and a clinical professorship at the medical school. He retired from practice in 1964, his 81st year, and died in Minneapolis in 1974 at 90 years of age.

He is remembered by one of his medical students in this way:

> One feature of the first two medical school years, however, still comes vividly to mind. Moses Barron, an internal medicine practitioner in Minneapolis, would come to the University Hospital as a clinical instructor and 8:00 a.m. on Friday mornings, he would meet for the first time, and then examine, a patient in front of the entire freshman class. The interns would have looked through the roster of hospitalized patients in order to select what they regarded as the most difficult diagnostic case. Dr. Barron would demonstrate how to take a history, do a brief physical examination, and then discuss the diagnosis. One morning, the patient was described as an unmarried, 51-year-old white female who was complaining about an abdominal tumor. Dr. Barron examined her and came to the correct diagnosis: pregnancy. That greatly surprised many of us who had thought pregnancy impossible for a woman of such an age. Moreover, in the course of the examination he pulled down the lower eyelids, inspected the conjunctivae, and announced that the hemoglobin level was 51 percent. Turning to the intern standing with the chart, he asked what the laboratory had found. The intern thumbed through the chart and responded that the laboratory report showed 53 percent hemoglobin, whereupon Dr. Barron informed us that one always had to allow 2 percent for laboratory error.

Ahh, for the good old days!

References

1. Barron M: The relation of the islets of Langerhans to diabetes with special reference to cases of pancreatic lithiasis. *Surgery, Gynecology, and Obstetrics* 1920; 31: 437–48.
2. Banting F: The story of insulin, Unpublished manuscript, the Banting Papers, University of Toronto.
3. Bliss M: *The Discovery of Insulin*. Chicago, IL: University of Chicago Press, 1982.
4. Barron M: Carcinoma of the lung: a study of its incidence, pathology, and relative importance. *Arch Surg* 1922; 4(3): 624–60.

This chapter has been reproduced from Loriaux, D. Lynn: Moses Barron: 1883–1974. *The Endocrinologist* 2009; 19(5): 203–4.

CHAPTER 52

Frederick Grant Banting (1891–1941)

The Discovery of Insulin

The isolation of insulin and its introduction into clinical use is one of the most riveting stories in the history of science. The intensity of the story derives from the medical impact of the discovery, the unlikely backgrounds of two of the central figures, and the bitter controversy that arose over credits for the work. At the center of the drama is Frederick Banting.

Frederick Banting was born the youngest of five children on November 14, 1891 in northern Ontario, Canada. From an early age, his family intended him for the ministry. In the local school system, he was known as a good athlete and a mediocre scholar. He enrolled in Victoria College in 1910 with the intention of becoming a Methodist minister, but was disillusioned and, in 1912, enrolled in the University of Toronto Medical School. In 1915, he enlisted in the royal Canadian Army as a private in the Medical Corps. He received the MC degree in 1917, and was promoted to Captain. Promptly dispatched to France, he was wounded in the right arm by shrapnel and received the Military Cross for valorous conduct in combat. He was discharged in 1919 and returned to Canada as a trainee in surgery at the Toronto Hospital for Sick Children. There he focused on orthopedics, and completed his training in 1920. Banting was not offered an appointment on the staff of the Hospital for Sick Children at this stage, probably because of a "willful" personality. Depressed, he decided to set up a practice in London, Ontario a few miles distant.

It was traditional for young physicians to enter practice by joining an older man, or purchasing an active practice from a retiring physician. Banting did neither; he borrowed the money to buy a house and hung out a shingle on July 1, 1920. His first patient was seen on July 29 and he made a $2.00 charge for baby feeding [1]. He made $37.00 in August, $48.00 in September, and $66.00 in October. Although the practice was growing, it was not fast enough to support it. To fill his time and make a few more dollars, Banting took a job as a demonstrator in anatomy and surgery at Western University Medical School. He was paid $2.00 an hour. On Monday, November 1, 1920, Banting was scheduled to give a talk on the pancreas to one of his classes. He

A Biographical History of Endocrinology, First Edition. D. Lynn Loriaux.

This work is a co-publication between the Endocrine Society and John Wiley & Sons, Ltd.

spent most of Sunday preparing the talk, mainly by reviewing the subject in standard textbooks. Preparations complete, he went to bed, intending to read himself to sleep with the latest issue of *Surgery, Gynecology, and Obstetrics.* His attention was captured by the first article, "The relation of the islets of Langerhans to diabetes with special reference to cases of pancreatic lithiasis" [2]. The paper described the effects of pancreatic duct obstruction leading to atrophy of the exocrine pancreas with apparent preservation of the endocrine pancreas. It failed to have the intended soporific effect. It proved to be a sleepless night. The combined anxieties of the coming lecture and the disappointing progress of his professional and personal affairs led to insomnia. Twenty years later, Banting recalled the night this way [3]:

> It was one of those nights when I was disturbed and could not sleep. I thought about the lecture and about the article and I thought about my miseries and how I would like to get out of debt and away from worry.
>
> Finally, about two in the morning, after the lecture and the article had been chasing each other through my mind for some time, the idea occurred to me that by the experimental ligation of the duct of the pancreas, that one might obtain the internal secretion separate from the external secretion. I got up and wrote down the idea and spent most of the night thinking about it.

The notebook into which the entry was made is preserved in the Toronto Academy of Medicine. It is dated October 30, changed to the 31st with the realization that it was 2.00 a.m.

> Diabetes. Ligate pancreatic ducts of dogs. Keep dogs alive till Acini degenerate leaving islets. Try to isolate the internal secretion of these to relieve glycosuria.

This idea had occurred to others, but Banting was unaware of it. Lydia De Witt had tried it in 1906 and tested the extract in an in vitro system without measurable effect [4]. Ernest Lyman Scott, a graduate student in physiology at the University of Chicago, wrote in 1912 [5]:

> It was hoped that the presence of the digestive enzymes could be eliminated by the atrophy of the gland which follows complete ligation of the ducts; but after several attempts in the dog which proved futile so far as complete atrophy was concerned, this method was abandoned as impractical. In subsequent work these enzymes were rendered inactive at once by a high percentage of alcohol and were later killed by long-continued contact with strong alcohol.

Anton J. Carlson, Scott's thesis advisor, discouraged him from pursuing this line of investigation, and it was abandoned. In 1923, Carlson offered the following apology [6, as presented in 7]:

> I feel that I personally have to shoulder a great deal of blame for discouraging you from going ahead with that work. I was more impressed with the fever and the unfavorable reactions secured than the undoubted lowering of the urine and blood sugar that you obtained.

Knowing none of this at the time, Banting determined to pursue his idea. Looking for ways to do the necessary experiments at Western met with frustration and failure. Banting was advised to present his ideas to J.J.R. Macleod, an expert in carbohydrate metabolism and professor of physiology at the University of Toronto. Their first meeting on November 8 did not go well. Banting was ill prepared and it was obvious that his scientific background was impoverished, as was his knowledge about diabetes, the pancreas, and its internal and external secretion.

> At one point early in the interview Macleod began reading some of the letters on his desk, a sometimes unconscious and common gesture bound to offend a sensitive visitor to anyone's office. Macleod's first comments on Banting's presentation, delivered in a tone that could only be seen as formal and patronizing (Macleod was chillingly formal to most strangers because he was a shy man) were to the effect that this kind of research was a serious matter. Dr. Banting would have to realize that many eminent scientists had spent many years in some of the world's best-equipped laboratories trying to isolate the internal secretion of the pancreas. None had succeeded [7].

Was Banting prepared for this kind of venture? He said he was, and with that, Macleod agreed that the idea was worth trying. If Banting was prepared to make the commitment, Macleod would provide the animals and the laboratory space. Sobered by the tenor of this interaction, Banting hesitated, but with the spring he was ready to begin. "On Saturday morning, May 4, 1921, Banting locked up his house, supervised a final examination for the fourth year medical students at Western, and then caught the noon train for Toronto" [7].

Macleod was leaving to spend the summer in Edinburgh. Before going, he provided Banting with a small laboratory and the money to buy "an adequate number" of dogs. Most importantly, he provided him with an experimental plan and with Charles Best. Best was 21 years old and had just graduated from the physiology and biochemistry course at the University of Toronto. He was looking for summer work. On the toss of a coin, he was paired with Banting. Best brought a contemporary knowledge of biochemistry to the project: in particular, he brought the technology for measuring urine and blood sugar, the technology necessary for success. The work began on May 17. As always, it went badly in the beginning. The pancreatectomized dogs died, and the ligatures around the pancreatic ducts failed to cause pancreatic atrophy. Catgut ligatures were used, and they dissolved to the extent that recanalization occurred. In the first seven weeks, Banting and Best operated on 19 dogs. Fourteen were dead, and the remaining five, all with pancreatic duct ligatures, showed no signs of pancreatic atrophy. Seven weeks had gone by.

By this time, most of the budget supplied by Macleod had been expended. Banting sold his Ford automobile to buy more dogs. Then, on July 30, an atrophic pancreas was identified in one of the five living dogs from the first phase of the project. An extract of the pancreas was made in iced Ringer's solution. That extract successfully lowered the blood and urine sugar of a pancreatectomized dog. By mid-August, the two investigators had shown that the extract could keep a pancreatectomized dog alive and in apparently good health. They called the active principle "isletin."

Macleod returned in late September to find the experimental work surprisingly promising. He succeeded in changing the name of the material to "insulin" and, most importantly, introduced J.B. Collip to the project. Collip had a PhD in biochemistry from the University of Toronto and had been appointed professor and chairman of the Department of Biochemistry at the University of Toronto. He played a pivotal role in isolating and purifying insulin from bovine pancreas for clinical application. As a result of this team effort, Leonard Thompson, a 12-year-old boy admitted to the Toronto General Hospital in ketoacidosis, was treated with insulin on January 11, 1922. Treatment was begun with insulin extracted from fresh beef pancreas. Improvement was dramatic, and the treatment was stopped after 3 days. As might be expected, the boy's condition deteriorated as a consequence, and the treatment was begun again with good effect. This first successful treatment of a diabetic human being with insulin happened less than eight months after the initial experiments had begun on May 17!

> The potential impact of these simple yet elegant experiments was recognized immediately. In keeping with the wishes of the will of Alfred Nobel (i.e. that the prize be given annually to those who during the preceding year had conferred the greatest benefit on mankind), the Nobel Prize in Medicine and Physiology was awarded to Banting and Macleod in 1923. The omission of Best, and for that matter the inclusion of Macleod, as a co-recipient of the award is a controversy regarding the judgment of the Nobel committee that rages to this day [8].

Banting immediately announced that he would share his prize with Charles Best, and Macleod countered that he would share his prize with J.B. Collip. A rift developed between Banting and Macleod that never healed. Banting believed that Macleod had contributed little to the work and had usurped the credit due Charles Best. Within a few years, Macleod accepted a position as regius professor of physiology in Aberdeen, Scotland; Banting refused to attend the farewell celebration. Wherever justice lies, it seems odd to punish Macleod for the decision of the Nobel committee. And in defense of the committee, how many "distinguished" professors would take a chance on a young orthopedic surgeon with no scientific background? In all probability, the success of the venture can be traced directly to Macleod. Putting Best with Banting was a masterstroke, and involving Collip paved the way for early clinical application. In fact, Macleod did not seek the recognition that came his way; he declined to be an author on the first paper announcing the isolation of insulin and did not allow his name to be on any paper until the eighth in the series, published in 1922 [9].

Charles Best became professor of physiology at Toronto in Macleod's stead. Collip went on to a distinguished career, pioneering the isolation of parathormone, ACTH, and the gonadotropins. Premarin®, was one of his products and is still much with us today. Banting was made the first professor and chairman of the Banting and Best Department of Medical Research. The Canadian Government awarded him a lifelong annuity of $7500.

Banting's life ended in the grip of the same forces that so strongly molded his character at the beginning of his career. With the outbreak of the Second World War, Banting took a keen interest in the physiology of flying, and developed one of the first pressurized flying suits. He was to take the suit to England for testing and the sense of urgency dictated that he take it on a transatlantic flight in a Lockheed-Hudson twin engine bomber. Banting was the only passenger on the plane with a crew of three. Flying out of Gander, Newfoundland, the plane was airborne only 12 minutes when it developed engine trouble. Turning back, the plane ran into a heavy February snow, and the remaining engine failed. The pilot crash-landed the plane and was thrown clear of the wreckage, unharmed. Returning to the plane, he found both crewmen dead and Banting alive but grievously injured. Banting died 20 hours later. He was 50 years old. A rescue crew arrived at the site 3 days later and the pilot was saved.

This is one of those rare true stories in which truth is, in fact, stranger than fiction. Who would "buy" this story line? An orthopedic surgeon with no scientific background and no laboratory experience presents himself to one of the leading scientific luminaries of the day with an idea that explains the workings of an obscure gland and will cure a dread disease. He is believed and supported with a laboratory, an assistant, and money for supplies. Running out of money, the young surgeon sells his car to keep the project going. Finally, in eight months, all predictions come true and the dread disease is stamped out, at least for the time being. Even Errol Flynn wouldn't take this one on.

It would not happen today. The project would never be funded (too risky, no preliminary data). The material could never be used in humans (no rat studies, no primate toxicity, no phase 1 studies, and no way to avoid hypoglycemia, too dangerous). But it did happen then, and thankfully so.

References

1. Bliss M: Dr. Frederick Banting: Getting out of town. *Can Med Assoc J* 1984; 130: 1215–32.
2. Barron M: The relation of the islets of Langerhans to diabetes with special reference to cases of pancreatic lithiasis. *Surg Gynecol Obstet* 1920; 31: 437.
3. Banting FG: The Story of Insulin. Unpublished Manuscript, Banting Papers, University of Toronto.
4. DeWitt L: Morphology and physiology of areas of Langerhans in some vertebrates. *J Exp Med* 1906; 8: 193–239.
5. Scott EL: On the influence of intravenous injections of an extract of the pancreas of experimental pancreatic diabetes. *Am J Physiol* 1912; 29: 306–10.
6. Carlson to Scott. 15 November 1923. Ernest L Scott Papers, National Library of Medicine, Bethesda, MD.
7. Sawyer WA: Frederick Banting's misinterpretation of the work of Ernest L. Scott as found in secondary sources. *Perspec Biol Med* 1986; 26: 611–18.
8. Morris JB, Schirmer WJ: The "Right Stuff": Five Nobel Prize-winning surgeons. *Surgery* 1990; 108: 71–80.
9. Editorial Note: New light on the insulin controversy. *Ann Intern Med* 1973; 91: 311.

This chapter has been reproduced from Loriaux, D. Lynn: Frederick Grant Banting (1891–1941). *The Endocrinologist* 1993; 3(5): 307–10.

CHAPTER 53
James Bertram Collip (1893–1965)
Isolation of Insulin

"Bert" Collip was born in Belleville, Ontario on November 20, 1892. He was the only son of Mary and James Dennis Collip, a florist. A younger sister, Rita, was born 8 years later.

Bert's early schooling was in a one-room schoolhouse in Belleville. He attended Belleville High School and then matriculated into Trinity College of the University of Toronto in 1908, at the age of 15. Bert worked in the honor course in physiology and biochemistry and graduated at the head of his class in 1912. He was not a dull boy. He participated in most of the undergraduate societies, played tennis, ran the University steeplechase, and skated with the girls from St. Hilda's School at Victoria College. It was there he met Miss Ray Ralph, whom he married in 1915. Bert then enrolled in the graduate school and, under the guidance of Professor A.B. Macallum, earned the PhD degree in physiological chemistry in 1916 [1]. He was given an immediate appointment in the Department of Biochemistry at the University of Alberta in Edmonton, where he shouldered a majority of the teaching duties for an academic staff much depleted by the First World War. In this period, he published 25 papers on the blood chemistry of vertebrates and invertebrates, focusing on acid–base exchange and osmotic pressure.

With the end of the War, Collip sought a period of renewal and applied for, and received, a Rockefeller Traveling Fellowship. He decided to journey back to the University of Toronto and work in the laboratory of J.J.R. Macleod on the effects of pH on blood sugar. This was an auspicious time in Toronto, the time that Banting and Best were in the midst of isolating insulin from dog pancreas. These two investigators had a crude extract of the "active principle," but it was too toxic to deploy in the treatment of human beings. Macleod asked Collip to help in the purification of the crude insulin, and thus Collip entered into the first of several controversies that were to dog his scientific career.

The seminal paper in this saga was published in March of 1922 by Banting, Best, Collip, Campbell, and Fletcher: "Pancreatic extracts in the treatment of diabetes

A Biographical History of Endocrinology, First Edition. D. Lynn Loriaux.

This work is a co-publication between the Endocrine Society and John Wiley & Sons, Ltd.

mellitus" [1]. The work was awarded the Nobel Prize in 1922, catalyzing a conflict and dispute about the relative contributions to the work that continues to this day. Banting describes the events in the following way [2]:

> On December 12th the whole pancreas of a cow was chopped in 3% hydrochloric acid in 95% alcohol, macerated, filtered, evaporated, emulsified in saline, and given subcutaneously to dog #35. Blood sugar fell from 28 to 11 in four hours. This was the first whole gland extract of beef pancreas. Dr. Collip had from time to time asked me if there was anything he could do. I was very anxious that the work advance more rapidly. I asked Professor Macleod three or four times if Dr. Collip could do portions of work, but he advised against it. I was very anxious to find out if glycogen could be stored in the liver of a depancreatized dog if extract were administered. I formulated an experiment and Best and I depancreatized two dogs in the surgical research, gave them extract and glucose, and Dr. Collip did glycogen estimates. He told Professor Macleod the results. This occurred about one week before Christmas Holidays. Collip began working on the biochemistry of the extract about this time. Before he commenced, Best and I were using alcohol extracts of whole beef pancreas.
>
> Shortly before January 25, 1922, Dr. Collip, who had been working in the laboratory of Dr. Harding, in the Pathological Building, announced that he had developed a process by which he could obtain an extract which contained no proteins and no lipase. On being asked his methods of preparation he refused to tell them. This was a breach of a gentlemen's agreement among Dr. Collip, Mr. Best, and myself, as we had agreed among ourselves to tell all results to each other. Dr. Collip discussed this new preparation with Professor Macleod and secured the consent of Professor Macleod to keep the process secret. I believe that Dr. Collip at this time endeavored to patent this process, and was only prevented from doing so by Professors Macleod, Hunter, and Henderson.
>
> Dr. Collip refined extract which was made by Mr. Best, sending the refined extract to the wards for clinical tests.
>
> Dr. Collip, although placed in charge of the production of Insulin in the Connaught Laboratory, did not work in the Connaught Laboratory but dabbled in the physiological properties of the extract. He reported results to Professor Macleod as his own which were not his own.
>
> In writing the joint paper that appeared in the March issue of the Canadian Medical Association Journal, Dr. Collip claimed that he was the first to make extracts from the whole gland by the use of alcohol. He also claimed to have made the first extract that was administered to a human diabetic. Professor Fitzgerald pointed out that these statements were not correct, and forced Dr. Collip to correct them.
>
> On February 19th, Dr. Collip found that he was unable to refine extract by his method, and was unable to keep up his supply to the Wards. During the following six weeks, or longer, no extract was available for clinical tests. I believe the reason for this to be that Collip, wishing to keep his process a secret, had not kept careful records. The whole investigation was thus held up, and after securing the consent of Professor Macleod, Mr. Best and myself commenced where we had left off in January to work on the refining of the extract.

Collip remembers it thus [2]:

> The contribution made by J. B. Collip to the Development of Insulin while he was in Toronto in 1921–1922.
>
> 1. The production of a state of hypoglycemia in normal rabbits following administration of a potent pancreatic extract. First experiment December 12, 1921.

2. The preparation of crude but potent extracts of pancreas, as follows:
   Fresh pancreas was ground and mixed with an equal volume of 95% alcohol. The mixture after thorough agitation was strained through cheese cloth and then filtered. The filtrate was concentrated in a vacuum still to 1/5 its volume either with or without the addition of 1 drop of glacial acetic acid per 100 cc. of filtrate before the concentration process was started.
3. The observation (December 1921) that little or no effect was produced in anaesthetized dogs by the administration of pancreatic extracts. The observations suggested the liver as a seat of action of the potent principle.
4. The storage of glycogen in the liver of a depancreatized dog following the administration of potent pancreatic extract. (The demonstration of this phenomenon was first made on December 22, 1921). The experiment was planned and carried out by Banting, Best, and Collip.
5. The observation that ketosis is abolished in depancreatized animals by use of potent pancreatic extracts.
6. The discovery of a method of preparing insulin in semi-pure form suitable for human administration.
7. The use of normal rabbits as a means of assay of the insulin used in treating the first clinical cases.
8. The observation that insulinated rabbits develop characteristic symptoms when the blood sugar has fallen to a low level.
9. The observation that these symptoms can be antedoted to a degree by adrenalin and can be controlled by glucose.
10. The observation that marked hypoglycemia was manifested in an etherized dog following the administration of highly potent insulin.
11. The production of a large part of this insulin preparation used by various members of the enlarged collaborating group during the early months of 1922.

Whatever the truth, it is clear that Collip brought a degree of biochemical expertise to the project that was previously lacking, and that the experience in the Macleod group determined the course of Collip's future research in the purification of hormones. He returned to Edmonton in 1922 as professor of biochemistry and immediately undertook the course of studies leading to the MD degree. This was awarded to him in 1926. His research now focused on the purification of parathyroid hormone. In December of 1924, Collip announced at a meeting of the American Physiological Society that he had successfully prepared an active extract of parathyroid hormone. He did not mention that the year before, Adolph Hanson reported a similar accomplishment in the *Military Surgeon* [3]. A second controversy, as unpleasant as the first, ensued.

Adolph Hanson was a medical practitioner who pursued science at his own expense, without modern tools or the backing of an institute or university, out of a love of discovery and a covenant to find new therapies for his patients. Hanson received his MD degree from Northwestern University in 1911 and trained in neurosurgery at the University of Pennsylvania. During the First World War, he served in France as a surgeon under Harvey Cushing at the famous Evacuation Hospital No. 8. Home from the war, he settled into private practice in the small town of Faribault, Minnesota. In parallel, he earned a bachelor and a master of arts degree in chemistry from St. Olaf's College in the neighboring town of Northfield.

Having built a small laboratory in his basement, Hanson then set out to isolate the active principle in parathyroid glandular tissue. He chose an unorthodox approach, boiling the glands in a weak solution of hydrochloric acid, and an unorthodox vehicle in which to report his findings, *Military Surgeon* [4]. What ensued was a struggle for priority, for patent rights, and for recognition. Ultimately, Hanson's extract was championed and then marketed by the Parke-Davis Laboratory as Paroidin, and Collip's extract was marketed by Eli Lilly as Para-Thor-Mone. Collip moved on to other venues of research, but Hanson jousted with the windmill until, in 1932, exhausted and bitter, he won an empty patent victory and his product was granted priority. It was marketed for a time by Lilly, Parke-Davis, and Squibb. It was, however, only legal recognition. The scientific community always associated Collip with the discovery, and Hanson's moment on the stage came to an unhappy end.

Collip was appointed professor of biochemistry at McGill University in 1928, succeeding the same Professor Macallum with whom he had started his scientific career. Here he recognized that ovarian hormones could be found in water-soluble form and, hence, could be orally active [5]. He named this estrogenic extract Emmenin, which, in collaboration with Wyeth Ayerst, came to market as Premarin.

Collip was among the first to isolate ACTH [6] and he characterized the molecules that neutralize hormones after repeated administration as antihormones, now known as antibodies [7].

In 1947, Collip left active science and became dean of the Faculty of Medicine at the University of Western Ontario. He held this job until 1961, when he retired at 69 years of age.

Collip was a shy man. He disliked conversation with strangers. He disliked even more the rigors of public speaking, and to the best of his ability he avoided teaching and lecturing. He was one of the great leaders in endocrinology of this century and he put the science of hormone isolation and bioassay on a sound and scientific foundation, doing more than most others to bring endocrinology out of its "glandular therapy" period and into the era of modern medicine.

He died of a stroke in London, Ontario on June 19, 1965 at the age of 72.

References

1. Keys DA: James Bertram Collip, an appreciation. *Can Med Assoc J* 1965; 93: 774–5.
2. Bliss M: Banting's, Best's, and Collip's accounts of the discovery of insulin. *Bull Hist Med* 1982; 56: 554–68.
3. Hanson AM: An elementary chemical study of the parathyroid glands of cattle. *Mil Surg* 1923; 53: 280–4.
4. Hanson AM: Notes on the hydrochloric X of the bovine parathyroid. *Mil Surg* 1923; 53: 434.
5. Collip JB: The ovary-stimulating hormone of the placenta: preliminary paper. *Can Med Assoc J* 1930; 22: 216.
6. Collip JB: Chemistry and physiology of anterior pituitary hormone. *Tran Cong Am Physicians Surgeons* 1933; 15: 47–64.
7. Collip JB: Inhibiting hormones and the principle of inverse response. *Ann Intern Med* 1934; 8: 10–13.

This chapter has been reproduced from Loriaux, D. Lynn: James Bertram Collip (1893–1965). *The Endocrinologist* 1996; 6(1): 1–3.

CHAPTER 54

Frederick Madison Allen (1879–1964)

The Diabetic Diet

Frederick Allen developed the most successful treatment for diabetes mellitus in the years leading up to the availability of insulin in 1923. Elliott Joslin referred to this period in the development of therapies for diabetes as "the Allen era" [1].

Allen was born in Des Moines, Iowa, March 16, 1879. He earned both the BA and MD degrees from the University of California. He was an intern in the University of California hospital in 1907 and 1908. He then went to Harvard Medical School for 3 years as a research fellow. He was supported by a small grant to study diabetes mellitus. These 3 years led to the 1913 publication of his encyclopedic text *Glycosuria and Diabetes*. The publication of the book, 1179 pages in length, was financed by his father. It contained what was known of the disease at the time with a bibliography of over 1200 references. It also contained his own research on the subject, 200 dogs, 200 cats and assorted experiments on rabbits, guinea-pigs, and rats. The book was an instant success and quickly became the "zeitgeber" to the field.

Allen's thesis was that diabetes was usually not associated with complete β cell failure and the key to effective management was to optimize the metabolic status of the patient to allow life to continue until the β cell failure was no longer compatible with life.

He championed a dietary regimen that would minimize glucosuria and ketones and, thus, maximize length of life. His diet was characterized by caloric restriction, severe enough to necessitate weight loss. The caloric restriction was balanced between protein and fat, carbohydrates being more severely restricted.

On the basis of his book, *Glycosuria and Diabetes Mellitus* [2], Allen was offered a position at the Rockefeller Institute in New York City. This position gave him access to a small ward of diabetic patients and laboratory space adequate for the chemical characterization of his experiments on animals and humans. Four years later, Allen and his associates published a second tome, *Total Dietary Regulation in the Treatment of Diabetes* [3]. This book contained extensive records of 76 of his patients treated with dietary therapy. His work was both heralded as an impressive advance in the treatment

A Biographical History of Endocrinology, First Edition. D. Lynn Loriaux.

of diabetes, and as a desperate attempt to keep diabetics alive at the expense of inanition and death from starvation. Allen understood this very well and made the case that on his diet, life was more tolerable for most diabetics and life was extended measurably. In the end, the Allen diet became the standard of care, at least in most academic centers.

No matter how one looked at this approach, all agreed that hundreds, if not thousands, of diabetic patients were kept alive long enough to benefit from the newly available insulin therapy, patients that otherwise would have perished before this great advance could be made available to them.

In 1919, Allen left the Rockefeller Institute. It is said that the reason for his departure was internecine controversy over the "ethics" of his total dietary treatment. The inanition, in the end, was very severe. Adults weighing 65 pounds were not an unusual occurrence, and many physicians condemned the therapy because it seemed to them merely a substitution of one disease for another. In 1919, Allen moved to Morristown, New Jersey and bought a palatial mansion. In this building he founded the Physiatric Institute, an institute intended to be a sophisticated center devoted entirely to the treatment of diabetes. It was divided into areas appointed according to the ability and desire of the patient to pay, much like first class and economy on an airplane flight. The rich paid handsomely for upscale rooms, which supported the care of the poor. The institute flourished and, with the advent of insulin therapy, branched out into the treatment of arterial hypertension. In the early 1920s Allen conceived of the relationship between salt intake and arterial hypertension. He began treating patients, with some success, using severe salt restriction. His basic approach to these patients can be seen today in the treatment of difficult hypertensive patients.

Frederick Allen was a tireless worker, 16-hour days Monday through Friday. On Saturday, he would take a few hours for tennis. He was a relentless, if not considerate, mentor of the young people who came in great numbers to work with him.

His interests finally took him into the field of cancer. In 1960, he wrote a forward-looking manuscript on the pathophysiology of cancer titled, *Anti-Tumor Defenses* [4]. His life ended at the Pondville Cancer Hospital in Massachusetts where he worked into his final days. He died in his 85th year.

References

1. Joslin E: Biography journal article. *Diabetes* 1964; 13: 318–19.
2. Allen F: *Glycosuria and Diabetes Mellitus*. Boston: WM Leonard, 1913.
3. Allen F, Edgar S, Fitz R: *Total Dietary Regulation in the Treatment of Diabetes*. New York: Rockefeller Institute for Medical Research, 1917.
4. Allen F: *Anti-Tumor Defenses*. Vienna: Austrian Cancer Research Institute, 1960.

This chapter has been reproduced from Loriaux, D. Lynn: Frederick Madison Allen, MD: 1879–1964. *The Endocrinologist* 2009; 19(3): 93.

CHAPTER 55

Elliott Proctor Joslin (1869–1962)

Insulin and the Treatment of Diabetes

Elliott Joslin was born on June 6, 1869. He grew up with an older half brother and sister in the small Massachusetts town of Oxford, just north of the Connecticut border. The town was situated in productive farmland and had an established manufacturing economy. Joslin's father, Allen, was a partner in the Joslin Shoe Factory. His mother, Sara Proctor, was a distant relative of the family that founded the Procter and Gamble Company. Elliott grew up with a reverence for the environment steeped in the liberal teachings of the Congregational Church. He went to boarding school, the Leicester Academy, at an early age. This was followed by Yale College and Harvard Medical School. He graduated as valedictorian of his class in 1895, and immediately embarked on the "tour of the Continent" that was required of ambitious young American medical graduates, visiting the leading medical clinics in Berlin, Freiberg, and Vienna. Returning to the United States in 1897, Joslin spent a year as an intern at the Massachusetts General Hospital. It was during his European tour and his year at "the General" that his interest in metabolic diseases was firmly established.

Joslin set up his practice in Boston's Back Bay at 81 Bay State Road. He had a townhouse and an adjacent building that soon filled to capacity with his growing practice. Joslin practiced at this site until the current Joslin Diabetes Center opened near the Harvard Medical School in 1956. Joslin's first encounter with a diabetic patient occurred during his internship year:

> Mary H, an unmarried woman, 26 years of age, was seen in the Outpatient department of the Massachusetts General Hospital on August 2, 1893. Her mouth was dry and she was "drinking water all the time, and was compelled to rise 3 or 4 times each night to pass her urine." She "felt weak and tired." Her appetite was variable, the bowels constipated, and she had a dizzy headache. Belching of gas, a tight feeling in the abdomen, and a burning in the stomach followed her meals. She was short of breath [1].

Joslin treated her with a strict diet of protein and fat. The polyuria decreased immediately, pruritis was eased, and she could almost sleep through the night. This was Joslin's "Case No. 1." Two more patients found their way to Joslin in short order. The

A Biographical History of Endocrinology, First Edition. D. Lynn Loriaux.

This work is a co-publication between the Endocrine Society and John Wiley & Sons, Ltd.

first was his Aunt Helen. She had increased thirst, weight loss, and weakness associated with a "healthy appetite." "Joslin again employed dietary therapy (a diet virtually free of carbohydrates) and fresh air and exercise." Helen declined over the following 18 months and, in March of 1899, developed a sore throat, languor, "peculiar respirations," delirium, coma, and death. Three weeks later, Joslin's mother, Sara, became Case No. 8. When she was found to have 5% glucose in her urine, she too was managed with a strict diet. In her case, it was more effective; she died of a stroke 13 years later at the age of 74.

It was about this time that Joslin dedicated himself to the study of diabetes. There was not a lot to help him at this juncture. There was the classic description of the disease by Aretaeus of Cappadocia [2]. There was the work of Von Mering and Minkowski, who showed that diabetes followed pancreatectomy in the dog, and that pancreatic transplant could correct the glycosuria [3]. Eugene Opie had found that β cells were replaced by scar tissue in people dying of diabetes [4]. Joslin knew of the work of Frederick Allen, a postdoctoral fellow working at the Harvard Medical School, who showed that a diet radically reduced in calories could improve the metabolic state of diabetic animals and prolong life. People also seemed to benefit from this intervention, and it was soon referred to as the "starvation diet" [5].

Joslin focused on dietary therapy for diabetes. He believed that the "starvation diet" was beyond the capacity of most patients to sustain. Working with Francis Benedict of the Carnegie Institution, he developed the "Joslin Diet," low in fat, moderate in carbohydrates, and overall restricted in calories. The diet was easier to tolerate and gave some measure of satiety. The treatment attracted attention and Joslin's practice increased geometrically. He collaborated with the New England Deaconess Hospital and admitted patients to "cottages" on the hospital grounds for extended periods of metabolic recovery and diabetes education [1].

When Joslin had treated 1000 patients with his diet, he concluded that his treatment was better than the alternatives. He described an approximate 20% reduction in mortality over the first year of treatment. He codified his approach in 1916 with his book, *The Treatment of Diabetes Mellitus* [6]. This text defined a new standard of practice in diabetes, and forever linked Joslin's name with the disease. Overnight he became the "consensus leader" in the treatment of diabetes. The book went through 10 editions in his lifetime.

Joslin published a companion volume in 1918 titled *Diabetic Manual–for the Doctor and Patient*, which focused on patient education and encouraged patients to take control of their disease management. It was an instant success. Still, therapeutic success was far from satisfactory.

The management of diabetes then took a huge step forward. In 1923, insulin became commercially available. The Joslin Clinic, as it is now called, became a mecca for the treatment of diabetes mellitus. The result was another exponential growth in the number of patients waiting to be seen. A generous gift from the philanthropist George F. Baker enabled the clinic to diversify its work into the emerging complications of diabetes such as peripheral vascular disease, renal disease, neuropathy, and proliferative retinopathy. This latter complication, leading to blindness in many cases, was the focus of studies by William Beecham, the Joslin Clinic ophthalmologist, who showed in a beautiful study that blindness can be prevented by laser ablation of early proliferative retinopathy. Joslin believed that the complications of diabetes were the result of poor diabetic control and elevated blood glucose levels. Highly debated in the 1960s and 1970s, the powerful "Diabetes Control and Complications Trial," published in the *New England Medical Journal* in 1993, validated his hypothesis and set targets for glycosylated hemoglobin that can largely prevent these complications [7].

On December 21, 1961, Joslin wrote his annual Christmas message to the staff of the Joslin Clinic. In this message he reminded his colleagues of how medical science and the dedication of doctors, nurses, and students had changed the lives of patients with diabetes everywhere. In describing the effects of insulin therapy, he refers to the 37th chapter of Ezekiel:

> And behold, a rattling and the bones came together, bone to its bone. And as I looked, there were sinews on them, and flesh had come upon them, and skin had covered them .... And the breath came into them, and they lived, and stood on their feet, an exceedingly great host.

A month later, after a full day's schedule, attending morning services at Old South Church, and corresponding with patients and friends, Joslin died at home in his sleep, 93 years of age.

References

1. Feudtner CJ: *Bittersweet: Diabetes, Insulin, and the Transformation of Illness.* Chapel Hill, NC: The University of North Carolina Press, 2004.
2. Loriaux DL: Diabetes and the Ebers Papyrus. *The Endocrinologist* 2006; 16: 55.
3. Loriaux DL: Oskar Minkowski. *The Endocrinologist* 2006; 16: 1.
4. Opie EL: The relation of diabetes mellitus tolesions of the pancreas. Hyaline degeneration of the islands of Langerhans. *J Exp Med* 1900; 5: 527–40.
5. Medvei VC: *The History of Endocrinology.* Lancaster, U.K.: MTP Press, 1982, p. 457.
6. Joslin EP: The treatment of diabetes mellitus. *Can Med Assoc J* 1916; 6: 673–84.
7. The Diabetes Control and Complications Trial Research Group: The effect of intensive treatment of diabetes on the development and progression of long-term complications in insulin-dependent diabetes mellitus. *N Engl J Med* 1993; 329: 977–86.

This chapter has been reproduced from Loriaux, D. Lynn: Elliott Proctor Joslin (1869–1962). *The Endocrinologist* 2006; 16(3): 123–4.

CHAPTER 56

J.J.R. Macleod

(1876–1935)

Discovery of Insulin

For most people, the discovery of insulin at the University of Toronto in 1921–1922 is an exciting story of the near-miraculous isolation and application of insulin leading to the first life-saving treatment for diabetes. The 1923 Nobel Prize in Physiology or Medicine was awarded for this great achievement. Unfortunately, the award left a legacy of continuing controversy because one of the Nobel laureates, Frederick Banting, believed that his student assistant, Charles Best, should also have been honored. Banting divided his share of the Nobel Prize money equally with Best. His co-laureate, J.J.R. Macleod, divided his money with a fourth member of the team, J.B. Collip. Then, as the discovery passed into medical history, with first Banting and then Best retelling their versions of the story many times, Macleod's role in these events became clouded and confused and somewhat blackened. The notion got about that Macleod had not really deserved to share in the prize awarded for the research. Particularly in Canada, Macleod's role in the discovery of insulin was almost forgotten. The University of Toronto, which possesses many monuments to Banting and Best, has no remembrance whatever of the presence and achievements of the university's greatest professor of physiology.

The research that led to my book *The Discovery of Insulin* [1], and the televised dramatization based on it, *Glory Enough for All*, has gone a considerable way to locate Macleod's true role in the discovery of insulin. In this paper I discuss these events with a stronger focus on Macleod as a physiologist of his time. His deep conservatism as a scientist, I suggest, leads to the irony that a co-discoverer of insulin was never particularly interested in either the pancreas or the endocrine system of the body. On the other hand, it was exactly his vast knowledge of the complexities of his subject and his commitment to the scientific vocation that made it possible for him to play a vital role in the discovery of insulin. Behind the highly televisual fights of passionate, flawed scientists in the labs at Toronto and the near-resurrections that insulin really did effect, there stood a gentle, learned physiologist doing his job with dignity and diligence as he orchestrated one of the great achievements in the history of medicine.

A Biographical History of Endocrinology, First Edition. D. Lynn Loriaux.

This work is a co-publication between the Endocrine Society and John Wiley & Sons, Ltd.

John James Rickard Macleod was born at Cluny, Scotland, in 1876. A minister's son, he was educated at Aberdeen Grammar School, and studied medicine at Marischal College, University of Aberdeen, graduating with honors in 1898. He further studied at Leipzig and Cambridge and held brief appointments at the London Hospital Medical College. In 1903 he left the United Kingdom to become professor of physiology at Western Reserve University in Cleveland, Ohio, where he taught and did research for the next 15 years. He was a prolific researcher, a professor deeply learned in his discipline, and an accomplished scientific writer at both advanced and introductory levels. His research interests evolved from early work with Leonard Hill on intracranial circulation to a concentration on metabolism with special emphasis on the body's use of carbohydrates. In 1907, he began publishing papers entitled "Studies in experimental glycosuria," and in 1913 he summarized the work in a monograph, *Diabetes: Its Pathological Physiology*.

While later events made this early research of little more than antiquarian interest, it reveals much about Macleod as an investigator and about the historical unfolding of the problem of diabetes. Specifically, it reminds us that both the pancreas and the idea of endocrine secretions were latecomers in the evolution of knowledge about diabetes. Macleod had been trained in the 1890s in the mainstream of physiology. This meant that he had absorbed conventional wisdom about the primacy of the nervous system in the control of physiological functions generally and also followed Claude Bernard's emphasis on the central role of the liver in carbohydrate metabolism. Macleod's concept of diabetes was the traditional one of a condition of hyperglycemia and/or glycosuria that could be created experimentally by cerebroventricular puncture, phlorizin poisoning, or asphyxiation. His studies seemed to confirm the view that the primary functional disorder in diabetes was hepatic, involving a failure of glycogen production from glucose, indeed a flooding of the system with it. It seemed important to Macleod to investigate the triggering mechanism of this process, which seemed related to nerve impulses acting on the liver.

As a chemical physiologist, Macleod took little interest in diabetes as a clinical condition; in the only comment I have found about the causes of clinical diabetes in his early writing, he attributes the disease, revealingly, to excessive nervous stimulation, writing in 1914 that "Diabetes is common in locomotive engineers and in the captains of ocean liners, that is to say in men who in the performance of their daily duties are frequently put under a severe nerve-strain. It is apparently increasing in men engaged in occupations that demand mental concentration and strain, such as in professional and business work" [2].

Speculative flights like this are mercifully rare in Macleod's writing, because the normal hallmark of his work was a conservative empiricism, which caused him seldom to be out of touch with recent research findings, particularly those of a negative variety, and also seldom to speculate without solid empirical data on hand. The problem with this caution was that the more Macleod learned about carbohydrate metabolism, the more baffling its physiology seemed to become–particularly because of the way that the pancreas and new ideas of hormonal action kept inserting themselves into the familiar and comfortable models of diabetes as a nervous and hepatic disorder.

The pancreas had made a somewhat sudden, somewhat unexpected and belated appearance in the diabetes story with the discovery by von Mering and Minkowski in 1889 that its extraction leads to the development of severe, fatal diabetes [3]. At first, no one knew or could intelligently speculate why that should be so, but by the turn of the century other discoveries involving ductless glands made it conceivable to speculate about the pancreas releasing some kind of internal secretion or (after the coining of the term at the instigation of Bayliss and Starling [4]) some kind of hormone that played a vital role in the regulation carbohydrate metabolism. But both the existence of that hormone and its mode of action remained hypothetical as Macleod and other researchers probed the mysteries of the supply of sugar in the body [1, 4]. Indeed, the role of the pancreas in metabolic events remained more obscure and appeared less important than that of the adrenal medulla, for the isolation of adrenaline (epinephrine) in the late 1890s soon led to the discovery of its hyperglycemic effects and the necessity of integrating an apparently hormonally induced form of diabetes into more traditional models of the disease. In his studies of glycosuria, Macleod was able to do this more or less to his satisfaction by highlighting the role of the sympathetic nervous system in releasing adrenaline to work on the liver. So the new organ and its secretion had been fitted into the neural–hepatic model; indeed, it was Walter Cannon's pioneering studies in emotional states and the release of adrenaline that supported Macleod's belief in stress as a principal cause of diabetes.

But always there remained the pancreas and its hypothetical hormone, at the center of the puzzle. By about 1914 the idea that the pancreas produced an internal secretion was the most logical explanation of its function, but Macleod knew that scores and scores of attempts to isolate this hormone had gone nowhere. No one had been able though pancreatic feeding or injection of pancreatic extracts, to demonstrate that they had captured the active principle that seemed to be lost in pancreatic diabetes.

As Macleod himself noted in reviewing some of the most recent attempts to find the elusive pancreatic hormone, there were "extreme technical difficulties" in tackling the problem [2]. For decades it had been next to impossible to trace the behavior of sugars in the blood because measuring techniques were so primitive, thus forcing researchers to concentrate on the study of glycosuria where they were gravely handicapped by the effects of renal intermediation. And even though recent improvements in techniques, which greatly interested Macleod, now facilitated study of the blood sugar, there remained the baffling problem of the relationship of blood glucose to glycogen and hepatic function generally. In other words, there was ongoing confusion about the course of physiological events in diabetes. As a cautious researcher, Macleod tended to favor the traditional view of hyperglycemia as the result of excess sugar production in the liver, but again there was a growing body of evidence suggesting that the real problem might lie in the inability of the tissues to burn sugar. Here was another and even more difficult problem of measurement which led Macleod and others into elaborate attempts to estimate the oxidation of sugars in the cell as measured through studies of respiration.

Macleod's work in experimental glycosuria established his reputation and that the problem was too complex to be unraveled with the experimental techniques then available. He cut back his work on carbohydrate metabolism, wrote what became a famous textbook in physiology (*Physiology and Biochemistry in Modern Medicine*), and became increasingly unhappy with the United States' non-participation in the First World War and with his position at Western Reserve. In 1918, he returned to British soil by accepting the chair of physiology at the University of Toronto. His main research interest now centered on attempts to explore centers of respiration (again seeing the problem as a study in the relations of nervous and chemical factors), but he did maintain a watching brief in the field of carbohydrate metabolism. While preparing this paper, I found in the University of Toronto archives evidence that in 1921 Macleod was preparing his students to undertake new studies in puncture-induced diabetes. These were interrupted, however, by the arrival in Macleod's life and laboratory of Frederick Banting and his ideas for work on pancreatic diabetes.

Macleod knew that Banting's proposal to ligate pancreatic ducts in the hope that intact islet cells and their secretion would survive had been tried before. As a liver man, rather than a pancreas expert, Macleod may have been a little fuzzy in his knowledge of the exact state of research on atrophy of the pancreas after duct ligation, and he may not have expressed an opinion on Banting's notion that this procedure would be a way of frustrating the supposed destruction of the "internal secretion" of the pancreas by its powerful "external" secretion. This seems to be a logical explanation of what some have seen as surprising gaps in Macleod's knowledge and/or shortcomings in the advice he gave to Banting, and underlay Sir Henry Dale's patronizing–and not envious–remark that insulin could only have been discovered in a lab whose director was slightly stupid [1, pp. 208 and 278]. He apparently did realize that no one had succeeded in following Banting's exact proposal before (unfortunately, Banting's exact proposal is not fully clear from the documents; it seems to have been a double surgical procedure, aimed at showing that a graft of atrophied pancreas would restore normal metabolism in a depancreatized animal; in fact, this would be what we now recognize as an islet cell transplant), and for this and other reasons involving the underutilization of his facilities and the desirability of encouraging all kinds of medical research at Toronto, he agreed to open his lab to Banting in the summer of 1921 and give him appropriate support and direction. Much direction was required because Banting, a dabbler who had worked out his idea after reading a journal article one night, was woefully ignorant of the field, inexperienced at research, unsure of his methods, and ignorant of the testing procedures he would have to use.

Macleod's support for Banting included giving him the help of his student assistants, notably Charles Best, advising him on the plan of the research, including methods of pancreatectomy (which he demonstrated to Banting), suggesting a research plan moving from transplants through the injection of extracts of atrophied pancreas, and explaining to Banting how to prepare an extract. After setting Banting and Best to work and consulting with them during the first several weeks of their research, Macleod left Toronto for Scotland for the balance of summer of 1921. When Banting and Best reported to him their initial success in lowering the blood sugar of a depancreatized dog with their extract in late July, Macleod gave instructions for controls, suggested problems with their findings, and outlined other experiments to make the results more convincing. There is no evidence that at any time Macleod developed much regard for Banting as a scientist or as a man. In fact, in September, when Macleod returned to Toronto, the two of them quarreled bitterly about research facilities–but he did gradually become convinced that the favorable pattern of Banting and Best's blood sugar readings suggested the presence in their extract of an active principle (i.e., the internal secretion of the pancreas). In the autumn of 1921, he gave Banting and Best better facilities and encouraged the work to continue.

The problem was how to complete the proof by producing something that would be conclusively recognized as the internal secretion. Other researchers, including Kleiner in the United States [5] and Paulesco in Romania [6, 7], had gone as far as Banting and Best and had, from time to time, cleared up glycosuria or hyperglycemia with pancreatic extracts. But blood sugar could go down for many reasons after administration of pancreatic extract. What would count as indisputable evidence that these extracts contained the internal secretion? "There is one experiment," Macleod had written, "and it consists in seeing in seeing the symptoms which follow pancreatectomy are removed, and a normal condition reestablished, when means are taken to supply the supposed missing internal secretion to the organism."

We do not know the exact details of his discussions with Banting and Best that autumn. We do know that Banting was dissuaded by someone from dissipating his energies in pancreas grafting experiments, and we know that Banting independently managed to find that extracts of fetal pancreas, and then fresh chilled pancreas were as effective as the earlier extracts of ligated, atrophied pancreas. We know that it was another member of Macleod's department who suggested to Banting and Best that a longevity experiment on a diabetic dog would be helpful in proving the extract's ability to supply the missing secretion. We know that it was Banting who asked Macleod to add to the team the biochemist J.B. Collip, who was in Toronto on sabbatical that year from the University of Alberta to work with Macleod. After Collip joined the team in December 1921, the group met daily for lunch. Macleod was supervisor and organizer of the work, suggesting improvements in the preparation of extract (alcohol was now being used as an extractive, possibly on Macleod's suggestion) and outlining the new experiments that should be tried. He saw the need to explore the extract's effect in other kinds of experimental diabetes and, above all, wanted to know what it did to the liver and glycogen formation.

While Banting and Best ran into great difficulties in the preparation of their extraction. Collip went from strength to strength, applying standard experimental techniques to the problem. His most exciting result, which took place just before Christmas 1921, was his discovery that pancreas extract enabled a diabetic liver to store glycogen [8]. This proved that the group had much more than a blood sugar reducer, and that the extract acted at what Macleod believed was the center of glucose metabolism. His finding were quickly supplemented by Collip's discovery that the extract also cleared up ketoacidosis–and all of this in the context of Banting and Best's apparent success with their longevity experiments. This was the evidence Macleod cited to his associates in the American Physiological Association at its New Haven meeting that Christmas holiday during the discussion of the paper [9] given by Banting, after Banting had failed to respond adequately to critical questioning about his and Best's experiments. However, it was precisely that intervention in the discussion which convinced Banting, who had never liked Macleod or felt comfortable in his presence, that both the work and the glory were being taken out of his hands by Macleod and Collip.

In January 1922, the young men moved forward in an atmosphere fouled by rivalry and paranoia. Collip was attempting to purify the extract for what would surely be the ultimate test on a human diabetic. Banting and Best had already tried such a test, apparently without telling Macleod, and it had failed. Macleod did consent to Banting and Best's extract being the first to be tested formally, on a 14-year-old boy named Leonard Thompson, in Toronto General Hospital on January 11, 1622. That test failed [10]. Twelve days later, however, Collip developed a process by which he could remove the toxic contaminants from the extract while holding it in solution, and then precipitate out relatively pure active principle. Collip's extract worked on Leonard Thompson [11].

Macleod was the man in charge of a situation of intense, almost unimaginable pressure, excitement, challenge, and potential. The research team had found its way to a Holy Grail and now they had to present it to humanity, and to a skeptical scientific community. The packaging and presentation of the discovery would not be easy. The team desperately needed to learn more about the substance they had, its impact on the body, its chemical composition, even its origin in the pancreas. Macleod organized this ongoing research and did much of it himself (e.g., [12, 13]). They had to explore its clinical impact on diabetes, work that Macleod coordinated with his fellow professor of medicine, Duncan Graham, and the appropriate clinicians, notably Walter Campbell. They had to organize production of much larger quantities of the extract, a process Macleod assigned to Collip, until Collip, using primitive apparatus and working with more variables than he could control, lost the ability to make it. Macleod had to orchestrate the second search for the metabolic Grail. While it was being found, Macleod had to hold together a team of researchers who had literally clawed at each other's throats (Banting twice attacked Collip); had to organize their publications to present the discovery to the world (he suggested they follow what I'm told had been a Scot's practice and publish alphabetically); and had to give the substance a name (it was Macleod who suggested insulin from the Latin root for islet, and only late did they realize that at least two previous researchers had suggested the same name for the internal secretion). They had to carry on the delicate, pioneering negotiations with an American drug company, Eli Lilly and Company, and various patent attorneys, for a licensing arrangement that would bring Lilly's resources to bear on the production problem without sacrificing the group's control of the extract. He also had to protect himself from Banting's bitter, malicious attacks on his integrity as a scientist and as a man.

This was J.J.R. Macleod's finest hour, a time when he employed all of his experience and skills as a scientist, an administrator, and a wise human being to keep the lid on a tremendously volatile situation, keep the work going steadily forward, organize insulin production, testing, and research, and generally carry on the elaboration of discovery in such a way that the world of science and diabetes quickly realized that Macleod's physiology lab at Toronto was giving it a very important, very precious gift.

While Banting raged and sulked, drank himself into oblivion, conspired for credit, and finally forced himself back into the picture as a clinician giving insulin to patients, Macleod carried an enormous burden of work and responsibility with immense patience, professional surefootedness of the first order, and quiet dedication.

By the summer of 1922, insulin was performing those wonderful miracles with dying diabetics and the glory was being showered on the insulin man, the brilliant Dr. Banting, who was never shy about telling people how he and Best had struggled against Macleod's stinginess and disparagement and intellectual dishonesty. Macleod, on the other hand, was in a lab in Atlantic Canada, trying to nail down the hypothesis that insulin actually was produced in the islet cells of the pancreas (he did this by drawing on much earlier research done in Aberdeen by Rennie and Fraser [14] using species of fish whose islet cells are anatomically separated from the rest of the pancreas [12]). When he returned to Toronto that autumn, he faced more attacks from Banting. At the invitation of the chairman of the Board of Governors of the university, Macleod wrote his only personal statement about these events, a 5000-word "History of the researches leading to the discovery of insulin." It was not made public until 1978. It is a dry, factual, carefully composed document, stressing the collaborative nature of the work. Perhaps Macleod's pride in his achievement is evident in the final paragraph, where he writes, "Through concentrated effort, for the co-ordination of which I have been responsible, we have given to Science in little more than one year a practically completed piece of research work. We have proved the value of Insulin" [15].

Macleod was not self-effacing to the point of abdicating his rightful claim to credit for his contribution. In his private and public accounts of the discovery of insulin, he was very careful to credit Banting with having initiated the work and having confirmed the hypothesis that the pancreas contained an internal secretion. But he then insisted that the isolation and investigation of that secretion had been a collaborative effort under his direction in which Collip had played a particularly important role. This was the view adopted by the Nobel Committee, which was particularly influenced by the great Danish physiologist, August Krogh, who, as the result of a visit to Toronto in the autumn of 1922, had nominated Banting and Macleod jointly, arguing that each was indispensable to the discovery process (see [1], drawing on the Nobel archive). I agree with this view, although I would be inclined to have added Collip's name to the prize, for his breakthrough in purifying the extract to the point where clinical success was unambiguous seems to have been the single achievement separating Toronto's work from the failures of predecessors. It was the product of hard work by a well-trained biochemist using the most advanced techniques in a very well-equipped laboratory.

Macleod's Nobel address, given in Stockholm in 1925, began with a tribute to the "numerous investigations over many years" by "workers in various fields of medical science" which had preceded the Toronto research. His lecture was entitled "The physiology of insulin and its source in the animal body," and Macleod used the opportunity to discuss the follow-up work his lab had been doing on insulin since 1923. After having proved insulin's source in the islet cells, Macleod left the pancreas, and in a sense left the exploration of insulin itself (the next important step in its story was

Abel's crystallization of insulin in 1926), to go back to what for him was the key physiological problem, which was how insulin worked in the body to facilitate the metabolism of sugar.

Macleod's interest still centered not on the pancreas but on the liver, for he was certain that insulin lowered blood sugar by stimulating glycogen formation and storage. It was "a great surprise" he acknowledged in perhaps his most emotional statement in a scientific paper, when he and his students found that this hypothesis was not correct [16]. By the time of his Nobel lecture, Macleod understood, as a result of his own and others' research, that insulin's principal action was in facilitating the passage of sugar into the cells. At that level he came upon, as it were, a brick wall: "we know nothing of the fate of the glucose which disappears [into the cell]," he wrote. He concluded his Nobel lecture not with a summary of past accomplishments, but with a scientist's simple look forward: regarding "the perplexing problem of [insulin's] action in the animal body," he wrote, "Facts of importance in this regard come almost daily to light and it is to be anticipated that, as these accumulate, a great advance will become possible in our knowledge of the history of carbohydrates in the animal body."

After 1928, Macleod's role in developing this knowledge diminished. In that year he decided to leave Toronto to return to Aberdeen as holder of the chair in physiology. In Aberdeen he would not have facilities for research comparable to those he commanded in Toronto, but this was perhaps the one time in Macleod's life that he acknowledged a stronger pull than physiology. He was coming home to Scotland and to Aberdeen. He was also leaving a city and a university whose splendidly equipped laboratories could no longer hold him in a climate spoiled by the ongoing rancor of his fellow Nobel laureate, Banting, with whom he did not speak. Sitting in the club car as the train was about to take him from Toronto for the last time, Macleod told a friend that he was shuffling his feet "to wipe away the dirt of this city" [1, 17].

Macleod may have loved his home in Scotland beyond reason, for, after returning to Aberdeen he began to suffer from crippling arthritis, which was not helped by the North Sea climate. Nonetheless he continued to lead a busy and by all accounts a reasonably happy life, furthering medical education at the university, working to improve its research facilities, carrying on research himself with the aid of students drawn to the university by his fame, including a young refugee from Hitler's Germany named Hans Kosterlitz. Macleod was one of Aberdeen's most famous sons, honored in his native land for his distinguished career in physiology, and apparently untroubled by the disgraceful campaign against him that occasionally rippled across the north Atlantic from Toronto. He died in Aberdeen in 1935. In his last research he was still trying to locate the center in the brain where nervous control of carbohydrate metabolism originated. The co-discoverer of insulin was never comfortable with the endocrine system. On the other hand, it may not be too fanciful to suggest that there is at least a tenuous link between this conservative physiologist's belief in the primacy of the nervous system and the ongoing work related to neural transmission by Kosterlitz and his students, which led to Aberdeen's central role in the discovery of the endorphins some 40 years after Macleod's death.

When laymen, and even some scientists, promulgate an image of scientific development as miraculous breakthroughs made by passionate geniuses engaged in cut-throat competition, there is a real danger of competition; there is a real danger of getting the business backwards. When we cut away the undoubted drama, passion, and tensions of the insulin story, at the center of things we find, in J.J.R. Macleod, a professional physiologist and hard-working, conservative, cautious, even unimaginative man, but one who was deeply studious and devoted to his calling, without whom the Toronto research would have fallen apart or dribbled away in blind alleys. Macleod's mastery of his discipline, his strength of character, and his dedicated professionalism were essential in Toronto's presentation of what was indeed a great and sensational gift of medical science to humanity. He has been dead for over half a century now. I am sure he would be pleased to realize that his contribution to science is now understood by history. But if he could return today, Macleod would probably not be particularly interested in learning about the longevity of some of those early insulin-dependent diabetics or in John Woodvine's portrayal of him in the movie *Glory Enough for All.* He would probably be most intrigued by what his fellow physiologists could now tell him about insulin receptors and "the history of carbohydrates in the animal body."

References

1. Bliss M: *The Discovery of Insulin.* Toronto: McClelland & Stewart; London: Macmillan, 1982.
2. Macleod JJR: *Physiology and Biochemistry in Modern Medicine.* London: Henry Kimpton, 1918.
3. Von Mering J, Minkowski O: Diabetes mellitus nach Pankreasextirpation. *Arch Exp Pathol Pharmakol* 1890; 26: 371–87.
4. Medvei VC: *A History of Endocrinology.* Lancaster: MTP Press, 1982.
5. Kleiner IS: The action of intravenous injections of pancreas emulsions in experimental diabetes. *J Biol Chem* 1919; XL: 153–70.
6. Paulesco NC: Action de l'extrait pancreatique injecte dans le sang, chez un animal diabetique. *C R Séances Soc Biol* 1921; LXXXXV: 555–8.
7. Paulesco NC: Influence de la quantite de pancreas employee pour l'extrait injecte dans le sang chez un animal diabetique. *C R Séances Soc Biol* 1921; LXXXV: 558–9.
8. Collip JB: History of the discovery of insulin. *Northwest Medicine* 1923; 22: 267–73.
9. Banting FG, Best CH, Collip JB, Macleod JJR: The preparation of pancreatic extracts containing insulin. *Proceedings and Transactions of the Royal Society of Canada, 3rd Ser* 1922; XVI (section V): 27–9.
10. Banting FG, Best CH, Macleod JJR: The internal secretion of the pancreas. *Am J Physiol* 1922; LIX: 479.
11. Collip JB: The original method as used for the isolation of insulin in semi-pure form for the treatment of the first clinical cases. *J Biol Chem* 1923; LV: xl–xli.
12. Macleod JJR: The source of insulin. A study of the effect produced on blood sugar by extracts of the pancreas and principal islets of fishes. *J Metab Res* 1922; 2: 149–72.
13. Best CH, Macleod JJR: Some chemical reactions of insulin. *J Biol Chem* 1923; LV: vvvix–xxx.
14. Rennie J, Fraser T: The islets of Langerhans in relation to diabetes. *Biochem J* 1907; II: 7–19.

15. Macleod JJR: History of the researches leading to the discovery of insulin, September 1992. *Bull Hist Med* 1922/78; 52: 295–312.
16. Barbour AD, Chaikoff IL, Macleod JJR, Orr MD: Influence of insulin on liver and muscle glycogen in the rat under varying nutritional conditions. *Am J Physiol* 1927; LXXX: 243–72.
17. Bliss M: *Banting: A Biography*. Toronto: McClelland & Stewart, 1984.

Sources

University of Toronto Libraries: Manuscript collections in the Fisher Rare Books Library and the University of Toronto Archives include substantial private correspondence by Macleod, Banting and Best as well as the complete notebooks of Banting and Best.

Banting FG, Best CH: The internal secretion of the pancreas. *J Lab Clin Med* 1992; VII: 251–66.

Banting FG, Best CH, Collip JB, Campbell WR, Fletcher AA: Pancreatic extracts in the treatment of diabetes mellitus, Preliminary Report. 1922. *Can Med Assoc J* 1991; 145: 1281–6.

Banting FG, Best CH, Collip JB, Macleod JJR, Nobel EC: The effect produced on diabetes by extracts of pancreas. *Trans Assoc Am Physicians* 1922; XXXVII: 337–47.

Bliss M (Ed.): Banting's, Best's and Collip's accounts of the discovery of insulin. *Bull Hist Med* 1982; 56: 554–68.

Donhoffer C, Macleod JJR: Studies in the nervous control of carbohydrate metabolism. I – The position of the centre. *Proc R Soc B* 1932; CX: 125–71.

Macleod JJR: Studies in experimental glycosuria – I. On the existence of afferent and efferent nerve fibers, controlling the amount of sugar in the blood. *Am J Physiol* 1907; XIX: 388–407.

Macleod JJR: Studies in experimental glycosuria – II. Some experiments bearing on the nature of the glycogenolytic fibers in the great splanchnic nerve. *Am J Physiol* 1908; XXII: 373–409.

Macleod JJR: Studies in experimental glycosuria – IV. The cause of thehypeglycaemia produced by asphyxia. *Am J Physiol* 1909; XXIII: 278–302.

Macleod JJR: Various forms of experimental diabetes and their significance for diabetes mellitus. *J Am Med Assoc* 1910; LV: 2133–8.

Macleod JJR: *Diabetes: Its Pathological Physiology*. London, New York: Edward Arnold, 1913.

Macleod JJR: *Carbohydrate Metabolism and Insulin*. London, New York, Toronto: Longmans, Green, 1926.

Macleod JJR: The physiology of insulin and its source in the animal body. In *Nobel Lectures, Physiology of Medicine 1922–1941*. Amsterdam: Elsevier, 1965, pp. 71–81.

Macleod JJR, Fulk ME: Studies in experimental glycosuria – XI. Retention of dextrose by the liver and muscles and the influence of acids and alkalies on the dextrose concentration of the blood. *Am J Physiol* 1917; XLII: 193–213.

Macleod JJR, Hoover DH: Studies in experimental glycosuria – XII. Lactic acid production in the blood following the injection of alkaline solutions of dextrose or of the alkaline solutions alone. *Am J Physiol* 1917; XLII: 460–8.

Macleod JJR, Pearce RG: Studies in experimental glycosuria – V. The distribution of glycogenolytic ferment in the animal body, especially of the dog. *Am J Physiol* 1910; XXV: 255–91.

Macleod JJR, Pearce RG: Studies in experimental glycosuria – VI. The distribution of glycogen over the liver under various conditions. Post mortem glycogenolysis. *Am J Physiol* 1911; XXVII: 341–65.

Macleod JJR, Pearce RG: Studies in experimental glycosuria – VII. The amount of glycogenase in the liver and in the blood issuing from it, as affected by stimulation of the great splanchnic nerve. *Am J Physiol* 1911; XXVIII: 403–21.

Macleod JJR, Pearce RG: Studies in experimental glycosuria – VIII. The relationship of the adrenal glands to sugar production by the liver. *Am J Physiol* 1912; XXIX: 419–35.

Macleod JJR, Pearce RG: Studies in experimental glycosuria – IX. The level of blood-sugar in the dog under laboratory conditions. *Am J Physiol* 1915; XXXVII: 415–24.

Macleod JJR, Pearce RG: Studies in experimental glycosuria – X. The sugar-retaining power of the liver in relationship to the amount of glycogen already present in the organ. *Am J Physiol* 1915; XXXVIII: 425–37.

Macleod JJR, Ruh HO: Studies in experimental glycosuria – III. The influence of stimulation of the great splanchnic nerve on the rate of disappearance of glycogen from the liver, deprived of its portal blood supply or of both its portal and systemic blood supplies. *Am J Physiol* 1908; XXII: 397–409.

This chapter has been reproduced from Bliss, Michael: J. J. R. Macleod and the discovery of insulin. *The Endocrinologist* 1994; 4(2): 85–91.

CHAPTER 57

Frederick L. Hisaw
(1891–1972)
Relaxin

In the early 1920s, the field of endocrinology was in an unsettled state. It was 30 years since thyroid extract had first cured myxedema, a remarkable treatment that led to a multiplicity of organ extracts being used to treat many disorders with the expected mixed results (the positive ones were, of course, published). There was, in fact, some science mixed in with this clinical activity. Once the idea took hold that some tissues contained active materials, now called hormones, a wide range of scientists, including anatomists, physicians, and biochemists, tried to figure out what these unknown substances were. But until the 1920s, there was little success and the successes were thus all the more remarkable. There was the adrenal hormone adrenaline or epinephrine. It was not clear until the late 1930s, however, that corticoids were the more important hormones. There was thyroxin, with its known chemical structure, which was shown to be wrong in 1926. In 1921–1922, a pancreatic extract called insulin gained worldwide acclaim when it kept young children from dying of diabetes mellitus. There was pituitary extract that made rats grow large due to a presumed growth hormone. Nothing was known of the chemistry of these hormones in the mid-1920s except that they might be protein like in nature. Crude though these efforts were at chemical identification, they did begin to change the public impression of endocrinology from the work of somewhat shady physicians, the "gland doctors," to a discipline based on scientific investigation.

Clearly, sex differences called for inquiry into what it was that the ovaries and testes secreted. Those gland extracts were the most widely used clinically. The results were ambiguous. Sometimes dried or crude extracts seemed to help patients and sometimes they did not. In 1921, the United States National Research Council formed one of the earliest grant-giving agencies, the Committee for Research in Problems of Sex. The Committee funded several scientists who immediately attacked the problems of ovarian and testicular hormones as well as other possible hormones of pregnancy.

One early result was the discovery of "oestrin" or "estrin," which turned out to be estrone. It was the ovarian hormone of estrus, discovered by Edgar Allen and Edward

A Biographical History of Endocrinology, First Edition. D. Lynn Loriaux.

This work is a co-publication between the Endocrine Society and John Wiley & Sons, Ltd.

A. Doisy, who were the leaders in this field in 1923. The story of these two early "hormonists," the chance meeting that started them working together, their discussions of what to do as they rode to work in Doisy's Model T Ford, and their lifelong friendship is well told by Arthur T. Hertig [1]. Hertig's personal description gives context and flavor to the bare facts of the published paper. In the same vein, there was another, less well-known endocrine pioneer, Frederick L. Hisaw, who found and named the hormone relaxin, and made major contributions to the physiology of the corpus luteum and the understanding of the pituitary control of the ovary.

Hisaw grew up on a farm and had limited schooling in his early years. His intelligence, however, impressed a local schoolteacher who lived with the Hisaw family and tutored the young boy. He was able to get into the University of Missouri Preparatory School at age 18 years, and went to the University proper the next year. Biology became his passion. By 1916, he had not only graduated but had acquired a master's degree. He joined the Army when the United States entered the First World War. When the War ended in 1918, he went back to the family farm, but was soon offered a job at Kansas State University. The Agricultural Experiment Station was bustling with experiments.

Beginning in about 1921, Hisaw got the task of figuring out how to eradicate the pocket gopher (*Geomys bursartus*), a burrowing mammal considered a pest by farmers (his funding was for the "study of injurious animals"). His entry point was to study the animal's seasonal breeding habits with the hope of interfering with its reproduction. Careful anatomic analysis showed that there were variations in the pubic bones. The symphyses pubis of young adults of both sexes was completely ossified. Hisaw measured the pelvis opening and compared it with the size of the fetuses. The opening was simply not big enough to allow a fetal passage. Then he noticed that in mature females the bony symphysis was partly resorbed and that in pregnancy the resorption continued so that the pubic bones had almost disappeared by the end of gestation and were replaced by a thin fibrous band. Here was the solution to the problem of the narrow birth passage. The pocket gopher solved it by getting rid of the obstructing bone.

At this point, estrin had not yet appeared on the scene but there were reasonable suspicions of such an ovarian substance. Because pelvic resorption did not occur in male pocket gophers, Hisaw was convinced that the ovaries were the cause of the resorption in the females. He extracted dried pig ovaries with warm saline and injected this quite crude extract into castrated male gophers. He got pelvic bony resorption just as in the pregnant females and resorption occurred whether or not the extracted ovaries contained corpora lutea. He concluded that "the loss of the pubic symphysis seems to be due to a hormone secreted by the ovary" [2].

While he completed his work with the pocket gopher in Kansas, Hisaw spent the summers at the University of Wisconsin as a graduate student. He earned his doctorate in 1924 and stayed in Madison as a member of the faculty. He began the study of the pelvis at birth in the guinea-pig. The guinea-pig does not resorb the pelvic bones in pregnancy but does relax the ligamentous symphysis so that the fetuses can pass through. He tried the crude ovarian extracts in castrated males, but with no success.

Because the guinea-pig's pelvic ligaments relax only at the end of pregnancy, he injected pregnant rabbit blood into female guinea-pigs. The choice of rabbit was critical. No other animal would have sufficed, some, but not all of the female guinea-pigs had "spectacular relaxation" of the symphysis. It turned out that the ones that did not respond were anestrus; if the injections were made at estrus, all responded. Using Allen's estrin, he was able to reproduce the relaxation even if the animal was an anestrus female or male, provided it was first prepared with injections of estrin. He concluded that there was a circulating substance in pregnancy that relaxed the symphysis but that its action depended on priming by an ovarian hormone. He was unsure of the origin of the relaxing substance but, in the rabbit, he thought that the fetal placenta was a possible site [3].

Hisaw's 1926 publication marks the discovery of relaxin. He had, in fact, found a new hormone. The finding was novel and clearly worth pursuing. Next, he chose to look for this new substance in the corpus luteum of the guinea-pig. Just why he made this choice instead of pursuing placental extracts is not known. In any case, Hisaw was quite lucky. The pregnant sow's corpus luteum has the highest known concentration of the relaxing hormone of any tissue yet studied.

In 1927 Hisaw recruited a chemist, Harry Fevold, to help with the work isolating this new hormone. They found that an acid–alcohol extract of the corpus luteum contained "very little protein," and still had both the relaxing activity and was able to induce ovulation. By 1928, he specifically called his relaxing hormone the "corpus luteum hormone" [4].

Work to purify this "hormone" intensified. Others were pursuing the same target. More corpora lutea were needed. To get them, Hisaw recruited many of his graduate students to make weekly visits to the Oscar Meyer abattoir to "snip corpora lutea out of the tubful of half-frozen sow ovaries" [5]. The students could not get a whole ovary to take back to the laboratory for processing, because the non-luteal portions had been contracted to Lydia Pinkham's company to enrich her famous and widely sold "Vegetable Compound." It was famous during this time of Prohibition because it contained a great deal of alcohol. Its ovarian material was of doubtful use but the buyers may not have cared. Hisaw got the corpora lutea at no cost.

Hisaw was able to get funds from the Committee for Research in Problems of Sex (the "Sex Committee") and continued to get the committee's support for the next decade, after which his funds came directly from the Rockefeller Foundation [6]. In the later 1920s, Hisaw still thought that he and his colleagues had isolated "the" corpus luteum hormone and said so in two papers–in 1929 and 1930 [7, 8]. The chemistry, however, did not support that conclusion. Later in 1930, his team reported that the corpus luteum extracts actually contained two hormones, one that caused pelvic relaxation and was water-soluble [9] and another that brought about what is now called progestational effects and was more soluble in lipid solvents [10]. Hisaw's group went on to purify both substances and reported their techniques in the *Journal of the American Chemical Society* [11, 12]. Others were ahead of them and succeeded in isolating the lipid-like hormone, which we now call progesterone. Hisaw called his hormone "corporin" and was unhappy that his scientific colleagues and competitors called it "progesterone." He finally gave the relaxing substance a name after realizing that it had, in fact, no progestational action. He called it "relaxin."

The chemistry of these hormones was elusive. No one knew the chemical nature of any peptide hormone. And there was no such thing as a steroid hormone. The elucidation of cyclopentanoperhydrophenanthrene structure came in 1934. The efforts of Hisaw and his associates, though they only came close to purifying progesterone, were not in vain. His laboratory became one of the centers of hormone research as Hisaw himself moved on to the pituitary gland and its gonadotropin. His group was able to show that there was not just one gonad-stimulation hormone in the anterior pituitary gland but two: one for the follicle and another for corpus luteum. This "two-hormone" concept was contested in the 1930s but has stood the test of time [13]. After he moved to Harvard in 1935, Hisaw continued with his efforts to purify these two gonadotropins [14]. The genial "Pappy" (to his friends and colleagues) settled into the elite eastern academic world with ease.

By now, Hisaw's work had brought him worldwide fame, as one of the major reproductive endocrinologists of the middle twentieth century. He trained about 60 graduate students, published over 300 papers, was offered the presidency of his alma mater (but refused), received the highest award of the Endocrine Society, and was elected to the National Academy of Sciences in 1947. He retired from Harvard in 1962 but stayed on for a few years to carry on some of his endocrine studies. He finally left Harvard when his health failed in 1970 and died in 1972 in Atlanta, Georgia [15].

For a time, there was controversy over whether or not relaxin actually existed. Some said the effect was all due to estrogen. Hisaw pointed out that that could not be, nor could the effect be a result of progesterone [16]. Some tried to use relaxin as a pregnancy test, but the available assays were simply not sensitive enough [17]. Later attempts to increase the bioassay's sensitivity had some success [18]. Drug companies took a look at relaxin to see if it was possible to get enough of it to study, test, and market, either in the field of obstetrics or rheumatology. Nothing came of this either [19].

Up until the 1970s, relaxin did not seem to do much. Some texts had no entry at all for this hormone. Assays were hard to do, some animals did not seem to have it, and clinical effects were inconsistent at best. Hisaw had always worked with clinicians as he tried to find practical application for his basic work. In the case of relaxin, however, he found no place in the clinic. In the late 1970s, Relaxin was more highly purified, and the assays were improved and more sensitive. Development of an immunoassay was the critical step. When the peptide structure was defined, relaxin's secondary structure was reminiscent of insulin. It was soon found that besides acting on the symphysis, there were effects on the myometrium, endometrium, and breast [20]. Relaxin was "in" again with major presentations at the Laurentian Hormone Conference and at the New York Academy of Sciences.

Because there is, as yet, no defined therapeutic role for relaxin, few obstetricians know much about it and almost none know who Hisaw was. Women who suffer pregnancy-associated separation of the symphysis are certainly a reasonable target, but clinical articles almost never mentioned Hisaw's hormone [21]. A certain minimum level of awareness does exist in the speculations that relaxin might be involved in pelvic relaxation or back pain in pregnancy [22, 23].

Relaxin is, in fact, present in women [24]. Blood levels rise in the luteal phase and the ovary is, as Hisaw speculated, the major source. Relaxin may enhance cervical softening at term and decrease the time to delivery once labor begins. But, curiously, the complete absence of relaxin in some women seems not to be associated with difficulty in delivery. There may be, in the future, a pharmacologic place for this elusive hormone. Time will tell.

References

1. Hertig AT: Landmark perspective. Allen and Doisy's "An ovarian hormone." *J Am Med Assoc* 1983; 250: 2684.
2. Hisaw FL: The influence of the ovary on the resorption of the pubic bones of the pocket gopher, *Geomys bursarius* (Shaw). *J Exp Zool* 1925; 42: 411.
3. Hisaw FL: Experimental relaxation of the pubic ligament of the guinea pig. *Proc Soc Exp Biol Med* 1926; 23: 661.
4. Hisaw FL, Meyer RK, Weichert CK: Inhibition of ovulation and associated histological changes. *Proc Soc Exp Biol Med* 1928; 25: 754.
5. Greep RO: Reflections on the life and works of F. L. Hisaw and H. B. van Dyke: two pioneers in research on the reproductive hormones. *Horm Prot Pept* 1980; 8: 199.
6. Aberle SD, Corner GW: *Twenty-five Years of Sex Research. History of the National Research in Problems of Sex 1992–1947*. Philadelphia, PA and London: W.B. Saunders, 1953.
7. Hisaw FL: *The corpus luteum hormone*. I. Experimental relaxation of the pelvic ligaments of the guinea pig. *Physiol Zool* 1929; 2: 59.
8. Hisaw FL, Fevold HL, Meyer RK: The corpus luteum hormone. II. Methods of extraction. Physiol Zool 1930; 3: 135.
9. Fevold HL, Hisaw FL, Meyer RK: Isolation of the relaxative hormone of the corpus luteum. *Proc Soc Exp Biol Med* 1930; 27: 604.
10. Fevold HL, Hisaw FL, Meyer RK: Purification of hormone of corpus luteum responsible for progestational development and other reactions. *Proc Soc Exp Biol Med* 1930; 27: 606.
11. Fevold HL, Hisaw FL, Meyer RK: The relaxative hormone of the corpus luteum. Its purification and concentration. J Am Chem Soc 1930; 52: 3340.
12. Fevold HL, Hisaw FL, Leonard SL: Hormones of the corpus luteum. The separation and purification of three active substances. *J Am Chem Soc* 1932; 54: 254.
13. Velardo JT: Induction of ovulation in immature hypophysectomized rats. *Science* 1960; 131(3397): 357.
14. Kroc RL: Rememberance: excerpta memorabilia. *Endocrinology* 1992; 131: 1587.
15. Editor: Frederick Lee Hisaw (1891–1972). *Endocrinology* 1973; 93: 273.
16. Hisaw FL, Zarrow MX, Money WL, Talmage RVN, Abramowitz AA: Importance of the female reproductive tract in the formation of relaxin. *Endocrinology* 1944; 34: 122.
17. Abramason D, Hurwitt E, Lesnick G: Relaxin in human serum as a test of pregnancy. *Surg Gynecol Obstet* 1937; 65: 335.
18. Kliman B, Greep RO: The enhancement of relaxin-induced growth of the pubic ligament in mice. *Endocrinology* 1958; 63: 586.
19. Kroc RL: Relaxin–a perspective of personal andecdotal recollections. *Ann NY Acad Sci* 1982; 380: 1.

20. Schwabe C, Steinetz B, Weiss G, et al.: Relaxin. *Rec Prog Horm Res* 1978; 34: 123.
21. Snow RE, Neubert AG: Peripartum pubic symphysis separation: a case series and review of the literature. *Obstet Gynecol Surv* 1997; 52: 438.
22. Maclennan AH: The role of the hormone relaxin in human reproduction and pelvic girdle relaxation. *Scand J Rheumatol* 1991 (Suppl); 88: 7.
23. Kristiansson F, Svardsudd K, von Schoultz B: Serum Relaxin, symphyseal pain, and back pain during pregnancy. *Am J Obstet Gynecol* 196; 175: 1342.
24. Weiss G, Goldsmith LT: Relaxin. In *Reproductive Endocrinology, Surgery and Technology*, Vol. 1, edited by EY Adashi, JA Rock, Z Rosenwaks. Philadelphia, PA: Lippincott-Raven, 1995, p. 827.

This chapter has been reproduced from Ziel, Harry K. and Sawin, Clark T: Frederick L. Hisaw (1891–1972) and the discovery of relaxin. *The Endocrinologist* 2000; 10(4): 215–18.

CHAPTER 58

Henry S. Plummer (1874–1936)

Toxic Nodular Thyroid Gland

"The best brain the clinic ever had." So said William J. Mayo, the well-known surgeon at Minnesota's Mayo Clinic, when asked about his junior colleague, the internist, Henry Stanley Plummer. Yet, Plummer's main contribution to endocrinology, the successful use of iodine to prepare patients with active Graves' disease for surgery and so decrease the mortality of the operation by 75%, was based on a mistaken theory.

Plummer came to the Mayo Clinic almost by accident. He had graduated from Northwestern University's medical school in 1898, and then returned to Racine, Minnesota to join his father, Albert, who was in general practice in that small town. Three years later, the senior Plummer asked William W. Mayo, to come to Racine to consult on one of his patients (in those days, the consultant traveled to the patient). William W. Mayo was the founder of the famous Clinic and the father of William J. (William J. was known as "Dr. Will" to distinguish him from his equally famous brother, Charles H. Mayo, known later as "Dr. Charlie"). At that time, the senior Mayo was away and could not come, so his son, William J., went to Racine in his father's place. When he got to Racine, the senior Plummer was ill and could not attend the patient. So, Dr. Will set out to see the patient. The elder Plummer suggested that his son, Henry, might go along with Dr. Mayo. The patient had leukemia (although the Mayos were known mainly for their surgical skill, they saw many kinds of patients in their earlier years and were considered quite expert). On the trip in a horse-drawn wagon to and from the patient, Mayo and the young Plummer talked about leukemia and a wide range of other topics as well. Unusual for the time, Plummer owned, and brought with him, a microscope. Henry's talk and knowledge about the blood so impressed Dr. Will that, when he got back to the Clinic in Rochester, he told his brother how impressed he was and they agreed to offer Henry Plummer a job to run the laboratories at the Clinic. A few weeks later, Plummer was on the Clinic's permanent staff. Over the next decade, he became one of the leaders of the rapidly expanding Mayo partnership.

Plummer's task was to run the diagnostic laboratory. He found some diagnostic procedures in place but, on the whole, the role of medical diagnosis was not high in

A Biographical History of Endocrinology, First Edition. D. Lynn Loriaux.

the largely surgical atmosphere. The laboratory was weak even for its time. He also took on the management of the primitive radiographic facilities, apparently little more than a closet. He also began to see general medicine patients and developed an interest in esophageal diseases. During this time, he noticed that some patients had an esophageal obstruction that seemed to be benign rather than malignant. He pursued this and found that dilation helped what we now call achalasia. He is also the Plummer of the Plummer–Vinson syndrome, an odd combination of iron-deficiency anemia and a "web" in the upper esophagus. The result is apparent in his publication record. His first seven papers are on diseases of the esophagus. After 1912, however, all but one of his published papers are on some aspect of the thyroid gland.

During Plummer's first years with the Mayo Clinic, it became clear that he was one of the brightest minds to come to the Rochester practice. He was a perfectionist as well. He was seen by many as an eccentric. The perfectionist attitude led him to write fewer papers than most. Everything needed just a bit more and nothing was ever finished (his lifetime total was only 31 papers, including book chapters). His intensity led to anecdotes about his focus. Once he sold his car to a colleague, forgot he had sold it, and drove it to his own house later that day. Needless to say, his colleague thought someone had stolen his newly bought car and there was confusion until Plummer looked in his garage. Plummer also married during these years. The laboratory assistant he married in 1904 was a niece of the Mayo brothers. Here, too, there were stories of the absent-minded physician. For instance, one day, while in his office, he agreed to take his wife shopping in Minneapolis. He left his office, jumped in his car, drove off, and was halfway to Minneapolis before he realized that he had left his wife behind.

Organizational issues captured Plummer's interest. How could he enhance the ability of the expanding medical group to work together to the patients' benefit? He helped establish the principle that the partnership was an entity, not just a group of physicians with independent practices. The key was specialization combined with cooperation. Plummer put a structure into place that embodied this principle. He invented one of the first centralized medical record systems, based on the idea that a patient's record belonged not to a particular physician but to the clinic as a whole. His system, put in place in 1907, replaced records held in individual offices and a now historic set of ledger books that were never cross-indexed. After his plan was in place, every patient had a unique assigned number, each case was cross-indexed by disease and pathologic findings, and all patients had an appointment time to come to the Clinic. In those days, patients came to the office and just waited to be seen. He introduced follow-up questionnaires for patients so as to find out the results of their treatment. Plummer wound up as chief of the division of general medicine, a position he held for more than 20 years.

Plummer's interest in diseases of the thyroid gland began when he was a boy, but was clearly stimulated by the huge numbers of thyroidectomies being done by Charles Mayo. Most of these were "simple" goiters due to iodine deficiency. A sizable minority of goiter patients, however, had the more serious exophthalmic goiter. Surgery in these patients was sometimes lethal. With care, multistage surgery, and prolonged hospitalization, the Mayos were able to bring the surgical mortality in this odd type of goiter down to about 4–5%, but no further. In the first decade of the twentieth century it was still not entirely clear that the symptoms of this disease were due to excess secretion of thyroid hormone. In the latter part of that decade, however, "hyperthyroidism" became the accepted name.

Plummer found that, while most patients with clinical hyperthyroidism had hyperplastic glands (provided one examined the entire gland), about 20% did not have hyperplasia. Plummer called these "nonhyperplastic goiter" [1]. By 1913, he had analyzed the clinical status of these hyperthyroid patients and concluded that, whereas the ones with hyperplastic glands had a fairly rapid onset of clinical disease, those who had nonhyperplastic glands had goiter for some 15 years before they became thyrotoxic. He also thought he detected a clinical difference in the two types of hyperthyroid patients. Those with the hyperplastic glands seemed to be more toxic than those without hyperplasia. Incidentally, in keeping with the current thinking in 1913, he also thought that "the administration of iodine could cause the sudden appearance of those symptoms." Iodine was then thought to be clearly contraindicated in patients with hyperthyroidism.

Plummer then developed the purely theoretical idea that the two types of hyperthyroidism he detected clinically were based on a difference in the hormonal cause of the hyperthyroidism. The nonhyperplastic type was due to excess secretion of the normal, but unknown, product of the thyroid gland, while in the hyperplastic type there was, in addition, the secretion of a "perverted thyroid hormone" caused by a "dyshormonogenesis." He speculated that this abnormal hormone was a toxic substance (hence, "thyrotoxicosis") and that it was the cause of the nervous phenomena and the exophthalmos in Graves' disease [2].

Plummer had always pushed the reluctant Mayo brothers to have the Clinic more involved in research. Together with Louis B. Wilson, the head of anatomic pathology, in late 1913 they convinced the brothers that it would be to their mutual advantage to hire Edward C. Kendall. Kendall's task was to isolate the normal thyroid hormone and search out the abnormal toxic variant. Kendall succeeded brilliantly at the first task; he became literally world-famous within a year of his arrival in Rochester in February, 1914, by isolating pure crystals of thyroxin on Christmas Day, 1914. Kendall did not succeed at the second task, however. The second thyroid hormone, long-acting thyroid stimulating substance, was isolated about 40 years later. Kendall went on to pursue the structure of thyroxin and was convinced by 1919 that he had it. He thought it was a tryptophan derivative with three iodine atoms in the molecule. He claimed he had synthesized it. Here, Kendall was wrong on both counts. Thyroxin is a tyrosine derivative and has four iodine atoms per molecule, facts which were shown by Charles R. Harington in 1926 and 1927. In the decade from 1915 to 1925, Kendall's postulates were accepted by all; Plummer still believed in a perverted thyroid hormone that was some variant of Kendall's incorrect molecule.

After Kendall's discovery, Plummer developed the idea that the abnormal product secreted in Graves' disease was a thyroxin relatively deficient in iodine compared to thyroxin itself. This idea was based on findings of David Marine who, few years before, had shown that the thyroid gland in patients with Graves' disease had a lower concentration of iodine than did the thyroid of normal persons. Marine actually thought that the symptoms of Graves' disease amounted to a form of *hypo*-thyroidism. Plummer had no easy way to prove his idea, however, and so matters stood.

By the 1920s, Plummer had risen high in the Mayo hierarchy. In 1915, he was one of six incorporators of the Mayo Foundation for Medical Education and Research and, in 1919, he was one of nine members of the newly formed Mayo Properties Association which, by deed from the Mayo brothers, controlled most aspects of the Clinic. After 1919, his practice was almost entirely made up of patients with thyroid disease.

In the early 1920s, the concept of "dysthyroidism," or the secretion of an abnormal thyroid hormone or toxin in Graves' disease, had won some acceptance, but there was also a good deal of skepticism because of the lack of supportive evidence [3]. It was still an attractive idea for Plummer. In 1922, he was asked to write the section on the functions of the normal and abnormal thyroid gland for *Oxford Medicine*, a compendium of medicine published and updated periodically by the Oxford University Press. It occurred to him that if the secreted toxic product in Graves' disease was iodine deficient, perhaps giving iodine to the patient would help. He was well aware of the dictum that iodine was to be avoided in Graves' disease. Had not the famous thyroid surgeon, Theodor Kocher, said so? Was not iodine itself one of the causes of hyperthyroidism, as in "iod-Basedow"? Iodine-induced hyperthyroidism was actually first published by J.F. Coindet in 1821. It was the first instance of a hyperthyroid state, although it was not then known to be hyperthyroidism. So, beginning in March, 1922, Plummer gave patients with Graves' disease awaiting operation 10–30 drops of Lugol's solution per day [4]. The results were startling. Patients' symptoms often disappeared in a few days, surgery was made easier, and surgical mortality dropped from the range of 4–5% to less than 1%.

Plummer thought these results supported his "two-product" theory of what was secreted in patients with Graves' disease and hyperthyroidism. Still, in keeping with his reluctance to publish his data on the preparation of Graves' disease patients for surgery with iodine, it never appeared in a major medical publication. The key references to his discovery are in local medical journals in Illinois and Iowa which were published because they were transcripts of his lectures. Although the reason for trying iodine was, in retrospect, erroneous, it was a true success and deserved widespread publication.

Plummer did note his discovery, somewhat belatedly, at the annual meeting of the Association of American Physicians (AAP), an elite group of internists, in 1924. Even here, he did not present his results in a formal talk but rather as part of the discussion of another presentation. He simply said that there were "some very definite reasons" for not reporting to the group earlier and then said that there was no time to say what the reasons were [5]. He had, however, become clearer in his terminology. The "nonhyperplastic" glands were now called "adenomatous" and he noted that the iodine pretreatment did *not* work in these patients. It was only in the patients with hyperplastic thyroids and hyperthyroidism (i.e., Graves' disease) that the iodine therapy was so effective. He elaborated these ideas further in 1928 in a formal talk to the AAP, by which time Kendall's errors had been pointed out and the correct structure of thyroxin, now termed thyroxine, was published.

Strictly speaking, Plummer was not the discoverer of the successful iodine treatment for Graves' disease. Others, dating back to the 1860s, had done it before him. But Plummer was unaware of these precursors (or at least he never referred to them) and, in any case, the dictum of "no iodine in hyperthyroidism" held sway [6]. One of the keys to his therapy's success in reversing the prevailing opinion and ensuring its widespread adoption was his own reputation as well as that of the Mayo Clinic. Of course, once tried with clear success, the therapy would likely have spread on its own momentum. An example of the change in practice brought by Plummer's finding is that the 1920 (9th) edition of *Osler's Principles and Practice of Medicine* makes no mention of the use of iodine in hyperthyroidism, whereas in the 1925 (10th) edition, iodine is a clear boon, although the idea of an abnormal secretion persists: "Iodine ... is often useful in cases of dysthyroidism. There may be marked improvement with its use and a trial of it is advisable before operation" [7].

In the early 1930s, Plummer gathered honors and moved toward retirement although he was still relatively young. In 1932, both he and Charles Mayo retired from active control of the Mayo Clinic. In 1933, Plummer was President of the American Association for the Study of Goiter (now the American Thyroid Association) and in 1935 he received an honorary degree from his medical alma mater, Northwestern University.

Plummer developed progressive bulbar paralysis, a variant of amyotrophic lateral sclerosis (ALS), in 1936 and, after carefully noting the clinical progress of his disease, died on the last day of that year. Curiously, his thyroid legacy is the eponym for hyperthyroidism due to thyroid nodular disease ("Plummer's disease") but his real contribution was in the treatment of the other kind of hyperthyroidism, Graves' disease. His theories were wrong, but it didn't matter to the pre-op Graves' disease patient waiting for thyroidectomy.

References

1. Plummer HS: The clinical and pathological relationship of simple and exophthalmic goiter. *Am J Med Sci* 1913; 146: 790.
2. Wilson LB: The pathology of the thyroid gland in exophthalmic goiter. *Am J Med Sci* 1913; 146: 781.
3. Howard CP: Dysthyroidism. In *Endocrinology and Metabolism*, edited by LF Barker, RG Hoskins, HO Mosenthal. New York: D. Appleton and Co., 1924, Vol. 1, p. 299.
4. Plummer HS: The function of the thyroid gland. In *Thyroid Gland*, edited by : CH Mayo, HS Plummer. Detroit, MI: Beaumont Foundation, 1925, p. 74.
5. Plummer HS: Discussion. *Trans Assoc Am Physic* 1924; 39: 178.
6. Kohn LA: The Midwestern American "epidemic" of iodine-induced hyperthyroidism in the 1920s. *Bull NY Acad Med* 1976; 52: 770.
7. McCrae T: *Osler's Principles and Practice of Medicine* (10th edn.). New York: D Appleton and Co., 1925 (1927), p. 901.

This chapter has been reproduced from Sawin, Clark T: Henry S. Plummer (1874–1936), iodine for hyperthyroidism, and Plummer's disease. *The Endocrinologist* 2003; 13(3): 149–52.

CHAPTER 59

Henry H. Dale
(1875–1968)
Catecholamines

On August 31, 1925, the Second International Conference on the Standardization of Biological Products held its first session in Geneva, Switzerland, at 9:45 a.m. Henry H. Dale, then 50 years old, presided. In attendance were 18 other scientists. Two of these were Nobel laureates who were almost Dale's age: J.J.R. Macleod, who had won for his work in developing a successful insulin preparation, and S.A.S. Krogh, whose prize was for his work on capillary function. The Conference's purpose was to bring some consistency into the manufacture and use of several biological preparations then used in research and clinical care: posterior pituitary extract, insulin, desiccated thyroid, digitalis, salvarsan (then the best therapy for syphilis), and several others. Decisions on the relatively new parathyroid extract and ovarian extract were put off as needing further investigation. Still, most of the discussions centered about hormonal "drugs." The thrust of the meeting was on bioassays because none of these preparations were what we would now call hormones for the simple reason that none of the relevant chemical structures were known. All they knew for certain was that these "hormones" had definite biological effects and that both patients and research studies suffered because of the confusion that arose because of the variations in potency among the available preparations. Who was Henry Hallett Dale, and what was his role in the developing world of endocrinology?

Henry Hallett Dale was born in London. His father was the manager of a pottery firm and, though not poor, there was little excess income in the family. As a schoolboy he had an interest in natural science, largely stimulated by a teacher who was an expert on insects. That teacher insisted that Dale rewrite everything so that anyone could understand it. Dale later thought that this was the best thing he could have learned in school and that this discipline was a clear benefit when he came to be a scientist. Still, there was no animus to drive him to a scientific career. At age 15, the end of school for most children, he planned to go into his father's business. This decision was delayed for a year when the schoolmaster asked him to stay on. Then, during this last school year, a chance meeting of his father with the Head of Leys

A Biographical History of Endocrinology, First Edition. D. Lynn Loriaux.

This work is a co-publication between the Endocrine Society and John Wiley & Sons, Ltd.

School led to Dale's taking a "stewardship" examination for the school. The school functioned as a preparatory school for Cambridge University, with an emphasis on Trinity College. Dale did well in the examination and received a scholarship to Leys, which he attended for the next 3 years. Without the scholarship he could not have afforded the school. At Leys, Dale studied a great deal of science, including a rigorous course in physiology. He had Foster's *Textbook of Physiology*, a rigorous text even at the university level, with full experimental details. He learned of new discoveries such as Von Mering and Minkowski's discovery of the connection between the pancreas and diabetes mellitus and Murray's successful therapy of myxedema with thyroid extract. He competed for another scholarship, now to Cambridge, and again succeeded.

Dale spent the next 6 years, 1894–1900, at Cambridge as a scholarship student of Trinity College. He was an excellent student, took both parts of the Natural Science Tripos (a peculiarly Cantabrigian institution), got a "First" in the end of his 3rd year, and managed to get further scholarship support for his last two Cambridge years as a College Fellow. These were research years. Dale spent them with J.N. Langley, one of Foster's protégés (Michael Foster was still the professor of physiology at Trinity and Cambridge). Although Langley was an expert on the autonomic nervous system and had shown nicotine's effects on sympathetic ganglia, Dale's work during this time was on the electro- and chemo-taxis of unicellular organisms. Dale later thought that Langley could have given him better direction, but the project did force Dale to think of his own experiments and carry them to conclusion.

Dale became enamored of the academic life, but had no money. The answer was a fellowship which, if he could get one, would give him an endowed career. He put his research in the form of a thesis to compete for one of the few fellowships available at Trinity. Although Dale was strongly recommended, the election committee tied, and the tie was broken by the College Master in favor of the other candidate.

Dale then took another examination for a scholarship, this one for attendance at St. Bartholomew's Hospital and open only to Cambridge graduates, to complete work for a medical degree. He won, attended Bart's for the next 2 years, and qualified to practice medicine. Although he did not think much of the intellectual atmosphere of medical training, he did well and was offered an entry-level position that could have sent him into academic medicine; his hospital mentor thought Dale could help make medicine scientific. It did not happen.

Dale's choice of career was forced by the sudden opening of a vacancy in the George Henry Lewes "Studentship." This was not a minor position for a young scholar. Endowed in 1879 by Lewes' "close companion" Marian Evans, known to most as the writer and novelist George Eliot, the Studentship was the equivalent of a well-funded postdoctoral fellowship. It was one of the few sources of funds for further training in physiology, although it focused almost entirely on Cambridge University. Awarded for up to 3 years, the awardee should be someone "who otherwise would be unable to devote themselves to physiological enquiry." Dale had to decide immediately whether or not to compete. This meant, in essence, that he had to choose between medicine and physiology as a career because the Studentship would not be open later and there was no such thing as a delayed acceptance. He decided to compete and, with the help of his Cambridge professors, won. The award allowed him to pick where he would spend his time and he chose to work in Starling's laboratory at University College London for the next 2 years, 1902–1904.

E.H. Starling was a leader in the world of physiology. In 1902 he had demonstrated, for the first time, the existence of a circulating hormone, secretin, in collaboration with his brother-in-law and colleague, W.M. Bayliss. Dale, now 27 years old, decided to look into the effect of secretin on the pancreatic islet cells, using histologic end-points, and to study the autonomic innervation of the gall bladder. The first project, Dale's first venture into endocrinology, led to a publication, but it turned out to be wrong. He thought that prolonged stimulation with secretin converted pancreatic exocrine cells to endocrine ones. Nevertheless, Dale learned from the experience about the interpretation of data. The second project, though minor, was a successful prelude to his later "neural" studies.

No great results came of his time in the Studentship, but he was developing into a mature scientist who could think for himself, come to experimental conclusions, and take advantage of unexpected findings. Starling's laboratory had other, less apparent, advantages. It was a mecca for physiologists who came from many parts of the world. Dale first met Loewi here when Loewi visited for a few months in 1902. A life-long friendship grew from this visit. Dale also was able to travel during the Studentship, and he visited the Frankfurt laboratory of Paul Ehrlich, another Nobelist (1908) and a world-famous immunologist. Dale did little research during these few months but came away with a clear picture of the need to standardize biologic materials used in science and medicine. Once Ehrlich had developed diphtheria antitoxin, there was a clear need to be sure that all preparations had a known amount of activity; Ehrlich set up a program that allowed the potency of a preparation to be measured against a standard preparation of known activity.

As the Studentship came to an end, Dale was still unsure of what to do with his career. He still wanted the "academic life." When the Sharpey Studentship opened up in March under Starling's aegis, Dale looked at it. It was the lowest rung on the academic ladder and paid less than the Lewes Studentship that he already had, but it was an entry point to medical teaching and a possible future professorship. The position required doing Starling's teaching during the summer session, 1904, and Dale took it. As it happened, his future was not in academic medicine after all.

Dale was now 28 years old and wanted to marry but could not do so with his current income of $150 per year. While Dale was teaching in that summer session of 1904, Starling had an inquiry from Henry S. Wellcome, the principal of what was then Burroughs, Wellcome and Company. Wellcome had established the Wellcome Physiological Research Laboratories 10 years before, and wanted someone truly qualified to run them. Starling had such a person: Dale. Wellcome and Dale discussed the job. It was one of independent research at more than twice the salary Dale had at the time. There would be periodic increases in salary (within 3 years, Dale's salary was $1000; the average full professor's salary then was about $600). Dale's friends in the sciences said he would be selling his soul. Dale took the job in August, 1904, and married in November. He remained there for the next 10 years.

Despite his academic brilliance, Dale had no particular idea about what to study. Wellcome himself gave Dale his first idea: study the active components of ergot, a fungus that contained alkaloids that were helpful in medicine, particularly in obstetrics. Dale's physiological training stood him well, and he started immediately. He was fortunate. The laboratory was one of the best equipped in the country. More importantly, there were competent chemists there with whom he could work. The work was not the pure science he had been led to believe it was, however. There was a continuing demand for routine bioassays of medical products. This did not bother Dale. He felt that he always learned from the problems that arose, and his later career suggests that he was right. Certainly he had the time and talent to turn out a large number of what can only be termed basic research papers and at the same time became an expert on bioassay.

Over the next several years he worked on problems stimulated by ergot. His background enabled him to see physiological questions in the pharmacologic work. His was "the prepared mind." He referred later in life to a series of lucky accidents. For example, among his first studies on ergot was an examination of the interaction of the effects of ergot extracts with adrenaline and the sympathetic nervous system. Unexpected results led Dale to join forces with the chemist George Barger. Barger made more than 50 catecholamine analogues in an attempt to shed some light on the mediator of sympathetic nerve activity. Dale and Barger recognized that, of all the synthetic amines, noradrenaline was the one that most closely mimicked natural sympathetic activity. However, at that time, a synthetic compound that was not known to exist in vivo was not thought to be of any physiologic relevance. Thus, they did nothing further along this line (they had in fact defined the actual physiologic transmitter but did not know it). Adrenaline was considered to be the hormone of the adrenal gland. Dale had made the connection between an endocrine gland and the nervous system. He invented the word "sympathomimetic."

The work on adrenalin also shows another side to Dale's personality. The policy at the company regarding publication was quite clear. Nothing could be published without the approval of Wellcome himself. The rule applied to any work, whether done in the Laboratories or not. Dale submitted one of his papers on adrenalin to Wellcome and immediately became embroiled in an internal controversy over the use of the word "adrenalin." Wellcome and others objected to its use, in part because it too closely resembled the trade name "Adrenaline," copyrighted by a rival firm. They preferred "epinephrine." Dale resisted and argued strongly to keep "adrenalin." He felt that "adrenalin" was the accepted term among the physiologists to whom the paper was directed and that "epinephrine" was the term for an impure chemical preparation. Wellcome dithered for a while. The possibility of a lawsuit from the other company and the chemists pushed him toward "epinephrine." Dale and the British physiologists insisted on "adrenalin." Dale, probably fearful of losing his job without other prospects, went so far as to make a not-so-veiled written threat to Wellcome: "the position I am striving for ... would be seriously imperiled by a breath of suspicion that the publication of my work was hampered or modified by other than scientific considerations." Wellcome agreed with Dale, and the paper was published with "adrenalin." There seemed to be no hard feelings on Wellcome's part. He promoted Dale, that year, to the directorship of the laboratory.

Another "lucky" break was Dale's discovery that the posterior pituitary contains something that stimulates uterine contraction. The vasopressor effect had been well-described for a decade. It was only because Dale was studying the effect of another ergot extract on smooth muscle, in this case a strip of cat uterine muscle, and used a pituitary extract as a control that he stumbled onto the oxytocic effect of the posterior pituitary.

The work on ergot, which in Dale's hands seemed to be a cornucopia of physiologically important agents, led to his discovery of histamine in ergot and the recognition that histamine's biologic effects resembled anaphylactic shock. This trail of work continued for some time, into and including the First World War; the analogy between histamine's vasodilator and vasodepressor effects and wound shock led to another series of papers. And then there was acetylcholine.

Dale was well-versed in the pharmacology of muscarine and nicotine. Others had found that something like muscarine seemed responsible for parasympathetic action in some tissues. When Dale found a muscarine-like substance in another strain of ergot, he and his chemical colleague found that it was in fact acetylcholine, a synthetic compound first made in the nineteenth century. This was the first demonstration that acetylcholine existed in a living organism. This, too, was a "lucky" stroke because Dale never found it again in any strain of ergot. Once again, because it was not known to occur in vertebrate tissue, acetylcholine, like norepinephrine, was not thought to be a natural compound in vivo. To claim so would require much more proof, but the clues were there. Dale stayed with this problem in one form or another for the next three decades, along with his work on the catecholamines.

All of this work had suitably impressed his scientific colleagues, even though it was all done from a "commercial" laboratory. Dale was first proposed for election to the Royal Society in 1910 and elected in 1914 at the age of 39 years. This year was a good and bad year for Dale. His election to the Royal Society meant real recognition. He was offered, but turned down, several professorships. Then, he was offered a position at the newly proposed National Institute for Medical Research (NIMR), which was to be developed under the auspices of the Medical Research Committee. It was an impressive offer but not without problems. Dale needed assurance that he would have a laboratory equal to the one he now had. Things were settled, and Dale signed on to begin in July, 1914. The first thing he and Barger did was to go to Germany and learn what they could about setting up new laboratories in the to-be-refurbished vacant Mount Vernon Hospital in Hampstead. They barely made it back to England before the First World War broke out the next month. Plans for the Institute were put on hold for the next 5 years. Dale went to work on problems related to the War in the nascent "Institute," which was temporarily put in London at the Lister Institute.

After the War, the NIMR finally opened at the Hampstead site. Dale become the de facto director and then, in 1928, the actual director. By now he was internationally renowned and gave invited lectures in the United States. The Rockefeller Institute asked him chair a department. Johns Hopkins University did the same. He liked

American audiences who "showed an interest and a real enjoyment," in contrast with the typical British audience who evinced "polite toleration." But he stayed where he was in Hampstead. That same year, he began a program of biological standards. It was based on his recollection of Ehrlich's work on the need to standardize diphtheria antitoxin and on his years of experience in bioassays at the Wellcome laboratories.

First Dale wanted to standardize posterior pituitary extracts. By the 1920s they had become widely used in obstetrics. Unexpected variations in strength, however, led to some tragic obstetric outcomes. He found that some preparations were as much as 80-fold more potent than others of supposed similar strength. The key to his program was not to set up standard assays but rather to prepare a standard preparation. The preparation then could be used as a standard in any assay an investigator wished to use. Because the extant preparations were not defined chemicals, the bioassays had to be defined in arbitrary units; thus, the defined standard would have a certain number of units per weight and all other preparations would, once assayed against the standard preparation, have the unitage defined as well. Dale's ability to convince others of the necessity of this approach, and his political skills, resulted in the passage of a law in 1922 requiring this approach to the standardization of posterior pituitary extracts. This facilitated the later switch to a more stable American standard.

Dale's stature and expertise led him, in 1922, to the University of Toronto to look into the new phenomenon of "insulin." The British Medical Research Council had been offered the British rights to the patent held by the Canadians. He found the manufacturing plant primitive but effective and realized again that there was no clearly defined standard against which to judge the merits of the several available bioassays. The need was clear. The next year Dale attended a preliminary conference on biological standardization in Edinburgh. He had his chemist at NIMR prepare a dry, stable, powder sample of reasonably pure insulin as the hydrochloride. Discussion about an insulin standard, however, got nowhere. All in attendance, including both Macleod and Krogh, argued for one or another bioassay to be adopted as the "standard." Dale said that they needed a standard preparation, not a standard assay. Macleod agreed but said it was not possible. Where would they get a stable preparation of insulin? Dale took his sample from his pocket, "Well, there it is." This sample became the first international insulin standard.

All of this was in preparation for a formal conference on standardization 2 years later, which brings us to August in Geneva in 1925. Dale was president of the Association for the Standardization of Biological Products because of his expertise in bioassay or because of his chemist's abilities. He saw a reasonable and balanced solution that fit the need. He was also adaptable. The standard for the posterior pituitary extract was a case in point. The first standard was one of his laboratory's making, but it had become clear between 1923 and 1925 that Carl Voegtlin had a better preparation. His was adopted after Dale convinced the group that a unit based on the oxytocic effect would be the best way to refer to the standard (it was still unsettled then whether there was more than one biologically active entity in the extract). Dale got both Macleod and Krogh to make the final proposal for the insulin standard, a nice maneuver considering their previous behavior. They agreed that Dale's preparation would be the standard; it was given 8 units/mg. There was similar harmony for the thyroid standard; here there was enough chemical information to define a proper thyroid preparation as containing 0.2% of iodine, even though the structures of neither thyroxine nor triiodothyronine were known. They all recognized that the only reason for a bioassay was to ensure that there was in fact biologic activity. A chemical standard was preferable but not possible for chemically undefinable substances. They applied the same approach to the other materials being considered: digitalis, salvarsan, a few antihelminthics and, of course, ergot. The meeting was a clear success and Dale's reputation grew again. His approach to international standardization of biologics is still the essential one used today and it is no accident that the NIMR, where Dale remained until 1942, became the repository for the various standards chosen.

Dale's work at the Geneva Conference was perhaps his most important contribution to endocrinology despite his discoveries in the catecholamine and posterior pituitary areas. Without some sort of agreed common standard, scientists and commercial firms and, ultimately, patients, would hardly work on the same problem. His work on biological standards continued. In the 1930s he chaired the three conferences on the Standardization of Sex Hormones in 1932, 1935, and 1938 (the chemist Girard seemed to have taken a page from Dale's book at the 1932 conference when he pulled 20 grams of a rare steroid from his pocket and asked if it would help). The 1932 conference focused on estrone, estriol, and estradiol as the three estrogens commonly found in mammals. The 1935 conference, also in London, settled on "progesterone" for the luteal hormone. At the 1938 conference, now in Geneva, there was agreement on standards for prolactin and chorionic gonadotropin but not for FSH or LH. The preparations were too crude.

Through all of this, Dale continued to direct the NIMR and pursue his laboratory work. By the late 1920s, the assay for acetylcholine was perfected and there was another explosion of papers. He and many others at NIMR studied the parasympathetic and central nervous systems as well as the motor end-plate at the neuromuscular junction; they proposed the essential role of acetylcholine in neural transmission. Along with parallel work on the sympathetic nervous system and the adrenal medulla, they helped define autonomic and peripheral nerve function. By 1936, the year he became a Nobel laureate, Dale's group was soaring, producing more than 25 papers in a single journal and others elsewhere, all on neural function. In 1933 Dale realized that to continue to refer to specific anatomic nerves as having one or another function was unnecessarily complex. He decided that functional terms were needed and proceeded to invent them, which is why we now call them cholinergic and adrenergic neurons. And he invented what came to be called "Dale's principle," that is, a given neuron releases the same transmitter from all its terminals. Thus, an adrenergic neuron releases only norepinephrine wherever its terminals may be.

Dale's stature continued to rise. He was knighted in 1932. He was secretary of the Royal Society for 10 years and then its president from 1940 to 1945, the worst years of the War, and received many honors and honorary degrees. He has more than a dozen publications listed in Garrison and Morton's medical bibliography as classic. His "principle" guided neuroscientific research for decades, although it is no longer strictly true. We now know that a single neural secretory vesicle can contain two neurotransmitters. Dale's later years were spent back in Cambridge where he lived so many of his formative years. He died there in 1968, aged 93.

Dale was a true polymath and seemed to excel at whatever he chose–or perhaps he chose what he was likely to be good at. In his day there really was no such thing as an endocrinologist; the field of science was more open. He can be seen as a neuroscientist or a pharmacologist, or an endocrinologist. His contributions to our field are clear. As is fitting, the Society of Endocrinology of the United Kingdom in 1959 named its highest honor, the Dale Medal, for him. As a reflection of Dale's efforts to foster international science, the Medal can be awarded to anyone in the world.

Sources

Dale HH: George Barger. 1879–1939. *Obituary Notices of Fellows of the Royal Society* 1940; 3(8): 83.

Feldberg WS: Henry Hallett Dale. 1875–1968. *Biog Mem Fell Roy Soc* 1979; 16: 77.

Medvei VC: *A History of Endocrinology*. Lancaster, UK: MTP Press, 1982.

Nicoll RA, Malenka RC: A tale of two transmitters. *Science* 1998; 281: 360.

Tansey EM: George Eliot's support for physiology: the George Henry Lewes trust 1879–1939. *Notes Rec Roy Soc Lond* 1990; 44: 221.

Tansey EM: What's in a name? Henry Dale and adrenaline, 1906. *Med Hist* 1995; 39: 459.

Tansey T: Sir Henry Dale and autopharmacology: the role of acetylcholine in neurotransmission. In *Essays in the History of the Physiological Sciences*, edited by C Debru. Amsterdam: Rodopi, 1995.

This chapter has been reproduced from Sawin, Clark T: Henry H. Dale (1875–1968) and early endocrinology. *The Endocrinologist* 1998; 8(6): 395–400.

CHAPTER 60
Robert McCarrison (1878–1960)
Iodine Deficiency and Goiter

In January 1901, a 22-year-old, newly qualified physician from the north of Ireland took the competitive examination to join the Indian Medical Service (IMS), a branch of the British military, at the first opportunity. He passed the IMS examination with ease and, within a year of his medical graduation, embarked for Imperial India. Although he made frequent trips to the United Kingdom and Europe over his lifetime, he spent his entire military career in the subcontinent.

Robert McCarrison was a man of determined and independent mind. Qualified as he was to practice general medicine, he had no training in research, either in the laboratory or in epidemiology. Yet, within a few years, he had established a clear reputation for his work on the endemic Himalayan goiter and proposed, based on his own investigations, a theory as to its origin that was widely accepted in its day.

After he arrived in India, his first venture was to look into typhoid fever in Gurkha soldiers. They were thought to be immune but were not. Shortly after, he was able to delineate sandfly fever as a separate disease. His post had taken him to northern India, in what is now the high mountains of the northern Afghan border, and Gilgit, about 150 miles due east of Chitral. Both are riven with valleys that are surrounded by "hills" 10 000–15 000 feet high. He later moved to Kasauli, about 100 miles south of Gilgit near Srinagar, in the Himalayan foothills. His duties were to provide medical care to the military in these isolated garrisons. His active intellect, however, went much further afield.

Two observations in particular intrigued him. One was the excellent physical condition, despite the hard winters and primitive living conditions, of almost all the people living in the local Hunza valleys. McCarrison thought that their diet was the key: grains, vegetables, fruits, and dairy products. He would later contrast this with the poor nutrition and poverty of much of the Indian population and spend much of his later career investigating the country's nutritional needs. His second observation was the many pockets of goiter in the Himalayan villages and, to a lesser degree, cretinism. By 1902, a year after his arrival, he had put together a smattering of

A Biographical History of Endocrinology, First Edition. D. Lynn Loriaux.

This work is a co-publication between the Endocrine Society and John Wiley & Sons, Ltd.

laboratory facilities, primitive even for the time, that consisted of a microscope from this student days, microscope slides, and bacterial culture media all packed in over the mountains. He had an incubator and sterilizer made from kerosene cans. With these, he determined to find out what caused endemic goiter.

At the time, in the first decade or two of the twentieth century, the predominant view was that endemic goiter was likely an infectious disease. The use of iodine to treat goiter in Switzerland in the early nineteenth century had fallen into disfavor by mid-century, largely because of toxic side effects from overdosing, and because there was no known physiologic underpinning to its use. No one knew then that there was iodine in the thyroid gland or that it was an integral component of thyroid secretion. Iodine was simply a drug and it was given up as dangerous. With the rise of the germ theory of disease in the later nineteenth century, germs, usually bacteria, were sought as a cause of most illnesses. A surprisingly large number were found to be causal. It took some years, and the strict application of Koch's postulates to bring this about. In the meantime, the cause of other disorders remained in a state of limbo. Endemic goiter was one of these. Although iodine deficiency had been a proposed cause of endemic goiter in the mid-nineteenth century, it was not taken seriously by most, mainly because the proposal could not be confirmed with the analytic techniques available and, more importantly, because the whole concept that a deficiency could cause a disease was then completely foreign to medical thinking. "Everyone knew" that no such thing occurred. The idea that endemic goiter–or, for that matter, any disorder–was due to infection or some form of "parasite" was so common that it was the standard teaching at leading medical schools (e.g., Johns Hopkins), at the end of the nineteenth century.

McCarrison had learned his medicine in this milieu. Further, though highly intelligent and curious-minded, he himself wrote that, he "knew nothing" about the cause of goiter. His "few books of reference, limited to student's manuals, had little to say of it. Probably my ignorance was no bad thing." This meant that he lacked a real knowledge of the nineteenth-century European work on goiter (though he learned it later). Even more, because of the obscurity of the journals and the poor medical indexing of the era, he was unaware of many of the observations of Himalayan goiter made by his own countrymen decades before, including the fact that many had been treated with iodine 80 years earlier.

He essentially copied some experiments done in a goitrous area of northern Italy, on the presumption that there was an infectious agent in the water that caused goiter. He gave five dogs in Chitral local drinking water and five others the same water after boiling. One dog given unboiled water had thyroid swelling; none given boiled water did so.

His next approach was epidemiologic. He noticed that goiter was prevalent in the people of Chitral and Gilgit and he was able to discern a particular pattern in Gilgit. He noted that the prevalence of goiter in several villages of Gilgit rose from 12% to 46% as one followed the stream that supplied the villages' drinking water down the mountainside. He also noted that the stream was visibly dirtier and more polluted as one went from upstream to downstream. He concluded that it was reasonable to suppose that something added to the water as a result of human habitation was the cause of goiter.

This observation almost exactly parallels the slightly later work of David Marine in river trout. McCarrison never claimed priority, but it is clear that the phenomena were the same except for the species studied. Marine, too, felt that the cause of fish goiter was something added to the water upstream from the fish "houses" and that it was related to dirt or an infectious agent. Marine also was quite specific at the time (the 1910s) that the goiter was specifically not due to iodine deficiency.

McCarrison tried the dog experiment again, but used puppies and gave them the water from the Gilgit village with the highest prevalence of goiter. Nothing happened to either the test animals or the controls. Nothing if not stubborn, he went on to do the experiment again in young men and monkeys. For three months he gave five prisoners and three monkeys the same drinking water from the goitrous village; five controls got boiled water and four controls got filtered water. Again, nothing happened. But McCarrison was indeed a man of conviction. He decided to concentrate whatever it was in the water by filtering the muddy drinking water. He took the residue remaining after large amounts of the water was filtered and added the residue to the drinking water. Over the course of 2 or 3 years, he gave this residue to 36 men, including himself. Ten of the 36 developed thyroid swelling, in six of whom it was transitory (he was one of the six). He discovered that some of the men in his area had goiter that disappeared when they left Gilgit but returned a few weeks or months after they returned to the district. He knew that visibly clean drinking water from a nearby stream that supplied his own village was not associated with goiter, and that boiling the residue from the filtered water abolished its goitrogenic action (studied in six men for a month). He felt certain that an infectious agent was the cause. As, he put it, "I am convinced that endemic goiter is due to a living excitant of disease."

Because of his conclusions, he focused on the living habits of the people. If something living in the water is the cause of goiter, and it is not present well upstream above the villages, then the villagers must put something into the water. Naturally, he decided that that something must be fecal material. His immediate approach, as a physician, was not a public health approach but an individual approach. He did not try to improve local hygiene but rather chose to feed goitrous patients thymol, an extract of oil of thyme, on the hypothesis that this antibacterial agent would disinfect the intestinal tract, the origin of the goitrogen. For reasons unclear, he stopped using controls but simply operated on his disinfection hypothesis. He collected 82 cases that he was able to follow after treatment with oral thymol; "of these eighty-two, sixty-eight were cured, or so markedly benefited as to be practically so."

He also tried a series of "vaccinations" as a cure. Vaccination here was simply the subcutaneous injection over some days of sterilized stool cultures without any attempt to "isolate any particular organism." He claimed success with this therapy in several patients, as was the case with vaccines derived from *E. coli* and staphylococci.

By now, in the later part of the century's first decade, it was not possible to ignore iodine. He agreed that iodine was likely effective as a therapy but that it was effective because of its intestinal antiseptic action.

McCarrison continued to look for an animal model of the disease and aimed at transmitting the disorder from man to beast. He had failed to induce goiter in dogs and so turned, for some reason, to goats. He found goats from a nongoitrous site in the high mountains above Gilgit. He fed them vegetation so as to minimize contamination with the presumably infected ground. He made an apparatus that filtered clean water through a box filled with soil to which he added feces of patients with goiter. The filtered water, now contaminated, was the goats' drinking water. Half the goats developed goiter with histologic hyperplasia. He knew by this time (1913), from his contacts overseas, that not all agreed with him. Still, given the knowledge of the time, it was reasonable for him to conclude, as he did, that "incomplete as our knowledge of its [goiter] causation is, we know enough to make it certain that good sanitation ... and the provision of water-supplies which are not fouled by excreta of man and beast are measures which promise an extermination of the disease."

McCarrison was no shrinking violet; he did not do his work out of the limelight and did not simply publish occasionally in obscure journals. He made frequent trips to Europe and lectured on his thyroid work to London's Medical and Chirurgical Society, the Royal Society of Medicine, and gave the invited Milroy Lectures to the even more prestigious Royal College of Physicians. By the time of the Milroy Lectures, he had written 12 papers on endemic goiter and published 11 more before the outbreak of the First World War. Despite the initial resistance by his superiors to his spending time on these investigative efforts, he was promoted to Major in the IMS by 1913; that year he was officially assigned to continue his research.

His next station was Kasauli. Here he chose a public health application of his ideas. He found that at a local boarding school with 500 students, 22% had obvious goiter. When he investigated, he found that the water supply was polluted. So he purified the water for the boys but not for the girls. Within six months the prevalence of goiter in the boys had fallen by half while there was no change in the girls. This led to the construction of a purer water supply to the school, after which goiter never reappeared. He dismissed the idea that iodine deficiency might be a cause because he had analyzed the iodine in the old and new water systems and found that the purer water, which did not cause goiter, actually had less iodine in it than did the old system.

Curiously, he used this story to support his contention of a contagium vivum as the cause of endemic goiter, but there is clear bias in the story. In summing up his career after his retirement from the IMS (1937), he never mentioned that the initial means used to purify the water at Kasauli was Nesfield's reagent, which contains potassium iodate. In fact, McCarrison had antedated Marine's famous study of using iodine to prevent goiter in Akron school children by 5 years. Either he did not realize it, or was so wedded to his theory of infection that he could not consider the possibility of iodine as a preventative. By the 1930s he was well aware of Marine's work. Nevertheless, he felt, correctly, that too many people were exposed to low iodine but never developed goiter for the iodine deficiency idea to be completely explanatory. That problem remains with us today.

McCarrison made his reputation based on his goiter studies from 1902 to 1914. When the First World War came, and he went on active military duty in the Middle East, he became ill and returned to India to recover in the more salubrious environs of Coonoor in the southern part of India, more than 1500 miles from his Himalayan haunts. There, after a year or so, he returned to work at the Pasteur Institute of South India, still with rank in the IMS. He established a Nutrition Research Laboratory, studied beri-beri, and became an expert on nutrition, no doubt stimulated by his early observations in the Himalayas on the strength and physique of the Hunzas, which he presumed were due to a healthy diet. His work was widely recognized. Meals and honors and lectureships came his way. According to his colleagues he remained a true individual, which is probably a polite way of saying that he was not easy to get along with, a characteristic that may have lain behind his occasional administrative difficulties in running his research laboratory. He was an excellent and persuasive speaker, which may have helped in his European contacts. In his own work, however, he followed his own lead and seems to have taken direction reluctantly. His research co-workers saw him as "remote and rather aloof."

By the time he retired from the Coonoor Nutrition Research Laboratories, 57 years of age, he had been knighted and promoted to Major-General in the IMS. After retirement, he settled in Oxford, England, became a churchwarden, assisted in the Emergency Medical Service during the whole of the Second World War and, in his late 60s, became the first director of post-graduate medical education at Oxford, a position he held for 10 years. He died in 1960, aged 82 years.

McCarrison's work is only occasionally remembered today. In his time, it was seen as truly novel and explanatory of a major world health problem. His epidemiologic observations were correct and his experiments largely, but not consistently, controlled, reasonably done or interpreted. His persistence, even stubbornness, allowed him to get results that might have escaped a less willful person. His willfulness, however, led him away from iodine even though he had iodine data in his hands. Marine's work overtook his and the world accepted iodine deficiency as the cause of endemic goiter, as it still does. Still, Himalayan goiter persists to this day, though less than common it was, and we are still trying to explain his findings.

References

1. McCarrison R: *The Etiology of Endemic Goiter*. London: John Bale, 1913.
2. McCarrison R: *The Thyroid Gland in Health and Disease*. New York: William Wood, 1927.
3. McCarrison R: *The Simple Goitres*. London: Ballière, Tindall and Cox, 1928.
4. Mile M: Goitre, cretinism and iodine in South Asia: historical perspectives on a continuing scourge. *Med Hist* 1998; 42: 47.
5. Sawin CT: David Marine and the prevention of goiter [historical comment]. *Endocrinologist* 1996; 6: 423.
6. Sinclair HM (Ed.): *The Work of Sir Robert McCarrison*. London: Faber and Faber, 1953.
7. Trail RR (Ed.): *Lives of the Fellow of the Royal College of Physicians of London*. London: Royal College of Physicians, 1968, Vol. 5, p. 250.

This chapter has been reproduced from Sawin, Clark T: Historical Note: Robert McCarrison (1878–1960) and the cause of goiter: dirt and infection. *The Endocrinologist* 1999; 9(6): 409–12.

CHAPTER 61

Hakaru Hashimoto (1881–1934)

His Disease

When Hakaru Hashimoto published his lengthy paper on a new type of goiter in 1912, he could not have known that the disease he described would eventually be named after him. Modesty and cultural self-effacement would have prevented such "bragging" in any case, even had he been so ambitiously selfish as to encourage such naming. On the contrary, he gave the disorder a technical name, struma lymphomatosa, that simply described the histologic characters that he found. He died of typhoid fever at the early age of 52 years. Only after his death was his description of struma lymphomatosa, more than two decades earlier, widely recognized by the medical and thyroid communities and consistently given the eponym Hashimoto's disease or Hashimoto's thyroiditis.

Hashimoto was born in a village in Mie prefecture, southeast of Kyoto and east of Nara and Osaka. He was the son and grandson of physicians. Although he was the third son in his family, he was treated as the eldest son because the two older boys died before Hakaru was born. He attended local schools at first but then went to Tsu, the major city in the prefecture, for Junior High School (the equivalent of an American high school). In 1900 he attended the National High School in Kyoto, the equivalent of college in the United States. He graduated from the High School in 1903 and decided to go to medical school, influenced by family tradition but also by the recent death of his physician father. He chose to enter the first class at the new Fukuoka Medical College more than 300 miles from his home (the College was then part of Kyoto Imperial University but later became a part of Kyushu University). We know little of his medical student years but he seems to have been quietly competent and graduated in 1907.

Soon after graduation from medical school, Hashimoto decided on a career in academic surgery. His professor of surgery at Fukuoka, Hayari Miyake, invited him to stay on and he did. He completed his surgical training in 1912. During this training, Hashimoto needed a topic for his MD thesis. The topic he chose, probably suggested by Miyake, was the careful study of an odd type of goiter that did not have the histologic

A Biographical History of Endocrinology, First Edition. D. Lynn Loriaux.

This work is a co-publication between the Endocrine Society and John Wiley & Sons, Ltd.

or clinical characteristics found in most goitrous persons and that seemed to be quite rare: only four cases were seen in Miyake's clinic over the course of 4 years. There was some resemblance to another rare type of goiter, Riedel's struma, but–at least to Hashimoto–the patients he studied had a disease quite different from those with Riedel's disease. Hashimoto set to work on the four patients. It is not clear whether he actually saw these patients before their operations. At least one of the four was operated on while Hashimoto was still a student. It is clear that he was responsible for the careful follow-up examinations done 2–6 years after surgery. He also had the thyroid tissue for histologic study. His results were published in 1912 in a long paper–almost a small monograph–in a German journal and in the German language. Most likely, this was because of Miyake's previous training in Germany, then the academic mecca for scientific medicine, and because the paper would more likely be seen and read by the international community than if it had been written in Japanese and published in a Japanese journal. However, the result was that Hashimoto's work was not particularly well known in his own country.

The four patients, all women over age 40 years, had been seen initially between 1905 and 1909. All four were treated by partial thyroidectomy, which was done without much difficulty. There was no problem in freeing the goiter from the surrounding tissue as there might have been in patients with Riedel's disease. Histologically, however, the goiters were unusual. Instead of the colloid goiter so commonly found, these goiters had a "massive overgrowth of lymphatic elements." Hashimoto recognized the similarity between this histology and that of Graves' disease, but ruled out Graves' disease on clinical grounds, something that other commentators often failed to do. One of the four, and perhaps two others, had hypothyroidism, at least postoperatively.

Hashimoto then reviewed what was known about diseases that had excess lymphatic tissue. Such illnesses had already been termed inflammatory even though they were not associated with anything resembling the classic signs of acute inflammation. They were thought to be chronic inflammatory disorders. His review was thorough and the references he found were, as one might expect, almost entirely in German. First, he considered whether there might be some form of chronic infection. It is important to note here that goiter in general, at that time, was thought by many to be due to infection. He was unable to find any convincing evidence that there was a chronic infection in these patients, such as tuberculosis or syphilis. When Hashimoto compared his patients to those with Riedel's thyroiditis, he found some histologic similarities. The thyroid gland in Riedel's disease had far more fibrosis than did that from Hashimoto's patients. The principal difference was clinical. His patients simply did not have the rock-hard thyroid seen in Riedel's patients and the surgery was fairly straightforward while in those with Riedel's surgery was difficult due to the adherence of the thyroid tissue to its surroundings. He decided that the two diseases were separate entities and that what he was describing was, in fact, a new and separate disease.

Hashimoto thought that Mikulicz' disease, a lymphocytic infiltration of the salivary and lachrymal glands that causes enlargement of both, looked quite similar to his new thyroid disorder. Since all he had to work with were the histologic findings, he was not able to do more than speculate on the similarities of the two conditions and finally wrote that, despite the similarities, there was no known cause of either disease nor was there an explanation of why one affected the thyroid gland and the other affected salivary and lachrymal glands. In the absence of a discrete cause, he felt the only name that could be given to the thyroid disease was the title of his paper: lymphomatous goiter.

He did make one important observation. Because the entire thyroid gland was involved in the infiltrative process that resulted in growth of the gland and clinical goiter, there must be some external stimulus to the gland as a whole: "we can assume that... the lymphocytic elements are stimulated by some factor." This, however, was speculative and he finally concluded that "at present we cannot say anything definite about the cause."

Thus, Hashimoto combined the clinical findings with the histological features of the disease to draw conclusions, an effort that was not that common at the time. He also made reasonable speculations while clearly defining what was speculation and what was not.

When Hashimoto finished his training in 1912, he went to Europe for further training. His family pleaded with him to come home and carry on the family tradition of practicing in his home community. His prime interest in Europe was in the pathology of genito-urinary tuberculosis. He worked for 2 years in Göttingen. However, plans for further study in Europe were cut short with the outbreak of the First World War. Japan and Germany were on opposite sides and Hashimoto had to leave Germany. He went to England for a short time and then returned to Japan. It is not clear whether or not he went back to Fukuoka but, if he did, it was only for a short time because, by April of 1916, he had been prevailed upon to return to his home village and set up his medical practice in the small community hospital doing both general practice and surgery. In 1917 he was finally awarded the MD degree from his alma mater, now Kyushu University. He remained in practice in his home town for the rest of his life, an honored physician carrying on the commitment of the previous generations of his family to the community.

If Hashimoto's description of this unusual thyroid disease was so new, one might expect rapid acceptance by the medical community, particularly among the Germans who were so adept at lengthy and complete descriptions of new entities. Such was not the case. The War certainly impeded recognition. That he was Japanese, and not European, almost certainly slowed recognition. Surprisingly, there was little recognition in Japan. Several papers on the topic were published in Japanese over the subsequent years by colleagues at Fukuoka. The fact that Hashimoto did not remain in an academic setting also limited his opportunity to discuss findings. However, his work did not sink into a "black hole" and disappear entirely from view. Others, particularly in Germany, did take note of his 1912 paper. Most simply did not know what to make of it. Even when they knew of the work, there seemed to be no framework into which it fit, making it difficult to think about it in a constructive way. In the long view, however, it was recognized that Hashimoto had uncovered something of value. Even by the end of the decade of the 1910s, however, there was no mention of Hashimoto in major texts devoted to the thyroid gland. There was some mention of Hashimoto's paper in the early 1920s, often by Germans who did not think there was anything special about Hashimoto's work. Thyroid surgical texts remained blissfully unaware of lymphoid goiter. By the mid-1920s, Hashimoto's work was generally either unknown, forgotten, or thought unoriginal in the world of western medicine.

A prime example of this is the study of a "new" disease reported by a British pathologist, George Scott Williamson, as part of his MD thesis; Williamson's "discovery" of the new disease, "lymphadenoid goiter," was, of course, identical to Hashimoto's description. Williamson had simply not reviewed the available literature (in fact he managed to ignore all the publications in German on the topic). Even when writing at the end of the 1920s, Williamson was unaware of Hashimoto. Another problem was that some who did know of Hashimoto's work confused his disorder with Riedel's thyroiditis, or considered it an early stage of Riedel's, despite his clear distinction between the two diseases.

The 1930s brought a change in attitude. Allen Graham, a Cleveland surgeon, not only referred specifically to Hashimoto but forcefully pointed out what Hashimoto had said in the first place: lymphomatous goiter was in fact a separate disease and it is not a phase of Riedel's struma. Allen wrote in popular surgical journals and his message was heard–but even here the dissemination of the message took some time. An example of this further delay comes in the text on thyroid diseases written by the British thyroid surgeon Cecil Joll (1885–1945). Joll quoted Williamson but never mentioned Hashimoto. By the time of Joll's second edition of his text, all was corrected: Hashimoto was clearly referenced and the chapter heading changed to read: "The pathology, diagnosis, and treatment of Hashimoto's disease (struma lymphomatosa)." Joll was honest enough to admit in print that he simply had not known or read about Hashimoto in the early 1930s. An American surgeon at about the same time was equally explicit and wrote that the disorder was "first accurately described by Hashimoto and commonly designated by his name" and that "to confuse the two (Hashimoto's and Riedel's) seems to me to be preposterous." Thus, by the end of the 1930s, the disease Hashimoto wrote about more than two decades earlier was finally recognized and his original work given its due.

This recognition was expressed at the Third International Goiter Conference held in Washington, DC, in 1938 with Allen Graham himself chairing the program committee. A full paper discussed Hashimoto's disease with the term being easily and commonly accepted.

Today, the term, "Hashimoto's disease," is more widely used than ever. In part, the eponym reflects the realization that what Hashimoto described is actually a form of autoimmune disease–another story in itself–that can present not only as goiter but also as a shrunken, poorly functioning thyroid gland. The eponym also recognizes that in another respect we are no further along than was Hashimoto himself. We still have no clear pathophysiologic understanding of why goiter occurs in those who, like Hashimoto's patients, have goiter in the first place. One could argue that despite our burgeoning knowledge of autoimmunity, we really do not know why some persons get autoimmune thyroiditis and others do not, even when both have thyroid antibodies. Food for thought and honor and remembrance to Hakaru Hashimoto.

Sources

Graham A: Riedel's struma in contrast tostruma lymphomatosa (Hashimoto). *West J Surg* 1931; 39: 681.

Graham A, McCullagh EP: Atrophy and fibrosis associated with lymphoid tissue in the thyroid. Struma lymphomatosa (Hashimoto). *Arch Surg* 1931; 22: 548.

Hashimoto H: Zur Kenntniss der lymphomatösen Veränderung der Schilddrüse (Struma lymphomatosa). *Arch Klin Chir* 1912; 97.

Hashimoto K: Hakaru Hashimoto–a family memory. In *80 Years of Hashimoto Disease*, edited by S Nagataki, T Mori, K Torizuka. New York: Excerpta Medica, 1993, p. 7.

Heineke: Die chronische Thyreoiditis. *Deut Zeit Chir* 1914; 129: 189.

Joll CA: *Diseases of the Thyroid Gland with Special Reference to Thyrotoxicosis*. London: William Heinemann, 1932.

Simmonds M: Über lymphatische Herdein der Schilddrüse. *Virch Arch* 1913; 211: 73.

Tanaka M, Akita H: Hakaru Hashimotoat Kyushu University. In *80 Years of Hashimoto Disease*, edited by S Nagataki, T Mori, K Torizuka. New York: Excerpta Medica, 1993, p. 11.

Volpé R: The life of Dr. Hakaru Hashimoto. *Autoimmunity* 1989; 3: 243.

Williamson GS, Pearse IH: The pathological classification of goitre. *J Pathol Bacteriol* 1925; 28: 361, 219.

This chapter has been reproduced from Sawin, Clark T: Hakaru Hashimoto (1881–1934) and his disease. *The Endocrinologist* 2001; 11(2): 73–6.

CHAPTER 62

Eugene F. DuBois (1882–1959)

Basal Metabolism and the Thyroid

Eugene F. DuBois (1882–1959) (his last name is generally pronounced "doo boyce," perhaps because most of his ancestors were of English extraction) grew up on Staten Island and went to private schools there and in Milton, Massachusetts before going on to Harvard College. He graduated cum laude in only 3 years (although, as he said, "without distinguishing himself"). During the summer before finishing at Milton Academy he and his brother volunteered as orderlies in the Army Hospital at Montauk Point on Long Island. The patients were mainly soldiers who had returned from Cuba during the Spanish American War and were quite ill with typhoid, malaria, and dysentery. That summer was a powerful experience for him and was the principal stimulus for him to go into medicine [1].

After Harvard, he went on to Columbia University's College of Physicians and Surgeons, graduated in 1906, and was accepted as an intern at New York's Presbyterian Hospital. The internship then was 2 years long and was essentially the first real exposure to ill patients. The medical school had low standards, teaching was almost entirely by lecture, and there was little or no experience in hospital, seeing and caring for sick patients (that all changed, of course, a few years later). In fact, he thought his training in physiology was inadequate in both college and medical school [2]. He finished medical school six months before the internship began so he went to Europe to study pathology in Berlin (this was just at the end of the era when ambitious medical graduates–at least those who could afford it–went abroad to learn what could not be learned in the United States with usually an emphasis on pathology). DuBois' aim, though never clearly stated as such, was to become a teacher, certainly an unusual career goal for a medical graduate of that era.

Two years of internship completed, in 1909 DuBois went back to Europe again to study bacteriology, then a branch of pathology. But, just before he was to leave, one of his teachers in pediatrics, John Howland (1873–1926), later to become the chief of pediatrics at Johns Hopkins and one of America's leading academic pediatricians, told DuBois that the thing to do was to study human metabolism in Berlin. DuBois and a

A Biographical History of Endocrinology, First Edition. D. Lynn Loriaux.

This work is a co-publication between the Endocrine Society and John Wiley & Sons, Ltd.

colleague, Borden Veeder (later a professor of pediatrics at Washington University in St. Louis) did exactly that. The logical person to study with would have been Adolf Magnus-Levy (1865–1955) who, not so coincidentally, was, in the 1890s, the first to show the high metabolic rate in persons given thyroid extract or who had hyperthyroidism. Unfortunately, the two Americans and Magnus-Levy did not get along so they went instead to the Charité Hospital in Berlin to work under Theodor Brugsch. Here the two resurrected an old metabolism machine, put it in good repair, and flipped a coin as to which of the two should go first into the rejuvenated machine (it was big enough to hold a person but not big enough to move about–something like a modern MRI machine). DuBois "lost" and so became the subject for normal observations (later, he would always do experiments on himself before asking others to do so). Sometime during this period, Graham Lusk (1866–1932) stopped by for a visit; Lusk was then the professor of physiology at Cornell Medical College and, importantly later for DuBois, the scientific director of the Russell Sage Institute of Pathology (Russell Sage [1816–1906] was a wealthy financier in nineteenth-century America who invented the Wall Street practice of "puts and calls" in the stock market and left an estate of about $70 million). One of Lusk's interests was overall metabolism in animals; he saw the possibility in DuBois' work of extending these studies to humans.

In Berlin, DuBois studied patients with diabetes mellitus to determine their energy requirements. He and Veeder wrote up the data into what Lusk called a "confused" paper that Lusk recalculated and rewrote. It appeared in 1910 [3].

The two Americans returned to the United States in 1911 after 2 years in Berlin. DuBois joined the department of pathology at Presbyterian to which he was committed before going to Berlin but now, thoroughly ensconced intellectually in the field of calorimetry and metabolism, he found that there were no facilities to do such research. In the meantime, Lusk had been able to get the Sage Institute to pay for, and the authorities at Bellevue to provide space for, a human calorimeter which was much larger than the one in Berlin and was in essence a small room. Lusk then offered the two intrepid young investigators positions at Cornell. DuBois accepted while Veeder did not. So Lusk put DuBois in charge as medical director of the Institute. The calorimeter was located next to a small metabolic ward and required the services of a full-time mechanic, hence, it was a fairly expensive proposition, well beyond most research budgets of the day.

One of the first things DuBois studied in New York was metabolism in disease, particularly febrile illnesses like typhoid fever, the disease that had gotten him interested in medicine in the first place. Note here that "metabolism" was not what we now think of as intermediary metabolism, that is, what goes on inside the body and is the basis of modern biochemistry, but rather the study of calorimetry (i.e., human heat production and its relationship to foodstuffs eaten). In this sense, the metabolizing body is a "black box" that burns calories by whatever mechanisms exist inside the body. The human calorimeter measures the heat given off. DuBois then engaged in a long series of these measurements and learned, for example, that patients with typhoid really need food, in contrast to one of the medical dicta of the time that one should not feed these patients.

Nevertheless, what DuBois was doing was clearly research, albeit clinical research. His studies could not easily be translated into an easily used clinical test. The human calorimeter was a large machine, finicky in its performance without the continuous attention of the mechanic, and required the subject or patient to be inside the "box" which was uncomfortable for people who were sick. If the measurement of calories could be done indirectly (the large calorimeter that measured heat production was a form of direct calorimetry), that is, by assessing the amount of oxygen used over time and calculating the presumed amount of heat generated, one would then have a much simpler approach to testing patients. Others had thought of this but had never standardized the procedure by testing enough normal persons so as to determine what was normal and what was not. Further, only if the direct and indirect measurements could be shown to correlate well with each other would the indirect method make sense to use in a clinical context. DuBois and his colleagues accomplished both of these tasks. They went even further to standardize the indirect method by assessing it against a standard body surface area and so decreased the variance of the method (which created some controversy on theoretical grounds). So, by the mid-1910s, he had created reference standards for oxygen consumption at rest (the so-called "basal metabolic rate" or BMR which is not really basal as no one is actually at complete rest, least of all a patient undergoing a test). The result was that he was able to offer a mean normal value for the BMR with a range of normal that was only 15% above and below the mean value.

As an echo of his time in Berlin when he almost settled in to work with Magnus-Levy, DuBois turned briefly to the study of the BMR in patients with disorders of thyroid function. Perhaps surprisingly to us as endocrinologists, but not if one's focus is on a more general view of life, DuBois wrote only 2 or 3 papers on metabolism in thyroid disease. The main one is a 50-page paper on hyperthyroidism that studied in exquisite detail 11 patients with hyperthyroidism and one unfortunate patient with cretinism [4]. Another is his "paper" that was the entire section on thyroid disease in Russell Cecil's textbook of medicine; DuBois wrote this section from the inception of the textbook in 1927 until the sixth edition in 1943, after which one of his successors as chief of the Medical Service at New York Hospital, David Barr, took it over. DuBois' work on standardizing the BMR, however, was his true contribution. With the standardizing completed, others could then use the much simpler indirect method of calorimetry to convert the BMR from an investigative research tool to a clinically useful test that could be done in a relatively short time rather than the hours it took for a thorough metabolic calorimetry study.

As an example of the clinical use of the BMR as a test, DuBois himself noted that the use of the BMR in thyroid dysfunction "was best demonstrated by Means in Boston" and "the first extensive studies in which a large number of patients were followed for a considerable period of time were published by Means and Aub" [5, 6]. James Howard Means (1885–1967) was the leader of the Medical Service at Boston's Massachusetts General Hospital for several decades in the early to mid-twentieth century and the originator and guide of its Thyroid Clinic and Laboratory [7]. The BMR became widely used by endocrinologists because at the time there was almost nothing else that provided an objective measure of thyroid function (this remained so until well after the Second World War when blood tests such as the protein-bound iodine (PBI) and the measurement of serum thyroxine and thyroid-stimulating hormone (TSH) became accurate and sensitive enough to use clinically). The BMR was for more than three decades the mainstay of thyroid diagnosis (Means, incidentally, dedicated his book on thyroid diseases to DuBois, and called DuBois a "pioneer in clinical calorimetry and a generous teacher and friend") [8].

Most of DuBois' work in the next decade or so focused on further refinements of the normal BMR and on the effects of food and disease. His attention to the physiology of heat exchange (as well as his wide reputation) is seen in his thin book that encompassed Stanford University's Lane Medical Lectures on heat loss and temperature regulation [9] as is his continued interest in febrile illness in his small book on fever that he wrote near the end of his career [10].

During the First World War, he was on active duty in the U.S. Navy and became an expert on the effects of submarines on human physiology and on the proper ventilation needed (he thought that the ventilation problem in a submarine was essentially the same as that in the calorimeter). One episode in a submarine during the War led to his being awarded the Navy Cross: he set up a rapid ventilation process to absorb gaseous chlorine that might have poisoned the crew during a rapid dive when sea-water could have gotten into the batteries.

While he remained as medical director of the Russell Sage Institute for almost 40 years (1912–1950), his work brought him local, national, and international acclaim. From 1919 to 1932, he directed the Cornell Medical Service at Bellevue and was professor of medicine beginning in 1930. In 1932 the entire calorimetry operation moved from Bellevue to the New York Hospital and DuBois became chief of the hospital's Medical Service. This lasted until 1940 when he shifted his department completely and became chairman of Cornell's physiology department, thus filling Lusk's former position (Lusk had died in 1932).

The Second World War started shortly after he assumed the physiology chair and DuBois once again joined the Navy, now as a Captain involved mostly with the safety of pilots. He did everything that pilots had to do: he flew at high altitudes, went on dive-bombing runs, and went under fire at the front so as to see the effects of stress on the human body [11]. Because the military was interested in turning out physicians during the War, the Navy, perhaps uniquely, allowed DuBois to be on active duty for six months, then to be inactive for the next six months while he taught physiology, and then to go back to active duty again for another six-month rotation.

After the War he returned to his physiology department where he stayed until he retired in 1950 at age 68 years. Four years later he suffered a major stroke and was wheelchair-bound for the remaining 5 years of his life.

Honors came his way as well. DuBois was elected to the National Academy of Sciences in 1933. He had been elected to the Association of American Physicians in 1921 (the same year as Means) and was the Association's president in 1939 as well as the recipient of its highest honor, the Kober Medal, in 1947.

DuBois was able to become a physician and further his training in Europe not only because of his intelligence and drive but also because he had the wherewithal to do so. Then, when the time came for a career choice, he had the backing of a mentor (Lusk) and the funding that went with Lusk at the Sage Institute. Note that this was at a time when there were few dollars for research and when most investigators got their research funds, if any, from a small departmental budget (even when a grant came from an external source such as a foundation, grants of $300–500 were not uncommon). DuBois' contribution to endocrinology was clearly an important one: he turned his resources into a clinically important and useful test that was quantitative, standardized, and repeatable. Few have done as much.

References

1. Aub JC: Eugene Floyd DuBois. June 4, 1882–February 12, 1959. *Biogr Mem Natl Acad Sci* 1962; 36: 125.
2. DuBois EF: Fifty years of physiology in America. *Annu Rev Physiol* 1950; 12: 85.
3. DuBois EF, Veeder BS: The total energy requirement in diabetes mellitus. *Arch Intern Med* 1910; 5: 37.
4. DuBois EF: Clinical calorimetry. XIV. Metabolism in exophthalmic goiter. *Arch Intern Med* 1916; 17: 915.
5. DuBois EF: *Basal Metabolism in Health and Disease* (2nd edn.). Philadelphia, PA: Lea and Febiger, 1927, Vol. 21, p. 294.
6. Means JH: Studies of the basal metabolism in disease and their importance in clinical medicine. *Boston Med Surg J* 1916; 174: 864.
7. Stanbury JB: *A Constant Ferment. A History of the Thyroid Clinic and Laboratory at Massachusetts General Hospital: 1913–1990*. Ipswich: The Ipswich Press, 1991.
8. Means JH: *The Thyroid and Its Diseases*. Philadelphia, PA: JB Lippincott Co., 1937.
9. DuBois EF: *Lane Medical Lectures: The Mechanism of Heat Loss and Temperature Regulation*. Stanford, CA: Stanford University Press, 1937.
10. DuBois EF: *Fever and the Regulation of Body Temperature*. Springfield, IL: Charles C. Thomas, 1948.
11. Means JH: Eugene Floyd DuBois. 1882–1959. *Trans Assoc Am Phys* 1959; 72: 23.

This chapter has been reproduced from Sawin, Clark T: Eugene F. DuBois (1882–1959), basal metabolism, and the thyroid. *The Endocrinologist* 2003; 13(5): 369–71.

CHAPTER 63

Herbert McLean Evans (1882–1971)

Pituitary Hormones

On December 28 and 29, 1936, in New York City, the pituitary gland was the topic of two days of intense discussion by almost every North American scientist with an interest in this gland. Hormones were then seen as a key to understanding much about how animals worked and behaved. The pituitary, the "master gland," was yielding some of its mysteries to these investigators. But it was not yielding all that quickly.

One serious problem, which in retrospect seems obvious, was a lack of knowledge about how many pituitary hormones there were and what each one did. Herbert McLean Evans had come by train from the University of California at Berkeley, where he had chaired the Department of Anatomy for 21 years. He was also professor of biology at the adjacent Institute of Experimental Biology, endowed only 6 years earlier. He had come to assert his belief that growth hormone was a discrete substance of the anterior pituitary and to defend this position against attack, particularly from Oscar Riddle. Riddle was a past president of the American Society for the Study of Internal Secretions (later the Endocrine Society) and a long-established investigator at the Carnegie-supported Station for Experimental Evolution at Cold Springs Harbor, Long Island. Riddle and Robert Bates had made a fairly pure preparation of prolactin and studied it primarily in pigeons. Riddle felt that all pituitary-related growth could be accounted for by the combined action of prolactin and thyrotropin.

Evans had data to the contrary of course, but equally as important was that growth hormone was "his" hormone. Fifteen years before, in 1921, he had astonished the world when he created a giant rat by injecting it with a crude extract of bovine anterior pituitary glands. Sometimes referred to as the "discovery" of growth hormone – implying recognition of a specific substance and its isolation – it was not. But it had focused Evans on the pituitary as a research object. He and his enormous laboratory and staff spent much of the intervening years trying to define separate pituitary hormones. Evans was a forceful man, then near the peak of his powers and reputation, who brooked little or no opposition when he thought he was right (which seems to have been almost always) and suffered fools (read: anyone who

A Biographical History of Endocrinology, First Edition. D. Lynn Loriaux.

disagreed with him) not at all gladly. Riddle was a much quieter man, but also confident and able to express his ideas and data well.

The clash between the two was intentional. Letters between them show the exaggerated politeness and deference to data which they knew was demanded of scientists, but it is clear that each simply thought the other was wrong. Each presented a paper at the New York meeting and the discussion was as expected; neither gave way. The somewhat expurgated version printed in the proceedings of the meeting in 1938 retains some of the flavor: Evans: "I regret that whereas Doctor Riddle has brought us valuable new data on avian physiology, he has also nevertheless tended to confuse the issue" and Riddle: "Of course, the existence of an individual growth hormone would be very simply indicated if Dr. Evans could hand us a preparation of 'growth hormone'."

In a major way, the confrontation was precipitated by Evans' personality. Clearly bright, probably brilliant, he attended medical school in large part because of family expectations, beginning at the University of California in San Francisco in 1904 (the pre-clinical years did not move to Berkeley until after the 1906 earthquake). Unhappy with the lecture-based curriculum, perhaps driven by the need to escape parental pressure, concerned about his upcoming secret marriage in the face of parental disapproval on both sides, and clearly ambitious, he sought to transfer to an eastern school. Harvard got low marks. It had too many lectures as well, and no time for investigation. Johns Hopkins, however, had a schedule which permitted quarter-time independent study. He applied and they took him. Using some of his wife's funds to help finance his education, he moved to Baltimore in 1905, ensconced his wife in an apartment far from the school (medical students were then not to be married), skipped any class he was not interested in, and spent a large part of his time in the anatomy department. Its chairman, Franklin P. Mall, was an eminent anatomist in an eminent department. He took Evans under his wing. By the time Evans graduated, he had published seven papers, one a classic done with the head of surgery, William S. Halsted, on the vascular supply of the human parathyroid glands. He did no internship but was offered, and immediately accepted, a position in the Hopkins Department of Anatomy, where he stayed for the next 7 years until 1915, rising to associate professor. He taught, traveled to Germany in the summers, where he learned about dyes and vital staining, and continued his research, publishing nine papers in 1914 alone. He now had a national reputation. His ambitions were being served.

The critical offer in his life–although there were others later–came in 1915, when the president of the University of California offered him the chairmanship of anatomy at the Medical School, the department now in Berkeley. The department had had an acting chair since 1907, was not well-equipped or funded, and did little research. The president wanted to develop a more academic department. Evans, then aged 33 years, bartered a deal that doubled the department's budget, recruited two of the staff at Hopkins to come with him, and left a well-endowed, prestigious, and established department to return west to a school that had more opportunity than resources; "The die is cast... I am going home."

Evans thought of anatomy as a set of fixed structures to be memorized and then used as a structurally based way of understanding how organisms worked. If physiology or biochemistry could help, so much the better. He had little patience for gross anatomy; it bored him. But histology, with various dyes staining different structures, was a set of clues to function. Reading anatomic changes in terms of function stayed with him for most of his career; this was the basis for his entry into endocrinology and for his development of the many bioassays needed in the next several decades in his pituitary work. He never really saw himself as other than an anatomist.

Evans' arrival at Berkeley was explosive. This tall, large man with a salary twice that of anyone else in the department had a lot of new ideas. He also had the energy and the budget to go after them. He supported the one member of his department engaged in research, Philip E. Smith, with a meager budget of a few hundred dollars per year. Evans, single-minded if nothing else, thought the research budget, including several thousand dollars provided by the university, was his personal budget. He proceeded to explore dyes and what they could tell him. Some readers may recall the measurement of blood volume with Evans blue dye.

Because of changes in ovarian staining during luteinization, Evans studied the estrous cycle in the rat. He needed many rats. With his collaborator from the zoology department, Joseph A. Long, he crossed a white Wistar rat with a wild rat caught at a nearby creek. The resulting strain became the well-known Long–Evans rat. To get reliable data, he helped put in place the idea of standard rats on standard diets. Long had discovered, probably before Stockard and Papanicolaou, that the vaginal mucosa of the rat becomes cornified in a rhythmic manner. The estrous cycle is reflected by periodic cornification easily seen in intact animals with periodic vaginal smears. Although no paper was ever written, the resulting 1922 monograph is a classic, used for decades by anyone studying mammalian ovarian function. The use of the phenomenon as a bioassay played a key role in the isolation of various estrogens in the 1920s and 1930s. Evans wrote the monograph but, as Long had made the original observation and done most of the work, Evans surprised Long by putting Long's name first. Evans may have been bombastic and arrogant, but he tried always to be fair. He was not always sensitive to others' feelings, nor did he find it easy to see things from another's viewpoint.

He was adept at picking up anomalies and finding out why they occurred. By the 1920s his laboratory was probably the best-funded anatomical research laboratory in the country. He used hundreds of rats per month, soon to rise to a few thousand rats per month. He noted that on some diets, fertility was not what it should be. The result was dietary experiments that led to the discovery and, later isolation, of vitamin X, later called vitamin E.

The other thread to his work is that which led to the confrontation with Riddle about the hormones of the anterior pituitary. It is not clear how he got onto this area. Partly, it was due to the influence of Harvey Cushing, his teacher and colleague at Johns Hopkins until 1912. A more direct influence was probably Smith in his own department. Smith's work had focused on the amphibian pituitary and the effects of its removal. Smith's publications flowed as Evans freed up time for Smith's research and raised his salary past that of those who simply taught. Whatever the direct stimulus, Evans was led to his "giant rat" experiment and stayed with pituitary hormones for the rest of his life. One would have thought that he and Smith would have had a wonderful collaboration, particularly as Smith worked on, and eventually perfected, hypophysectomy in the rat as well as in the frog. But it was not to be. Evans' overbearing and dominating personality, which meshed well with the quiet and unambitious Long, did not fit at all well with the quiet and reserved but intensely ambitious Smith. Sometime in the early 1920s, Smith thought Evans had taken unwarranted credit for some work that Smith had done. There is no record of just what happened, but the story in Smith's family is one of hostility. The two never co-authored a paper, either before or after the episode. Their only work together was two abstracts in the early 1920s.

Smith left in 1926 to go to Stanford. Probably, once again, Evans' personality got in the way. He may well have done something without bad intentions but with little sensitivity to another's feelings. And so it went throughout Evans professional life. Combative, and often arrogant in public, colleagues around the country seemed to love him or hate him (he could be quite charming). He was certainly no politician.

Still, he attacked the pituitary with skill, vigor, a large staff, thousands of rats, and a large budget from many sources, even through the economic depressions of the 1930s. He knew the need for chemical assistants and had several. The most prominent, who joined him in 1938, was Chao Hao Li, whose work resulted in purification of several of the pituitary hormones, including growth hormone and ACTH.

Those who could stand Evans learned to adapt to his ways, despite his personal characteristics. Evans did want his colleagues and students to do well. He was among the first at Berkeley to recruit women as staff and not as technicians. Those who did adapt often stayed for years or even decades. His work was not always correct. He and Olive Swezy determined, in 1929, that humans have 48 chromosomes, partly on the basis of work done on the testes of just-hanged criminals at San Quentin Prison. It took several decades to correct this error. He was clearly able to admit error. His mind and view were broad and eclectic. Stimulated early on by William Osler when a medical student in Baltimore, he was fascinated by the history of science, biology, and medicine. He organized and ran for years a history dinner club in Berkeley, collected and sold and collected again major books in his fields of interest and taught an outstanding course in the history of medicine after his retirement.

His "acerbic wit, sarcasm and... gratuitous insults" mellowed somewhat with age, but his "high-flown literary style" did not. This complex, difficult, brilliant man left a legacy of more than 600 publications. He was one of the dominant figures in American endocrinology throughout most of the first half of the twentieth century. Had he been easier to get along with, he would certainly have been president of the Endocrine Society and probably won at least one Nobel Prize. But then, not many American scientists have been elected to both the U.S. National Academy of Sciences and to the Royal Society. He died in 1971 at the age of 88 years old.

Sources

Amoroso EC, Corner GW: Herbert McLean Evans. 1882–1971. *Biogr Mem Fellows R Soc* 1972; 18: 83–136.

Bennet LL: Endocrinology and Herbert M. Evans. In *Hormonal Proteins and Peptides*, Vol 3, edited by Li CH. New York: Academic Press, 1975, pp. 247–72.

Corner GW: Herbert McLean Evans. 1882–1971. *Biogr Mem Natl Acad Sci* 1972; 45: 153–92.
Grumbach MM: Herbert McLean Evans. Revolutionary in modern endocrinology: a tale of great expectations. *J Clin Endocrinol Metab* 1982; 55: 1240–7.
Parkes AS: Herbert McLean Evans. Foreword and interview. *J Reprod Fertil* 1969; 19: 1–49.
Raacke ID: "The die is cast" – "I am going home": the appointment of Herbert McLean Evans as head of anatomy at Berkeley. *J Hist Biol* 1976; 9: 301–22.
Timme W, Frantz AM, Hare CC: The pituitary gland: an investigation of the most recent advances. *Assoc Res Nerv Ment Dis* 1938; 17: 188–90, 295–6.

This chapter has been reproduced from Sawin, Clark T: Herbert McLean Evans (1882–1971). *The Endocrinologist* 1993; 3(6): 382–4.

CHAPTER 64

Philip E. Smith (1884–1970)

Trophic Hormones of the Pituitary

In a sense, Philip Edward Smith "invented" the pituitary gland for modern endocrinologists. His major work, done in Berkeley, California and at Columbia University during the 1910s and 1920s, solidly established this gland as essential for the control of skin color in amphibians, and later for the control of gonadal and thyroid function in mammals. The key was the ability to perform a hypophysectomy without damage to the hypothalamus in larval amphibians and, later, in rats and other mammals. By the end of the 1920s, this led to the use of the hypophysectomized animal as the standard model for assessing the activity of various pituitary extracts which were, at the time and for some decades to come, quite impure.

Smith was born in DeSmet, a small town on the Chicago and Northwestern Railroad in the lake country of eastern South Dakota. His father was a Protestant missionary to the American Indians. He was descended from New England forebears. One ancestor was Josiah Bartlett, a physician and signer of the Declaration of Independence. The family moved to Nebraska and then to Moorpark in southern California when Smith was a young child. His father bought and ran an apricot farm. In his teens, Smith had to work on the farm but hated the work, although he was later an excellent gardener.

Smith's father was remembered as stern and authoritarian. The family was well educated (both parents attended Oberlin College) and encouraged Philip and the other children to finish school at a time when most Americans did not go on to college. Smith attended Pomona College, which was a several days' bicycle ride from home. Tall and thin, the young Smith, nicknamed "Slats," played both football and tennis.

After graduation from college in 1908 and a year working for the state of California as an entomologist, Smith went east to Cornell for graduate training in entomology. He received his MSc in this field in one year, but had been attracted by histology and embryology, and he went on to get his PhD in anatomy in 1912. By now his interest had definitely focused on the development of the amphibian nervous system with a particular interest in the pineal and pituitary glands.

A Biographical History of Endocrinology, First Edition. D. Lynn Loriaux.

This work is a co-publication between the Endocrine Society and John Wiley & Sons, Ltd.

After graduation, he returned to California and took up a position in the Department of Anatomy at the University of California (UC), then at Berkeley. Within a year he met and married Irene Patchett, who had been a graduate student working on the frog pituitary gland. For years afterward she helped him, without pay, both in the field and in the laboratory. She was a co-author on several publications. Their research focus in the 1910s and early 1920s was on amphibians, which they collected in Muir Woods and carried back on the train in coffee cans.

Early on, Smith showed that removal of the developing pituitary gland in the frog embryo stopped metamorphosis. He met Bennett M. Allen, then teaching at the University of Kansas, and learned that he, too, was working on the same problem with the same result. They arranged to submit their manuscripts to *Science*, where both were published in 1916. Smith's amphibian work led to a monograph on disturbances in growth, pigmentation, and endocrine function in 1920. By this time he realized that it would be important to show the same effects in mammals, so he began work with the rat. Success was not immediate. In fact, it took several years, but by 1923 he had data showing that the rat pituitary could be removed without damaging the hypothalamus, thus avoiding the obesity sometimes attributed to pituitary deficiency. He showed that crude extracts of ox pituitary glands could temporarily replace the loss of the rat's pituitary gland. All of this culminated in a classic article in 1930 that summarized years of work and formed the groundwork knowledge for pituitary function. He went on, producing paper after paper, until, in 1963, at the age of 79 years, he wrote his last paper on the effects of homotransplanted pituitaries into the rat pituitary portal system.

While Smith is remembered by endocrinologists for his research, there was more to him than just working in the laboratory. He viewed teaching as a major responsibility. His perfectionist approach brought on severe headaches when he was to lecture, but he seems always to have shown up. He was clearly not a dynamic speaker – his medical students in histology at Columbia called him "whispering Phil" – but he knew what he was talking about. Few realized that he had been president of his college's debating society. In the 1930s, he was responsible for a major revision of a standard textbook of histology, a task he took on because he felt responsible for the quality of the material he taught. He was at his best with graduate students and fellows, with whom he was friendly and attentive. He was seen as a loner, not given to "big science" but preferring to work with a small group at what he knew best. He was liberal-minded but never talked politics; ambitious but never overweening; and he never drew conclusions that overreached the data.

In later life his colleagues elected him president of the American Association for the Study of Internal Secretions (later the Endocrine Society). He was also a member of the American Association of Anatomists, the Society for Experimental Biology and Medicine, and the Harvey Society. He was elected to the National Academy of Sciences and received the Dale Medal of Great Britain's Society of Endocrinology.

Despite all of this success, life was not all smooth sailing for Smith. Three years after starting his first job, the UC Department of Anatomy got a new chairman, Herbert McLean Evans. Evans, only a year older than Smith, was a native Californian whose physician father had sent him to Johns Hopkins Medical School. He was a recognized and innovative functional histologist and had invented Evans blue dye. Evans' and Smith's personalities could not have been more different: Evans was large, gregarious, boisterous, and even bombastic. In terms of science, Evans and Smith were of equal stature, but Evans was an early proponent of large experiments, large laboratories, and large budgets. He saw early on the need for a standardized strain of laboratory rat and developed the Long–Evans rat, breeding them by the hundreds. He also appropriated to his research any funds in sight.

Evans recognized Smith's talent, and promoted him and raised his salary faster than other more senior department members. Nevertheless, by the early 1920s Smith resented Evans. Despite the apparent common interest of their work, there is no paper co-authored by them. At the least, Smith did not care for Evans' style nor for his habit of continually looking over Smith's shoulder. Further, Smith had little or no research funds of his own. As an example, when the National Research Council's Committee for Research in Problems of Sex began to make grants to investigators in 1922, Evans received money from the beginning, being granted $24 750 from 1922 to 1926, while Smith got nothing. Yet, when Smith left Berkeley, he was granted funds immediately and continued to receive them for the next decade. It is unclear whether the root of the problem was style and attitude, or resentment over independent funding, more likely it was an episode in which Evans published some of Smith's data, prematurely and on his own.

By 1926, Smith was ready to move, possibly precipitated by the university's refusal to grant him a sabbatical leave. He refused a professorship of physiology at UC because he felt he was an anatomist. Instead, he accepted a lateral move to become associate professor of anatomy at Stanford. The move was a happy one but short. After buying a house and settling in, he was asked to be a professor of anatomy at Columbia University's College of Physicians and Surgeons. He accepted, got an agreement for several months' sabbatical leave abroad, uprooted the family once again, and began work at Columbia in early 1928. He carefully avoided becoming chairman of his department. He continued to publish on the functions of pituitary and gonadal hormones, trained his graduate students and fellows, and then retired from Columbia in 1954 at 70 years of age. In fact, he had become emeritus in 1952 after a severe leg injury from a rototiller accident in 1951.

Retirement, however, lasted only 2 years. In 1956, he decided to go back to the laboratory. He wrote a former Columbia graduate student, who had become a professor of anatomy at Stanford, and asked if he could work in a corner of the laboratory with a few monkeys. The department took him on as a research associate and, at the age of 72 years, he got a National Science Foundation grant and went west again. The arrangements for monkeys never worked out so he returned to the study of the rat pituitary, combining as always the functional and anatomic. He worked for 7 more years until 1963. Failing vision finally halted the career of this remarkable man.

Smith and his wife tried retirement homes in Carmel and Oakland, California. However, in part because of the right-wing views of his neighbors, the couple decided to go back to Massachusetts. There he lived until he died of carcinoma of the colon in

1970, not quite 87 years old. His wife survived him by nearly two decades, dying at the age of 101 years.

There are many styles in science as well as personalities in life. Smith's style was quietly ambitious. He picked a topic that was fruitful and persevered until it bore results. While resources were limited, there was no pressure for instant publication. The results spoke for themselves; conclusions were strictly limited to what was before one's eyes without speculation as to what might be. Smith's caution and manifest integrity, as much as the clear design of his experiments, were an inspiration to endocrinologists struggling to separate fiction from fact. Evans was brilliant, but his flamboyant manner attracted criticism and distrust; Smith balanced this style with his own brand of brilliance: quiet, restrained, clear, steady, and convincing. Science needs both.

Sources

Aberle SD, Corner GW: *Twenty-Five Years of Sex Research*. Philadelphia, Saunders, 1953, p. 127.

Agate FJ Jr.: Philip Edward Smith. *Dict Sci Biog* 1975; 12: 472–7.

Grumbach MM: Herbert McLean Evans, revolutionary in modern endocrinology: a tale of great expectations. *J Clin Endocrinol Metab* 1982; 55: 1240–7.

Raacke ID: Herbert McLean Evans (1882–1971). A biographical sketch. *J Nutr* 1983; 113: 929–43.

Severinghaus AE: A memorial resolution for Philip Edward Smith. *Am J Anat* 1971; 135: 159–64.

This chapter has been reproduced from Sawin, Clark T: Philip E. Smith (1884–1970). *The Endocrinologist* 1992; 2(4): 213–15.

CHAPTER 65

Edward C. Kendall (1886–1972)

Structures of Cortisol and Thyroxin

When he looked through his microscope on Christmas Day, 1914, in Rochester, Minnesota, Edward Calvin Kendall finally saw the crystals of thyroxin he had sought since 1910. This was a major achievement for the 28-year-old biochemist. Yet, while a time of triumph, it was also a time of frustration. Although Kendall made his name with this "discovery" of thyroxin and eventually became president of the American Society of Biological Chemists (ASBC), he never found the correct structure. A reminder of his proposed, but incorrect, structure still exists as the "in" in thyroxine.

Although seen in retrospect as another step in the steady progression of endocrine discovery, Kendall's work grew out of a widely recognized problem which he attacked with skill and persistence, even stubbornness. It was fraught with uncertainties and perplexing difficulties. His persistence was clearly needed, but it led him to stick with an incorrect structure longer than he should have.

After George R. Murray described the successful treatment of myxedema with thyroid extract in 1891, many chemists tried to isolate the active principle. The most striking advance was Eugen Baumann's discovery, in 1895, that the thyroid contained iodine. He made a brownish preparation that he thought was the active material. It did ameliorate hypothyroidism and he called it thyroiodin (later iodothyrin). Still, not everyone could confirm that the active material contained iodine and, despite fairly intensive work by several chemists, there was little further progress for almost 20 years.

When Kendall ("Nick" to close friends but "Dr. Kendall" to most) finished his PhD work on pancreatic enzymes, in June, 1910, after 2 years of work at Columbia University, he did not know that the thyroid gland contained iodine. His first job in Detroit was with Parke, Davis and Co., where he was assigned to work on isolation of thyroid hormone. He stayed only a few months, but continued with the problem for 20 years. At St. Luke's Hospital in New York City, the atmosphere was less commercial, but few physicians saw any merit in his work. There was already an effective thyroid therapy. But Kendall had made three key decisions on what was, after all, a high-risk venture: (1) to stick with the problem; (2) to regard iodine as so critically important to

---

A Biographical History of Endocrinology, First Edition. D. Lynn Loriaux.

This work is a co-publication between the Endocrine Society and John Wiley & Sons, Ltd.

thyroid hormone's action that it could be used as a tracer in the hormone's isolation; and (3) to improve the sensitivity of the iodine assay. He spent the better part of 2 years on this last.

By 1912–1913, Kendall had isolated what he thought were at least two hormones. Still, he felt unappreciated. He learned that the Mayo Clinic, a bastion of thyroid surgery, was interested in extending its research work to the biochemistry of the thyroid. He applied and got the job, beginning in February 1914.

Now his only task was to work on finding thyroid hormone in an institution that wanted him to do just that. By the end of 1914, he had isolated various fractions after harsh alcohol–alkaline hydrolysis of hundreds of pounds of animal thyroid tissue provided by the Parke, Davis Company. These fractions were whitish powders and crusts which had up to 47% iodine by weight. He had submitted an abstract to the ASBC on two of his isolated fractions, A and B. The meeting was on December 28, 1914, in St. Louis. He was hard at work to get the best data possible for the meeting. Whatever he said would be noticed as there were only 19 abstracts on the entire ASBC program that year. On December 23, he accidentally boiled off all the alcohol from a preparation containing 60% iodine, leaving an insoluble white crust. Rather than throw it out, he worked it over the next 2 days. Finally, he dissolved the crust in sodium hydroxide, added sulfuric acid, and boiled it. On cooling he saw, for the first time, sheaves of needle-shaped crystals. His presentation went well. On the same ASBC program at a joint session with the American Physiological Society was a paper by the physiologist Walter B. Cannon on hyperthyroidism induced in cats by connecting the phrenic nerve to the cervical sympathetic nerves. The work was never confirmed. In May 1915, Kendall published a picture of his crystals in the widely read *Journal of the American Medical Association* and presented his work to the prestigious Association of American Physicians, making his mark on a national audience. Ironically, during the entire year of 1915, he was able to make his crystals only one more time. He made 125 mg. As you would predict, he lost the knack in the midst of acclaim.

Because of World War I, there was no competition from Europe. Failure to get more crystals did not mean he would "lose the race." Finding the structure and synthesizing the compound were the "real" goals of the biochemist. In early 1917, he was again consistently able to get crystals of the material. When he had 5 or 6 g on hand, he hired an organic chemist, Arnold Osterberg, to help with structural analysis and synthesis. In September 1917, Kendall spoke to the American Chemical Society in Boston and announced the structural formula of "the thyroid hormone" as well as its synthesis. He thought the structure was a triiodooxyindol derivative. He and Osterberg, while waiting for a train in Chicago earlier that year, searched for a simpler name than the cumbersome "thyro-oxy-indol"; Osterberg suggested the contraction "thyroxin" in which the "in" was the remnant of "indol," and so it was for the next 10 years.

Kendall gave many presentations and wrote many papers on thyroxin, including long, definitive papers in the *Journal of Biological Chemistry*. He probably knew there was something amiss when he claimed a synthesis he never actually published as such. He was convinced that the structure was correct and that it explained the hormone's biologic actions.

The structure was neither correct nor explanatory. Kendall had made a small error when he did not realize that iodination changes the chemical reactions of tyrosyl residues, something known since the 1890s. He stuck with his structure for 10 years, continuing to synthesize a wide variety of indole derivatives in an attempt to get a biologically active compound, even though others had told him that there was something wrong with the structure. His fame was undiminished.

Kendall applied for a patent on his product in 1916. He applied again in 1919 and only after a third application, in 1921, now including the "structure," was the patent granted. Kendall's intent was to protect the isolated product's purity and effectiveness from less careful manufacturers (the processing of tons of thyroid tissue included many steps and was tedious in the extreme). With the active support of William J. Mayo, the older of the two Mayo brothers then in charge of the Clinic, Kendall tried to assign the patent to the American Medical Association (AMA), provided any profits were used for medical research. Incredibly, the AMA would not accept the proviso. The American College of Surgeons was more enthusiastic but also eventually refused. The pending patent was finally assigned to the University of Minnesota, whose Board of Regents had sole power over the distribution of any profits accruing to the university. A small fraction of the university's share (no more than 10%) might be awarded the discoverer (Kendall) or his heirs. The university licensed E.R. Squibb and Sons as exclusive manufacturers and, by 1920, thyroxin was offered for sale. Unfortunately, however, it was expensive and turned out to be only erratically effective. No one realized that although the sodium salt is well absorbed, the free acid is not. By 1931, accumulated sales were only a few thousand dollars.

Kendall stopped trying to synthesize thyroxin in 1926 when he learned of Charles R. Harington's success. Harington's work was "a severe test" for Kendall, who wrote, "The failure to synthesize thyroxin was a bitter disappointment." Harington changed the name to "thyroxine" with the terminal "e" to conform to the current nomenclature for amino acids; Kendall readily accepted the change in name by 1928 and entitled his 1929 book, *Thyroxine*.

Kendall moved on to the adrenal cortex. Once again he isolated crystals in 1934 and determined a tentative structure which he refused to give in public. The adrenal-derived crystals contained more than one substance. Kendall kept on through World War II. There was a flurry of interest in adrenal hormones when the military thought that it would allow aviators to fly higher and longer. With Phillip S. Hench, he gave cortisone to patients with rheumatoid arthritis. The dramatic results were the introduction of corticoids as a treatment for a host of inflammatory diseases and led to a shared Nobel Prize for Kendall and Hench.

Kendall's role in the discovery of thyroxine was its isolation as crystals. His thyroid work did not directly change therapy but gave great credibility to the infant field of endocrinology and, not coincidentally, helped put the Mayo Clinic on the map as a center of research. His career is an example of science advancing in fits and starts rather than progressing smoothly to ever-higher achievements. This was perhaps a result of choosing only the hardest problems to solve.

Sources

Ingle DJ: Edward C. Kendall. *Biogr Mem Natl Acad Sci* 1975; 47: 249–90.
Kendall EC: *Cortisone*. New York: Charles Scribner's & Sons, 1971.
Sawin CT: Defining thyroid hormone: its nature and control. In *Endocrinology: People and Ideas*, edited by SM McCann. Bethesda, MD: American Physiological Society, 1988.

This chapter has been reproduced from Sawin, Clark T: Edward C. Kendall (1886–1972) and thyroxine. *The Endocrinologist* 1991; 1(4): 291–3.

CHAPTER 66
David Marine (1880–1976)
Iodine and Goiter

During his long life of 96 years, David Marine was often honored. He gave a Harvey Lecture in 1924, received the Squibb Award of the Endocrine Society (1953), the Kober Medal of the American College of Physicians (1960), and a special award from the American Thyroid Association in 1968 when he was 88 years old. J. Howard Means, one of the foremost clinical thyroidologists in the United States in the first half of the twentieth century, called Marine the "Nestor of the Thyroid." Marine's reputation rests on two accomplishments. The first is his work on the experimental pathophysiology of the thyroid gland, particularly his efforts to find a rational explanation for the midwestern United States goiter epidemic. The second is his role in demonstrating that iodine could prevent goiter.

Marine was born on a farm in Whitleysburg, Maryland. He was orphaned at age 7 and raised by an aunt. He never finished high school, but was admitted to Western Maryland College. The college had only one course of study consisting of languages, the classics, and some science. When he graduated in 1900 at 20 years of age, he enrolled in the graduate biology program of Johns Hopkins University. That program, under William Keith Brooks, was one of the few in the United States that granted a doctorate in biology.

Marine stayed in the program for only one year. A fellow student, Edward H. Richardson, interested him in medical school and so it was arranged. He began his medical course the same week that he made out his application. It seems that he was admitted before he formally applied. The requirements for admission, at least to Hopkins Medical School, were quite different from those of today. The student needed to demonstrate the ability to read both French and German and be able to list the Latin works he had read in the original.

There is no evidence that Marine did research during medical school or was otherwise a "star," although he graduated well up in his class. Later in life, Marine recalled the influence of his professor of surgery, William Halsted, on his thyroid studies. Halsted had investigated dog thyroid glands in an attempt to better understand Graves'

A Biographical History of Endocrinology, First Edition. D. Lynn Loriaux.

This work is a co-publication between the Endocrine Society and John Wiley & Sons, Ltd.

disease. Not much came of this work in terms of understanding Graves' disease, but one thing did stick in Marine's mind. It was clear that the histologic changes of the dog's thyroid gland, when it regrew after partial resection, looked much like those of the thyroid hyperplasia of Graves' disease in humans.

Marine was not selected as a house officer at the Johns Hopkins Hospital. So, when he graduated in 1905 (future Nobel laureates Peyton Rous and George Whipple were classmates), he left Maryland for Cleveland and a residency in pathology. This was a common path for those planning to train in internal medicine. The chief pathologist at Cleveland's Lakeside Hospital was a Hopkins trainee, so there was a connection.

When Marine arrived in Cleveland in 1905, there were few paved roads, no neon lights, and no movie theaters. Not much was known about thyroid physiology despite the decade or so of fairly intense study that followed George Murray's discovery of the successful treatment of myxedema with thyroid extract (1891) and Eugen Baumann's finding of iodine in the gland (1895). Marine's new job allowed half-time for research. On his first day, June 30, he was walking to the hospital for his first meeting with his new professor and saw in the streets of Cleveland women and dogs with enlarged thyroid glands. At the hospital, the bacteriology professor asked Marine what he wanted to work on, and he said "the thyroid." And so, a lifelong career was set in motion.

It is worth noting that at that time there was no clear agreement on what was wrong with patients who had Graves' disease. Whether or not there was hypersecretion of thyroid hormone was not universally agreed upon. Further, non-toxic goiter, the so-called "simple" goiter, was not common along the United States east coast where Marine had lived all his life. Yet, in 1905, he had seen several examples of the malady simply walking to work. Some experts thought that the cause was an unknown "parasite" (i.e., an infectious disease). It was not thought to be due to iodine deficiency, a theory that had been raised in mid-nineteenth century France and later discarded. So Marine's proposal to his professor of bacteriology that he study the thyroid gland and goiter was not unsurprising.

Marine was a hard worker. He began by studying the histology of the dog thyroid gland. By the end of his second year of residency, he had submitted for publication four papers and had presented one of these at a national meeting. More importantly, the end of his residency coincided with the opening of a new Department of Experimental Medicine at the affiliated Western Reserve School of Medicine. The department had its own independent endowment that guaranteed a departmental income of $13 000 per year, quite a large sum at the time. There were few such departments in the United States. George Stewart, Western Reserve's former professor of physiology, came back to Cleveland to head the new department and immediately appointed Marine to work with him. Marine now had a job that was "free of routine teaching" and had a "minimum of administrative detail." He worked even harder. His former classmate, George Whipple, said that Marine published earlier and faster than anyone else in his medical school class.

Marine began studying dogs because they were cheap. He was able to use animals that had already been used in other experiments. There was a wide range of histologic changes in the thyroid glands of these dogs, and they were quite different from the

Baltimore dogs. Ninety percent of the Cleveland dogs had thyroid hyperplasia and under the microscope they looked much like the glands of patients with toxic goiter. Marine thought that this microscopic picture meant that the thyroid was reacting to some kind of deficiency by analogy with Halsted's partial resection experiments. His idea was that the gland became hyperplastic because it was trying to grow larger to overcome the deficiency. This concept that a hyperplastic thyroid gland was a deficient one, no matter what the clinical circumstance, is a thread that runs through Marine's work over the next several decades.

His initial approach was to repeat some of Halsted's work by showing that partial thyroid resection led to hyperplasia. His problem was that all the Cleveland dogs, experimental or control, had hyperplasia. He next studied the effects of iodine, an idea that "naturally ... suggested itself [because] it is generally accepted that iodine compounds benefit the majority of simple goiters" He showed in a single dog that hyperplasia seemed to change to "colloid goiter" after treatment with iodine. He speculated that iodine content might be low when there was hyperplasia, but he had no data. He needed to measure the iodine and so recruited a colleague from the pharmacology department to do assays. He gave the dog a combination of iodide and desiccated thyroid. Measuring iodine in a piece of the dog's thyroid, he found that it was low, which meant that the "lack of iodine was the essential deficiency." He concluded that the low iodine concentration of the enlarged simple goiter and of the goiter in Graves' disease showed that both conditions were due to the same problem. For Marine, the iodine deficiency of the thyroid gland was caused by an internal misallocation of the elements, and the element was iodine.

Marine's idea for remedying the problem in dogs was straightforward: give iodine to the dog with the expectation that some of it would end up in the thyroid gland. When he did this, he consistently got conversion of hyperplasia to colloid goiter. This was a major discovery and made his reputation as an investigator. There was now a glimmer of pathophysiologic sense as to what was happening.

Intellectually, he transferred this idea to the problem of Graves' disease in humans, but he struggled to fit the similar histology and low thyroid iodine concentration of Graves' and simple goiters with the widely disparate clinical picture of the two conditions. He concluded that the Graves' glands "have a hyposecretion physiologically, yet quantitatively they have a hypersecretion." The problem in toxic goiter was too much of a weakly acting hormone that caused the "toxic" symptoms. Graves' disease was simply another disorder of local tissue iodine deficiency. Few others agreed. Those who disputed Marine's conclusion included Charles Mayo, Henry Plummer, and George Crile, all nationally known experts on the thyroid gland.

One would have thought that this concept would have come to a definite dead end. But it did not. It was, in fact, the stimulus for one of Marine's successes which was recognized at the time and then lost. He gave iodine to patients with Graves' disease in an attempt to replace their deficiency. Remarkably, he found that "as a rule, the symptoms become less marked." No one adopted this as a treatment for these patients because no one believed him. It took another decade for Henry Plummer to rediscover the phenomenon and make thyroid surgery safer as a result.

Marine continued to believe that the source of the iodine did not matter. He found that "commercial thyroid [is] often beneficial" in Graves' disease, a recommendation that hardly would have helped the patients clinically. And as one might expect, he did not use the term "hyperthyroidism" in his writings about Graves' disease.

Because Marine never thought of iodine deficiency as a global problem, he never measured iodine in the drinking water or in patients' or dogs' urine, even though the sensitivity of the available assays allowed these measurements. Marine did do an important clinical experiment though. He gave iodine to the schoolchildren of Cleveland hoping to cure, or even prevent, goiter. The city heartily disapproved of such a radical idea. The great thyroid surgeon E. Theodor Kocher had already stated that the worst thing a physician could do to a goitrous patient was to give iodine. That pronouncement was good enough for the physician advisor to the Cleveland School Committee. Marine later recalled that he then "made a hasty retreat and at once decided to go back to the laboratory and stay there." He was 29 years old and only 5 years out of medical school.

He continued in the laboratory and was one of the first to perfuse a thyroid gland in vitro. His purpose was to deal with the gland in isolation so that he could see what it would do if given iodine directly. He was able to show that the thyroid gland took up iodine from the perfusate and that, after a time, the tissue concentration of iodine was clearly higher than in the perfusate. He showed for the first time that one of the major functions of the thyroid gland was the concentration of iodine, which he did without the aid of radioiodine.

Marine's failure to get the Cleveland schools to allow him to give iodine to the students still rankled. He never asked the city of Cleveland to reconsider. He did, however, treat goitrous patients with iodine at the Lakeside Hospital Medical Dispensary. He must have mentioned the idea to medical students in his lectures. One day, a third-year medical student came to Marine to find out why the idea of giving iodine to children had not been carried out. Marine told him the story and the student, Oliver Perry Kimball, mentioned that he had taught school in Akron before coming to medical school. Perhaps Akron would be more receptive. They both went to Akron and met with school superintendent H.V. Hotchkiss, yet another Hopkins graduate. He thought it was a good idea and gave his approval.

It was 1917. World War I had been going on in Europe for 3 years, and the United States was about to be drawn into the conflict. In fact, the United States declared war two weeks before Hotchkiss approved the project. Marine went on active duty in the U.S. Army less than two months later. Kimball carried the ball. He went to Akron several times over the course of 1917, first to do a survey of schoolgirls (we would call it establishing a baseline), then to distribute small bottles of iodine to the schools, and later to repeat the survey to see what happened. Marine and Kimball did the first survey in April 1917, and Kimball did the follow-up survey in November of the same year. Meanwhile Marine was on active duty at Camp Custer, Michigan.

In April 1917, 50% of the 3872 girls examined had some thyroid enlargement and 7% had a moderate to marked degree of goiter. The peak seemed to occur in the early teen-age years. The girls were given a total of 2–4 g of sodium iodide over the course of 10 days. Either the teacher or the school principal gave each day's dose and recorded it on a card. The dose was to be repeated at six-month intervals. Some of the girls took the iodine and some did not, but there were no randomized controls in the modern sense. What determined whether or not a girl got iodine was whether or not the girl's parents agreed to the study. Those whose parents approved got it, and those whose parents did not approve did not. The results were striking: "not a single pupil in whom the thyroid was normal last year [April, 1917] and who took iodine, showed any enlargement, while of those not taking iodine, 26 percent showed definitely enlarged thyroids."

The study design would have appalled modern statisticians. There was no committee approval for the study, there was no committee. The parents made the decisions. Nothing was randomized and no one was blinded to either the treatment or the results. There was enormous potential for selection bias which was essentially ignored. There were no progress reports because at first there was no grant and no one to report to. Yet, somehow, a fourth-year medical student and a professor on active duty elsewhere in the military managed to carry out an important study. The results were clear-cut.

Marine became famous and moved to Montefiore Hospital in the Bronx where he spent the rest of his medical career. Kimball graduated from medical school and practiced general medicine. He spent much of his time trying to get salt manufacturers to put iodine in salt and to get the U.S. Congress to pass a law mandating iodized salt. The law never passed. To this day, salt in the United States need not be iodized. However, iodized salt is available and is widely used. Marine's and Kimball's work is not yet done. The challenge is no longer in the United States but in the many other parts of the world where iodine remains deficient in the diet. The Akron experiment has gone worldwide, fostered by the International Council for Control of Iodine Deficiency Disorders (ICCIDD). Their work will not be done until they put themselves out of business by seeing that all have enough iodine and that these preventable diseases are, like smallpox, banished from the human condition.

Sources

Harvey AM: David Marine: America's pioneer thyroidologist. *Am J Med* 1981; 70: 483.

Kimball OP: History of the prevention of endemic goitre. *Bull World Health Org* 1953; 9: 241.

Kimball OP, Marine D: The prevention of simple goiter. Second paper. *Arch Intern Med* 1918; 22: 41.

Marine D, Kimball OP: The prevention of simple goiter in man. A survey of the incidence and types of thyroid enlargements in the schoolgirls of Akron (Ohio), from the 5th to the 12th grades, inclusive – the plan of prevention proposed. *J Lab Clin Med* 1917; 3: 40.

Matovinovic J: David Marine (1880–1976): Nestor of thyroidology. *Persp Biol Med* 1978; 21: 565.

Rawson RW: David Marine. 1880–1978 (sic). *Trans Am Assoc Physicians* 1978; 41: 38.

This chapter has been reproduced from Sawin, Clark T: David Marine, iodine and goiter. *The Endocrinologist* 1996; 6(6): 423–6.

CHAPTER 67
George Washington Corner (1889–1981)
Progesterone

George Washington Corner was born in Baltimore, Maryland, on December 12, 1889. At the time of his birth, the family business, the shipping firm of James Corner and Sons, had been established for more than a century at the foot of Central Avenue on Corner's Wharf. Corner's father had not joined the family firm, but continued to live near the focus of family activities. The family was Methodist and teetotal; George was in his early 20s before he ever saw a stage play, and more than 30 before he sampled his first alcoholic beverage. He and his brother Harry grew up in a happy home. Corner went to public schools until he was 14 and then enrolled in the Baltimore Boys' Latin School. The curriculum was the traditional one and focused on Latin, English, and mathematics. Corner, however, had an interest in the natural sciences which he pursued on his own by reading the *National Geographic, Scientific American*, and *Johnson's Universal Encyclopedia*, all of which were in the family reading room.

In 1906 Corner was accepted at Johns Hopkins University. At the time, it was a small school of 750 students, of whom more than 600 were in the graduate schools. Still interested in the natural sciences, George obtained permission to drop Latin in his second year and substitute for it general biology and comparative anatomy. This was an important step. It revealed Corner's extraordinary abilities in the biological sciences and cast the initial seeds of his *oeuvre* to come.

Corner's growing interest in the sciences led to postgraduate study, and he opted for medical school. He entered the Johns Hopkins Medical School in 1909. He was a good student and enjoyed these years immensely. In particular, he enjoyed the adventure of the summer terms. One summer was spent in Freiburg attending the lectures of the famed German pathologist Ludwig Aschoff (Aschoff's node; the atrioventricular node) "Aschoff was a man evidently of intense energy, he had a military haircut and two deep scars from one corner of his mouth to the ear, relics of his student days in one of the aristocratic fraternities (*Korps*) that maintained the custom of dueling with swords" [1]. Two summers, 1912 and 1913, were spent in Labrador as a volunteer with the Grenfell Society at the Battle Harbor Hospital. It was there, in 1912, that

A Biographical History of Endocrinology, First Edition. D. Lynn Loriaux.

Corner met Betsy Copping of Acton, Massachusetts. She was the volunteer teacher for the summer term at the Battle Harbor Schoolhouse. This chance meeting led to courtship and a marriage that lasted for 60 years, ending with the death of Betsy at 85 years of age.

Corner graduated from Hopkins in 1913. Still attracted to the basic sciences, he spent the next year at Hopkins as an assistant in anatomy. His mentor, Dr. Franklin Mall, was the most distinguished morphological embryologist in the world. Other luminaries in the department included Florence Sabin, "whose fame as a teacher became all but legendary, (and) was well known for her work on the origin of blood cells" [2], and Herbert Evans, pioneer in the study of pituitary function. Corner served as a teaching assistant to Dr. Sabin's histology course and began his research career in the field of mammalian reproduction. Mall was interested in finding ways to date the age of embryos, and he believed that the histological appearance of the corpus luteum might serve as a marker of gestational age. Corner's project was to correlate the stages of embryonic development with the appearance of the corpus luteum under the microscope. Corner was able to define seven stages in the 115 days of porcine gestation (hence the title of Corner's later autobiography, *The Seven Ages of a Medical Scientist*), but was unable to correlate the appearance of the corpus luteum in the very early stages of development. Unfortunately, that period was Mall's primary interest in the project.

Corner spent the next year working as a house officer in the Department of Obstetrics and Gynecology at Hopkins. It was during this tumultuous year that he decided that the "call of laboratory was stronger than that of the clinic." In the throes of deciding how to act on this conclusion, he received a visit from Herbert Evans who had accepted a professorship in the Department of Anatomy at Berkeley. He invited Corner to join him in the move. The salary was $1500 per year. This generous remuneration would permit him, at last, to marry Betsy Copping, and the deal was struck.

Corner arrived in California in September of 1915. Evans and Philip Smith were well into work on pituitary function and both, in their separate ways, proved to be valuable collaborators and role models for Corner in his work on the reproductive cycle of the sow. Corner stayed in the Berkeley lab for 4 years and then moved back to the anatomy department at Hopkins and his beloved Baltimore. Work on the porcine reproductive cycle continued uninterrupted, however, and it was soon established that ovulation in the pig occurs on the second day of estrus, and that the corpus luteum is derived from both granulosa cells and the cells of the theca interna. A monograph on the subject in 1921 [3] brought the whole picture together for the first time:

> [I]mmature follicles up to five millimeters (1/3 inch) in diameter are always present in mature sows. At intervals of about twenty-one days, several follicles suddenly enlarge to a diameter of eight to ten millimeters. On the second day of estrus, they rupture and discharge their ova into the oviducts. On the fourth day after ovulation the ova reach the uterus where, if they are not fertilized by mating with a boar, they degenerate and disappear. I could find no ova later than six days after ovulation. Meanwhile the discharged follicles are converted into corpora lutea which, reaching full development about ten days after ovulation, put forth progesterone to condition the endometrium (uterus) to receive and nourish the embryos. The preparation for pregnancy is characterized by a great increase in complexity of the endometrial glands. I have

> called this changed state "progestational proliferation." As seen in women, gynecologists have named it the premenstrual stage. If the ova are not fertilized, the corpora lutea degenerate, beginning on about the fifteenth day. The endometrium, no longer supported by progesterone, reverts to its original state, and another estrous period soon sets in. If the ova are fertilized, however, the corpora lutea persist, maintaining the uterus until the end of the pregnancy.

Studies were extended to the rhesus monkey and it was shown that ovulation occurred on the 14th day of the menstrual cycle, with the remainder of the events much the same as detailed in the sow [4]. This description has served as the template for our understanding of the events of the reproductive cycle since its publication. Thus, Corner produced the first clear picture of the normal events of the reproductive cycle in mammals, probably his most important scientific contribution.

Corner was recruited as chairman of anatomy to the new medical school in Rochester, New York, in 1923. His research now focused on the active principle of the corpus luteum that had such powerful effects on the endometrium. What was its chemical nature and structure? Corner's problem at this juncture was akin to that faced by Banting in his search for the active principle of the pancreatic islet: he did not have the chemical background to permit substantive progress on the problem. Corner solved his problem in a way remarkably similar to the solution found by Banting: he turned to a first-year medical student for help [1].

> Willard Allen, a very likeable young man, was close at hand and ready to join me. That I chose a twenty-three year old first-year student for so important a venture may at first seem rash, but Bill had high qualifications, too. Born on a farm at Macedon, New York, twenty miles from Rochester, he won his B. S. degree at nearby Hobart College at Geneva, New York, in June 1926, and in September of that year enrolled in the second class that entered our new school of medicine. At Hobart, he was a star student, especially in chemistry. Once, on a written examination, he told me, he had earned a grade of 110 percent. The professor had included one question so difficult that he made it optional but promised a 10 percent bonus to any student who answered it correctly. Bill solved that hard one and also answered all the other questions accurately, so the professor had to rate his paper 110 percent. At Rochester in 1926–27 Allen led his class in Anatomy and Biochemistry. I had at my disposal a fellowship for him if he would drop out of his class for a year to assist us in teaching microscopic anatomy and collaborate with me in research. As willing as I to take a long chance, he became the first student at Rochester to receive such a fellowship, and we began work in October 1927 [1].

The approach to the problem was systematic and carefully planned. Sow ovaries were purchased from the slaughterhouse in 5 pound lots. Corner picked out all of the ovaries containing a corpus luteum. The rest were discarded. The corpora lutea were shelled out with a scalpel and minced. Corner then made an aqueous extract of the tissue and Allen followed with an ethanolic extract. The test of potency was the ability of the extract to induce proliferative change in rabbit endometrium. The alcoholic extract contained the active principle. The two investigators quickly showed that the extract could support pregnancy in rabbits castrated 18 hours after mating. The race was on to see who could first provide a chemical characterization of the material. It was Allen's task to purify the hormone. In the process, he learned that a chemist at Eastman-Kodak had a high-vacuum fractional distillation apparatus that could fractionate oils and waxes. He fractionated the extract into three parts, and found all of the activity in one. From that fraction he crystallized the material. He showed the crystals to Corner for the first time on May 5, 1933:

> "This is it," he said. "It's a steroid." We were almost too happy to talk [1].

Working with Oskar Wintersteiner at Columbia University in New York, the structure was deduced in the following year, 1934. Allen had achieved this *tour de force* in his spare time from the medical school curriculum and house officership in obstetrics and gynecology. As Corner put it, he worked "afternoons and weekends."

At the time, several biochemical discoveries had been patented with the rights of patent assigned to the university in whose laboratories the work had been done. Progesterone was not patented, and Corner stated: "The opinion at the University of Rochester, led by Dean George Whipple (with whom I agreed), was that discoveries useful in medicine, supported by academic funds, should not be commercially restricted, even for the benefit of the university" [1] – an enlightened position unfortunately much eroded in recent times.

Corner continued to study the physiologic effects of progesterone and clarified its role in menstruation and its role in lactation. From the latter studies came the most compelling evidence for the existence of a pituitary hormone affecting lactation, and Corner's studies were an important stimulus for the discovery and chemical isolation of prolactin.

As with most successful careers in science, Corner became more and more in demand as an administrator. He was appointed director of the Carnegie Institution in 1940 and, in 1960, at the age of 71, became the executive officer of the American Philosophical Society, a post he held for 16 years, handing it to his successor in his 88th year.

In this latter period of his life, Corner became a medical historian of some renown.

> Corner's historical publications in quality and number might easily satisfy a professional historian, bringing tenure, promotion, grants, and a reduced teaching load. They were, however, only a fraction of his total output of 15 books and more than 250 articles and reviews. There is no secret about his prodigious productivity. Corner rose early, even in his 80s. He wrote and read for several hours at home before coming to his office at 9 o'clock; he worked steadily, with great concentration, and he laid out in his mind the essential structure of his paragraphs and pages before putting pen to paper. He planned his projects, estimating what time they required, and he started nothing he could not see his way clear to complete. A few weeks after his death, a younger colleague and admirer inquired whether there might be some notes he might put in order, some uncompleted manuscript to prepare for the press out of friendship and respect. There was nothing of the sort. Corner completed everything he set out to do even to making the index to his autobiography and a list of those to whom copies were to be sent and left no loose ends [5].

This life of steady accomplishment and constructive effort was not without its moments of sorrow and occasional despair. Corner's wife of 60 years spent the last 10 years of her life in a state of senile dementia in a sanatorium where he visited her weekly until her death. They had two children. George Jr. graduated from Hopkins and did an internship and residency in obstetrics and gynecology there, following in his father's footsteps. Hester Ann completed all of the requirements for the PhD degree in English literature at Yale University. While writing her dissertation, she wrote to her father saying that:

> She was slightly ill and was entering the Yale infirmary. She thought that she might have monocytosis, a debilitating sickness that had recently been prevalent in New Haven.
>
> In my office ... the telephone rang and a man's voice said: "Dr. Corner, I am an intern at the Yale infirmary. Your daughter is a patient here. We think you ought to know that her leucocyte count is two hundred thousand." Appalled, I could only query, "Leukemia?" "Yes," he said gently. "You may want to take her home. She is strong enough to travel." I said that her mother and I would come to New Haven the next day and asked that the Yale Professor of Medicine Francis Blake be requested to see Hester Ann. Then I hung up and sat there in a daze, wondering how I could break the news to my wife.
>
> ... [T]he Hopkins specialist on leukemia, Dr. James Conley, came to our home and took blood samples, calling the next day to confirm the diagnosis of acute myelogenous leukemia. He suggested a stay in the hospital to try one of the new experimental drugs which had shown some power to stay the disease. At our daily visits we saw her rapidly fail and pass into a coma as the swarming leukocytes invaded her brain. Eleven days after that telephone call, as I walked into the ward where she lay, an intern came up to me to say that in the small hours of the morning she had ceased to breathe. I think that for me never a day has passed since then without a pang of sorrow for the loss of my daughter. As I grow older I feel more and more what I have lost. To have her with me in my old age, a mature experienced, understanding woman, what a blessing that would have been [1].

George Washington Corner died quietly in his home in the 91st year of his life.

References

1. Corner GW: *The Seven Ages of Medical Scientist; An Autobiography*. Philadelpia, PA: University of Pennsylvania Press, 1981.
2. Zukerman S: George Washington Corner. *Biogr Mem Fellows R Soc* 1983; 29: 93–112.
3. Corner GW: Cyclic changes in the ovaries and uterus of the sow, and their relation to the mechanism of implantation. *Contr Embryol* 1921; 13: 117–46.
4. Corner GW: The relation between menstruation and ovulation in the monkey: its possible significance for man. *J Am Med Assoc* 1927; 89: 1838–40.
5. Bell WJ: George W. Corner (1889–1981): Medical historian. *Bull Hist Med* 1982; 56: 93–103.

This chapter has been reproduced from Loriaux, D. Lynn: George Washington Corner 1889–1981. *The Endocrinologist* 1995; 5(2): 87–90.

CHAPTER 68
Henry H. Turner
(1892–1970)
Gonadal Dysgenesis

Henry Turner was born August 28, 1892, in Harrisburg, Illinois. He went to St. Louis University, and earned his MD degree from the University of Louisville School of Medicine in 1921. He became one of this country's leading clinical endocrinologists. He played a pivotal role in launching the *Journal of Clinical Endocrinology*. He was secretary-treasurer of the Endocrine Society for about 20 years and president of the Endocrine Society in 1968. Turner is primarily remembered for his landmark article in 1938, describing infantilism, webbed neck, and cubitus valgus.

Turner's classic article, entitled "A syndrome of infantilism, congenital webbed neck, and cubitus valgus," appeared in *Endocrinology* in 1938 [1]. Although he referred to prior reports of short neck (as described by Klippel and Feil [2]), he differentiated his patients on the basis of webbing of the neck and lack of fusion or limitation of motion of the cervical spine.

He did, however, note a report by Funke in 1902 of a 15-year-old girl with a height of 132 cm, sexual infantilism, and webbing of the neck [3]. She also had congenital lymphedema of the hands and feet, low-set and posteriorly displaced ears, hypoplasia of the nipples, ptosis, micrognathia, and a high-arched palate. Although she had no evidence of cubitus valgus or other skeletal deformities, she otherwise closely resembled the seven cases reported by Turner 36 years later. She could, as suggested by Wiedemann and Glatzl, be considered the first illustrated case report of this condition [4].

In fact, it is likely that the syndrome described by Turner had been identified several times before his report. In 1768, Giovanni Battista Morgagni [5], according to two referenced sources, credited by some with being the father of the scientific theory of medicine, described an autopsy of a small woman, "yet much larger than to be classed with the species of dwarfs," who had died of peritonitis in her mid-fifties. Autopsy revealed renal malformations, an extremely small uterus, and no identifiable gonadal tissue. Although this description might also fit a diagnosis of hypopituitarism, the failure of a skilled anatomist, such as Morgagni, to identify any gonadal tissue is more consistent with the diagnosis of gonadal dysgenesis: "I looked upon the upper

A Biographical History of Endocrinology, First Edition. D. Lynn Loriaux.

This work is a co-publication between the Endocrine Society and John Wiley & Sons, Ltd.

edges of these ligaments, to see what kind of testes (gonads) this woman had been furnished with; but I looked to no purpose ... . I very clearly perceived that she had never had any testes, nor even the most obscure beginning of them."

Morgagni's description was largely ignored for the next 150 years. In 1883, Kobylinski [6] described a patient with webbing of the neck, but this individual was a phenotypic male. Both Turner and Ullrich subsequently cited Kobylinski's case (possibly Noonan syndrome), thereby ushering in decades of confusion about terminology for such cases. Funke's illustrated report is a more convincing case of gonadal dysgenesis [2, 3]. The patient was a 15-year-old phenotypic female, with a history of normal intrauterine growth. She had congenital lymphedema of the hands and feet. She was noted at birth to have redundant skinfolds at the back of the neck which, over time, evolved into lateral webbing, which Funke termed "pterygium colli." Other features consistent with a diagnosis of classical gonadal dysgenesis included short stature (135 cm), absence of secondary sexual characteristics, low-set and posteriorly angulated ears, hypoplasia of the nipples, and a narrow, high-arched palate [3, 7].

The Russian literature also includes an early report [8] of apparent gonadal dysgenesis, with many of the classical phenotypic features, including an adult height of 132 cm [8], which led to the occasional use of the term, "Seresevskij syndrome," or "Seresevskij–Turner syndrome" [9]. In the 1940s, Seresevskij subsequently reported five additional cases, all of which are consistent with a diagnosis of gonadal dysgenesis [10].

It was left to Ullrich [11] to provide a definitive description of gonadal dysgenesis. His first report of an 8-year-old girl was made on December 12, 1929, at a meeting of the Munich Pediatric Society. It was published with illustrations in 1930, 8 years before Turner's initial article. The patient was the 2850 g product of a normal pregnancy, but was noted at birth to have pitting lymphedema and severe redundancy of the skin of the posterior neck. This did not begin to resolve until 2 years of age. At 8 years of age, her height was 9 cm below average. Additional features included pronounced webbing of the neck bilaterally, ptosis, micrognathia with an anterior cervical web, a high, narrow palate, low-set years, low posterior hairline, and hypoplastic, inverted nipples. She was studied again in 1987 at the age of 66 years [4]. She had a graduate degree in chemistry and worked as an industrial chemist. She had never entered puberty and had received no hormonal therapy. Her adult height was 144.5 cm. Cytogenetic analysis of peripheral lymphocytes revealed a 45 X karyotype.

In his 1930 publication concerning this patient, Ullrich cited the reports of Funke and Kobylinski, the former almost certainly representing a classical case of gonadal dysgenesis. Ullrich, however, has the first report of a case supported by karyotypic analysis, even if performed almost 60 years after the initial publication.

Henry Turner was an internist in Oklahoma City, specializing in "internal secretions." Much of his scientific productivity concerned thyroid and testosterone replacement therapy. He went on to establish, in the 1950s, one of the first radioisotope laboratories in the United States. For over 20 years, he was secretary/treasurer of the Endocrine Society, and eventually became its president in 1968.

It is for his 1938 publication, "A syndrome of infantilism, congenital webbed neck, and cubitus valgus" [1], however, that Turner will be remembered. A non-pediatrician (unlike Ullrich), he did not even mention short stature in the title, although the growth abnormalities are amply discussed in the article itself. He described seven patients, who ranged in age from 15 to 23 years. A footnote to the text briefly mentions three additional cases observed between the writing and the publication of the manuscript. This multiplicity of cases added greatly to the definition of the clinical syndrome. In addition to the characteristic phenotypic features, Turner emphasized the lack of sexual development and the ovarian dysgenesis. Turner was probably the first to treat such patients with exogenous sex steroids, ushering in estrogen replacement for gonadal dysgenesis. Sex steroid replacement represented a major breakthrough and was the first therapy directed at normalizing endocrine function in affected women. In subsequent publications, Turner emphasized the clinical differences between gonadal dysgenesis and pituitary dwarfism and stressed the importance of primary gonadal failure.

There is one aspect of gonadal dysgenesis in which Turner's precedence goes unquestioned: he was the first to employ growth hormone therapy. In his 1938 article, he writes: "Treatment with pituitary growth hormones has been unsatisfactory."

Ultimately we are left with the question of which eponym to attach to this syndrome. Funke appears to have the first modern description, amply illustrated and cited by both Ullrich and Turner. Seresevskij appears to have identified several cases with classical features. Ullrich's description is beautifully detailed and had the advantage of 60-year follow-up and karyotypic confirmation. Turner described multiple cases and properly emphasized the importance of primary gonadal failure. Ultimately, it is Morgagni, with his description of a small woman with no visible gonadal tissue, who probably deserves credit for first describing this syndrome.

It seems unlikely, however, that the eponyms of Turner syndrome in the United States and Ullrich syndrome in Europe will be easily replaced. A better alternative might well be to progress beyond eponyms, and describe cases pathophysiologically: gonadal dysgenesis associated with an abnormal sex chromosome.

References

1. Turner HH: A syndrome of infantilism, congenital webbed neck, and cubitus valgus. *Endocrinology* 1938; 23: 566–74.
2. Klippel M, Feil A: Un cas d'absence des vertébres cervi- cales avec cage thoracique remontant jusqu à la base du crâne *Nouv Iconogr Salpétrière* 1912; 25: 223–4.
3. Funke O: Pterygium colli. *Dtsch Z Chir* 1902; 63: 162–7.
4. Wiedemann HR, Glatzl J: Follow-up of Ullrich's original patient with "Ullrich-Turner syndrome." *Am J Med Genet* 1991; 41: 134–6.
5. Morgagni GB: *Epistula anatomica medic* 1768; XLVI: Art 20.
6. Kobylinski O: Ueber eine Flughautahnliche Ausbreitung am Halse. *Arch Anthropol* 1883; 14: 343–8.
7. Opitz JM, Pallister PD: Brief historical note: the concept "gonadal dysgenesis." *Am J Med Genet* 1979; 4: 333–43.
8. Seresevskij NA: In relation to the question of a connection between congenital abnormalities and endocrinopathies. The Russian Endocrinological Society, November 12, 1925.

9. Lonberg NC, Neilsen J: Seresevskij-Turner's syndrome or Turner's syndrome. *Hum Genet* 1977; 38: 363–4.
10. Seresevskij NA: *Annu Rev Soviet Med* 1944; 1: 337–9.
11. Ullrich O: Uber typische Kombinatiosbilder multiplier Abartungen. *Z Kinderheilk* 1930; 49: 271–6.

This chapter has been reproduced from Rosenfeld, Ron: Morgagni, Ullrich, and Turner: The discovery of gonadal dysgenesis. *The Endocrinologist* 1995; 5(5): 327–8.

CHAPTER 69

Ernest Basil Verney (1894–1967)

Vasopressin is a Hormone

Until the 1670s, patients with diabetes could have the potential diagnosis of diabetes mellitus confirmed with a urine "taste-test." Patients with voluminous urine flow simply provided a sample, and the diagnosing physician tasted it. A sweet taste meant diabetes mellitus. But a few patients had polyuria without a sweet-tasting urine; their urine was tasteless, the far less common "diabetes insipidus." Diabetes insipidus was distinguished from diabetes mellitus in 1674 by the English physician Thomas Willis. What might be the specific cause of diabetes insipidus was not thoroughly resolved until the early twentieth century.

The first physiologic work that showed a biologic action of the pituitary gland was done in 1894. Edward Schafer, England's premier physiologist found, almost by accident, that a crude extract of the whole gland raised the blood pressure. A bit later, others found that this hypertensive effect was localized to the posterior portion of the pituitary gland. In the course of the next decade or two, other biologic effects of crude posterior pituitary extract were uncovered, such as effects on stimulating uterine contraction and milk ejection.

In 1901, Schafer studied the effect of posterior pituitary extract on the kidney, particularly on urine flow. The result was clear-cut: posterior pituitary extract increased urine flow. It was in fact a diuretic. Schafer's prestige in his field was so high that this diuretic action was taken as a given for the next two decades. In the late 1910s and early 1920s, for example, major endocrine and physiology texts noted this diuretic action and speculated that the cause of diabetes insipidus was an "irritation" or injury of the posterior pituitary with the resulting excessive release of the diuretic substance. This physiologic idea was powerful enough to override the clinical observation that injections of posterior pituitary extract, already in wide clinical use, reduced urine volume in patients with diabetes insipidus, an effect that physiologically minded authors thought "somewhat paradoxical" and "still awaits explanation." This beneficial effect could be written off as an example of a pharmacologic effect of a tissue extract that had no necessary relationship to a true endocrine function.

A Biographical History of Endocrinology, First Edition. D. Lynn Loriaux.

This work is a co-publication between the Endocrine Society and John Wiley & Sons, Ltd.

Thus was the level of knowledge or, better, of confusion when Ernest Basil Verney, "Basil" to his colleagues, decided on an academic career in experimental medicine rather than on clinical practice. A farmer's son, Verney had both a classical and scientific education, unusual in middle-class England at the time. Though not particularly good at chemistry, he did quite well at Cambridge and won a scholarship to complete his medical education at St. Bartholomew's Hospital in London. Once qualified as a practitioner, he joined the British Army, then still fighting World War I, as a Medical Officer in 1918. After the war, he finished his clinical training and was in practice for several months in 1921. When he experienced having two boys die in renal failure, he decided that he would try for an academic career and investigate diseases of renal function.

In the summer of 1921, Verney sought out Ernest H. Starling, professor of physiology at University College London (UCL), to discuss his aims. Starling was impressed enough to offer him a position on the spot at the princely salary of £200 per year (the British pound was worth much more then than now but the salary was still not much to live on). He immediately began work on the kidney with his main tool being the heart–lung–kidney preparation derived from Starling's earlier studies. Over the course of his 3 years with Starling, Verney published two major papers on the regulation of urine volume in this preparation. He was able to show that the blood pressure and the composition of the blood (e.g., the nature of the solutes and the amount of protein) were the principal determinants of urine flow. As an aside, he noted that the urine formed by this isolated preparation could maintain a fairly high flow rate over several hours and was always hypotonic. He thought this last finding might be due to acidosis.

By 1925, Verney had completed a long series of experiments with Starling. Most were examinations of glomerular and tubular function. He showed, for example, that the tubules probably resorbed water, chloride, and glucose, and probably secreted urea, sulfate, and phenol red. More to our interest here, he attacked directly the problem of why the isolated kidney secreted a hypotonic urine. Starling's textbook said that posterior pituitary extract induced diuresis. However, both Starling and Verney knew of the apparently contradictory antidiuretic effect of this extract when given to patients with diabetes insipidus. The key experiment was to inject pituitrin, the name now given to the posterior pituitary extract, into the blood perfusing the isolated kidney. Their results were clear: pituitrin caused a rapid fall in urinary flow and a parallel rise in urinary solute concentration. Further, and perhaps equally important, the antidiuretic effect could occur with no change in blood flow or perfusion pressure, which meant that the antidiuresis was a specific and separate effect of the pituitrin and unrelated to vasopressor effect. The action was thus renal and not vascular.

The cause of the prior observation of the diuretic effect was not clear to them although they speculated that it might have been due to the vascular effect of pituitrin. Others later thought the diuretic effect might have been due to the anesthesia used in the intact animals. Verney's data showed that the effect was directly on the kidney and not secondary to pituitrin's actions elsewhere in the body. They concluded that the original problem they faced, the hypotonic urine of the isolated kidney preparation, was almost certainly due to the absence of an antidiuretic substance.

But is an effect of an exogenous substance enough reason to say that the active substance is an endogenous hormone? Verney thought not. There were enough instances of effects of tissue extracts that did not, in fact, reflect an endogenous physiologic function. The "diuretic" effect of pituitrin itself was an example. In his 1925 paper, he did think that a true antidiuretic hormone from somewhere in the body was a likely possibility. He also raised the opposite question: how does water load generate a rapid diuresis? Could it be by stimulating the release of a hormone that blocks the action of pituitrin? Or perhaps "some slight blood change ... inhibits the formation of the pituitrin-like hormones." Prescient words, indeed.

Verney had held research fellowships of one sort or another from 1921 to 1923. In 1924 he was also appointed to be an assistant in medicine at University College Hospital with a few clinical duties. His work, however, had so impressed his colleagues that in 1926 he was named to, and accepted, the chair in pharmacology at University College London, recently vacated by A.J. Clark. Now, for a few months, he was a fellow professor with his mentor, Starling, who died later that year.

In his last year or so as a fellow and just before assuming his professorship, Verney completed work on his next question: was pituitrin, or something like it, secreted in vivo? He now used an elaborate variation on the isolated perfused kidney that involved an isolated perfused heart, and a dog preparation that allowed blood flow from the head (or other parts) to flow into the renal perfusate. In essence, Verney used the perfused kidney not to study its function but as a bioassay. The results were clear-cut: blood from the head inhibited urinary flow while blood from the pelvis or lower legs did not. Further, blood from the head lost its power if the pituitary were removed during the course of an experiment. Verney concluded that "an antidiuretic ... principle or principles are contributed by the pituitary body to blood."

Verney was now reasonably fixed on the main research work of his life and was widely recognized for the clarity and quality of his work and for the way it answered important physiologic and clinical questions. He next addressed another confusing issue of posterior pituitary function, this time without such clear success. The proximate cause of diabetes insipidus was by now agreed to be a lack of pituitrin or the antidiuretic substance pituitrin contained; it was a hormonal deficiency. But what caused the deficiency? One thought was that it was due to a lesion of the posterior pituitary gland. The problem was that removal of this gland did not always cause the disorder. Other data pointed to the hypothalamus as the site of lesions that could cause the disease, so was it a pituitary problem or a hypothalamic one? Verney gave the Goulstonian Lectures to the Royal College of Physicians in 1929 (these are usually given by the most recently elected member of the College and are considered a high honor) on the topic of polyuria. With the physiologic techniques then available, it was probably not possible to decide between the two; Verney leaned toward the pituitary hypothesis which we now know is usually incorrect.

A hard and conscientious worker, Verney often worked into the late hours. His experiments were all thought out in advance and done with precision and great surgical skill (few, for example, could consistently exteriorize the renal artery in vivo). In the early 1930s, his health failed, perhaps as a result of overwork. He nevertheless returned to an earlier problem in water balance, namely, the reason why a water load induces a clear diuresis. He reasoned in 1933 that the endogenous antidiuretic hormone must be shut off in some way but wanted to figure out where this occurred. One possibility was that a rise in the water concentration of the blood ("dilution") acted directly on the posterior pituitary gland. Another idea, the one he preferred, was that the higher water concentration acted somewhere in the nervous system, which in turn caused the hormonal secretion to shut off. If the latter were so, there had to be a neural receptor to bring about the effect, an "osmoreceptor." Some thought that other nerves, such as renal nerves, could be the mediator while others postulated an intestinal hormone as the intermediate cause. Again, Verney was unable to provide iron-clad proof, at least to his own critical satisfaction, that he was right. This was the direction for further study.

Perhaps because of his illness, Verney resigned his chair at UCL in 1934 and moved to Cambridge, his old haunts, as an associate professor of pharmacology and remained such until promoted to the chair of that department in 1946, a position he held until his partial retirement in 1961. He continued to gain recognition, however, and was elected as Fellow of the Royal Society in 1936.

In the 1930s and 1940s he continued with the problem of the osmoreceptors. He did experiment after experiment in an attempt to locate precisely where in the brain these receptors were. The pace was slow. The controls he needed were many and difficult to create in the experimental animal. His idea was that they were somewhere in the brain but to locate them one needed to control blood flow to many different brain loci and, furthermore, to isolate a large number of specific brain areas in the attempt to locate the postulated receptors as specifically as possible. It is also important to note that the only way to assay for the antidiuretic hormone was by bioassay (in Verney's case, in the intact animal) and that modern neurosurgical techniques simply did not exist. In 1942, he studied the effects of stress on the hormone's release to further the idea that the central nervous system was part of the process. One method was to have a dog chase a ball on the roof of the physiology building and then study the animal. He later employed an indoor treadmill which gave the same results and avoided the rain that so commonly interrupted his studies. By the time of his Sharpey-Schafer lectures in 1945, he was able to show that hypertonic solutions injected directly into the carotid artery caused a rapid fall in urine flow; the effect had to act somewhere in the brain. He was now quite comfortable in considering a water diuresis the equivalent of a functional diabetes insipidus.

But where were the osmoreceptors? Verney continued with more experiments. Finally, in 1957, he published an enormous paper, 130 pages long, that summarized his work on the problem over 14 years (few funding agencies today would tolerate this "lack of productivity"). This was his masterwork on antidiuretic hormone. His conclusion was one that we today accept without thinking as it appears so obvious. But it now appears obvious in large part because of Verney's work. The osmoreceptor does in fact exist. It is located in the hypothalamus, probably, in the anterior or preoptic areas. Connections with the paraventricular and supraoptic nuclei must be intact in order for the hormone to be released. Thus, Verney's conclusions have held true, a reflection of the careful, conscientious, and unrushed method that he insisted on.

Verney did occasionally touch on other areas of endocrinology. In the 1930s, for example, he did several studies on the neural control of ovulation mediated by the anterior pituitary gland, similar to experiments that started Geoffrey Harris on his path to the elucidation of major areas of the neuroendocrinology of anterior pituitary hormones. In 1961, at the age of 67 years and just before his retirement from his Cambridge chair, he turned to the isolated, but in vivo, perfused dog adrenal gland. He showed that the changes in cortisol secretion were almost entirely due to secreted ACTH. He did this by removing the pituitary gland in the course of the experiment. He also showed that the effects of ACTH are directly on the gland and not due to changes in blood flow to the gland. He still remains best known as the definer of the hormonal control of water balance.

Those who do not know of Verney's work might well be forgiven for this omission, for his studies were so fundamental as to become the fabric of our knowledge. Did we not always know this? No. Did someone really have to determine that these facts were so? Yes, and we are in Verney's debt.

Sources

Daly IdeB, Pickford LM: Ernext Basil Verney, 1894–1967. *Biogr Mem Fellows R Soc* 1980; 16: 523.

Frank E: Ueber Beziehungen der Hypophyse zum Diabetes insipidus. *Klin Wochenschr* 1912; 49: 393. [Frank was the first to associate the posterior pituitary gland with the presence of diabetes insipidus.]

Greenway CV, Verney EB: The effect of tadrenocorticotrophic hormone on the secretion of corticosteroids by the isolated perfused adrenal gland of the dog. *J Physiol* 1962; 162: 183.

Jewell PA, Verney EB: An experimental attempt to determine the site of the neurohypophysical osmoreceptors in the dog. *Phil Trans Roy Soc Lond* 1957; 240: 197.

Kivela T, Pelkonen R, Oja M, et al.: Diabetes insipidus and blindness caused by a suprasellar tumor. Pieter Pauw's observations from the 16th century. *J Am Med Assoc* 1998; 279: 48.

Klisiecki A, Pickford M, Rothschild P, Verney EB: The absorption and excretion of water by the mammal. Part II. Factors influencing the response of the kidney to water ingestion. *Proc Roy Soc Lond B* 1933; 112: 521.

O'Connor WJ, Verney EB: The effect of the removal of the posterior lobe of the pituitary on the inhibition of water-diuresis by emotional stress. *Quart J Physiol* 1942; 3: 393.

Sawyer WH: A short history of neurohypophysical research. *Ann NY Acad Sci* 1993; 689: 1.

Verney EB: The secretion of pituitrin in mammals, as shown by perfusion of the isolated kidney of the dog. *Proc Roy Soc Lond B* 1926; 99: 487.

Verney EB: Polyuria. *Lancet* 1929; 1: 539, 645, 751.

Verney EB: Absorption and excretion of water. The antidiuretic hormone. *Lancet* 1946; 2: 739, 781.

Verney EB, Starling EH: On secretion by the isolated kidney. *J Physiol* 1922; 56: 353.

Von den Velden R: Die Nierenwirkung von Hypophysenextrakten deim Menshen. *Klin Wochenschr* 1913; 50: 2083. [The first use of posterior pituitary extract to treat diabetes insipidus.]

This chapter has been reproduced from Sawin, Clark T: Vasopressin is a hormone: The work of Ernest Basil Verney (1894–1967). *The Endocrinologist* 2000; 10(2): 79–82.

CHAPTER 70

Gerty and Carl Cori (1896–1957) (1896–1984)

Glucose Metabolism and Lactic Acid

Arthur Kornberg, a senior biochemist who shared the Nobel Prize for Physiology or Medicine in 1959, said of Carl F. Cori that, "I didn't know that I'd ever match Cori in his intellectual breadth and capacity, and, maybe, I haven't" and of Cori's wife, Gerty that "Gerty liked me and helped me. She was a most remarkable scientist and woman" [1]. Kornberg also noted that "in the later years Cori mellowed a lot."

Carl Cori was born in Prague near the end of the nineteenth century when it was in the Austro-Hungarian empire. His father, also named Carl, earned both an MD and a PhD in zoology but did not practice medicine. He became a lecturer at Prague's Zoological Institute. When the young Carl was only 2 years old, the senior Carl was appointed director of the Marine Biologic Station in Trieste. Young Carl grew up in Trieste. His high school education was a mix of classic Greek and Latin and some science. He was not a particularly good student but did well on final examinations. The summer he finished school, he went on a marine expedition to the Adriatic. While he was at sea, the First World War broke out. In 1914, he decided to go to medical school and enrolled at the Carl Ferdinand University in Prague. Rather than follow the usual custom of attending several universities in the course of his medical curriculum, he took all of his courses in Prague, largely because of the War. There he met and "dated" a fellow medical student who was a few months older than him [2].

In his third year of medical school, he was drafted into the Austrian army and assigned to the ski troops. Having nearly been killed in action, he transferred shortly afterward to a bacteriologic laboratory in the army's sanitary corps, but contracted typhoid fever and took some time to recover. When clinically better, his chief thought he was reporting too many cases of typhoid so he sent Cori to set up a bacteriologic laboratory in the Trieste Marine Station. Cori managed to survive the war, although at one point had to stay for several days on the roof of a freight car during the sudden dissolution of the Austrian Army at the end of the war. He returned to medical school in 1918, completed his studies in 1920, and went to Vienna for postgraduate work in

A Biographical History of Endocrinology, First Edition. D. Lynn Loriaux.

This work is a co-publication between the Endocrine Society and John Wiley & Sons, Ltd.

internal medicine and pharmacology. That summer (1920) he married the woman he had dated before the war, Gerty Radnitz.

Gerty had remained in Carl's medical school class and she, too, had received her MD in 1920. In Vienna, she studied pediatrics and took, as one of her research projects, the control of temperature in patients and rabbits with hypothyroidism. In his pharmacology work, Carl was able to publish a paper on the effects of epinephrine and vagal stimulation on the cardiac sinus node using frogs sent to him by his father. Times were hard in Eastern Europe and in Vienna in 1920–1921 with the complete collapse of the Austro-Hungarian Empire and the formation of entirely new countries. Food was scarce. The one free meal a day that the Coris got at Carl's clinic was the only payment they received. Nutrition was poor; Gerty got xerophthalmia, which was cured only by her temporary return to Prague. Carl's superior in the Viennese clinic was "strongly anti-Semitic," which reflected the Austrian tone of the time; Carl spent a few months in Graz, but had to "prove his Aryan descent" to get the appointment. Prospects for a permanent job in research were slim, not only because of the economic conditions, but because of the anti-Semitism. Gerty was of Jewish ancestry [3].

Things looked up a bit in the summer of 1921 when Harvey Gaylord came to Europe to interview candidates for a clinical biochemistry position at Buffalo State Institute for the Study of Malignant Disease, later the Roswell Park Memorial Institute. Gaylord was the director of the institute. His background included a monograph on thyroid carcinoma in trout, wherein he mistook thyroid hyperplasia for cancer [4] and stated his firm belief that parasites were the cause of cancer. Gaylord was interviewing Austrians because he thought they would be more acceptable in the United States than Germans. Cori was interviewed twice, once in a moving automobile and once in his laboratory while performing urinalyses [5]. He thought nothing would come of it but, in fact, he was offered the position, accepted it, and moved to Buffalo in 1922. Gerty followed six months later.

Carl's new position was not precisely defined. He needed to do routine clinical laboratory work, but once that was done he could do whatever he wanted. During the few months he had spent in Graz, he had decided to study how glucose was handled in the mammalian body, probably influenced by the discovery of insulin in 1921–1922.

The first year at Buffalo, the Coris were studying carbohydrate absorption and metabolism, and began to assess the effects of epinephrine and insulin on glucose metabolism. They also learned and developed several micromethods that were new at the time and quantitative enough to provide accurate measurements of tissue glucose and glycogen. The home institution was there to study cancer and, in fact, the Coris began the study of lactate production.

With accurate measurements of glycogen now possible, they showed that epinephrine decreased muscle glycogen, raised the blood lactate level and induced, at the same time, a modest increase in the level of liver glycogen. They already knew that the breakdown of muscle glycogen did not raise blood glucose, so there had to be another mechanism by which a decrease in muscle glycogen led to a rise in the glycogen in the liver. They discovered that the blood lactate produced by muscle was reformed into glycogen. They showed that half or more of the lactate from muscle was converted to hepatic glycogen. This was a remarkable set of findings. The Coris called it the "cycle of carbohydrates," wherein muscle glycogen breaks down, raises the blood lactate level, which is then converted to liver glycogen, which breaks down and is released into the blood as glucose, part of which in turn appears in the muscle as glycogen, thus completing the "cycle." Others called it "the Cori cycle" and as a result the Coris became famous in the world of biochemistry [6].

The Coris stayed in Buffalo for 9 years, during which time they both became naturalized U.S. citizens. They were increasingly concerned that their work was not in line with the primary mission of the Institute – cancer – and began to think of moving elsewhere. They had then published more than 90 papers: 80 by Carl, 50 of which were with Gerty, and 11 others by Gerty alone.

In 1931, the chairman of the Department of Pharmacology at Washington University School of Medicine in St. Louis, Herbert Gasser, left for Cornell. Carl was asked to replace him (Gasser shared the Nobel Prize in Physiology or Medicine in 1944 for his work in neurophysiology). Cori accepted the position in St. Louis.

The move to a university medical school from a state-funded institute resulted in Gerty receiving only a token salary as a research associate. Nevertheless, she accepted the change and their work continued.

The main direction they set was to build on another of their findings in Buffalo. They showed that when epinephrine broke down muscle glycogen to lactate, there was a marked increase in the muscle content of hexose monophosphate (HMP). This was associated with a clear decrease in the muscle content of inorganic phosphate. The change in HMP could account for the decrease in muscle glycogen that was not accounted for by the release of lactate. They also showed that the process was reversible: the HMP could go back to glycogen without first being converted to lactate. They knew that glycogen breakdown led to the production of a hexose phosphate (i.e., a phosphate residue esterified with a hexose). One such hexose phosphate was glucose-6-phosphate (G-6-P) (i.e., one with the phosphate attached to the 6 position on the glucose molecule). They had other evidence, however, that there was an "intermediate" between glycogen and G-6-P.

By the mid-1930s they had done a good deal of work to isolate this purported intermediate, but the work led nowhere and they were about to give up. Cori attributed what happened next to luck. They found that the intermediate was glucose with a phosphate attached to a different position on the glucose molecule. It was glucose-1-phosphate (G-1-P). Thus, glycogen breakdown involved direct phosphorylation so that a terminal glucose residue in the glycogen chain had a phosphate added which, in turn, resulted in the release of the G-1-P. Further work led to the isolation and crystallization of the enzyme responsible, which was named phosphorylase. Another enzyme, a phosphomutase, converts the G-1-P to G-6-P and other enzymes change the G-6-P to lactate. Almost exactly the same mechanism occurs in the liver when glycogen breaks down. The difference is that the G-6-P loses its phosphate and the glucose enters the blood stream, thus maintaining the blood glucose level. The G-1-P was later named the "Cori ester" and was a critical finding in unravelling carbohydrate metabolism.

By now it was clear that enzymes were the key to further understanding how carbohydrates are metabolized. The Coris' laboratory became a mecca for enzymology. Cori believed that hormones act by changing enzyme activity in some way. This is true in the general sense but hormones, as we now know, do not act directly on these enzymes, but rather through sets of more complicated mechanisms often involving the cell membrane. Carl strongly believed, for example, that insulin directly stimulated the hexokinase reaction (i.e., the initial step in glucose metabolism by the liver in which blood glucose is itself phosphorylated to G-6-P before being used) [7].

Carl switched from pharmacology to the chairmanship of biochemistry. He remained in that position until his retirement in 1966 at age 70 years. Just a few months before they were presented the Nobel Prize, Gerty learned that the weakness and fatigue she had complained of for several months was caused by an incurable form of anemia (myelofibrosis). With the help of frequent transfusions, she lived and worked for another 10 years, dying in 1957. It took a Nobel Prize for her to gain a professorship in 1947. During the last decade of her life, she was the driving force behind the elucidation of the causes of several of the glycogen-storage diseases, showing that specific molecular–enzymatic defects were the culprits.

One mark of the quality of the Coris' laboratory is that six colleagues, in addition to the Coris themselves, won the Nobel Prize: Severo Ochoa and Arthur Kornberg in 1959, Luis Leloir in 1970, Earl Sutherland in 1974, Christian de Duve in 1974, and Edwin Krebs in 1992.

After Carl retired from Washington University, he and his second wife Anne moved to Boston, where he had a laboratory at the Massachusetts General Hospital and an appointment as visiting professor at Harvard. He continued to publish until the year before his death in 1984 at age 87 years.

No student of their lives, including those who worked closely with the Coris, has been able to decide which of the two was the intellectual leader. Likely that is because it was truly a shared lifetime in science and because neither was actually more important than the other. The question is, in any case, irrelevant. One expert noted that "very little was known of carbohydrate metabolism or its regulation when the Coris began their work and they were true pioneers" [8]; and so it was.

References

1. Hargittai I: *The Road to Stockholm. Nobel Prizes, Science, and Scientists.* New York: Oxford University Press, 2002, p. 163.
2. *Nobel Lectures including Presentation Speeches and Laureates' Biographies. Physiology or Medicine.* Amsterdam: Elsevier, 1964, p. 186.
3. *Nobel Lectures including Presentation Speeches and Laureates' Biographies. Physiology or Medicine.* Amsterdam: Elsevier, 1964, p. 184.
4. Gaylord HR, Marsh MC: *Carcinoma of the Thyroid in the Salmonid Fishes.* Washington, DC: U.S. Government Printing Office, 1914.
5. Cori CF: The call of science. *Annu Rev Biochem* 1969; 38: 1.

6. Kornberg A: Remembering our teachers. *J Biol Chem* 2001; 276: 3.
7. Cori CF, Sutherland EW, Cohn M, et al.: Purification of the hyperglycemic-glycogenolytic factor from insulin and from gastric mucosa. *J Biol Chem.* 1949; 180: 825.
8. Randle P: Carl Ferdinand Cori. 3 December 1896–20 October 1984. *Biogr Mem Fellows R Soc* 1986; 32: 67.

Sources

Larner J: Gerty Theresa Cori. August 8, 1896–October 26, 1957. *Biogr Mem Natl Acad Sci* 1992; 61: 111.
Lipmann F: Carl Ferdinand Cori, 1896–1984. *Bioessays* 1985; 2: 231.
Ochoa S: Carl Ferdinand Cori. 1896–1984. *Trends Biochem Sci* 1985; 10: 147.

This chapter has been reproduced from Sawin, Clark T: Gerty and Carl Cori and how the liver raises the blood glucose. *The Endocrinologist* 2003; 13(6): 441–4.

CHAPTER 71
Charles Robert Harington (1897–1972)
Synthesis of Thyroxine

In 1926, Charles Robert Harington solved a longstanding problem in biochemistry by synthesizing the principle thyroid hormone, thyroxine, for the first time. His paper, published in the following year, is a classic in endocrinology not so much for its immediate impact on therapy but rather because it showed that an imaginative, planned attack on a hormonal problem is more likely to bear fruit than a less soundly based, "shotgun" approach.

Harington was descended from a long line of English landed gentry with ancestors traceable to the twelfth century. Sir John Harington, a godson of Queen Elizabeth I and probably a collateral ancestor, was the only scientifically inclined member of the family. He invented the flush toilet and probably qualifies as an applied scientist. Charles Harington's father was a younger son. In England, that meant that he became a clergyman instead of inheriting the lands. The father was serving as a vicar in North Wales when the son, Charles, was born on August 1, 1897. At age 4, his family moved to Herefordshire, where he was raised. Many of his childhood years were spent at home because of tuberculosis of the hip that he contracted at age 10. The result was complete immobilization for 4 years, and another year or so of walking with crutches. The young man survived and adapted, returning to school in 1914. He was left with a permanent and severe limp. While this prevented him from playing in team sports or from serving in World War I, the disability did not stop him from taking long walks in the moors or fishing for trout in mountain streams. It certainly did not affect his mind.

In 1916 Harington went to the University of Cambridge, Magdalene College, after winning a prize in mathematics. His intent was to become an engineer. However, he was told to change and avoid any career requiring physical ability. After 3 years, he got a first class grade in Part 1 of the Natural Sciences Tripos (an honors examination peculiar to Cambridge and named after a medieval scholar's three-legged stool) covering several subjects including chemistry, physics, physiology, and zoology. For reasons unknown, he did not take Part II of the tripos but took his BA and left Cambridge to go to Edinburgh.

A Biographical History of Endocrinology, First Edition. D. Lynn Loriaux.

This work is a co-publication between the Endocrine Society and John Wiley & Sons, Ltd.

In Edinburgh, Harington joined George Barger's laboratory, where he spent the years 1919–1920. The choice of laboratory was almost by chance. The 22-year-old Harington was looking only for work in the general area of chemistry applied to pharmacology. George Barger was a fortunate choice. Almost a generation older than Harington, he, too, had received a first class grade in the Cambridge Natural Sciences Tripos in 1901. After working in the Wellcome Physiological Research Laboratories for some years, he entered academia in 1909. He spent the "War years" with the Medical Research Committee, which later became the National Institute for Medical Research. When Harington joined him in 1919, Barger had just been appointed to a new Chair of Chemistry in Relation to Medicine at the University of Edinburgh. By then, Barger was an eminent chemist working with biologic compounds. He spent years working on various ergot alkaloids and was among the first to isolate and identify histamine from animal tissue. It must have been an exciting time for both Barger and Harington, the one starting up a new department and the other, freshly graduated, looking for his way into the field.

After a year with Barger, Harington switched to the Department of Therapeutics and Clinical Medicine at Edinburgh's Royal Infirmary to work toward his doctorate under Jonathan C. Meakins, a Canadian who had just become professor in 1919. Harington finished his work in only 2 years and was awarded the PhD degree in 1922. His thesis was on "An aspect of the pathology of protein metabolism." Only one publication resulted from this. It was co-authored with his future wife, Jessie M. Craig. Dr. Craig was a physician and may have been partly responsible for Harington's interest in the thyroid gland. Barger may have discussed the problem of the structure of thyroid hormone with him as well. In any event, on Barger's strong recommendation, Harington was appointed lecturer in chemical pathology at University College Hospital Medical School in London. Before actually taking up his position, the Medical School sent him to the United States for further work during 1922–1923 and supported him financially during this time. He spent several months working with Henry D. Dakin, a well-known English biochemist who had settled in New York some years before and who worked in his own private laboratory north of the city. Dakin highly recommended Harington to a post at the Hospital of the Rockefeller Institute for Medical Research (RIMR), where he then spent several months. Harington's interest in the thyroid antedated his arrival in the United States. His application to RIMR noted that he had begun research on metabolic variation in "exophthalmic goiter." Dakin was an expert on amino acids, among other things, and Harington's only paper with him was on an attempted amino acid synthesis. At RIMR Harington worked with Donald D. van Slyke and A. Baird Hastings, learning, in the process, the use of gasometric methods. He co-authored two papers in the *Journal of Biological Chemistry.*

In the early 1920s, the structure of thyroxine (then called thyroxin) was thought to be settled within the small community of biochemists. Edward C. Kendall (1886–1972) had isolated the hormone in 1914, published an indole-derived structure in 1917, and claimed its synthesis that same year. Experts such as Barger and Dakin, however, had some misgivings about the structure because it was based on a nonspecific test and on possibly erroneous elemental analyses. Nonetheless, Kendall's structure was accepted in the United Kingdom as well as the United States. A British text on the chemistry of hormones noted that the "indole nucleus had been known for some considerable time." Although Harington published nothing on thyroxine before returning to London, it seems clear that his interest had been piqued not only by the prior influences of Craig and Barger but also, importantly, by Dakin, who had urged him to look closely at thyroxine's structure. Dakin also pursued the issue after getting a small amount (10 mg) of crystalline thyroxine indirectly from Kendall via Simon Flexner, the director of RIMR. Harington, 26 years old, also plunged into the chemistry of thyroxine on returning to London in 1923. The attack on Kendall's structure had begun.

In London, Harington got the necessary support for the project from his school and, in three papers published during 1926–1927, improved the process of isolating thyroxine from thyroid tissue, showed that Kendall's structure was wrong, determined the correct structure, and synthesized the hormone. To complete the picture, he had a friend in Edinburgh give synthesized thyroxine by injection to two myxedematous women and showed that it was effective in raising both the metabolic and pulse rates. Both Barger and Dakin were involved. Barger was actually a co-author of Harington's paper on synthesis. Although still in Edinburgh, Harington thought that Barger's advice by correspondence was so important that Barger, although reluctant, should be included. Dakin had come to the same general conclusions as Harington about the structure of thyroxine, but when his friend Barger wrote him of Harington's success, Dakin withdrew his own paper from the *JBC* and notified Kendall, who was, by his own admission, crushed.

The impact of Harington's synthesis was instantaneous. He was only 29 years old. A fellow biochemist wrote 50 years later: "I well remember the effect that this carefully executed work had on all of us who had been brought up to think of thyroxine as an indole derivative." In contrast to what happens today, neither Harington nor the school sought a patent. Anyone who wished could make it. Although the synthesis caught the eye of biochemists and endocrinologists, there was no effect on therapy as it was still too costly compared to desiccated thyroid. It did, however, pave the way to further understanding of thyroid physiology and opened the door to much of the work done over the subsequent 30 years.

Harington, though bright and ambitious, was a shy man and not easy to know. He was warmly supportive of colleagues and co-workers. He was not a good teacher. Students stopped coming after the first lecture in his course. Nevertheless, his talents were not limited to chemistry. He edited or co-edited the *Biochemical Journal* from 1930 to 1942, a task that required vigor, tact, and administrative ability. In 1931, at age 33 years, he was promoted to professor and elected to the Royal Society. In 1942, he became director of the National Institute for Medical Research, the premier scientific appointment in the United Kingdom, succeeding Henry H. Dale (1875–1968), its first director and an old friend and colleague of Barger. Harington led the Institute for 20 years and was able to build it into a world-class research organization. From 1962 to 1967, he worked as an adviser to the Medical Research Council and then, limited by arthritis and coronary heart disease, retired. Still active in retirement, he relearned the classical Greek of his youth. He died of heart disease in 1972.

Harington combined his quiet ambition and an astute, "chemical" brain to achieve major success in a biologic area while still a young man; he went on to further quiet success as an organizer and supporter of others' research.

Sources

Barger G: The thyroid gland and throxine. *Pharmac J Pharmacist* 1927; 65: 609–14.

Himsworth H, Pitt-Rivers R: Charles Robert Harrington 1897–1972. *Biog Mem FRS* 1972; 18: 267–308.

Neuberger A: Obituary notice. Sir Charles Harington (1897–1972). *Biochem J* 1972; 129: 801–4.

Pitt-Rivers R: The thyroid hormones: historical aspects. In *Hormonal Proteins and Peptides*, edited by CH Li. New York: Academic Press, 1978, pp. 391–422.

Sawin CT: Defining thyroid hormone: its nature and control. In *Endocrinology: People and Ideas*, edited by SM McCann. Bethesda: American Physiological Society, 1988, pp. 149–99.

This chapter has been reproduced from Sawin, Clark T: Charles Robert Harington (1897–1972). *The Endocrinologist* 1992; 2(2): 81–4.

CHAPTER 72

Dorothy Price and Carl Moore (1899–1980) (1892–1955)

Regulation of Gonadal Hormone Secretion

In 1930, no hormone of the ovary or testis had been isolated. In fact, the steroid structure of these hormones was yet to be discerned. But extracts of the gonads had been made and, with the help of crude bioassays, the physiological activities of "male hormone" from the testes, and of two ovarian hormones, later termed "estrogen" and "progestin," were being sorted out. Most of the work in this area in the 1920s focused on attempts to figure out what these hormonal activities were.

The time was early in the development of endocrine concepts and of the definition of what a hormone was. The reliance on bioassays was forced on investigators because there was no way of assessing these obscure substances chemically. Experimental anatomists, either in zoology or medical anatomy departments, were the ones who worked on the problem. The bioassays depended on their expertise with animals and their ability to use various animal tissues as markers for the hormone activity. It was also the time when, as never before, there were substantial funds available to perform the work. The funds might seem minuscule today, but at that time, they were strikingly generous.

Into this setting came, in 1932, a classic and lengthy article that defined the relationship between gonadal hormones and the pituitary gland and laid out the broad concept of negative feedback control of the pituitary gonadal axis.

Carl R. Moore and Dorothy Price had been engaged in a series of studies on the effects of gonadal extracts on rats. They were looking for hard evidence for a demonstrable antagonism between the effects of ovarian and testicular extracts. The data, in part, did show such an antagonism, but other experiments did not. Finally, it became clear. If one shifted one's thinking from a mindset of hormonal antagonism to a mindset in which the pituitary gland was a mediator of some of the effects, all made sense. Reciprocity of effect between the gonads and the pituitary was the explanation, and direct antagonism of estrogens and androgens had little to do with it. In their own words: "Gonads function only when they are forcibly stimulated by

A Biographical History of Endocrinology, First Edition. D. Lynn Loriaux.

This work is a co-publication between the Endocrine Society and John Wiley & Sons, Ltd.

certain secretions that are normally provided by hypophysical activity. Hypophysis activity, on the other hand, is to some extent controlled by gonadal secretions."

Moore grew up in the Ozark county of Missouri. He attended a one-room school as a child and attended a small local college, where he paid his tuition by working a variety of odd jobs. At college, he had an influential biology teacher who affected his entire career. There he developed a remarkable work ethic, often being in the laboratory nights and weekends, and learned to perform experiments with minimal resources. After graduation in 1913, medical school was the goal but was out of the question. There was no money. So, he stayed at Drury College for another year, with a salary of $100 for the year, and got his MS degree. A side trip to the University of Chicago during the summer of that year, his first trip ever away from home, took him to the University of Chicago's Department of Zoology for a short course. He went there because of his curiosity about Frank R. Lillie (1870–1947), the author of the then-dominant text on the embryology of the chick. Entranced by Lillie's department, Moore chose the University of Chicago's Department of Zoology for his graduate training after he finished at Drury College, and the University of Chicago offered him a fellowship.

Moore's thesis at the University of Chicago was on the fertilization of the eggs of marine invertebrates, such as sea urchins. He finished in good time, got his PhD in 1916, and was immediately hired by Lillie as a member of the department. He spent a large amount of his time teaching and was a mentor to many. However, in the spirit of the University of Chicago, he also engaged in research under Lillie's auspices. Moore's research took a sharp turn from the marine to the mammalian in 1918–1919, driven by one of Lillie's tangential but puzzling interests.

Between 1913 and 1919, Lillie was trying to understand the phenomenon of the bovine freemartin. A freemartin was recognized at that time as a female fetus, twin to a male fetus, with a poorly developed reproductive tract. Based solely on anatomic observation, Lillie concluded in a massive article in 1917 that sex hormones from the male fetal testis, via vascular connections in the cow's placenta, cause these effects in the female fetus. Ruminants have a cotyledonary placenta, in which the blood of twin fetuses can mix. Thus, the fetal testis could antagonize the fetal ovary. He then proposed that normal sexual differentiation, heretofore thought to be predetermined, was actually controlled by gonadal hormones and might not be predetermined after all. Because Lillie's data were all observational, however, he advised caution and made a "mild suggestion" that Moore should perform some experimental studies to help define the thing a little better. Moore attacked the problem with vigor. He tried transplantations of all types. Initially, none worked. He did, however, succeed in making testicular grafts work in female rats although he never got a model freemartin. We now know that Lillie was partly right. The freemartin is a result of secretions from the male testis, but it is anti-müllerian hormone rather than testosterone that causes it.

The somewhat different issue of the idea that male and female sex glands can antagonize each other, which might be part of the freemartin problem, was more amenable to experimental attack. By using his newfound expertise of gonadal grafts (including ovarian grafts to males and testicular grafts to females) Moore was able to show that there was no such thing as sex gland antagonism. In another series of studies he also was the first to show that the temperature of the testis was critical for proper spermatogenesis. His data showed that one of the functions of the scrotum was to decrease the testicular temperature by a few degrees. He also examined the claim that ligation of the testicular veins increased the secretion of male hormone. The so-called Steinach operation, performed on thousands of men in the 1920s in a sophomoric attempt at rejuvenation. He found no effect of vasoligation or vasectomy on testis function.

In 1923, an active ovarian extract was shown to induce vaginal cornification in rats. The excitement of the 1920s was the realization that one might be able to get active extracts of the gonads that brought about specific male and female actions. In 1927, Moore showed that a bull testis extract could cause capon comb growth. This discovery occurred in the University's Department of Physiological Chemistry, then chaired by Frederick C. Koch. The two chairmen, Lillie and Koch, agreed to work together to study male hormones and develop good bioassays for their activity.

In the 1920s, Dorothy Price was an undergraduate at the University of Chicago and got her BS degree in 1922. She began graduate work in embryology in the Department of Zoology but had to leave because of lack of money. Lillie heard of this and offered her a job – not as a graduate student but as a technician at $1000 per year. The pay and status were not what she had hoped, but she took the position with hopes of completing some thesis work. She never did finish that work but soon was "adopted" by Moore. Her main function was to prepare histological sections and then to assist in the development of the needed bioassays for the male and female hormone preparations. She worked with him for the rest of his career at the University of Chicago.

In 1927, when the testis extract was being studied by Lillie and Koch, the main goal was to develop bioassays that worked in mammals, not just capons, so that the results would seem to be more applicable to humans. Others were known to be working on the same problem. There was a race to see who could get crystals of the male hormone first. Price's part was to use the rat prostate as a bioassay. In Price's own words, the pace was "frenetic." They did not succeed in crystalizing the hormone. Crystals were not obtained by anyone until several years later in 1935 when Dutch investigators managed the feat. Even though pure hormones were not available at the end of the 1920s, lipid extracts containing both androgen and estrogen made it possible for Moore to attack, again, the old problem of gonadal hormone antagonism. Now, instead of having to laboriously graft the glands and interpret the results in light of possibly erroneous "takes," one could administer the actual hormonal preparations by injection in known "bioassayable" quantities and observe directly whether or not one antagonized the other.

Moore and Price began a set of studies that involved more than 300 rats, male and female, with or without ovaries or testes, and with or without injections of "oestrin" or "testis hormone." They did not like the term "testosterone." By the spring of 1930, they had accumulated enough data to become more confused. Their thesis was that there was a direct antagonism of oestrin on the testis and of testis hormone on the ovary. The castrate rat seminal vesicle and prostate had a good response to testis hormone injections, as expected. However, there was no inhibition of the effect by oestrin. So, the idea of a direct hormonal antagonism seemed incorrect. However, confusion arose because oestrin administered to an intact, non-castrate male rat shrank the prostate and seminal vesicles. Even more confusing, it also shrank the size of the testes. Here was evidence that there was, in fact, antagonism. Moreover, injections of the testis hormone into normal male rats also shrank the size of the animals' own testes, whereas the end organs maintained their size. How could this be explained?

Moore had designed the experiments and now was frustrated in their interpretation. Price "had a hand in every phase of the work" and was studying her own set of the histologic slides. Moore really needed to make sense of the evidence because he was scheduled to present his findings in July 1930 at the Second International Congress for Sex Research. In late May, he was still confused and asked Price to think about it as well. She did, and she shifted gears just a bit. She recalled the new information on gonadotropic effects of pituitary gland extracts. She tried to put that knowledge into the context of presumed hormone antagonism. The evening after Moore asked her to think about it, something clicked. If both the oestrin and the testis hormone had similar effects on the testis weight, there had to be some common denominator. The pituitary came to mind because if the testis depended on the pituitary, and if both injections suppressed the testis, it was likely that both hormonal preparations acted via the pituitary. And so the idea of "reciprocal influence" (or, later, negative feedback) was born.

The next day, Price "almost burst into Moore's office to tell him that I thought I had solved the riddle." He thought it was a brilliant idea and they promptly performed a few more studies with pituitary extracts, which confirmed the hunch. Moore went to London with his new idea, came back, and wrote a short article in 1930. Moore followed it with the long exposition in 1932 mentioned previously. The two had known a bit about possible neural control of ovarian function in the rabbit. Ovulation in response to coitus was widely recognized, but incorporation of that idea into the pituitary gonadal relationship was to come later. The two had solved part of the problem and established a solid experimental basis for the role of the pituitary in regulating gonadal function.

The concept became known as the "Moore–Price" theory, so termed by Price herself. Why was it called that if Price was the one who came up with the concept? She herself noted that Moore was an excellent teacher and was "almost unfailingly cheerful and amiable." Nevertheless, she also observed that "Moore was a male chauvinist, and women ... were not really to be considered scientifically equal to men. I think he did not realize the depth of his own prejudice." Further, whereas she remained in Moore's department and received her PhD in 1935, it was not until 1947 that she became an assistant professor, 25 years after she first entered the department. One senses the she accepted all this because she judged the net result to be more interesting and exciting. Evidence of this is seen in her obituary of Moore, wherein she never mentions her role in creating the solution to the puzzling data. This was in contrast to her own memoir, which is quite explicit. This tacit assignment of credit and delay in recognition would be intolerable today.

Moore never did figure out what caused the freemartin. In the 1950s, he thought wrongly that it had nothing to do with fetal hormones at all. He became a full professor in 1928 and chairman of his department after Lillie's retirement in 1934. Moore was elected to the National Academy of Sciences and was president of the American Association for the Study of Internal Secretions (now the Endocrine Society) from 1944 to 1946. For most of his career, he was supported by funds raised by Lillie from the Committee for Research on the Problems of Sex. Lillie's first grant from this Committee paid for Price's $1000 salary. It was no accident that Lillie was one of the first members of this Committee, or that Moore replaced him in 1938. Moore died of cancer in 1955 when he was only 62 years old, thus preventing him from retiring to the Ozark county he loved.

Price became full professor (finally) and retired from the University of Chicago in 1967. She did not stop there, but went on working and teaching in "retirement" while dividing her time between Chicago, Puerto Rico, and Leiden, The Netherlands, where she died in 1980, a full 50 years after she had her wonderful idea. She is remembered at the University of Chicago by the Dorothy Price Lecture in Reproductive Biology. Koch's widow gave a generous gift. The name of the Endocrine Society Medal was changed to the Koch Award, and it was won by Carl Moore in 1955, just a few months before he died.

Sources

Bern HA, Gorbman A: Dorothy Price. 1899–1980. *Gen Comp Endocrinol* 1982; 48: 530.

Foreman D: The concept of negative feedback Moore and Price. *Endocrinology* 1992; 131: 543.

Lillie FR: The free-martin: a study of the action of sex hormones in the foetal life of cattle. *J Exp Zool* 1917; 23: 371.

Moore CR, Price D: Gonad hormone functions, and the reciprocal influence between gonads and hypophysis with its bearing on the problem of sex hormone antagonism. *Am J Anat* 1932; 50: 13.

Price D: Carl Richard Moore. December 5,1892–October 16, 1955. *Biog Mem Natl Acad Sci* 1974; 45: 385.

Price D: Feedback control of gonadal and hypophyseal hormones: Evolution of he concept. In *Pioneers in Neuroendocrinology*, edited by J Meites, BT Donovan, SM McCann. New York: Plenum, 1975, p. 219.

This chapter has been reproduced from Sawin, Clark T: Dorothy Price, Carl Moore, and the regulation of gonadal hormone secretion. *The Endocrinologist* 2002; 12(1): 1–4.

CHAPTER 73
Fuller Albright
(1900–1969)
Uncharted Seas

Fuller Albright was born in Buffalo, New York, on January 12, 1900. His father, John Joseph Albright was a man of property, making his fortune in coal, steel, and automobiles. John's first wife, Harriet, died in 1895. He was left with three motherless children, Raymond, Ruth, and Langdon. To remedy this situation, he wrote to the president of Smith College inquiring if there was a recent graduate who might like the job of governess to the children. Susan Fuller accepted the job. She rapidly became one of the family, and she and John were married 2 years later. Together they had five children. Fuller, after his mother's maiden name, was the middle child and the second of two boys.

John Albright founded the Nichols School for boys and the Franklin School for girls. All of his eight children were educated in these two institutions. Fuller was a good student with a strong interest in sports. He was the captain of the football team. He went to Harvard College when he was 17. Eighteen months later he joined the Army and was sent to the Officer Candidate School in Plattsburg New York. It is during this year that he likely fell victim to the influenza pandemic. He recovered, but retained a proclivity for von Economo's encephalitis, which revisited him many years later in the form of post-encephalitic Parkinson's disease.

The end of the War found Albright an instructor in the Student Army Corps at Princeton University. Despite having attended only 18 months of college, he applied to Harvard Medical School, and was accepted. He was elected to Alpha Omega Alpha in 1923, and graduated in 1924. He took a 2-year internship at the Massachusetts General Hospital.

Albright and a co-intern, Read Ellsworth, became fast friends during this time. Ellsworth came from a wealthy family living in Coos Bay Oregon, at that time the timber capital of the western United States. He graduated from Reed College in Portland, Oregon, and was handsome, outgoing, musically talented, and could tell a good joke. Albright, on the other hand, was quiet, reserved, serious, and tone deaf. Together they made a famous team.

A Biographical History of Endocrinology, First Edition. D. Lynn Loriaux.

This work is a co-publication between the Endocrine Society and John Wiley & Sons, Ltd.

Albright and Ellsworth both developed an interest in endocrinology. Albright followed this interest as a fellow with Joseph Aub, a leading endocrinologist at the Massachusetts General Hospital, whereas Ellsworth returned to Johns Hopkins to work with John Eager Howard. Albright joined Ellsworth at Hopkins for a year in 1927. Thus began a fertile collaboration on the physiology and pathophysiology of disorders of calcium metabolism that endured until Ellsworth's death from tuberculosis in 1937.

Albright left Hopkins in 1928 to spend a year with Jacob Erdheim, the famed Viennese pathologist. Erdheim showed that parathroidectomy prevented calcification of the teeth in rats, an important insight into the regulation of calcium homeostasis. Albright described Erdheim as follows:

> "Was ist die ursacke dafür" (What is the cause of this?). These words meet our ears as we approach. They are spoken by the head gardener for the tree, the fruit of which can save lives. The appearance of the head gardener is so arresting that, for the moment, we turn our full attention to him. He has a huge frame. Although he is not excessively tall, his hips are as high as an average man's chest. The hands are large and deft. His eyes smile from behind gold-rimmed spectacles as he expostulates in a somewhat high pitched voice, "manche leute sehen sehr gut aber sie schauen nicht an" (many people see well but neglect to look) [1].

This was probably Albright's first introduction to the syndrome of hypogonadotropic hypogonadism. Albright returned to the Massachusetts General Hospital in 1929. He established the "Biological Laboratory" in order to offer the Ascheim–Zondek pregnancy test to the hospital clinical services. More tests followed, and the name was changed to the "Endocrine Laboratory." It was this laboratory that, in time, became the core of the world-famous "Endocrine Unit," of the Massachusetts General Hospital.

In 1930, Albright met Claire Birge of Greenwich, Connecticut, and they were married 2 years later. They had two sons – Birge and Read. As a wedding present, Fuller's father gave them a house in Brookline. The conductor Serge Koussevitzky was their next door neighbor.

At the annual Atlantic City clinical science meeting of 1936, John Eager Howard noted the beginnings of a "pill rolling" tremor in Albright's right hand. The Parkinson's disease advanced rapidly. By 1940, Albright could no longer write. By 1945, his speech was so impaired that he could be understood only by family and a few close associates. By 1950, Albright was sure that the disease was affecting his thought processes. Sometimes, he said, it could take him an entire evening to write a single paragraph. He resolved to do something about it.

A young neurosurgeon at New York University, Irving Cooper, had developed an operation that helped many patients with Parkinson's disease [2]. It was called "chemopallidectomy" (so-called because Cooper believed that the cannula tip was in the body of the globus pallidus, although subsequent postmortem studies showed that the successful operations ablated the posterior portion of the ventral nucleus of the thalamus). A burr hole was drilled, and a cannula advanced into the center of the globus pallidus by hand, without the aid of any stereotactic apparatus, at least in the early years when Albright was treated. A small balloon at the tip of the cannula was inflated and, if the tremor stopped, was in the right place. A small amount of ethanol was introduced through the cannula, killing the neurons surrounding the tip of the instrument. Every two or three days, another dose was given until maximum benefit was achieved in terms of a reduction in rigidity, tremor or both. Cooper had recently moved to St. Barnabas hospital in New York City. He agreed to see Albright as a patient, and the surgery was performed in June of 1956. The immediate post-operative results were favorable. Albright was free of tremor and rigidity on the left side. He could write better, and could perform useful acts with his left hand. The family, in a state of euphoria, returned to Boston. Only his son Read remained behind in order to accompany his father home. On the seventh post-operative day the cannula was withdrawn. About 3 o'clock in the afternoon, Albright was found, akinetic and mute, in his hospital bed.

> During the next two decades, on a least one hundred occasions, when my name was mentioned during an introduction at a dinner party or at a medical conference or at an airport or in a hotel lobby, the mention of my name was followed by the comment, "Oh you're the man who operated on Fuller Albright." On two occasions, when I was introduced at a dinner party, one of the doctors rose, stating he would not stay in the same room with the man who had destroyed Fuller Albright. It is a marvelous thing to behold a teacher of medicine held in such affection and respect that the surgeon considered to be his enemy could not be tolerated by some in the same room. It was a painful, irreversibly traumatic experience for me, a young surgeon, continuing even when I was no longer young [2].

Albright was moved back to the Lemuel Shattuck Hospital in Boston and then to the Massachusetts General Hospital. It was in this time that a young psychiatrist, Paul McHugh, was the attending neurologist responsible for many disabled patients suffering from advanced neuropsychiatric disorders. He rounded daily on Fuller Albright, and would comment on each occasion, that the team should be careful about what they said because it was possible that the patient could hear and perhaps understand them.

> So we were pleased to care for him. But this did not ease the task before me upon visiting his bedside each morning as I searched for something interesting to say to my jaded interns. Soon enough they began to grumble that I was repeating myself as I would note dutifully that, although Dr. A's apathetic state was profound and unchanging, occasionally such a patient might, if startled, give out a coherent response revealing some human consciousness. Looking at the man lying before them, they thought they had ample reason to doubt the applicability of my ideas to this case. A particularly bold intern challenged me one morning: "Enough of that, show us that he can respond." I knew perfectly well that I was being baited over a matter where I was unsure of my ground, but I moved briskly from the records cart to the bed, shook the patient by the shoulder, and asked in a sharp voice: "Dr. A, what's the serum calcium in pseudopseudohypoparathyroidism?" For the first time in my experience with him, he glanced up at me and, loudly enough for all the interns to hear, said: "It's just about normal."

> A full and complete sentence had emerged from a man who none of us had ever heard speak before. His answer was correct as he should know, having discovered and named the condition I asked him about. Subsequently, in all the months we cared for him, he would never utter another word. But what a difference that moment had made for all of us. We matured that day not only in matters of the mind but in matters of the heart. Somehow, deep inside that body and damaged brain, he was there and our job was to help him. If we had ever had misgivings before, we would never again doubt the value of caring for people like him. And we didn't give a fig that his EEG was grossly abnormal [3].

Over the years, others were convinced that Fuller Albright could understand their discussions with him, but as far as I know, he never spoke again. He died of pneumonia in 1969 in the Massachusetts General Hospital.

These years of progressive disability before the operation coincided with Albright's most fertile period of translational research. His CV contains 118 peer-reviewed papers. This was in the era before the "least-publishable" unit. A paper was written when something substantive could be said. You will see here the first American description of hyper- and hypoparathyroidism, the first description of pseudohypoparathyroidism, resistance to parathyroid hormone, and pseudo-pseudohypoparathyroidism. You will see the first descriptions of Klinefelter syndrome, the McCune–Albright syndrome, the first description of androgen resistance, Reifenstein's syndrome, the Forbes–Albright syndrome, renal tubular acidosis, vitamin D-resistant rickets, the first convincing explanation of the pathophysiology of congenital adrenal hyperplasia (if you want to feel the power of a tempered steel intellect, read this paper [2]), the second substantive paper on Turner's syndrome, and the best paper on Cushing's syndrome ever written. The list goes on.

How did he do this? First, but not foremost, he was blessed with the gift of inductive reasoning. He was homozygous for this trait. Second, he saw patients and reviewed laboratory results every day. He never lost touch with the patient, and depended upon his patients to teach him and propose topics for fruitful investigation. His strength was the "bedside to bench" limb of the translational research paradigm.

He insisted that problems chosen for study were ones presented by real illness in real patients. Albright knew that the best translational investigation happened when the investigator was the funded entity, not the problem. Unfortunately, this criterion is almost impossible to achieve in today's financial climate and from the funding mechanisms that are available. Mallinckrodt Chemical Corporation funded Albright to do as he wished. Albright was fond of saying that, in his unit, matters of budget were all discussed and decided on only one day each year. It was a good corporate decision. It is in the model used in one of the world's greatest institutions for clinical science, the NIH, where there is a plethora of clinicians and basic scientists, and translational research is the rule rather than the exception. NIH cannot seem to translate this model into the extramural world. If you are not an intramural scientist, you are dependent upon the RO1. No "true" translational investigator can compete for RO1s for very long. Their success depends upon the study of experiments of nature, not confined by "subspecialist" boundaries. This "lack of focus" is difficult for a "study section" to deal with. Study sections tend to value a longitudinal commitment to a single problem rather than a horizontal approach to clinical research focusing on the problems that present the fruitful hypotheses of the moment.

Can this ever change? Unlikely. The RO1 mentality is self-perpetuating, and too successful to change for a single group of scientists. I remember talking about clinical investigation with a very successful academic who wanted to be thought of as a clinical investigator. He had spent his life working out the details of one enzymatic disorder that was the cause of one of the glycogen storage diseases. One patient – one enzyme. He had been a clinician at one time, but now he was a laboratory scientist. Not a bad thing, in fact a good thing, but not to be confused with a bona fide translational investigator. We have a surfeit of laboratory investigators, and a penury of translational ones. It may always be so, at least for our time.

I propose that, pound for pound, Fuller Albright is the most successful translational investigator of the twentieth century. How did he do it? He saw patients every day. He worked in the laboratory every day. He found funding that allowed him to choose his own problems without asking permission. He was unbelievably "intuitive." He did not work to get rich.

I close with this, an eyewitness report of a talk given by Fuller Albright at one of the National Society Meetings in 1945:

> I had hoped [began the physician] that someone would tell you about the Albright lecture. ... Albright, that's it, Fuller Albright, professor of internal medicine at Harvard. Authority on adrenal glands and steroid chemistry ... I went early to be sure and get a good seat. I got there at 1:20, thinking I would find 200 or 300 others. That's the average for those addresses. But every seat was taken, even in the balcony, and they were standing six deep on all sides and in back and even sitting on the floor, where they could. There must have been 4,000 in that ballroom.
>
> At first all anyone could think of was his infirmity, for Albright has Parkinson's disease, degeneration of the central nervous system. It's characterized by a tremor. He is bent and stooped with it, although he is only 47. He has the masked face, too. Can't smile or change expression. Has difficulty enunciating. Had to use a throat mike to talk.
>
> Medical lectures are technical and heavy. The audience usually fidgets and yawns and reads the address later to find out what is what. Well, he stood up there and talked 45 minutes, and you could hear a pin drop. ... The Subject really was over the heads of almost every one, there, but he made it simple and graphic, and vital, interspersing his explanation of his intricate research with wry, funny remarks. All with never a smile or a change of tone. Just that dead voice, that mask-like face.
>
> I have never known a medical audience not to sleep during the lantern slides, but no one did this time. He illustrated with the line drawings of a child. An oblong for a man. Squiggles for extremities. A box or circle for whatever organ he was talking about at the time. Lines for the bones. At the final slide he stood back. Printed on it was something like this: "Result: I have told you more than I know myself. I hope I have told enough to make you want to learn more."
>
> Medical audiences are reserved and noncommittal, but when Mr. Albright stopped, every person there jumped to his feet. They cried "Bravo, bravo!" for what seemed an hour. I guess it was purely an emotional reaction on my part, a reaction to this brilliant and powerful mind which had overcome the wracked body, but I've never seen or heard anything like it, never [4].

References

1. Albright F, Ellsworth R: *Uncharted Seas*. Portland, OR: Kalmia Press, 1990.
2. Cooper IS: *The Vital Probe*. New York & London: W.W. Norton & Co., 1981.
3. McHugh P: *The Mind has Mountains*. Baltimore, MD: Johns Hopkins University Press, 2006.
4. Anonymous: *Annals of Internal Medicine*, 1995; 123, 46.

This chapter has been reproduced from Loriaux, D. Lynn: Fuller Albright and Read Ellsworth. Uncharted seas. *The Endocrinologist* 1991; 1(4): 349.

CHAPTER 74

Charles Brenton Huggins (1901–1997)

Androgen Ablation Therapy for Prostate Cancer

Charles Huggins was born on September 22, 1901 in Halifax, Nova Scotia. He graduated from Acadia University, in 1920, and in 1929 graduated from Harvard Medical School. He took an internship and residency in general surgery at the University of Michigan. Following a research fellowship at Michigan, Huggins became a research fellow in the Department of Surgery at the University of Chicago in 1927. Dr. Dallas Phenister, the first chairman of surgery at the University of Chicago, encouraged Huggins to specialize in urologic surgery, and he accepted the position of chief of urological surgery in 1929. He became a United States citizen in 1933 and professor of surgery in 1936. Over the course of his career, he gradually gave up his surgical practice to focus on research. He avoided burdensome administrative tasks and spent 60–70 hours a week in his laboratories with a small, dedicated research group. He had a plaque in his office that stated "Discovery is our Business." His modus operandi: "Don't write books. Don't teach hundreds of students. Discovery is our business. Make damn good discoveries."

Huggins' early work focused on the effects of androgens on the male urogenital tract, most importantly the prostate gland. He demonstrated the dependence of the prostate gland on androgen support, and was the first to recognize that withdrawal of androgen support could induce regression in the growth of prostate cancer cells. In a landmark series of papers in 1941 [1–3], he demonstrated conclusively that castration could induce remission in metastatic prostate cancer. Some of these remissions were so profound as to suggest cure. Four of Huggins' 21 patients with metastatic prostate cancer treated with castration lived more than 12 years after the procedure. This work was followed by the use of "estrogens" in these patients as an "androgen antagonist." This therapy was also successful and the combined approach defined the treatment of prostate cancer for half a century.

In a series of analogous studies, Huggins showed that ovariectomy was often beneficial in the treatment of metastatic breast cancer. In an effort to define which patients would respond to castration, Huggins encouraged his colleague, Elwood

A Biographical History of Endocrinology, First Edition. D. Lynn Loriaux.

Jensen, to develop a test for estrogen responsiveness, which he did by characterizing laboratory methods to measure estrogen receptor "positivity" or "negativity" as a predictor of the response to ablative therapy.

Dr. Huggins shared the Nobel Prize with virologist Peyton Rous in 1966. Huggins' work that revealed the hormone dependence of normal and neoplastic prostate cells was the basis of the prize. The committee noted that his work had "given many years of active and useful life to patients with advanced cancer over the entire civilized world – patients who would have been lost to other forms of therapy." [4].

Huggins founded the Ben May Laboratory for Cancer Research in 1951, an institution designed to provide collaboration across traditional disciplines in the study of cancer biology. He was named the William B. Ogden, distinguished service professor at the University of Chicago in 1962. In addition to the Nobel Prize, Huggins received more than 100 awards and honorary degrees, including membership in the National Academy of Sciences, the American Physiological Society and, finally, the chancellorship of Acadia University, his alma mater.

Huggins married Margaret Wellman, a nurse he met while working at the University of Michigan. They raised their family in Hyde Park, the neighborhood that is home to the University of Chicago. They had two children, seven grandchildren, and eight great-grandchildren. Margaret died in 1989, Charles in 1997.

Dr. Peyton Rous, who shared the Nobel Prize with Huggins, wrote: "The importance of this discovery far transcends its practical applications. Previous thoughts and endeavors in cancer research have been misdirected in consequence of the belief that tumors cells are anarchic" [5]. The course of research in cancer biology was forever changed by Huggins' discoveries.

References

1. Huggins C, Stephens RC, Hodges CV: Studies on prostatic cancer: 2. The effects of castration on advanced carcinoma of the prostate gland. *Arch Surg* 1941; 43: 209.
2. Huggins CB, Stevens RA: The effect of castration on benign hypertrophy of the prostate in man. *J Urol* 1940; 43: 105.
3. Huggins CB, Hodges CV: Studies on prostate cancer: 1. The effects of castration, of estrogen and androgen injection on serum phosphates in metastatic carcinoma of the prostate. *Cancer Res* 1941; 1: 203.
4. Professor G. Klein. Award Ceremony Speech, 1966. In *Nobel Lectures, Physiology or Medicine 1963–1970*. Amsterdam: Elsevier, 1972.
5. Peyton Rous, 1966. In *Nobel Lectures, Physiology or Medicine 1963–1970*. Amsterdam: Elsevier, 1972.

This chapter has been reproduced from Loriaux, D. Lynn: Charles Brenton Huggins (1901–1997). *The Endocrinologist* 2005; 15(6): 333–4.

CHAPTER 75

Vincent du Vigneaud (1901–1978)

Antidiuretic Hormone

Vincent du Vigneaud was born in Chicago, Illinois in 1901. His father, Alfred, was a mechanical engineer. The family was financially secure. Vincent went to the Carl Schurz High School and displayed an early interest in chemistry, especially sulfur-containing explosives. His early career goal was to be a farmer. He had worked on several farms during the summer vacation months and found that he loved working with the land and animal husbandry. He went to college at the University of Illinois at Urbana-Champaign and majored in chemistry. He married his college girlfriend, Zella Zon Forde, in 1924. He became very interested in Banting's discovery of insulin, and finally wrote a PhD thesis on "The sulfur in insulin."

He next did a post-doctoral fellowship on the synthesis of peptides with George Barger in Edinburgh. Returning to the United States, he accepted a position in the Chemistry Department of his alma mater. Three years later, he became chairman of the Chemistry Department at George Washington University in Washington, DC, 1932–1938. He then left George Washington for Cornell Medical College to chair the Department of Biochemistry. He stayed at Cornell for the remainder of his professional career, spending the last 4 years on the university campus at Ithaca.

Du Vigneaud's work on the protein chemistry of hormones began in 1932. Along with several other investigators he showed by acid hydrolysis the protein nature of insulin. It was believed at the time that insulin was not a protein, but a small molecule attached to a protein. He spent considerable energy in understanding the mechanism of cysteine formation and the metabolic relationships among methionine, cysteine, homocysteine, cystathionine, and choline. He labeled the underlying mechanisms as "trans-sulfuration" and "trans-methylation."

He received an invitation from Paul György to work on the chemical nature of "anti-egg-white injury factor in liver." This factor proved to be biotin. The structure was worked out by du Vigneaud and was verified by chemical synthesis at the Merck Laboratories.

Du Vigneaud started working on the chemistry of oxytocin and vasopressin in 1932, but the work was put off by the Second World War. He was assigned to work on

A Biographical History of Endocrinology, First Edition. D. Lynn Loriaux.

This work is a co-publication between the Endocrine Society and John Wiley & Sons, Ltd.

the chemistry of penicillin, and was able to synthesize small quantities of the antibiotic before the War's end.

Back from the War in 1947, du Vigneaud acquired a concentrated extract of posterior pituitary that had considerable oxytocic bioactivity. The bioassays for oxytocin and vasopressin were cumbersome. Oxytocin bioactivity was measured by blood pressure "depression" in white leghorn chickens. Injections were made into a cannulated wing vein, and blood pressure response measured in the cannulated ischiatic artery [1]. The bioactivity of vasopressin was found by measuring blood pressure rise in the phenobarbital anesthetized cat [2].

In this way, homogenous oxytocin was isolated. The amino acid content was cysteine, glutamic acid, aspartic acid, glycine, isoleucine, leucine, proline, and tyrosine in a molar ration of 1 to 1. The hydrolysates also contained 3 moles of ammonia. Added up, these constituent parts of oxytocin accounted for 97% of the hydrolyzed material. The amino acid sequence was quickly determined to be H-Cys-Tyr-Ile-Gln-Asn-Cys-Pro-Leu-Gly-NH_2. It was a cyclic nonapeptide based upon a cysteine–cysteine disulfide bond. Du Vigneaud next synthesized oxytocin and published his results in 1953 [3]. The journey from a concentration of posterior pituitary extract to the total synthesis of oxytocin took only 6 years. Everything fell into place. The structure of vasopressin followed in 1955 [4].

Du Vigneaud's work with oxytocin and vasopressin showed for the first time that changing the amino acid sequence of biologically active peptides can result in dramatic changes in biologic activity. For example, exchanging isoleucine for phenylalanine, and leucine for cystathionine in oxytocin changes the "oxytocic" molecule into a "vasopressin" molecule. In addition, his work set a very high bar for efficiency in isolating, purifying, and synthesizing hypothalamic/pituitary hormones. The exceptional quality of his work presented a substantial challenge for those investigators who followed du Vigneaud in identifying the hormones of the pituitary and hypothalamus.

Du Vigneaud won the Nobel Prize for Chemistry in 1955. He worked in the laboratory until he suffered a debilitating stroke in 1974. He died as a result of the stroke in 1978, aged 77 years [5].

References

1. Lloyd S, Pickford M: The persistence of depressor response to oxytocin in the fowl after denervation and blocking agents. *Br J Pharmacol* 1961; 16: 129–36.
2. Turner RA, Pierce JG, du Vigneaud V: The purification and amino acid content of vasopressin preparations. *J Biol Chem* 1951; 191: 21–8.
3. Du Vigneaud V, Ressler C, Swan CJM, et al.: The synthesis of an octapeptide amide with the hormonal activity of oxytocin. *J Am. Chem Soc* 1953; 25: 4879–80.
4. Du Vigneaud V: The isolation and proof of structure of the vasopressins and the synthesis of octapeptide amides with pressor-antidiuretic activity. *Proceedings of the Third International Congress of Biochemistry*, Brussels, pp. 49–54.
5. Hoffmann K: *Vincent du Vigneaud, 1901–1978. A Biographical Memoir.* Washington, DC: National Academy of Sciences, 1987.

CHAPTER 76
Russell Earl Marker (1902–1995)
The Mexican Yam

At the dedication meeting for the memorial plaque, October 1, 1999, Steven M. Weinreb, the Russell and Mildred Marker Professor of Natural Products Chemistry, Pennsylvania State University, said: "There are more stories told about Russell Marker than perhaps any other chemist. Although many of these stories are apocryphal, they are so fascinating that most of us cannot bear to stop repeating them" [1].

Russell Marker was born on a farm near Hagerstown, Maryland on March 12, 1902. Little is known of his boyhood. He went to college at the University of Maryland, and got his BS degree in chemistry in 1923 and a master's degree in physical chemistry in 1924. He began his work at Maryland on a PhD in chemistry with Morris Kharasch. It appears that Marker produced enough data to write a thesis in 1 year of work, but he was short two physical chemistry courses needed for the degree. He refused to take them. He noted he already had a master's degree in physical chemistry. As you would expect, the University was unmoved, and Marker left without receiving the degree.

He married Mildred Collins in 1926, and began work at the Ethyl Corporation, which was created in 1923 by General Motors and Standard Oil of New Jersey. The focus was the development of tetraethyl lead as an "anti-knock" agent in gasoline. It was Marker who invented the "octane" rating system as a derivative of his discovery that increased branching in hydrocarbons reduces "knock."

Marker moved to the Rockefeller Institute in 1928 to work with P.A. Levene. Here, Marker published 32 papers on basic organic chemistry in 6 years. He wanted to shift his work into steroid chemistry, but Levene was not interested. Marker accepted a Parke-Davis funded position at Pennsylvania State College in 1934.

By 1937, Marker had extracted enough pregnanediol from the urine of pregnant cows and mares to produce 35 grams of progesterone by established chemical reactions. Progesterone was the theoretical precursor of the naturally occurring androgens, estrogens, and glucocorticoids, molecules that were beginning to acquire powerful clinical applications.

A Biographical History of Endocrinology, First Edition. D. Lynn Loriaux.

This work is a co-publication between the Endocrine Society and John Wiley & Sons, Ltd.

Marker realized that a reliable source of progesterone would be a gold mine, and he began looking for plant steroids that could serve as precursors for progesterone production on a larger scale. He began his work with a steroid extracted from sarsaparilla root, sarsasapogenin. He showed that he could remove the complex side chain of sarsasapogenin and make progesterone in low yield. Sarsasapogenin was very expensive, $80/gram (7 times more than gold). He needed a better source.

He undertook the study of botany looking for a plant that contained steroids of the sapogenin class with a ring structure more like progesterone. Japanese chemists had isolated such a steroid from a yam of the Dioscorea family and named it diosgenin. The raw material was still too expensive.

Marker then hired a botanist and began extensive plant collecting trips in the American southwest, examining more than 400 species of yam-like plants and identifying a dozen or more new sapogenins. None really fit the bill.

Then in 1941, in an old botany book, Marker saw the picture of a dioscorea that grew in Vera Cruz near Orizaba. The root, called "cabeza de negro," was huge, often 200 pounds or more. Marker took a bus to Orizaba and, it is said, recognized the terrain in the photo of the "cabeza de negro" in the botany book as the bus passed. He stopped the bus and got off. He found a nearby *tienda* and, with the help of the proprietor, was able to harvest two roots. One was confiscated at the border. The larger 50-pound root, however, was "passed" on the strength of a bribe. Marker began his chemistry. The root was loaded with diosgenin, and Russell worked out the now legendary Marker degradation that led to synthesis of progesterone [2].

Marker tried to interest Parke-Davis in the process, but got nowhere. He decided to "do it himself." He returned to Vera Cruz and, with local hired help, harvested and dried 10 tons of "cabeza de negro." The roots were extracted, and the extract dehydrated to a syrup. Marker synthesized 3 kg of progesterone with a market value of $80/gram.

Marker resigned from Penn State in 1943, and kept his patents for the synthesis. In 1944, he started a new company in Mexico called Syntex (from synthesis and Mexico). Marker received 40% of the shares in return for his 2 kg of progesterone. Within 1 year, Syntex was selling progesterone for $50/gram.

Marker asked the finance people about the "profit line" for Syntex in 1945 and was told, to his surprise, that there were no profits. Marker immediately severed ties with Syntex and left with his "degradation" methodology still in his sole possession. He started another company, Botanica-mex, which was later restructured to Hormonosynth and, after Marker retired, Diosynth. All prospered making progesterone.

Marker retired from chemistry in 1949. He spent most of his time in Mexico City and at his house in State College, Pennsylvania. His new passion became the study of rare silver masterpieces produced by the eighteenth-century European silversmiths and their reproduction by contemporary Mexican silversmiths.

> Finally, Russell came to me one day and said he would like to contribute to the Penn State museum the reproductions he had kept. But the Penn State museum rejected them. They said they did not want copies of anything. The Philadelphia museum looked at three of them and

> assessed them at $450,000. In the end, he gave them to his sons. Our museum was crazy to have rejected those [3].

He left considerable money to his academic homes in the form of professorships and endowed lecture series. He never received the acclaim that was his due.

What does it all mean? The Marker degradation made possible the commercial production of androgens, estrogens, progesterone, and glucocorticoids. Enormous research activity was stimulated by his work that resulted in the oral contraceptive, and all of the clinical uses of glucocorticoids, including the treatment of inflammatory and neoplastic disorders. The end is not in sight!

References

1. Raber L: Steroid industry honored. *American Chemical Society News* 1999; 77: 78–80.
2. Fieser LF, Fieser M: *Steroids*. New York: Reinhold Publishing Corp, 1959 (second printing 1967, pp. 547–550).
3. *Penn State Sciences*. A former dean remembers Russell Marker, developer of the octane rating for gasoline and co-developer of the birth control pill, February 17, 2011.

This chapter has been reproduced from Loriaux, D. Lynn: Russell Earl Marker (1902–1995). *The Endocrinologist* 2008; 18(3): 107–8.

CHAPTER 77

Gregory Goodwin Pincus (1903–1967)

The Birth Control Pill

Gregory Goodwin (Goody) Pincus was born in 1903 in New Jersey, the son of Russian Jewish immigrants who lived on a farm colony founded by a German-Jewish philanthropic organization. Pincus was the oldest of six children and grew up in a home of intellectual curiosity and energy. His family regarded him as a genius.

Pincus graduated from Cornell and went to Harvard to study genetics, joining Hudson Hoagland and B.F. Skinner as graduate students of W.J. Crozier in physiology, receiving degrees in 1927. Crozier's hero was Jacques Loeb, who discovered artificial parthenogenesis working with sea urchin eggs. Most importantly, Loeb was a strong believer in applying science to improve human life. Thus Crozier, influenced by Loeb, taught Pincus, Hoagland, and Skinner – reproductive biology, neurophysiology, and psychology, respectively – to apply science to human problems. This was to be the cornerstone of Pincus's own philosophy.

Hoagland, after a short stay at Harvard, spent a year in Cambridge, England, then moved to Clark University in Worcester, Massachusetts, to be the chair of biology at the age of 31. Pincus went to England and Germany, and returned to Harvard as an assistant professor of physiology.

Pincus performed pioneering studies of on the meiotic maturation of mammalian oocytes in both rabbit and human oocytes. In 1934, Pincus reported the successful in vitro fertilization of rabbit eggs, earning him a headline in the *New York Times* that alluded to Haldane and Huxley. An article in *Collier's* depicted him as an evil scientist. By 1936, Harvard had cited Pincus's work as one of the University's outstanding scientific achievements, but it denied him tenure in 1937.

At Clark University, Hudson Hoagland was in constant conflict with the president of the University, Wallace W. Atwood, the senior author of a widely used textbook on geography. In 1931, the Department of Biology consisted of one faculty member and his graduate student, and their chair, Hudson Hoagland. Hoagland, upset and angry over Harvard's refusal to grant tenure to his friend (suspecting that this was fueled by anti-Semitism), invited Pincus to join him at Clark.

A Biographical History of Endocrinology, First Edition. D. Lynn Loriaux.

This work is a co-publication between the Endocrine Society and John Wiley & Sons, Ltd.

Hoagland secured funds for Pincus, enough for a laboratory and an assistant, from philanthropists in New York City. This success impressed the two men, especially Hoagland, planting the idea that it might be possible to support research with private money.

Min-Chueh Chang received his PhD degree from Harvard on an infamous day, December 7, 1941. He was drawn to Pincus because of his book, *The Eggs of Mammals*, published in 1936, a book that had a major impact on biologists at that time. The successful recruitment of M.-C. Chang by Hoagland and Pincus was to pay great dividends.

Hoagland put together a group of outstanding scientist but, because of his ongoing antagonism with President Atwood, the group was denied faculty status. Working in a converted barn, they were totally supported by private funds. By 1943, 12 of Clark's 60 faculty were in the Department of Biology.

Frustrated by the politics of academia, Hoagland and Pincus (who both enjoyed stepping outside of convention) had a vision of a private research center devoted to their philosophy of applied science. Indeed, the establishment of Worcester Foundation for Experimental Biology in 1944 can be attributed directly to Hoagland and Pincus, their friendship for each other, their confidence, enthusiasm, ambition, and drive. It was their spirit that turned many members of the Worcester society into financial supporters of biologic science. Hoagland and Pincus accomplished what they set out to do. They created and sustained a vibrant, productive scientific institution where it was a pleasure to work.

Although named the Worcester Foundation for Experimental Biology, the Foundation was located in the summer of 1945 across Lake Quinsigamond in a house on an estate in Shrewsbury. The Board of Trustees was chaired by Harlow Shapely, a distinguished astronomer, vice-chaired by Rabbi Levi Olan, and included three Nobel laureates and a group of Worcester businessmen. From 1945 to the death of Pincus in 1967, the staff grew from 12 to 350 (scientist and support people), 36 of whom were independently funded and 45 post-doctoral fellows. The annual budget grew from $100 000 to $4.5 million. One hundred acres of adjoining land was acquired and the campus grew to 11 buildings. In its first 25 years, approximately 3000 scientific papers were published.

In those early years, Pincus was the animal keeper, Mrs. Hoagland the bookkeeper, M.-C. Chang was the night watchman, and Hoagland mowed the lawn. During the years of World War II, Pincus and Hoagland combined their interests in hormones and neurophysiology to focus on stress and fatigue in industry and the military.

In the 1930s, producing sufficient amounts of the sex steroids was a major problem. The extraction and isolation of a few milligrams of the sex steroid required starting points measured in gallons of urine or thousands of pounds of organs. Edward Doisy processed 80 000 sow ovaries to produce 12 mg of estradiol.

The supply problem was solved by an eccentric chemist, Russell E. Marker. In 1935, working at Pennsylvania State University, Marker became interested in solving the problem of producing abundant and cheap amounts of progesterone. At that time it required the ovaries from 2500 pregnant pigs to produce 1 mg progesterone. Marker became convinced that the solution was to find plants containing sufficient amounts of plant steroids that could be used as a starting point for progesterone synthesis. He organized extensive botanical expeditions in the southwest and Mexico, sending home more than 100 000 pounds of material. In 1942, from the roots of the Mexican yam, he worked out the degradation of diosgenin to progesterone. United States pharmaceutical companies, however, refused to back Marker. Even the university refused, despite Marker's urging, to patent the process.

In 1943, Marker resigned his academic position and went to Mexico where he collected 10 tons of *Dioscorea mexicana*. In an old pottery shed in Mexico City, he was able to prepare several pounds of progesterone. With two partners, Marker formed a company called Syntex (synthesis + Mexico). But true to his eccentric nature, Marker had a falling out with his partners and sold his share of the company in 1947, retiring to Pennsylvania to devote the rest of his life to making replicas of antique masterworks in silver. Fortunately for Syntex, he had published a scientific description of his process, and Syntex recruited George Rosenkranz, a Hungarian refugee living in Cuba, to reinstitute the commercial manufacture of progesterone from Mexican yams. The task took Rosenkranz 2 years.

In 1949, it was discovered that cortisone relieved arthritis, and the race was on to develop an easy and cheap method to synthesize cortisone. Carl Djerassi joined Syntex to work on the synthesis, which was achieved in 1951. Soon after, an even better method of cortisone production using microbiologic fermentation was discovered at Upjohn. This latter method, however, used progesterone as the starting point, and Syntex found itself as the key supplier of progesterone in the world.

Djerassi and other Syntex chemists then turned their attention to the sex steroids. They discovered that the removal of the 19 carbon from yam-derived progesterone increased the progestational activity of the molecule. Ethisterone had been available for a dozen years, and the Syntex chemists reasoned that removal of the 19 carbon would increase progestational potency of this orally active compound. In 1951, norethindrone was synthesized, and 2 years later G.D. Searle & Company filed a patent for norethynodrel.

The initial discoveries that led to an oral contraceptive can be attributed to M.-C. Chang, who was also the first to describe the capacitation process of sperm. I remember listening to him talk in the classroom and in the hallway, and never understood much, if anything, that he said. In 1951, he confirmed the work of Makepeace who had demonstrated that progesterone could inhibit ovulation in rabbits. When norethindrone and norethynodrel became available, Chang found them to be virtually 100% effective in inhibiting ovulation when administered orally to rabbits.

Katherine Dexter McCormick was a very rich woman. In 1904, she married Stanley McCormick, the son of Cyrus McCormick, the founder of International Harvester. She was intelligent, the second woman to graduate from the Massachusetts Institute of Technology, socially conscious, and a generous contributor to family planning efforts. McCormick's husband suffered from schizophrenia, and she established the Neuroendocrine Research Foundation to study schizophrenia. This brought her together with Hoagland who told her of the work being done by Chang and Pincus.

Pincus attributed his interest in contraception to his growing appreciation for the world's population problem, and to a 1951 visit with Margaret Sanger, president of the Planned Parent Federation of America. At that visit, Sanger expressed hope that a method of contraception could be derived from the laboratory work being done by Pincus and Chang.

Margaret Sanger brought Pincus and Katherine McCormick together in 1952. During this meeting, Pincus formulated his thoughts derived from his mammalian research. He envisioned a progestational agent in pill form as a contraceptive, acting like progesterone in pregnancy. Sanger and McCormick provided a research grant for further animal research. By the time of her death, McCormick had contributed more than $2 million to the Worcester Foundation, and left another $1 million in her will. In his book, *The Control of Fertility*, published in 1965, Pincus wrote: "This book is dedicated to Mrs. Stanley McCormick because of her steadfast faith in scientific inquiry and her unswerving encouragement of human dignity."

It was Pincus who made the decision to involve a physician because he knew human experiments would be necessary. John Rock, chief of gynecology and obstetrics at Harvard, met Pincus at a scientific conference and discovered their mutual interest in reproductive physiology. Rock and his colleague pursued Pincus's work. Using oocytes from oophorectomies, they reported in vitro fertilization in 1944, probably the first demonstration of fertilization of human oocytes in vitro. Rock was interested in the work with progestational agents, not for contraception, but because he hoped the female sex steroids could be used to overcome infertility.

Sanger and McCormick needed some convincing that Rock's Catholicism would not be a handicap, but they were eventually won over because of his stature. Rock was a physician who literally transformed his personal values in response to his recognition of the problems secondary to uncontrolled reproduction. The first administration of synthetic progestins to women was to Rock's patients in 1954. Of the first 50 patients to receive 10–40 mg of synthetic progestin for 20 days each month, all failed to ovulate during treatment (causing Pincus to begin referring to the medication as "The Pill") and 7 of the 50 became pregnant after discontinuing the medication, which pleased Rock who, all along, was motivated to treat fertility.

Pincus and Chang decided to announce their findings at the International Planned Parenthood meeting in Tokyo, in the fall of 1955. Rock refused to join in this effort, believing that Pincus and Chang were moving too fast. Despite this disagreement (which apparently was spirited and strong), it was done and the Tokyo presentation generated worldwide publicity.

In 1956, with the help of Celso Ramon Garcia and Edris Rice-Wray working in Puerto Rico, the first human trial was performed. The initial progestin products were contaminated with about 1% mestranol. In the amounts being used, this added up to 50–500 μg of mestranol, a sufficient amount of estrogen to inhibit ovulation by itself. When efforts to lower the estrogen content yielded breakthrough bleeding, it was decided to retain the estrogen for cycle control, thus establishing the principle of the combined estrogen–progestin oral contraceptive.

Pincus, a long-time consultant to Searle, picked the Searle compound for extended use and, with great effort, convinced Searle that the commercial potential of an oral contraceptive warranted the risk of possible negative public reaction. Pincus also convinced Rock, and together they pushed the U.S. Food and Drug Administration for acceptance of oral contraception. In 1957, Enovid was approved for the treatment of miscarriages and menstrual disorders, and in 1960, for contraception. Neither Pincus nor the Worcester Foundation got rich on the Pill; alas, there was no royalty agreement.

The Pill did bring Pincus fame and travel. There is no doubt that he was very much aware of the accomplishment and its implications. As he traveled and lectured in 1957, he said: "how a few precious facts obscurely come to in the laboratory may resonate into the lives of men everywhere, bring order to disorder, hope to the hopeless, life to the dying. That this is the magic and mystery of our time is sometimes grasped and often missed, but to expound it is inevitable."

Pincus was the perfect person to bring oral contraception into the public world at a time when contraception was a private, suppressed subject. Difficult projects require people like Pincus. A scientific entrepreneur, he could plow through distractions. He could be hard and aggressive with his staff. He could remain focused. He hated to lose, even in meaningless games with his children. Yet he combined a gracious, charming manner with his competitive hardness. He was filled with the kind of self-confidence that permits an individual to forge ahead, to translate vision into reality.

Pincus died in 1967 (as did Katherine McCormick at the age of 92) of aplastic anemia. Some have argued that this was caused by his long-term exposure to organic solvents. The Foundation immediately felt the loss of Pincus, and a year later Hudson Hoagland resigned. The Foundation successfully weathered a transition to new leadership and direction, but the seeds of success were sown by the visionary Pincus.

Pincus met with Hudson Hoagland's son Mahlon (a protein chemist who identified transfer RNA) in 1965 and suggested that he move to the Foundation to develop a program in molecular biology. Three years later, a search committee chaired by Roy Greep asked Mahlon Hoagland to become the director of the Foundation. He accepted the challenge at a time of declining federal support for research. From 1970 to 1985, he engineered a move from physiology and biochemistry to molecular biology, beginning with the establishment in 1972 of a federally funded center for cancer research.

Pincus wrote his book, *The Control of Fertility*, in 1964–1965, only because "a break came in the apparent dam to publication on reproductive physiology and particularly its subdivisions concerned with reproductive behavior, conception, and contraception."

> We have conferred and lectured in many countries of the world, seen at first hand the research needs and possibilities in almost every European, Asiatic, Central, and South American country. We have faced the hard fact of overpopulation in country after country, learned of the bleak demographic future, assessed the prospects for the practice of efficient fertility control. This has been a saddening and a heartening experience; saddening because of the sight of continuing poverty and misery, heartening because of the dedicated colleagues and workers seeking to overcome the handicap of excess fertility and to promote healthy reproductive function. Among these we have made many friends, found devoted students [1].

In 1968, less than one year after the death of Pincus, I arrived in Shrewsbury as a student in the Steroid Training Program at the Foundation. I came to know many of Pincus's friends and colleagues, and through them, I realized what I had just missed: Goody Pincus was truly a great man.

Reference

1. Pincus G: *The Control of Fertility*. New York: Academic Press, 1965.

Sources

Chesler E: *Woman of Valor: Margaret Sanger and the Birth Control Movement in America*. New York: Simon & Schuster, 1992.

Djerassi C: *The Pill, Pygmy Chimps, and Degas' Horse*. New York: Basic Books, 1992.

Halberstam D: *The Fifties*. New York: Fawcett Columbine, 1993.

Hoagland M: *Toward the Habit of Truth: A Life in Science*. New York: W.W. Norton & Company, 1990.

Pincus G: *The Eggs of Mammals*. New York: Macmillan, 1936.

Pincus G, Enzmann EV: The comparative behavior of mammalian eggs in vivo and in vitro. I. The activation of ovarian eggs. *J Exp Med* 1935; 62: 665.

Pincus G, Saunders B: The comparative behavior of mammalian eggs in vivo and in vitro. VI, The maturation of human ova. *Anat Rec* 1939; 75: 537.

Rock, J, Menkin MF: In vitro fertilization and cleavage of human ovarian eggs. *Science* 1944; 100: 105.

Rock J, Pincus G, Garcia C-R: Effects of certain 19-nor steroids on the normal human menstrual cycle. *Science* 1956; 124: 891.

This chapter has been reproduced from Speroff, Leon: "Goody" was a great man. Gregory Goodwin Pincus (1903–1967). *The Endocrinologist* 1995; 5(4): 249–52.

CHAPTER 78

G.F. Marrian (1904–1981)

Isolation of Estrogens

Guy Frederic Marrian was born in London on March 3, 1904. His scientific career began early when, at the age of 18, he was appointed by Dr. (later Sir) Henry Dale to a laboratory technician's post at the National Institute for Medical Research in Hampstead, London [1]. The following year, he commenced undergraduate studies in chemistry at University College, London, graduating with second class honors in 1925. He then began work as a research assistant in biochemistry in the laboratory of Professor Jack Drummond. Initially he worked on the lipids of the adrenal cortex but, in 1928, he began collaborating with A.S. Parkes in work on the estrus-inducing principle, which they termed "oestrin" [2].

Marrian entered the field at a most exciting time, which has been referred to as the "heroic age of reproductive endocrinology" [3]. In 1923–1924, Allen and Doisy demonstrated that the cornification of vaginal cells, characteristic of estrus, could be reproduced in ovariectomized mice by the injection of porcine ovarian follicular fluid [4,5]. They proceeded to develop a reliable quantitative bioassay. Their attempts to isolate the estrogenic principle, however, were handicapped by the high cost and limited availability of sow ovaries [6]. When their collaboration ended in 1927, they still had not obtained a crystalline product. It was in this year, however, that Ascheim and Zondek showed that the urine of pregnant women was very high in estrus-producing activity. With this readily available source of estrogen and the bioassay developed by Allen and Doisy, "the stage was thus set for an intensive attack on the isolation and identification of the hormone" [7]. Four main groups were involved: Doisy and colleagues in St. Louis, Butenandt and co-workers in Gottingen, Laqueur's group in Amsterdam, and Parkes and Marrian in London [8].

The methods used by the four groups to isolate estrogen were similar. The first step was ether-extraction of the hormone from acidified pregnancy urine; this was followed by multiple purification steps using diffusion separation between immiscible solvents and fractional distillation and sublimation in a high vacuum. They all assessed the potency of the extracts in various modifications of the Allen

A Biographical History of Endocrinology, First Edition. D. Lynn Loriaux.

This work is a co-publication between the Endocrine Society and John Wiley & Sons, Ltd.

and Doisy bioassay. Marrian's first attempt at extracting the estrogen principle, in fact, resulted in the isolation, not of an estrogen, but of a compound later to be called pregnanediol. Butenandt subsequently isolated and characterized the compound independently, but it was not until 1937 that it was recognized as the major metabolite of progesterone [9].

Competition was fierce in the race to isolate the estrogenic hormone. In the fall of 1929, first Doisy and then Butenandt reported the isolation of crystalline estrogen [10, 11]. Laqueur published a similar report a few months later. All three groups had isolated the same hydroxyketone, now known as estrone, although the small amounts of the substance available initially caused some confusion about its nature (note that the four-ringed steroid structure was then unknown). Marrian then greatly increased the confusion in the field by reporting the isolation from pregnancy urine of a crystalline estrogen with a melting point considerably higher than the previously isolated estrogen, and which was chemically distinct from it in that it was a triol rather than a hydroxyketone [12, 13]. As Marrian later remarked, "At that time this was all very puzzling since the physiologist and biochemists of the period were reluctant to believe that the body could secrete chemically different hormonal substances possessing similar physiological properties" [9].

These discrepant findings caused some controversy, "with the odds apparently 3 to 1 against Marrian" [3]. In 1931, however, after further work and exchange of specimens, it was confirmed that both the hydroxyketone (estrone) and the triol (estriol) were present in human pregnancy urine as separate entities. In addition, Butenandt showed that, by dehydrogenation with potassium hydrogen sulfate, the triol could be converted to the hydroxyketone, an early indication of the metabolic relationship between the two substances. Doisy's group isolated the triol (which they called "theelol") independently a few months after Marrian's report [14].

According to Parkes, "This vindication of his work was rightly considered as a triumph for Marrian" [3]. Still only 26 years old, he received the degree of Doctor of Science from the University of London for his meticulous work on "The chemistry of oestrin." The research had been carried out virtually single-handedly and with facilities far inferior to those of his rivals.

A question that was resolved at the time was why Butenandt isolated estrone only, Marrian isolated estriol only, while Doisy isolated first estrone and then estriol independently. The answer seems to lie in the different biological half-lives of the two estrogens [15]. Butenandt used a single injection of hormone in his bioassays, effectively minimizing the relative activity of estriol to estrone. Marrian gave four injections over 36 hours, which had an opposite effect. Doisy used an intermediate method of three injections over 12 hours, which allowed good bioactivity of both estrogens in the assay, leading to the isolation of both [16].

By 1931, the molecular formulas of estriol and estrone had been established, but their structure remained to be elucidated. Rapid progress was made possible in this area by Zondek's discovery that pregnant mare's urine was an even richer source of estrogen than human pregnancy urine, and by the development by André Girard of new ketonic reagents for the isolation of crystalline estrogens from this source. The publication by Rosenheim and King of their ground-breaking work on the structural formula of cholesterol led to the attractive proposal that the sterols and estrogens might be chemically related, and subsequent work in the laboratories of Butenandt and Marrian presented at a League of Nations conference in 1932 gained wide acceptance, replacing a wide variety of names that had been in use up to then.

In 1933, Marrian was appointed associate professor of biochemistry at the University of Toronto. There he began work on the conjugated forms of estrogen present in pregnancy urine and placenta. The first step was to develop a reliable chemical assay for estrogen. With S.L. Cohen, then a graduate student, he modified a colorimetric test for estrogens that had been reported by Kober, who worked in Laqueur's laboratory in the Netherlands. The result was a colorimetric assay for estrogen that was at least as accurate and less laborious than the bioassays [17]. With later modifications, this assay was to form the basis of estrogen research for the next 40 years.

Cohen and Marrian in Toronto isolated the principal estrogen conjugate from human pregnancy urine and identified it as estriol glucuronide [18]. Concurrent with this work, Benjamin Schachter, also a graduate student, and Marrian identified the principal conjugated estrogen in pregnant mares' urine as estrone sulfate [19]. Estrone sulfate and other conjugated equine estrogens are pharmaceutical agents that remain the major estrogen products in use today.

In 1939 Marrian left Canada to take up the position of professor of chemistry in relation to medicine at the University of Edinburgh. There he carried out research into pregnanediol, adrenal steroids, the minor estrogens, and pathways of estrogen metabolism. He played an important part in the development of the Clinical Endocrinology Research Unit in Edinburgh, the first of its kind in the United Kingdom. In 1958 he was appointed director of research at the Imperial Cancer Research Fund, presiding over the expansion of this institution into a major research center until his retirement in 1968. He died on July 24, 1981.

Marrian was one of the first scientists to apply chemical techniques to the study of reproductive endocrinology, and there followed a period of remarkable achievement. As Parkes notes, "It is indeed remarkable that after so long a prelude, the chief naturally occurring estrogens and androgens, as well as progesterone, were all isolated and their biological properties extensively investigated within the seven years 1929–35" [3]. The principal circulating estrogen, estradiol, was isolated from porcine ovary by MacCorquodale, Thayer, and Doisy in 1935. Although Marrian was much honored during his lifetime, the Nobel Prize eluded him, unlike his rivals Doisy and Butenandt.

Acknowledgments

The research upon which this article is based was supported by the Wellcome Unit for the History of Medicine, University of Oxford.

References

1. Grant JK: Frederic Marrian. *Biogr Mem Fellows R Soc* 1982; 28: 347–78.
2. Walsh JP: The Scientific Work of Guy Marrian (1904–81). Mainly with Respect to Steroid Hormone. Bachelor of Arts dissertation, University of Oxford, 1985.
3. Parkes AS: The rise of reproductive endocrinology. 1926–1940. The Sir Henry Dale Lecture for 1965. *J Endocrinol* 1966; 34: xix–xxxii.
4. Corner GW: The early history of the oestrogenic hormones. The Sir Henry Dale Lecture for 1964. *J Endocrinol* 1965; 31: iii–xvii.
5. Allen E, Doisy EA: An ovarian hormone. *JAMA* 1923; 81: 819–21.
6. Doisy EA: Isolation of a crystalline estrogen from urine and the follicular hormone from ovaries. *Am J Obstet Gynecol* 1972; 114: 701–2.
7. Marrian GF: *The History of the Discovery of the Oestrogenic Hormones*. Berlin: Scientific Relations Department, Schering AG, 1972, p. 5.
8. Parkes AS: *The Offbeat Biologist*. Cambridge: Galton Foundation, 1985, p. 126.
9. Marrian GF: Early work on the chemistry of pregnanediol and the oestrogenic hormones. The Sir Henry Dale Lecture for 1966. *J Endocrinol* 1967; 35: vi–xvi.
10. Doisy EA, Veler CD, Thayer S: Folliculin from urine of pregnant women. *Am J Physiol* 1929; 90: 329–30.
11. Butenandt A: The discovery of oestrone. *Trends Biochem Sci* 1979; 4: 215–16.
12. Marrian GF: The chemistry of oestrin. III. An improved method of preparation and the isolation of active crystalline material. *Biochem J* 1930; 24: 435–45.
13. Marrian GF: The chemistry of oestrin. IV. The chemical nature of crystalline preparations. *Biochem J* 1930; 24: 1021–30.
14. Doisy EA, Thayer SA, Levin L, Curtis JM: A new triatomic alcohol from the urine of pregnant women. *Proc Soc Exp Biol Med* 1930; 28: 88–98.
15. Anderson JN, Peck EJ, Clark JH: Estrogen induced uterine responses and growth: relationship to receptor estrogen binding by uterine muclei. *Endocrinology* 1975; 96: 160–7.
16. Marrian GF: The chemistry of the oestrogenic hormones. *Ergeb Vitam Hormonforsh* 1938; 1: 419–54.
17. Cohen SL, Marrian GF: The application of the Kober test to the quantitative estimation of oestrone and oestriol in human pregnancy urine. *Biochem J* 1934; 28: 1603–14.
18. Cohen SL, Marrian GF, Odell AD: Oestriolglucronide. *Biochem J* 1936; 30: 250–6.
19. Schachter B, Marrian GF: The isolation of estrone sulphate from the urine of pregnant mares. *J Biol Chem* 1938; 126: 663–9.

This chapter has been reproduced from Sawin, Clark T: Historical Note: GF Marrian (1904–81) and the isolation of estrogens. *The Endocrinologist* 1996; 6(2): 76–8.

CHAPTER 79

Berta and Ernst Scharrer (1906–1995) (1905–1965)

Concept of Neurosecretion

In the first third of the twentieth century, endocrinology was a revolutionary field. Glandular structures, at first called "blood-glands" or "glands of internal secretion," and then "endocrine glands," were seen as providers of essential substances for the control of a multitude of bodily functions. Previously, no one knew what these structures did, if anything. These secretions were, in turn, controlled in several ways. Sometimes, the control was by another hormone, as these secretions came to be called. Or the control might be a neural mechanism, as in the case of the adrenal medulla where the autonomic nervous system directly impinged on the adrenal medulla to stimulate the secretion of adrenal catecholamines. The pituitary was the "master gland" and these glands as a whole constituted the "endocrine system" that coordinated most, if not all, functions of the body.

A heretical view arose in the late 1920s that some nerves were themselves secretors of hormones. Now a commonplace idea, best exemplified by the remarkable discoveries of hypothalamic hormones and factors over the last 40 years, the concept met strong resistance from the scientific community at first. Glands and nerves had always been separate. That nerves secreted hormones has no single "classic" experiment or observation that struck all as proving the concept. Rather, the idea had to grow slowly and erratically before reaching full acceptance in the late 1950s and 1960s.

In fact, the idea that nervous tissue secreted something that affected the rest of the body is old. It can be traced back to Theophile de Bordeu in 1722 who had only a vague speculation and no data whatsoever to offer. It was finally realized that neurohumors did exist, as shown by the release of catecholamines or acetylcholine from nerve endings close to effector organs of one sort or another. None of this, however, led to the concept of neurosecretion discussed here, namely the release of hormonal substances from neurons wherein the hormone acts on an effector at some distance rather than at an immediately nearby synapse or endplate.

Berta and Ernst Scharrer were key players in the neurosecretion story. Both came to the concept by the study of non-mammalian species: he by studying teleost fish and

A Biographical History of Endocrinology, First Edition. D. Lynn Loriaux.

This work is a co-publication between the Endocrine Society and John Wiley & Sons, Ltd.

she by examining insects (principally one or another species of cockroach). Eventually their work and ideas were accepted but only after several decades. There were good reasons for the delay. The fact that the concept was largely based for some years on histologic anatomy was a problem. The primary resistance was based on the more visceral reaction of "it couldn't possibly be true."

Both Scharrers (she, nee Vogel) were born in Munich, Germany, and attended the University of Munich where they met. Ernst proceeded to his PhD in 1927. When he was 21 years old, he observed with light microscopy that certain hypothalamic neurons had an unusual structure. Their cytoplasm had granules that suggested an endocrine function. He proposed in 1928 that these cells were actually true neurons and that these neurons had something to do with the control of pituitary hormone secretion [1].

Berta bucked the usual societal fashion by being a woman who attended the university in the first place and even more so by going on to graduate study, in this case with Karl von Frisch. He was well-known for his work on animal behavior and the language of bees, for which he won the Nobel Prize for Medicine or Physiology in 1973. She became expert in the study of insects and received her PhD in 1930. By this time, Ernst had spent a year in Vienna as an assistant in zoology and a year in New Haven at Yale University as a Sterling Fellow in Zoology. Times were not easy in the 1930s anywhere in the world, particularly in Germany if one were not a National Socialist (Nazi). After another year in Vienna, he returned to Munich in 1931 to work as a research investigator in the psychiatric institute for the next 2 years (it is not clear if he received a salary although he was able to continue his histologic studies). Berta had stayed at the University of Munich as a research associate, probably unpaid, after gaining her degree. In 1933, Ernst was appointed director of the Neurologic Institute in Frankfurt am Main. Now that he was ensconced in a "real job," Berta joined him the next year, 1934, and they married.

In Frankfurt, Berta continued as a research associate in the Institute that her husband directed and pursued her work with insects and other invertebrates. She and her husband continued to be enamored of the neurosecretion idea and decided to divide the work. He would focus on vertebrates and she would concentrate on invertebrates. The driving force behind this division of labor was the idea that if one could show the same histologic phenomenon in a wide range of species, then it could not be a species-specific quirk but must have a wider physiologic meaning. There was little acceptance of this idea. In Frankfurt, they met the young Wolfgang Bargmann who was intrigued by the neurosecretory concept and was to return to it and the Scharrers almost two decades later.

By 1937, they were becoming known for their work although their ideas seem not to have been any better accepted. They published a major review of their work before the scientific public in 1937 [2]. Politically, circumstances were changing in a serious and dangerous direction. Ernst applied for, and won, a Rockefeller Fellowship for a year's study at the University of Chicago. Although not Jewish, they elected not to return to Germany because of their hostility to Hitler's policies and the treatment many of their German colleagues had received. Their Chicago year was followed by a

2-year temporary appointment for Ernst at the Rockefeller Institute in New York. Berta went, as she notes, as a research associate. In fact she was not paid. The Rockefeller Institute lists her as a "volunteer worker." During that time, they were invited to present their work at the 1939 meeting of the Association for Research in Nervous and Mental Disease. This was a prestigious invitation engineered by John Fulton who chaired the editorial board of the Association and who wanted, it seems, to have a more open discussion of the neurosecretory idea. The Scharrers presented their case cautiously, with slides and plates to show the neural granules, some actually in the process of being extruded from their neurons, hence being secreted [3]. Their paper, apparently well-received, elicited none of the usual discussion (at least in print) that usually accompanied talks to the Association.

Ernst had his appointment at the Rockefeller Institute sponsored and arranged by Charles R. Stockard, who was chairman of the Department of Anatomy at Cornell Medical College. Apparently, there was an agreement for Ernst Scharrer to join Stockard when his term at the Institute was over. Stockard's death in 1939 obviated this arrangement. Ernst next moved to Cleveland to become assistant professor of anatomy. There they remained for the next 6 years, years that covered the entire Second World War. The Scharrers continued their work, stumped in part by their inability do the classic endocrine experiment: remove a gland, show a physiologic deficit, and repair the deficit by giving a glandular extract or a hormone. They did the next best thing: pursue the comparative anatomy approach and show how the neural structures that suggested secretion were present in all manner of animals. They visited the Marine Biological Laboratory (MBL) in Woods Hole, Massachusetts, to study even more species and published several more papers in the MBL's journal, including an article that specifically drew an analogy between the vertebrate hypothalamic–pituitary relationship and a similar pattern in insects [4]. Another well-regarded review, entitled simply, "Neurosecretion," appeared during their stay in Cleveland [5]. Perhaps other scientists were beginning to think the Scharrers had something after all.

The year 1946 saw yet another move for the couple, this time to the University of Colorado in Denver where he became associate professor of anatomy. She won a Guggenheim Fellowship, followed by a U.S. Public Health Service Special Fellowship, and finally a research assistant professorship in anatomy during their 9 years there. As she pointed out, she had finally gotten a job that paid her a salary. That year (1946) also saw the publication of an experiment by Carroll Williams, a well-known insect biologist, in which he was able to do the classic endocrine experiment. He transplanted a presumed neuroendocrine part of the insect brain to another insect in which that part of the brain had been removed and showed that the missing function was replaced. The concept had moved another step forward thanks to knowledge about insects, rather than about mammals.

Berta was now recognized as an expert on insect physiology. She was asked to write the section on insect hormones in the first encyclopedic endocrine compendium to appear since the War [6] and, naturally, included a complete review of neurosecretion in insects. It seemed that neurosecretion was fairly well accepted by insect physiologists.

In the meantime, Bargmann had several academic appointments. In 1942, he became professor of anatomy in Konigsberg, now a part of Russia. By 1944, conditions had worsened so much that all research stopped. In January of 1945, when the Russians were about to besiege the city, Bargmann escaped to Kiel as professor of anatomy. He started doing research again in 1948. In the past, Bargmann had looked for "neurosecretory" granules in the neurohypophysis but failed. In Kiel, he recalled the Scharrers' work from the early 1930s in Frankfurt, and put that together with the fact that there was an effective histologic stain for pancreatic islet cells, the Gomori stain. Perhaps this stain could be effective for endocrine cells in the brain. He tried it and it worked. The entire hypothalamo-neurohypophyseal system picked up the stain and was easily visible with its small granules attached to the neurons. The granules had been named the "Herring bodies." He had no difficulty getting his work published as he was the editor of the journal [7].

In 1950, Bargmann received a three-month travel grant from the Rockefeller Foundation and went to the United States. He showed his slides to Dr. Gomori, who was quite surprised at what this stain could do in the brain. He then moved on to Denver, where he renewed his acquaintance with the Scharrers after almost two decades [8]. Ernst Scharrer and Bargmann decided to write a paper together on the neurohypophysis, its staining for neurosecretory material, and the sequential motion of the granules down the neuron to the posterior pituitary [9]. The key observations were two. In one, when the neuronal axons were cut, the granules, instead of accumulating in the posterior pituitary, collected at the end of the neuronal stump, thus demonstrating that the granules moved down the neural portion of the pituitary stalk. In the other, dehydration caused the stainable material to disappear, thus suggesting strongly that the granules contain the hormone. This paper was later recalled as the one that caused "doubters [to] belatedly and often reluctantly accept that neurohypophyseal hormones were manufactured in the hypothalamus" [10]. Neurosecretion had arrived, at least for the posterior pituitary.

The switch in the attitudes of the endocrine scientific community toward the idea of neurosecretion is reflected in the texts of the time. For example, in 1948, a textbook of general endocrinology put the concept of neurosecretion in the chapter on invertebrates with a passing mention that the phenomenon may occur in mammals. It quotes the Scharrers and notes that "while most biologists ... view the concept of neurosecretion with some skepticism, future experiments may prove it to be a phenomenon of widespread importance" [11]. Seven years later, in the second edition of the same text, things had changed. We now read that "these older views can no longer be maintained and must be abandoned in favor of the neurosecretory origin of these [posterior pituitary] hormones" [12]. The major clinical textbook was a bit slower in acceptance but came around nevertheless. Thus, in 1950, it said that the posterior pituitary hormones were secreted by posterior pituitary cells that were stimulated by the hypothalamic neurons [13]. Five years later, in its second edition, it mentions, cautiously, that "these ... observations have been interpreted as indicating that ADH is formed chiefly in the hypothalamus and is transmitted in part to the neurohypophysis for storage" [14].

Another key indicator of acceptance was an invitation to the Scharrers in 1953 to present their findings to the annual Laurentian Hormone Conference in 1953. The title of their talk really says it all: "Hormones produced by neurosecretory cells." The paper, 58 pages long, was equally divided between Ernst and Berta, he covering vertebrates (especially mammals) and she insects. In the discussion that always took place after every presentation, Ernst was cautious and careful to note that "contradictory ... conclusions are frequent in this field, although people are seemingly doing the same experiments" and that "I am on very tenuous ground" [15]. This presentation, however cautiously worded, in fact made a clear impression on leaders in the field and almost certainly influenced the textbook authors.

The Scharrers' last academic move came in 1955 when they went back to New York to join the faculty of the brand new Albert Einstein College of Medicine, he as chairman of the Department of Anatomy and she as a full professor of anatomy, her first real academic appointment that paid a salary. Within a few years, the field of neuroendocrinology had become firm. The hypothalamus was being looked at for other neurosecretions that might control the secretion of the anterior pituitary hormones through the hypothalamo-pituitary portal system. The Scharrers' work clearly had an influence on this search, which culminated in the discovery of a full range of hypothalamic releasing factors or hormones and Nobel Prizes for two investigators.

Ernst and Berta Scharrer played a major role in the founding of the International Symposia on Neurosecretion beginning in 1953 and continuing for many years. They were both invited in 1960 to give the Jesup Lectures at Columbia University. The result was their book, *Neuroendocrinology*, that appeared in 1963 and nicely summarized the field and their life's work [16].

Ernst Scharrer died in 1965 in a swimming accident after 10 years as chairman of his department. Berta took over as acting chair for the next year and again in 1974–1975. She was elected to the National Academy of Sciences in 1967, was awarded 11 honorary degrees, and numerous other honors. One of these was the highest honor bestowed by the Endocrine Society, the Koch Award (1980). She became emeritus professor in 1978 and died in 1995. Her colleagues remember her elegance, modesty, and warmth.

Finally, one should note the absence of a sudden "discovery" in this saga. An idea with some but not strong evidence led the way. Evidence grew slowly over decades as other scientists rejected, considered, and then slowly accepted the possibility, and then the "reality," of the concept of neurosecretion.

References

1. Scharrer E: Die Lichtempfindlichkeit blinder Elrizen (Untersuchungen uber das Zwischenhirn der Fische). *Z Vergl Physiol* 1928; 7: 1.
2. Scharrer E, Scharrer B: Uber Drusen-Nervenzellen und neurosekretorische Organe bei Wirbellosen and Wirbeltieren. *Biol Rev* 1937; 12: 185.
3. Scharrer E, Scharrer B: Secretory cells within the hypothalamus. In *The Hypothalamus and Central Levels of Autonomic Function*, edited by JF Fulton, et al. Baltimore, MD: Williams and Wilkins, 1940, p. 170.

4. Scharrer B, Scharrer E: Neurosecretion. VI. A comparison between the intercerebralis-cardiacum-allatum system of the insects and the hypothalamo-hypophyseal system of the vertebrates. *Biol Bull* 1944; 87: 242.
5. Scharrer E, Scharrer B: Neurosecretion. *Physiol Rev* 1945; 25: 171.
6. Scharrer B: Hormones in insects. In *The Hormones. Physiology, Chemistry and Applications*, edited by G Pincus, KV Thimann. New York: Academic Press, 1948, p. 121.
7. Bargmann W. Uber die neurosekretorische Verknupfung von Hypothalamus und Neuroskeretorischerohypohypophyse. *Z Zellforsch* 1949; 34: 610.
8. Bargmann W, Marvelous region. In *Pioneers in Neuroendocrinology*, edited by J Meites, et al. New York: Plenum Press, 1975, p. 37.
9. Bargmann W, Scharrer E: The site of origin of the hormones of the posterior pituitary. *Am Scientist* 1951; 39: 255.
10. Sawyer WH: A short history of neurohypophysial research. *Ann NY Acad Sci* 1993; 689: 1.
11. Turner CD: *General Endocrinology*. Philadelphia, PA: W.B. Saunders, 1950, p. 66.
12. Turner C: *General Endocrinology* (2nd edn.). Philadelphia, PA: W.B. Saunders, 1955, p. 424.
13. Williams RH: *Textbook of Endocrinology*. Philadelphia, PA: W.B. Saunders, 1950, p. 66.
14. Williams RH: *Textbook of Endocrinology*. Philadelphia, PA: W.B. Saunders, 1955, p. 66.
15. Scharrer E, Scharrer B: Hormones produced by neurosecretory cells. *Rec Prog Horm Res* 1954; 10: 183.
16. Scharrer E, Scharrer B: *Neuroendocrinology*. New York: Columbia University Press, 1963.

Sources

Oksche A: In memoriam. Berta Scharrer. 1906–1995. *Cell Tiss Res* 1995; 282: 1.

Scharrer B: Neurosecretion and its role in neurosecretion and its role in neuroendocrine regulation. In *Pioneers in Neuroendocrinology*, edited by J Meites, et al. New York: Plenum Press, 1975, p. 527.

Scharrer B: The concept of neurosecretion and its place in neurobiology. In *The Neurosciences: Paths of Discovery*, edited by FG Worden, et al. Cambridge, MA: MIT Press, 1975, p. 231.

Scharrer B: Neurosecretion and neuroendocrinology in historical perspective. In *Hormones Proteins and Peptides*. Vol. 7: *Hypothalamic Hormones*, edited by C-H Li. New York: Academic Press, 1979, p. 279.

Scharrer B: Neurosecretion: Beginnings and new directions in neuropeptide research. *Annu Rev Neurosci* 1987; 10: 1–17.

This chapter has been reproduced from Sawin, Clark T: Berta and Ernst Scharrer and the concept of neurosecretion. *The Endocrinologist* 2003; 13(2): 73–6.

CHAPTER 80

Ulf Svante von Euler (1905–1983)

Neurosecretion of Norepinephrine

In December, 1970, the king of Sweden presented the Nobel Prize for Physiology or Medicine to three men: First was the American Julius Axelrod; second, the immigrant Englishman and secretary of London's Royal Society, Bernard Katz; and third was the king's countryman and chairman of the Nobel Foundation's board, Ulf Svante von Euler-Chelpin. Von Euler (he seems not to have used the last part of his legal surname) was the oldest of the three and won the prize because of his work in establishing that norepinephrine is the principal hormone secreted by adrenergic nerves. He also made original observations on substance P and the prostaglandins, the latter of which he had named, he later thought erroneously. There remains the suspicion of a bit of patronage in the award to him inasmuch as he had chaired the committee that awarded him the prize until 5 years before he won it.

Von Euler came to science with the equivalent of a silver spoon in his mouth. His father, Hans, was a well-known chemist who won the Nobel Prize for Chemistry in 1929 for work on what we would now call biochemistry. This is one of the few parent–child Nobelists and both have been honored with a Swedish postage stamp. In one sense, he was even better known than his son because the father is listed in the *Dictionary of Scientific Biography* (DSB) but the son is not (but then the DSB is weighted against biology and medicine). The paternal family had been established for generations in Bavaria, Germany. Hans moved to Stockholm in 1899 to become an assistant to another Nobelist and physical chemist, Svante Arrhenius. Hans became Swedish, was appointed successively to positions in physics, chemistry, and biochemistry at Stockholm's Hogscola (the University of Stockholm), and remained in Sweden for the rest of his life, during which he developed a major international center for biochemistry. The father's attachment to Arrhenius is clear. Ulf's middle name is after Arrhenius' first name, and Arrhenius was Ulf's godfather. Hans' attachment to Sweden was, however, not complete. While Sweden remained "neutral" in the First World War, as it did in the Second, Hans returned to Germany during WWI to fly and command in the nascent German air force for six months each year.

A Biographical History of Endocrinology, First Edition. D. Lynn Loriaux.

Ulf's mother, Astrid, nee Cleve, was also a scientist, as was her father, who was a professor of chemistry and the discoverer of two rare earth elements, holmium and thulium. Her father shifted his scientific interests in midlife to botany and the study of marine plankton, which he felt, when fossilized, could offer clues in the history of geology and oceanography. Astrid continued her father's later work until late in life. She wrote a lengthy monograph on diatoms in her late 70s.

Ulf's parents divorced in 1912; his father then remarried a Swedish chemist and raised another family. His mother taught school while the five children grew up on a farm outside Stockholm, supervised by a nurse with weekend visits from their mother. During the War years, food shortages affected Sweden as well as the belligerents, but the children did reasonably well with the added food from their mother's garden. Ulf, then 13 years old, went with his mother when she moved to head a research laboratory elsewhere in Sweden, in 1918, after the War was over.

When Ulf reached 17 years of age, he went to Stockholm to study medicine and live with his father. He attended medical school off and on for 8 years, receiving his degree in 1930. The delay, compared with the usual medical student, was not because of academic difficulty but rather because he was otherwise occupied. He was almost immediately involved in research. Following on his parents' careers, his first paper in 1922 was published with him as second author to his father. A remarkably authored paper in 1946 was written by three Nobelists; the two von Eulers and Gyorgy Hevesy. His father was a useful guide to other laboratories where Ulf could gain experience. Ulf recognized that the life of research after WWI was not an easy one. Facilities were, as elsewhere, almost laughably inadequate, with few positions and at best modest salaries. Yet, on recalling those days, von Euler felt that he was actually in a "privileged position."

In 1926, the 21-year-old von Euler, still a medical student, attended the 12th International Congress of Physiology in Stockholm. This was a formative experience for his future in science. The secretary was one of his own teachers, Goran Liljestrand. Others in attendance were the pioneers and leading lights of modern physiology: Ivan Pavlov, Ernest Starling, and Joseph Barcrof. Insulin had been in use for only a few years, and there was a demonstration of its physiologic action by one of its discoverers, Charles Best, and Henry Dale, in whose laboratory Best was spending a "sabbatical year." There was also a dramatic presentation by Otto Loewi on his "vagusstoff," later found to be acetylcholine (ACh). This was strong evidence that neuronal substances are released humorally to affect the tissues on which they act. The meeting had its moments of controversy. There was disagreement as to whether France or England were the best in physiology. There were also major disagreements on grafts of monkey testes into humans. Serge Voronoff claimed they were of clear value, but he was denounced as a charlatan by the classical American physiologist Anton Carlson. By then Ulf von Euler was fixed on a life of research. By the time he received his medical degree in 1930, he had published 18 papers. Ten of these were studies on the action of adrenaline (epinephrine), a clear premonition of the direction his career would take, and two were about insulin.

After von Euler graduated from medical school, he took an entry-level appointment in pharmacology at the Karolinska Institute. Liljestrand thought this was fine but that the opportunities were greater in physiology. So von Euler became an instant beneficiary of a Rockefeller Fellowship, one of the few well-funded programs that allowed scientists to learn from each other at an early stage in their careers. Von Euler went to Dale's laboratory for a few months in 1930, and by the end of the 2-year fellowship, he had visited laboratories in Birmingham, England; Ghent, Belgium; and Frankfurt, Germany. All were for von Euler to learn about physiology.

In Dale's laboratory at the National Institute for Medical Research in London, von Euler, then 25 years old, was assigned to work on Dale's principal interest, acetylcholine. Although Loewi had shown that there was a "vargusstoff," there was only speculation that it was acetylcholine because, although it mimicked the action of this "stoff," acetylcholine had never been found in the body, probably because of its short half-life. Dale remedied this situation in 1929, the year before von Euler's arrival. The laboratory was studying the substance intensively. Von Euler set to work to see whether he could show evidence of ACh in the perfusate of the electrically stimulated turtle and rabbit intestine. He failed. So he tried a simpler study: extract the intestine and see whether the extract had a substance that contracted another sample of intestine. This succeeded, but the substance could not be acetylcholine because its action was not blocked by atropine. Brashly, von Euler said that he had discovered a new biologically active substance. Few thought it so, but after some months more of work, aided by the experienced chemists at the Institute, some were convinced that he had discovered a new active substance. They called it substance "P" for preparation or, perhaps simply because the letter "P" was written on the bottle of the extract. "Substance P" it remains today. Then, of course, no one knew whether or not it had any physiologic role.

Some of von Euler's work in the early 1930s took up other issues in general of standard endocrinology. For example, he wrote several papers on the physiology and pharmacology of thyroxine and pituitary extracts. His main interest, however, continued to be adrenaline-like substances, and his curiosity was aimed at natural biologically active materials. Adrenaline was present, for example, in the sheep prostate. But the bioassays still showed activity after the adrenaline was destroyed. Could it be substance P in the prostate? The material from sheep prostate and human seminal fluid acted somewhat like substance P, but differed from it significantly when subjected to multiple bioassays. Purified preparations of the new substance showed it to be lipid-like. Thinking that the prostate gland was its principal source, von Euler named the substance "prostaglandin" and first used the name in a paper published in 1936. He was only 31 years old.

Von Euler pursued "prostaglandin," believing that it came from the prostate gland and that a similar material came from the seminal vesicles ("vesiglandin"). Only some years later did he realize that the main source was actually the seminal vesicles and not the prostate gland. Decades later, others realized that the apparently separate substances from the prostate and seminal vesicles were actually different mixtures of several prostaglandins. Over the course of the mid to late 1930s, von Euler continued his attempts to purify prostaglandin with the help of the Icelandic Slaughter Company, which provided large numbers of sheep seminal vesicles. He retained a life-long interest in this strange lipid that had no known physiologic function. After the War, some of his freeze-dried, semi-purified material left over from the 1930s still had activity. After a lecture on lipids by Sune Bergström, von Euler offered Bergström some of the material to study. So began another pathway that led to the elucidation of the chemical structure of the first prostaglandins and a Nobel Prize for Bergström in 1982. Von Euler's last paper, published in 1983, the year of his death, was a review of the prostaglandins.

By 1939, von Euler had been promoted to full professor and chairman of the Department of Physiology at the Karolinska Institute and was actively attacking the topic of adrenaline. In fact, he had never stopped. The hypothesis had been raised by several others that the active principle secreted by sympathetic nerves was adrenaline. Or maybe it was noradrenaline. But how could one tell?

There had been considerable interest in adrenaline as the hormone of the adrenal medulla for almost half a century. The interest began with the fascinating demonstration in 1893 of the blood pressure-raising effect of an adrenal extract. This was the result of a collaboration between a London clinician, George Oliver, and Edward Schafer, the professor of physiology at London's University College. The "active principle" was rapidly found to be adrenaline. By the end of the 1890s, its structure and chemical synthesis were complete. In fact, it was the first hormone to have a defined structure and the first to be made in the laboratory. For a time, adrenaline *was* the adrenal hormone because it took until the mid-1920s for everyone to realize that the anatomic distinction of medulla and cortex in the adrenal gland actually had physiologic meaning. The medullary extract did not, for example, successfully treat Addison's disease, whereas lipid extracts of the cortex did, at least in animals.

Although adrenaline might not be the adrenal hormone, physiologists of this era had improved in their study of the sympathetic nervous system. They now knew that the adrenal medulla, with its adrenaline, was a part of this system. The speculation arose that perhaps sympathetic nerves, at least at their postganglionic sites, might use adrenaline to bring about their actions on responsive tissues. The idea came to light as early as 1904 when the British physiologist Thomas Elliott first proposed that nervous transmission was a humoral event. During the 1920s and 1930s, the major proponent of this view was Harvard's professor of physiology Walter Cannon. There are differences between "sympathetic actions" and the actions of adrenaline itself. Because analogues of adrenaline were fairly easy to make in the laboratory, a wide range of compounds in this catecholamine class were available. It took a while for investigators to realize that these were often racemic mixtures of D- and L-versions of the same compounds. However, there was a suspicion in the 1930s that norepinephrine might be the neurotransmitter rather than adrenaline itself, mainly because its actions nearly mimicked those of sympathetic nerve stimulation.

Immediately after the Second World War, von Euler thought that this would be a good problem to study. He thought he could make a real contribution, in part, because of his extensive prior experience with adrenaline. His first step was to see whether there was any noradrenaline in the adrenal medulla. He found only adrenaline in rabbit adrenal glands. There was then no support for noradrenaline. However, others did find noradrenaline in the adrenal medulla of other species. The idea was in fact a sound one (von Euler had picked one of the few species in which the adrenal medulla contains mainly adrenaline). So he persisted. In the summer of 1945, he got some pure L-noradrenaline indirectly from Hermann Blaschko, then in Oxford, as well as another sample from New York. Now von Euler was able to compare, both chemically and physiologically, the known chemical, noradrenaline, with a sufficiently large amount of sympathomimetic substance directly extracted from bovine spleen. The chemical and the extract were the same. By 1946, von Euler had published these results.

The idea that sympathetic nerves made and secreted noradrenaline still was not acceptable to most physiologists. A few, including Nobelist Bernardo Houssay, were strong supporters. Von Euler was his own strongest supporter. By the late 1940s, there was a international interest in his work. He published a series of experimental papers in favor of the idea. Slowly, by the end of the decade, it seems that most physiologists were won over to the idea that noradrenaline was the sympathetic transmitter and also acted as a hormone. Physicians may have been more convinced by von Euler's, and other's, demonstration of large amounts of noradrenaline in the urine of patients with pheochromocytoma. It is fair to say that, by 1950, all were convinced.

Von Euler went on to deal with the puzzle of how such a metabolically labile substance as noradrenaline could survive in a neuron until it was needed, then to be released only on nervous stimulation. This led him and many others to look at the peculiar granules found in these nerves, now known to be storage granules, but that is another story.

Von Euler clearly recognized the role of informed luck in his work as well as the influence of context and environment. He knew well that scientific advance often is not a series of flashes of light but rather the culmination of "apparently lackluster and uninspired, tedious work." He experienced in his own work the phenomenon of others' initial resistance to his data, followed almost immediately by the criticism that, "well, it's probably true but isn't new." He also knew that all ideas that are readily acceptable are not necessarily correct, that sometimes ideas are "fashionable" and that to "turn the tide in such cases is often a slow and tiresome process." But, even so, he was comfortable with the state of affairs because it would "challenge the ingenuity ... of the proponents and lead to a quicker solution of the problem."

Von Euler retired as professor in 1971, loaded with honors and with an international reputation for the quality of his work. He died in Stockholm in 1983 at the age of 78 from the complications of open-heart surgery. The Nobel Prize in 1970 was probably his most prominent award, but endocrinologists saw him as one of theirs. In 1972, he was awarded the Dale Medal, named for one of his mentors, by the British Society for Endocrinology. For endocrinologists today, he is most remembered for his life in science as a physician–investigator.

References

Blaschko HKF: Ulf Svante von Euler. *Biogr Mem Fellows R Soc Lond* 1985; 31: 145.

Kyle RA, Shampo MA: Ulf von Euler – norepinephrine and the Nobel Prize. *Mayo Clin Proc* 1995; 70: 273.

Kyle RA, Shampo MA: Hans von Euler-Chelpin – Nobel laureate. *Mayo Clin Proc* 1996; 71: 596.

Manger WM, Gifford RW (Eds.): *Clinical and Experimental Pheochromocytoma*. Cambridge, MA: Blackwell Science 1996, p. xiii.
Von Euler US: Pieces in the puzzle. *Annu Rev Pharmacol* 1971; 11: 1.
Von Euler C: Curt von Euler. In *The History of Neuroscience in Autobiography*, Vol. 1, edited by LR Squire. Washington, DC: Society for Neuroscience, 1996, p. 528.
Whitteridge D: *One Hundred Years of Congresses of Physiology*. Oulu: International Union of Physiological Sciences, 1989.

This chapter has been reproduced from Sawin, Clark T: Ulf Svante von Euler (1905–1983) and the neurosecretion of norepinephrine. *The Endocrinologist* 1999; 9(5): 327–30.

CHAPTER 81

Saul Hertz
(1905–1950)
Radioactive Iodine and the Treatment of Graves' Disease

I was walking down the twelfth floor corridor in Building 10 of the NIH with Roy Hertz to look at his new laboratory. He had just been made a Scientist Emeritus and was anxious to get started. We were talking about the different places we had trained and when he learned that I had been a house office at the Peter Bent Brigham Hospital, he asked if I had liked the Harvard people I had worked with. I replied that I had liked them very much. "Why do you ask?" I said. "It is a long story that I will tell you sometime," he replied. "They destroyed my brother." The topic never came up again, but I looked into it myself to see if I could get a sense of what he was talking about. The story follows.

Saul Hertz, born in 1905 in Cleveland, Ohio, was the oldest of seven sons, hence Roy's "big brother." He attended public school and then went to the University of Michigan, graduating with a BS in biology and a Phi Beta Kappa key. He went to Harvard Medical School, and then a residency in internal medicine at Cleveland's Mount Sinai Hospital. He then returned to Boston to join the Thyroid Unit at the Massachusetts General Hospital. He began his academic career with Dr. Jacob Herman working on exophthalmic goiter and the effects of iodine on the disease. Some time between then and 1934, he became the director of the Thyroid Clinic under the supervision of James Howard Means. On November 12, 1936, the direction of his research took a new and unexpected turn. On that day, Karl Compton, the president of MIT, gave a lecture to a group of Harvard faculty entitled "What physics can do for biology and medicine." He mentioned the great potential that radioactive "tracers" had for helping to sort out the complex mechanisms of metabolism. It is said, and most of the principals agree, that in the question and answer period, Hertz asked if "Iodine could be made artificially radioactive." Compton said that he did not know, but would get back to him with an answer. On December 15, Compton wrote to Hertz that an iodine isotope with a half-life of about 25 minutes, I^{128}, could be made relatively easily.

During the next six months, Compton and Means developed a project to produce I^{128} and to understand its potential role in sorting out thyroid physiology and pathophysiology.

A Biographical History of Endocrinology, First Edition. D. Lynn Loriaux.

This work is a co-publication between the Endocrine Society and John Wiley & Sons, Ltd.

Robley Evans PhD, a junior faculty at MIT, was given the task of producing the radioactive isotopes of iodine. He gathered as many used radon needles as he could find and incorporated them into a small block of paraffin which became the neutron source used to bombard ethyl iodide. A small amount of I^{128} was created, enough to begin animal experiments. Hertz was given the responsibility, and he started with a measurement of iodine uptake into a rabbit's thyroid gland. The research progressed at a rapid pace. It was clear to everyone that isotopes with a longer half-life were going to be a necessity, I^{130} with a half-life of 2 hours, I^{126} with a half-life of 13 days, and I^{131} with a half-life of 8 days. For these isotopes, they were going to need a cyclotron, the money for which, $30 000, was provided by the Markle Foundation. This cyclotron, sited at MIT, was the world's first cyclotron built exclusively for biological and medical use. Its first product was I^{130} produced by deuteron (the deuterium nucleus, a neutron and a proton) bombardment of tellurium. Hertz's early animal studies rapidly evolved into the treatment of Graves' disease with I^{130}. Means worried that I^{130} treatment might lead to thyroid storm. He decided that patients treated with I^{130} also be given Lugol's solution as a "storm" preventative.

It was about this time that Joe Hamilton, a young MD physiologist and a member of the original Compton–Means group, decided to return to California. He had Means' blessing to continue the radioactive iodine studies on the West Coast. He developed a strong collaboration with the Radiation laboratories at Berkeley. Mayo Soley, a former MGH house officer, led the clinical activities of the initiative. They were the first to use I^{131} as a therapeutic agent. Using I^{131}, they replicated all of Hertz's studies with Roberts, except that they did not use concomitant treatment with Lugol's solution. This group worked on the I^{131} treatment of Graves' disease until Soley's untimely death in 1949. The work of this group seems to be the stimulus for creating a new specialty in nuclear medicine. At this juncture, it was clear that Saul Hertz had treated the first Graves' patient with radioactive iodine (I^{130}) in January of 1941. Hamilton had been the first to use I^{131} in October of 1941.

Hertz joined the Navy in 1943 and did not return until 1946. Means asked Earl Chapman to direct the Thyroid Clinic in Hertz's absence. There is no evidence that any commitment was made to Hertz about resuming his job, clinic chief, when he returned. Means then asked Rulon Rawson to direct the Thyroid Clinic. At the time that Hertz left, he and Roberts had treated 29 patients with Graves' disease, 20 with ancillary Lugol's solution. In Hertz's absence, Chapman and Robley Evans treated 22 more patients and none received Lugol's solution.

The subsequent events are well described by David Becker [1]:

> The next stage in this Saga occurred when Hertz entered the Navy in April 1943 and asked Earle Chapman to take over his radioiodine treated patients. Chapman soon discovered that many of Hertz's patients were taking potassium iodide making clinical evaluation difficult, and some were still hyperthyroid. Most of these patients had received KI – shortly after the radioiodine – apparently at Mean's insistence. This became a point of contention and controversy. Means commented somewhat defensively in a paper in 1949 that he felt it necessary to follow radioactive iodine with "ordinary iodine" … . To protect the patients against the mischief from thyrotoxicosis during a period in which treatment of unknown efficacy was being tried out.

> Early in 1946, Morris Fishbein then editor of the JAMA wrote to Means about two manuscripts he had received on the treatment of hyperthyroidism with radioiodine. They both came from the MGH Thyroid Clinic, both used the same I^{130}–I^{131} mixture from MIT, and both thanked Means for his support – but both had different authors. Fishbein – diplomatically asked Means for clarification. Means – also diplomatically – wrote back explaining simply that they were two different excellent series. Fishbein took the hint and so in the May 11, 1946 issue of the JAMA there were two papers on radioiodine treatment of hyperthyroidism from MGH. The first, on page 81, was a follow-up of 29 patients treated by Hertz and Roberts in 1941 and 1942 ... and the second on page 86 was a new series of 22 patients treated by Chapman and Evans.

The issue of the appropriate dose of I^{130} was never resolved. One week after the publication of these two papers, in the June 14 issue of *Science*, radionuclides in large quantities and of high purity were made immediately available from the Manhattan Project.

> That announcement opened the Modern Radioisotope Era. In the following year (1946), 407 shipments of radioactive materials for medical therapy were made from Oak Ridge, and by five years later, the number had risen tenfold – most of which was I^{131}.

John Stanbury sums up the episode like this:

> It may be interesting to interject a personal view of priorities in the introduction of radioiodine into medicine at this point. Hertz, Roberts, and Evans clearly were the first to report studies on animals. Just who verbalized the idea, whether Means or Hertz, of using radioactive iodine at that fateful luncheon at Vanderbilt Hall will remain a mystery, but the idea came from a joint discussion among Means, Chapman, Hertz and Lerman. Nevertheless, quite certainly it was Hertz who posed the question to President Compton. Means was familiar with radiation effects on the overactive thyroid gland from his work with Holmes in the 1920's, so that from the earliest discussions there was a consensus that radioiodine might be used for the treatment of Graves' disease. Hamilton and his colleagues began using radioiodine almost at the same time. Insofar as the therapeutic program is concerned, Hertz, Means, Evans, and colleagues did indeed interject an element of uncertainty by adding stable iodide after radioiodine, but the paper of Hertz and Roberts in the Journal of the American Medical Association in 1946 makes it perfectly clear that most of their patients were successfully treated by radioactive iodine alone. Thus my own view is that the priorities both for investigations of thyroid function and in therapeutics belong to Hertz, Means and Evans, and my additional perspective is that in these instances the issue of priority is not particularly important [2].

Coming back after the Second World War ended, Hertz did not assume his previous position as chief of the thyroid unit. The reason is not known, but the unravelling of things at the end of this glittering chapter in American medicine probably left no one feeling fairly treated.

Mayo Soley committed suicide in 1949, and Saul Hertz committed suicide in 1950. Joe Hamilton died of multiple myeloma, probably the result of radiation overexposure, as we see in so many radiologists of the time. This is probably what Roy Hertz was going to tell me, but we will never know. If it is of any consolation, I know of no other family in which the concentration of creative intellect was so high as it was in the Hertz family. We have a lot to thank the Hertz family for.

References

1. Becker DV: The early history of the use of radioiodine in thyroid disease. Presidential Address, American Thyroid Association, October 7, 1983, pp. 12–13.
2. Stanbury JB: *"A Constant Ferment." A History of the Thyroid Clinic and Laboratory at the MGH. 1913–1990.* Ipswich, MA: Ipswich Press, 1991.

CHAPTER 82

George Widmer Thorn (1906–2004)

The Treatment of Addison's Disease

George Thorn died on June 26, 2004, in Beverly, Massachusetts at the age of 98 years. He was one of the leading endocrinologists of our age.

Thorn was born in Buffalo, New York, on January 15, 1906. He attended the College of Wooster in Ohio followed by the University of Buffalo Medical School, earning the MD degree in 1929. He did his postgraduate training at the Johns Hopkins Medical Center and stayed on as a faculty member until he was appointed physician in chief at the Peter Bent Brigham Hospital in 1942. He held this post for 30 years.

Thorn was a pioneer in the diagnosis and treatment of Addison's disease. He devised the first useful clinical test for the diagnosis of this condition. The cortisol response to an ACTH challenge was assessed indirectly by the effect of cortisol on the eosinophil count, the "Thorn test." He was among the first to use synthetic glucocorticoids to treat the disease. The first preparation he used for this purpose was desoxycorticosterone acetate (DOCA). It was marginally effective and was associated with the unusual side effect of calcification of the pinna of the external ear, Thorn's sign. With the availability of cortisone acetate, he established the optimum dose of replacement steroid, devised the concept of giving two thirds of the dose in the morning and one third in the evening, still used by many endocrinologists, and proposed that stressful conditions such as surgery should be "covered" with increased doses of glucocorticoid in patients with adrenal insufficiency.

Thorn was among the first to propose and actively investigate organ transplantation. It was he who persuaded Willem Kolff of the Netherlands to bring his prototype "artificial kidney" to the United States for development. This work was done in the Peter Bent Brigham Hospital and was fundamental to the success of kidney transplantation. The first dramatic success in this effort occurred in 1954 with the successful transplantation of a kidney between identical twins under the direction of Dr. Joseph Murray. This effort led to the Nobel Prize in Medicine for Murray and to the transplantation of other organs, including the heart, liver, lungs, and pancreas.

A Biographical History of Endocrinology, First Edition. D. Lynn Loriaux.

This work is a co-publication between the Endocrine Society and John Wiley & Sons, Ltd.

One of Thorn's many influential patients was Howard Hughes. In the course of their physician–patient relationship, Thorn interested Hughes in endowing a fund to support medical research. Over the years, this grew into the Howard Hughes Medical Institute (HHMI), the most prestigious of the non-National Institutes of Health funding agencies. Thorn was affiliated with HHMI for more than 40 years as director of research, president, and chairman of the board from 1984 to 1990. He was also a founding editor of *Harrison's Textbook of Medicine*, the dominant medical text of the twentieth century.

I was a house office in Thorn's program at "The Brigham" in the final years of his tenure there. He was a remarkable chief: patient, kind, insightful, and without a scintilla of bombast or self-aggrandizement. In my time with him, he gave me two important gifts: insight into the mind of the complete physician and insight into the power of a committed mentor.

The first insight came through the medium of the "work-up" of his private patients. By and large these people were wealthy "movers and shakers" of society. They would come to see Dr. Thorn at regular intervals, usually annually. They would carry diagnoses such as "partial adrenal insufficiency" or "idiopathic hypothalamic dysfunction." They would enter the hospital exhausted, enervated, and discomfited, often unable to "go on." The house staff, as a rule, resented these patients for occupying a valuable hospital bed by virtue of wealth, fame, or celebrity. They were not sick as defined by tired interns and residents. They were, however, diseased in its literal sense. Thorn would see them and they would brighten. He would prescribe small, almost homeopathic doses of cortisol to "supplement" the axis and Dilantin (phenytoin) to "quiet" the hypothalamus. He was also fond of vitamin E. By the end of the week, the women were wearing make-up again, and the men were shaved. They could not wait to get out of the hospital and get back into the foray of life. Thorn always held them an extra day to ensure that the new regimen was "optimized." It was the "royal touch" in its purest form. I never saw it fail. I came late to the realization of what Thorn knew all along. It is always easier to restore "well" people to productive life than it is the chronically ill. I still often use a CT scan as a therapeutic intervention. Evidence-based medicine is mute on the subject.

Then I learned a lesson about the power of a committed mentor. The story goes like this. Two months into my internship, a community physician admitted, late one Friday evening, a man with advanced and rapidly progressing cirrhosis of the liver resulting from alcohol abuse. He was deeply jaundiced and had ascites, pleural effusions, and esophageal varices. The patient came into the hospital with a set of directions from his physician to do a number of tests and procedures, including a thoracentesis and paracentesis. I argued that these invasive procedures in a man with a very prolonged bleeding time were likely to lead to complications, but to no avail. Instructions from the chief resident were to get on with it, and so I did. The thoracentesis and paracentesis were done at approximately 9:00 that night. I was called back to the bedside at midnight. The nurse said that the patient was experiencing difficulty breathing. He was hypotensive and diaphoretic. I found a very tense but nonacute abdomen and suspected a hemoperitoneum. Not surprisingly, a second "tap" produced serosanguineous fluid with a hematocrit of approximately 15%. Luckily, he had been typed and crossmatched with 5 units of packed red cells in the blood bank. The blood bank was far from the patient's bedside, down a long corridor running the length of the hospital called "the Pike." The blood was kept in a large refrigerator in alphabetical order and could be signed out after hours by any physician needing it. I ran down the pike, signed out 1 unit, and ran back, instructing the nurse to give the blood under pressure from a blood pressure cuff. I ran back for a second unit and then a third. The pike was dimly lit at night, and returning with the third unit, I could hear, but not see, someone running toward me from the far end. Then I made out the nurse from my patient's bedside. "What is the man's name?" she shouted. Let us say his name was McGee. "McGee" I shouted. "Oh no," she said. "The band says McFee!" "Not possible" I said. "Let's look together." She was right. McFee. Wrong wristband, total ABO mismatch. The spun hematocrit was so hemolyzed that the meniscus of red cells could barely be discerned. The patient died a few hours later. I was stricken. What was I doing here anyway? Trying my best to do good, I had failed in the most flagrant way imaginable.

In the next few days I found it difficult to concentrate. I lost my appetite, and my thinking became solipsistic. I was asked to present the case to the assembled staff of the Brigham on Thursday morning at 8:00 a.m. I can take you to the spot I stood to make the presentation if you want to see it. I can tell you who sat in what seat in the first row. I am sure the presentation was halting in an unsure voice and that it was a brutal thing to watch. I cannot remember that part. The staff and most of my peers looked at their shoes or fiddled with their fingernails. Some beeped themselves out of the conference. What followed was a discussion akin to death by a thousand cuts. I was done, finished. I remember leaving the auditorium alone in a crowd of distinguished physicians and physicians to be. I can remember my visual fields constricting to tunnels and thinking that I cannot go on many more minutes – overmatched by place and task. I was trying to sort out how to leave the hospital quietly and to remember the number of the bus that would get me home. Then, I felt a tug on my coat sleeve. I looked around but saw no one. The tug came again and looking down I saw Dr. Thorn. "Here it comes," I thought, "the call to the office for the final chapter."

"Lynn" he said. I could only look at him. "If I ever need a blood transfusion, I want you to give it to me." "He is mocking me," I thought. He smiled. It was a smile like none I had ever seen before – understanding and empathetic at once – sincere, beatific. "Did you hear me?" he said. A few other people were now walking along in step with us. "If I ever need a transfusion, you better be here to give it to me. Do you understand what I am saying to you?" "I think I do," I stammered. He was saying that I had made a bad mistake, like most physicians will sometime in their lives, and that he knew it was an honest error of commission that I would not repeat. He was saying he still trusted me as a doctor and valued me as a person. It was the smile, however, that made the point. It would have been enough. "Good," he said. "Good, let's get on with it. It will be a long day." And so he walked on, and a few of my fellow interns gathered around and started talking about the things we would usually talk about, and I began my climb out of the darkest recess of my life. That was about 40 years ago. I think about it nearly every day. The world will remember him as a mentor in the finest sense of the word – a father unfettered by the ties that bind. Can a better thing be said about any man?

Sources

King N: George Thorn, 98, pioneer in Addison's disease, dies. *New York Times*, July 18, 2004.
Nathan D: George Widmer Thorn. *Trans Clin Climatol Assoc* 2005; 116: 64–6.

This chapter has been reproduced from Loriaux, D. Lynn: George Widmer Thorn (1906–2004) – The treatment of Addison's disease. *The Endocrinologist* 2004; 14: 305–6.

CHAPTER 83

Hans Hugo Bruno Selye
(1907–1982)
Stress and the Endocrine System

Hans Selye was born in Vienna on January 26, 1907. He was the son of a physician, Dr. Hugo Selye, an Hungarian. His early childhood years were spent in Komarno, Slovakia, where his father was stationed during the First World War. Sited at the confluence of the Danube and Vah rivers, Komarno was an Hungarian cultural center. Selye's basic education was received there. He began his medical studies with the medical faculty in Prague, and graduated from the German University in Prague in 1929. He obtained a position as assistant to the Institute of Experimental Pathology and remained there until 1931, when he won a Rockefeller scholarship to spend a year at Johns Hopkins University. In 1932 he moved to the Institute of Experimental Medicine and Surgery at the Université de Montréal, and remained there until 1976, 42 years. He was professor of histology from June 1941 to 1945, and director of the Institute thereafter. In 1979, in association with Alvin Toffler, he founded the Canadian Institute of Stress, and remained there until his death in 1982.

Selye's entire scientific career was based upon an experiment he did in 1935 at 28 years of age. He was looking for a new endocrine factor of ovarian origin and his experiments were based upon the injection of ovarian "extracts" into rats. To his great excitement, he found that this treatment resulted in adrenal hypertrophy, atrophy of the thymus, and gastrointestinal hemorrhage from mucosal ulcerations. The severity of the syndrome varied directly with the dose of the extract. He was sure that he was on the trail of a new endocrine factor. The "control" experiments, however, told a different story. He found exactly the same results with placental extract, pituitary extract, and formalin. His disappointment must have been great. On the other hand, Selye recognized a uniform response to homeostatic "threat," which he termed "stress." The stress response, regardless of the "stressor," had three phases. The first phase began 6–48 hours after the injury and consisted of a rapid decrease in the size of thymus, spleen, and lymph nodes, disappearance of fat, and acute hemorrhagic erosions in the gastrointestinal tract. The second phase began 48 hours after injury and was characterized by adrenal hypertrophy, thyroid atrophy, and gonadal atrophy.

A Biographical History of Endocrinology, First Edition. D. Lynn Loriaux.

This work is a co-publication between the Endocrine Society and John Wiley & Sons, Ltd.

The third phase occurred only if the noxious challenge was continued. In this phase, all of the affected organs returned to a relatively "normal" baseline level of function in spite of continuation of the "stress" stimulus. Selye termed this sequence of events as the "general alarm reaction" followed by the "general adaptation syndrome."

This work was published in *Nature*, Vol. 138, p. 32, 1936. The entire paper, "A syndrome produced by diverse nocuous agents," was five paragraphs long:

> Experiments on rats show that if the organism is severely damaged by acute nonspecific nocuous agents such as exposure to cold, surgical injury, production of spinal shock transection of the cord, excessive muscular exercise, or intoxications with sub-lethal doses of diverse drugs (adrenaline, atropine, morphine, formaldehyde, etc.), a typical syndrome appears, the symptoms of which are independent of the nature of the damaging agent or the pharmacological type of the drug employed, and represent rather a response to damage as such.
>
> The syndrome develops in three stages: during the first stage, 6–48 hours after initial injury, one observes rapid decrease in size of the thymus, spleen, lymph glands, and liver; disappearance of fat tissue; edema formation especially in the thymus and loose retroperitoneal connective tissue; accumulation of pleural and peritoneal transudate; loss of muscular tone; fall of body temperature; formation of acute erosions in the digestive tract, particularly in the stomach, small intestine, and appendix; loss of cortical lipoids and chromaffin substance from the adrenals; and sometimes hyperemia of the skin, exophthalmos, [and] increased lachrymation and salivation. In particularly severe cases, focal necrosis of the liver and dense clouding of the crystalline lens are observed.
>
> In the second stage, beginning 48 hours after the injury, the adrenals are greatly enlarged but regain their lipoid granules, while the medullary chromaffin cells show vacuolization; the edema begins to disappear; numerous basophiles appear in the pituitary; the thyroid shows a tendency towards hyperplasia (more marked in the guinea pig); general body growth ceases and the gonads become atrophic; in lactating animals, milk secretion stops. It would seem that the anterior pituitary ceases production of growth and gonadotropic hormones and prolactin in favor of increased elaboration of thyrotrophic and adrenotropic principles, which may be regarded as more urgently needed in such emergencies.
>
> If the treatment be continued with relatively small doses of the drug or relatively slight injuries, the animals will build up such resistance that in the later part of the second stage the appearance and function of their organs returns practically to normal; but with further treatment, after a period of one to three months (depending on the severity of the damaging agent), the animals lose their resistance and succumb with symptoms similar to those seen in the first stage. This phase of exhaustion being regarded as the third stage of the syndrome.
>
> We consider the first stage to be the expression of a general alarm of the organism when suddenly confronted with a critical situation, and therefore term it the "general alarm reaction." Since the syndrome as a whole seems to represent a generalized effort of the organism to adapt itself to new conditions, it might be termed the "general adaption syndrome." It might be compared to other general defense reactions such as inflammation or the formation of immune bodies. The symptoms of the alarm reaction are very similar to those of histamine toxicosis or of surgical or anaphylactic shock; it is therefore not unlikely that an essential part in the initiation of the syndrome is the liberation of large quantities of histamine or some similar substance, which may be released from the tissues either mechanically in surgical injury, or by other means in other cases. It seems to us that more or less pronounced forms of this three-stage reaction represent the usual response of the organism to stimuli such as temperature changes, drugs, muscular exercise, etc., to which habituation or inurement can occur [1].

It soon became clear that humans responded to "stress" much the same as rats do, and that almost every injury or systemic illness would be associated with a "general adaptive response." Clinical medicine took a step forward. Much of what clinicians were contending with at the bedside turned out to be the response to an illness, not the illness itself. A transformative insight.

All that Selye did after this seminal experiment was derivative to it, and he did a lot: 1700 publications, 40 books, thousands of presentations and addresses. He was the most celebrated endocrinologist of the twentieth century. He was a Doctor Honoris Causi 43 times, he was nominated for the Nobel Prize 10 times, he became a Fellow of the Royal Society of Canada, and an Honorary Fellow of 68 other scientific societies, an honorary citizen of more than a dozen countries, recipient of the Starr Medal of the Canadian Medical Association, the Prix de l'Oeuvre Scientifique, the Killam scholarship, the International Kittay Award, the Canadian Authors Association Literary Award for nonfiction, and a Companion of the Order of Canada.

Was he a genius? Not by my definition, which requires at least two "great insights" – Fuller Albright was a genius with only 116 papers. Selye, however, was brilliant, hard-working, articulate, and wedded to the basic science of human disease. Celebrity is only loosely linked to genius as everybody knows. Selye is a great example of this. None the less, he recognized the biologic consequences of stress for the first time, and brought order and structure to the concept. His idea is still going strong.

Reference

1. Selye H: A syndrome produced by diverse nocuous agents. *Nature* 1936; 138: 32.

This chapter has been reproduced from Loriaux, D. Lynn: Hans Hugo Bruno Selye (1907–1982). *The Endocrinologist* 2008; 18(2): 53–4.

CHAPTER 84

Jerome W. Conn (1907–1994)

Adrenal Mediated High Blood Pressure

Jerome Conn was born in New York City in 1907. He was the oldest of four children. His father, Joseph, owned and operated a luncheonette, and his mother, Dora, was a homemaker. Jerry was an excellent student and skipped a grade in elementary school. He went to Rutgers University and, after 3 years, went on to the University of Michigan Medical School. It was 1920, a year before "Black Tuesday." During the ensuing period of financial penury, his two sisters worked as secretaries and largely paid for his medical education [1].

Jerry graduated with honors and was elected to the Alpha Omega Alpha honor society. He became interested in clinical research, and married a like-minded student, Betty Stern. He started an internship in surgery at Michigan, but switched to medicine a year later. After residency was complete, Jerry and his wife joined the laboratory of Louis H. Newburgh, an expert in the areas of obesity, diabetes, and energy metabolism.

Jerry became an assistant professor in 1938, director of the Division of Endocrinology and Metabolism in 1943, and was named the L.H. Newburgh Distinguished University Professor in 1968. He spent his entire academic career at the University of Michigan, retiring in 1974. Conn's research focused on two areas – hypertension and diabetes mellitus. He is best known for his work in hypertension and his description of Conn's syndrome.

During the Second World War, Conn began a series of investigations focused on acclimatization to environmental heat. He made careful measurements of salt loss in sweat, saliva, urine, and feces and was able to show that acclimatization was dependent upon a rapid reduction in salt loss. He postulated that the mechanism of this reduction in salt loss was a "salt-active corticoid" from the adrenal glands. He attempted to identify these corticosteroids without much success. (Aldosterone was ultimately isolated and characterized by Simpson and Tait in 1950) [2].

But chance favored the prepared mind. A 34-year-old woman was admitted to Conn's care in 1954, complaining of episodic muscle weakness that could be so severe as to cause paralysis of her legs. The laboratory test revealed hypokalemia and alkalosis.

A Biographical History of Endocrinology, First Edition. D. Lynn Loriaux.

This work is a co-publication between the Endocrine Society and John Wiley & Sons, Ltd.

She had no signs of Cushing's syndrome. Sodium chloride balance studies showed her to be in the range of "heat acclimated" volunteers. Conn hypothesized that the cause of her disease was the hypersecretion of salt-active corticoid. David Streeten, a young associate at the time, demonstrated excess mineralocorticoid in her urine using a bioassay in adrenalectomized rats. Conn was convinced that she had a mineralocorticoid-secreting tumor. Surgical exploration revealed a 4-cm tumor, which was removed leading to resolution of the patient's complaints. This was "Conn's syndrome." Conn became the world's referral source for this disease, and most of what we know about mineralocorticoid disorders is provided by his research.

As the work of others clarified the role of renin as the trophic hormone for aldosterone secretion, Conn used plasma renin to clarify the various causes of mineralocorticoid excess, primary and secondary, and of mineralocorticoid deficiency, primary and secondary. He described one of the first cases of renin hypersecretion by a renal tumor.

Conn's other passion was "glucose tolerance" and insulin secretion. He was one of the first to recognize the effects of obesity on insulin resistance, and to show that weight loss could reverse the effect. He was one of the first to use the new radioimmunoassay for insulin and demonstrated the effectiveness of leucine and arginine in stimulating insulin secretion. He was one of the first to show excess glucocorticoid administration led to insulin resistance in much the same way as obesity.

Conn authored 284 scientific papers and book chapters. He received many honors, including the Claude Bernard Medal, the Banting Medal, the Henry Russell Award, the Gordon Wilson Medal of the American Clinical and Climatological Association, and the Elliot Proctor Joslin Award. He was elected to the National Academy of Sciences in 1969.

He left us an insightful picture of life as a translational investigator in his presidential address to the Central Society for Clinical Research in Chicago, Illinois in 1954 [3].

> Let us remember that we are all painting background. Regardless of how important or unimportant your contribution of today may seem, no sooner has it been expounded than it has become background. There is some solace in the fact that your brain child is not dead! The entire background is seething with life and motion, but acceptance of the idea of painting background is sufficient to remove the undesirable gusts of wind from many sails. Let us rejoice in the knowledge that to us has come the opportunity to paint background.

References

1. Daughaday WH: Jerome Conn. *Biographical Memoirs*. Washington, DC: National Academy of Sciences, 1997.
2. Simpson SA, Tait JF, Bush IE: Secretion of a salt retaining hormone by the adrenal cortex. *Lancet* 1952; 263: 226–8.
3. Conn JW. Presidential address. II. Primary aldosteronism, a new clinical syndrome. *J Lab Clin Med* 1955; 45: 3–17.

This chapter has been reproduced from Loriaux, D. Lynn: Jerome W. Conn (1907–1994). *The Endocrinologist* 2008; 18(4): 159–60.

CHAPTER 85
Frank G. Young
(1908–1988)
The Pituitary Gland and Diabetes Mellitus

The medical weekly, *The Lancet*, had a remarkable paper in its issue of August 14, 1939 [1]. Frank G. Young, a 29-year-old biochemist at London's National Institute for Medical Research, told of his success in causing permanent diabetes mellitus in dogs by the injection of a pituitary extract, and that he had done this without operating on the dog's pancreas. Not much remembered today, this result caused great excitement at the time in the medical world because it was the first demonstration that a physiologic substance, without accompanying pancreatectomy, could not only raise the serum glucose level but could do so permanently even after the injections were stopped. Yes, it muddied the waters for those struggling to explain the cause of diabetes mellitus, thought then to be mainly due to a defect in the pancreatic islet cells. But it brought together older clinical knowledge and fit better with the innate sense that such a disease was more likely a complex event that involved more than a single simple explanation. Diabetes mellitus remains to this day a complex disorder, although endogenous pituitary hormones likely have little to do with induction of the natural disease.

A connection between the pituitary gland and diabetes had been known since the 1890s. Many of the original cases of acromegaly had obvious glycosuria [2]. There was no good explanation for the relationship. Thirty years later, in the 1920s, laboratory investigation of the pituitary gland was underway in earnest. Arguments abounded as to what hormones there were in this small cranial organ thought to have no function at all as recently as 1900. Some thought that there was a single hormone ("one gland, one hormone"), while others found up to 10 or 12 hormones. Most agreed that there was at least a growth factor. Injections of crude extracts in the early 1920s caused the widely publicized "giant rat."

In Argentina, Bernardo Houssay had been studying the pituitary gland since 1910, mainly because of his interest in the posterior pituitary and diabetes insipidus. His studies were not widely noted at the time, both because Argentina was not in the mainstream of science and because he worked with frogs – most who studied mammals had trouble believing that what happened in a frog applied to their favorite

---

A Biographical History of Endocrinology, First Edition. D. Lynn Loriaux.

This work is a co-publication between the Endocrine Society and John Wiley & Sons, Ltd.

beasts (e.g., rats, cats, dogs, or human beings). By the 1920s, Houssay began to study the relationship of the pituitary gland to carbohydrate metabolism [3]. He was able to show that removal of the pituitary, now in dogs as well as frogs, made an animal much more sensitive to insulin than a normal animal. His initial thought was that this effect was due to a loss of the posterior pituitary, but, as a skeptic, he pursued the point. In frogs, one can remove just the anterior pituitary fairly easily; Houssay did this and was able to show that this part of the gland was the part responsible for the change. Somehow, the anterior pituitary did something that modulated the action of insulin.

Houssay then turned to the next obvious question: would removal of the pituitary improve diabetes mellitus? He invented what came to be called the "Houssay animal." This was a dog without a pancreas or a pituitary. Removal of the pancreas alone caused overt diabetes and death in a week or two, as expected. What was unexpected was that the same operation in a hypophysectomized dog resulted in a dog that lived for months. Something in the pituitary must allow diabetes to get worse. By 1930, Houssay reversed the idea to examine the effects of pituitary extracts, largely bovine, in dogs that were partially pancreatectomized and did not initially have diabetes. With these injections, the dogs became diabetic. This was not permanent, however. The diabetes disappeared after the injections were stopped. This was not a model of "natural" diabetes.

Houssay did not know what it was in the pituitary that caused diabetes and, given the uncertainties of the time, there was no way to know. Even so, his observations were not easily accepted and he had difficulty getting his work published in the English literature. He finally managed to get a summary of his work published in *Endocrinology* in 1931 [4]. One of the reasons for the lack of acceptance was that others had difficulty repeating his results. Houssay did not realize until 1936 that the main problem was that other investigators did not follow his directions as carefully as they should have. The technical detail of processing the pituitary extracts in the cold and keeping them cold until used turned out to be quite important. Houssay had mentioned this to Young in late 1935 and to others in the United States, but, as Houssay noted in 1943, "only Young followed our advice" [5].

Frank George Young was born in London, England, in 1908. There was no science or medicine in his family, but he was a reader and had access to books of all sorts. He recalled becoming interested in chemistry from reading the *Encyclopedia Britannica*, and, in fact, it was his major subject at University College of London (UCL). He graduated with high honors in 1929 at age 21 and decided to go into graduate work in biochemistry at UCL. Apparently a woman who knew Frank also knew the professor of biochemistry at UCL, Jack Drummond (1891–1952). She wrote Drummond, who then met and talked with Frank. Drummond's exuberance and enthusiasm seem to have done the trick and Young decided on biochemistry. (Tragically, Drummond was later murdered, along with his wife and child, while on vacation in the French Alps; Young wrote his obituary note [6].)

In 1929 Young won a Bayliss–Starling Scholarship for the year and a Sharpey Scholarship for the following 2 years (1930–1932), all spent at UCL. He worked to catch up in biology and began studies in Drummond's laboratory as well as in the physiology laboratories of Charles Lovatt-Evans (1886–1977). The result was a PhD in 1933 and nine papers, mainly on carbohydrate metabolism. Evans was likely the main stimulus to Young's interest in hormones.

The stage was set. Young was trained, directed toward the areas of carbohydrates, biochemistry, and physiology, and had won a prestigious Beit Memorial Fellowship. This allowed him to spend 4 years to do whatever he wanted wherever he wanted to do it. He spent 1 year at UCL to finish work he had started, and then the next 2 years with two of the four investigators who had discovered insulin a bit over a decade before: J.J.R. Macleod (1876–1935) in Aberdeen and C.H. Best (1899–1978) in Toronto. Despite the fame and prestige of these seniors, Young accomplished little; he returned to London for his final fellowship year. Now he really needed a position. Once again Drummond stepped in.

By this time, Young had made something of a name for himself, and in the mid-1930s he got several job offers, some as a chair of biochemistry (which then required a good deal of teaching), and thought he might emigrate to the United States or Canada. Drummond saw this as a loss to British biochemistry and so contacted Henry Dale (1875–1968), then the director of the National Institute for Medical Research (NIMR), to see whether there was anything for Young. Dale already had been asked to provide a recommendation for Young for one of the other positions; Dale spoke to Young and offered him a position himself at NIMR to begin in 1936. So Young stayed in London.

By Young's last year of the Beit Fellowship, he knew he wanted to do biochemical endocrinology but was unsure of what problem to take up. He was expert in carbohydrate biochemistry and physiology but needed focus. He got that focus from a colleague a few years his senior, Guy Marrian (1904–1981), well-known for his work on estrogens. They knew about Houssay's studies, and some time during 1935 they talked during a taxi ride about the diabetogenic effect of the anterior pituitary gland. Young decided to try to identify the responsible pituitary substance. He probably corresponded with Houssay himself; Houssay, as noted above, recalled advising Young to keep the pituitary extracts cold in late 1935.

Young took the broad view. He thoroughly studied the history of carbohydrate metabolism from Claude Bernard onward and concluded with an analysis of the causes of diabetes mellitus and the effects of the pituitary gland thereon. Given as lectures at UCL, his review was published in 1936 while still a Beit Fellow [7]. He then undertook his classic work in 1935–1936 [1]. He gave large doses of cold pituitary extract to three dogs. All became diabetic and two of the three remained so for more than 300 days, even after the extract was stopped [8]. The diabetes was permanent, and this was the first time this had been shown. The result was startling to scientists of the time as it indicated another mechanism for the generation of diabetes without touching the pancreas; it later was called "Young's diabetes." So Young's reputation was made, and in 1939 he gave a major lecture at Harvard Medical School on the anterior pituitary gland and diabetes [9].

By the time the studies were completed, Young had moved to the NIMR. His discovery was rapidly confirmed by several others. The discovery and its confirmation transformed Houssay's findings in the eyes of others from things to be viewed with skepticism to solid data (Houssay later acknowledged as much). Young pursued his original idea of identifying the pituitary factor. It was a difficult task. The controversies over the number of pituitary hormones and what they might be persisted through the 1930s and 1940s (in some cases, e.g., human prolactin, the problem persisted even into the 1970s). Young did as well as any, with one of his papers appearing in the first volume of the UK's *Journal of Endocrinology* [10].

There were suggestions in the 1930s, some by Young, that perhaps growth hormone was the diabetogenic agent. The difficulty was that, given the apparent impurity of the existing preparations, no one knew whether the effect was due to growth hormone or one of the "impurities." Young was able to show that the effect did not originate with TSH, prolactin, or one of the gonadotropins. He was not able to eliminate a possible effect of ACTH or of an as-yet unknown hormone. By the mid-1940s, purer preparations of growth hormone began to appear [11], and after 10 years of intermittent work, Young was able to use a fairly pure preparation of growth hormone and get the diabetogenic effect [12] even in the absence of the adrenal glands [13]. Young's work was, of course, slowed by World War II. He remained in England during the War and tried to show a benefit of pituitary extracts on wound healing, but the study was not a success [14].

Not all were satisfied with the idea that the answer was growth hormone. Growth hormone preparations became much purer in the 1950s, and by the end of the 1950s there was an acceptance that growth hormone was, in fact, the culprit [15, 16]. So it remains today.

What of Young's heritage? There were attempts by analogy to use Young's and Houssay's findings to treat severe retinopathy in patients with diabetes mellitus. The idea was that if excess growth hormone were removed, the retinopathy would improve. Studies done in the days before controlled trials became *sine qua non* of evidence led many to perform partial or total hypophysectomy, stalk section, or pituitary radiation to lower growth hormone and try to help the patients' retinopathy. Success was usually claimed [17–19] but never proven. Further, when measurement of growth hormone in serum became possible, there was a poor correlation between growth hormone levels and any improvement in retinopathy [20], thus undercutting the original rationale for the therapy. More studies are unlikely to be done to establish the point as photocoagulation has become the preferred treatment.

Is there a role for growth hormone in the ordinary patient with diabetes mellitus? Probably not. There are few data that indicate abnormal growth hormone secretion in patients with diabetes mellitus, although one always could speculate that the regulation of growth hormone has still not been as carefully studied in adults with type 2 diabetes mellitus. Young's real contribution was to point to the fact that there are factors other than insulin deficiency that can lead to, or contribute to, diabetes mellitus and that a broader view of the disease is needed to understand its pathophysiology and therapy. That principle is still valid.

Young went on to a distinguished career. He left NIMR in 1942 to be professor of biochemistry at St. Thomas' Hospital Medical School and then moved back to his origin, UCL, in 1945 as chair of biochemistry. His final position was at Cambridge, where he was appointed professor of biochemistry in 1949, the same year he was named to the Royal Society. His international recognition continued; he received the Banting Medal of the American Diabetes Association in 1950. After 1950, his time was taken up with teaching and the burdensome load of administration, mixed with the politics of a changing science of biochemistry (i.e., molecular and cell biology). He retired in 1975 after more than a quarter century in the position. While the newer biochemistry may have, in a sense, passed him by, he became an excellent facilitator of committees and smoothed the way for many colleagues. Thus he contributed to his science and his community.

Note: a major resource for this note is Young's biographical memoir by Philip Randle [21].

References

1. Young FG: Permanent experimental diabetes produced by pituitary (anterior lobe) injections. *Lancet* 1937; 2: 372.
2. Marie P, Souza-Leite JD: *Essays on Acromegaly*. London: New Sydenham Society, 1891, p. 53.
3. Sawin CT: Bernardo Houssay (1887–1971) and pituitary diabetes. *Endocrinologist* 1997; 7: 79.
4. Houssay BA, Biasotti A: The hypophysis, carbohydrate metabolism and diabetes. *Endocrinology* 1931; 15: 511.
5. Houssay BA: History of hypophysial diabetes. In *Essays in Biology in Honor of Herbert M. Evans*. Berkeley, CA: University of California Press, 1943, p. 247.
6. Young FG: Jack Cecil Drummond 1891–1952. *Obit Notices Fellows R Soc* 1954; 9: 99.
7. Young FG: Glycogen and the metabolism of carbohydrate. *Lancet* 1936; 2: 237, 297.
8. Young FG: Experimental investigations on the relationship of the anterior hypophysis to diabetes mellitus. *Proc R Soc Med* 1938; 21: 1305.
9. Young FG: The anterior pituitary gland and diabetes mellitus. *N Engl J Med* 1939; 221: 635.
10. Young FG: Anterior pituitary fractions and carbohydrate metabolism. I. The preparation and properties of diabetogenic extracts. *J Endocrinol* 1939; 1: 339.
11. Li CH, Evans HM, Simpson ME: Isolation and properties of the anterior hypophyseal growth hormone. *J Biol Chem* 1945; 159: 353.
12. Cotes PM, Reid E, Young FG: Diabetogenic action of pure anterior pituitary growth hormone. *Nature* 1949; 164: 209.
13. Lockett MF, Reid E, Young FG: The diabetogenic action of purified growth hormone in adrenalectomized animals. *J Physiol* 1953; 121: 28.
14. Young FG: The anterior pituitary gland and protein metabolism. III. The influence of anterior pituitary extract on the rate of wound healing. *J Endocrinol* 1941; 2: 475.
15. Young FG: The growth hormone and diabetes. *Rec Prog Horm Res* 1953; 8: 471.
16. Field JB: On the nature of the metabolic defect(s) in diabetes. *Am J Med* 1959; 26: 662.
17. Fager CA, Rees SB, Bradley RF: Surgical ablation of the pituitary in the treatment of diabetic retinopathy. *J Neurosurg* 1966; 24: 727.
18. Hardy J, Ciric IS: Selective anterior hypophysectomy in the treatment of diabetic retinopathy. *JAMA* 1968; 203: 73.
19. Munichoodappa CS, Rees SB, Bradley RF, et al.: Bragg peak proton bean irradiation of the pituitary gland for proliferative diabetic retinopathy. *Ann Intern Med* 1971; 74: 491.

20. Powell ED, Frantz AG, Rabkin MT, et al.: Growth hormone in relation to diabetic retinopathy. *N Engl J Med* 1966; 275: 922.
21. Randle P: Frank George Young 25 March 1908–20 September 1988. *Biogr Mem Fellows R Soc* 1990; 36: 583.

This chapter has been reproduced from Sawin, Clark T: Frank G. Young (1908–1988), the pituitary gland, and diabetes mellitus. *The Endocrinologist* 2001; 11(4): 255–8.

CHAPTER 86

Edwin B. Astwood (1909–1976)

Radioiodine Treatment for Thyrotoxicosis

At a meeting of the Middlesex County (Massachusetts) Medical Society in the late 1940s, an audience of more than 200 physicians heard about the various therapies for hyperthyroidism. Frank Lahey, the internationally renowned surgeon based in Boston at the clinic he founded, who had done thousands of thyroidectomies, spoke on the then-standard treatment, subtotal thyroidectomy. Earle Chapman, based at Boston's Massachusetts General Hospital, talked about radioactive iodine, a new treatment begun there by Saul Hertz and continued by Chapman during the years of World War II. Edwin B. Astwood – "Ted" to most at his own request – spoke about the new medical therapy he had devised a few years before, the thiourylene derivatives thiouracil and propylthiouracil (PTU) or, as he called them, anti-thyroid drugs (ATD). Lahey was highly complementary to Astwood for perfecting the medical therapy, but Lahey's view was that these drugs were useful only as an aid to surgery. They brought a patient from the hyperthyroid to the euthyroid state and so made the surgical risk much less. He did not think, as Astwood did, that some patients might be treated with drugs alone, either until the disease – usually Graves' hyperthyroidism – had run its course, or for as long as necessary so as to maintain euthyroidism. Lahey said as much and referred to "poor Dr. Astwood," for thinking that something other than surgery could be an appropriate definitive therapy. Astwood, a quiet and shy man not given to bombast was, nevertheless, as acute of mind as anyone in medicine. He rose in rebuttal. He made a few points, and then finished by noting that he could not refer to his critic, who had recently been listed by a Boston newspaper as having one of the ten highest incomes in Massachusetts, as "poor Dr. Lahey." He brought down the house and there was pandemonium for more than 5 minutes.

This episode points out the tension that arises when something new in science or medicine meets the old and well established. But whether or not the resistance is simply reluctance to adopt the new, or is more rationally based on the best available evidence, hinges on the details known at the time. How then did Astwood come upon this therapy and how did it fit into his life and career?

A Biographical History of Endocrinology, First Edition. D. Lynn Loriaux.

This work is a co-publication between the Endocrine Society and John Wiley & Sons, Ltd.

Ted was born in Bermuda on December 29, 1909. His father was a distant man, who nevertheless provided financial support to his son for some time; it was not easy to make ends meet early in a research career. His mother had become a Seventh Day Adventist (SDA) and Ted attended college at Washington Missionary College, an SDA school in Washington, DC. Mainly interested in mathematics, he decided on medicine as a career, in part because his family felt that mathematics was suitable for working in a bank and Ted wanted more. So he continued in the same line and matriculated at the only SDA medical school, the College of Medical Evangelists, then as now located in Loma Linda, CA, and now called Loma Linda University School of Medicine. He stayed for 2 years. Deciding to follow his growing "agnostic" bent, and he transferred to McGill University's medical program, and graduated in 1934.

Ted Astwood's internship at the Royal Victoria Hospital exposed him to endocrinologists such as J.S.L. Browne and Hans Selye, but he did not stay on for further training. A critical incident with the chief of medicine, where authority overrode fact, decided him on a research emphasis so that he could follow his innate curiosity in a scrupulously rigorous way. He chose endocrinology as the vehicle and moved to Johns Hopkins Medical School, where he worked in the surgical pathology laboratories on the hormonal control of the rat mammary gland and of color change in fish. During his 2 years there he was recognized as "up and coming" and won a Rockefeller Fellowship for further training, which he chose to do with Frederick Hisaw at Harvard's biological laboratories. Within 2 years he had his PhD degree and had become enamored of reproductive endocrinology. He had invented a rapid bioassay for estrogen, another for progesterone, and defined a new placental hormone which maintained the rat's corpus luteum.

The 29-year-old scientist–physician returned to Johns Hopkins in the Department of Obstetrics; he now had a "real job." It was not to last long. The Medical Service at the Peter Bent Brigham Hospital (PBBH) in Boston had just undergone a reorganization under its new chief, Soma Weiss. In 1940, Ted was recruited to join the staff as an associate in medicine at PBBH, in the Department of Pharmacology. He taught in the School's pharmacology course, saw some patients at PBBH as outpatients, and continued his endocrine research with a focus on ACTH and its regulation of adrenal function.

Some time in 1941, Astwood read a short report by Cosmo and Julia Mackenzie, who were working in Johns Hopkins' School of Hygiene and Public Health. It is not clear how he happened to see this report. Possibly it caught his eye because Julia knew Astwood's wife when the Astwoods were in Baltimore. In fact, the Mackenzies had attended the Astwoods' wedding. In any case, it was serendipity of the first order. The Mackenzies had found that sulfaguanidine, an antibacterial agent which they were using to change the flora of rats' intestines in nutritional experiments, caused the rats to develop an enlarged thyroid gland. Astwood and his colleagues pounced on this finding. They realized that the availability of a drug which would reliably enlarge the thyroid gland could provide a way of untangling problems in thyroid physiology and perhaps elucidate the pathophysiology of goiter.

This idea was reinforced by another paper from another group at Johns Hopkins, led by Curt Richter and entirely separate from the Mackenzies. He showed that phenylthiourea also caused goiter in rats. By 1943, Astwood wrote in *Endocrinology* that the effect of these sulfa drugs and, most importantly, of thiourea, did not occur if the rats were either fed desiccated thyroid or had been hypophysectomized. The goiter induced in rats by these drugs was in fact caused by pituitary stimulation. The goiter, with its attendant histologic hyperplasia, was an indirect, not a direct, consequence of the drugs. Astwood's conclusion as to the immediate action of these agents was clearly stated; they caused a "failure of thyroid hormone synthesis."

Meanwhile, the Mackenzies had continued their work during 1941 and 1942 and probably became aware of Richter's work some time in 1942. Their findings, which now included thiourea as well, also appeared in 1943 in *Endocrinology*. They were in the same issue and printed on pages immediately in front of Astwood's 1943 paper. In fact, Astwood's paper was officially submitted a few weeks before the Mackenzies' in October 1942, and was really ready for publication earlier. The editor, who was Astwood himself, held up his own paper so that both could appear simultaneously.

Richter did not pursue the issue, as his main interest was in animal behavior and helping Baltimore with its rat problem by looking into rat poisons. Clearly the problem interested both Astwood's group and the Mackenzies, hence their 1943 papers. However, while they were independently working on the problem, Astwood, in early 1942, felt that the Mackenzies did not have a clear idea of how these anti-thyroid drugs worked. He thought then that the Mackenzies did not agree that the mechanism was due to an inhibition of synthesis of thyroid hormone and recalled that, at the time, he said he would prove it by showing that the drugs could be used to treat spontaneously hyperthyroid humans. The Mackenzies recall it differently. They felt that there were other possible mechanisms and that caution should prevail pending better data. In any case, by the time their 1943 paper was written, they did conclude that these drugs "exert a depressing influence primarily on the functional activity of the thyroid." Certainly Astwood's simple statement was a clearer conclusion.

In 1942 Astwood obtained some thiourea and got another anti-thyroid drug, thiouracil, from the American Cyanamid Company (Lederle Laboratories, Inc.). Beginning in the spring of 1942, he gave one or the other to euthyroid persons and patients with hyperthyroidism at PBBH who were being prepared for surgical treatment. Not much happened in either group. Beginning in July 1942, he gave these drugs as the only treatment to three patients with hyperthyroidism. They clearly improved after several weeks. One, a diabetic patient taking insulin, became hypoglycemic during the course of ATD treatment and insulin was stopped altogether. Another got a rash and was successfully switched to the other ATD, and another developed agranulocytosis, which reversed a week after the ATD was stopped. Although preliminary, these results revolutionized the treatment of hyperthyroidism. They were published in the *JAMA* in May 1943, appearing shortly after the detailed work on rats mentioned above. By the next year, 1944, Astwood was able to publish a report on 62 patients treated with thiouracil with good effect and showed that some patients remained euthyroid when thiouracil was stopped, provided it had been given for at least six months. During its centennial in 1985, the editors of *JAMA* marked Astwood's 1943 paper as one of the Journal's 51 landmark articles in its 100 years.

Astwood and his colleagues never stopped. They pursued thyroid physiology and medicine and took full advantage of radioactive iodine when it became available as a physiologic marker and a treatment. They studied literally hundreds of anti-thyroid drugs in a search for the one with the most potent action and the least toxicity. This sort of screening of large numbers of compounds needed, of necessity, to be done in animals (rats and chicks). The results were transposed to humans on the assumption that potencies and toxicities would be about the same, but they were not. For example, PTU initially replaced thiouracil as the anti-thyroid drug of choice for hyperthyroidism because it was much more potent in animals. PTU turned out not to be more potent in humans, but did have many fewer side effects than thiouracil. Because of this, by the late 1940s PTU and the truly more potent methimazole became the standard anti-thyroid drugs in the United States. They remain so, perhaps because no one has developed a new anti-thyroid drug in the past 30 years.

Astwood's mind was ever curious. Over the next three decades, his laboratory attracted dozens of future leaders in endocrinology. While the laboratory's focus was on the thyroid gland, no endocrine problem was ignored if it sparked an interest. Astwood's style was about as non-directive as it was possible to be. He let his fellows and colleagues pick their own problems, occasionally giving advice as to which avenue to pursue and always offering a wise and informed comment if asked. Unless he personally took part in the work, his name was not to be on the paper. This style was not due to a lack of ambition. He was, in fact, intensely ambitious, but had in addition a strict code of behavior as to what one did or did not do – and followed it. His Lasker Award in 1954 and membership in the National Academy of Sciences reflect the esteem in which he was held, largely owing to his invention of the medical treatment of hyperthyroidism.

In 1972, Astwood retired to Bermuda at the early age of 62 and died of cancer in 1976. Most will remember him for the anti-thyroid drugs, but his style of work in science and medicine was equally as impressive, a style much needed in today's overtly competitive world

Sources

Astwood EB: Treatment of hyperthyroidism with thiourea and thiouracil. *JAMA* 1943; 122: 78.

Astwood EB: Thiouracil treatment in hyperthyroidism. *J Clin Endocrinol* 1944; 4: 229.

Astwood EB: Interview by D. Becker, 1971.

Astwood EB, Sullivan J, Bissell A, Tyslowitz R: Action of certain sulfonamides and of thioureaupon the function of the thyroid gland of the rat. *Endocrinology* 1943; 32: 210.

Greep RO, Greer MA: Edwin Bennett Astwood. *Biogr Mem Natl Acad Sci* 1985; 55: 3.

Mackenzie CG, JB Mackenzie: Effect of sulfonamides and thioureas on the thyroid gland and basal metabolism. *Endocrinology* 1943; 32: 185.

Mackenzie JB, Mackenzie CG, McCollum EV: Effect of sulfanilylguanidine on thyroid of rat. *Science* 1941; 94: 518.

Richter CP, Clisby KH: Toxic effects of the bitter-tasting phenylthiocarbamide. *Arch Pathol* 1942; 33: 46.

VanderLaan WP: Interview by C.T. Sawin, 1990.

VanderLaan WP, Storrie VM: A survey of the factors controlling thyroid function, with especial reference to newer views on antithyroid substances. *Pharmacol Rev* 1955; 7: 301.

This chapter has been reproduced from Sawin, Clark T: Historical Note: Edwin B. Astwood (1909–1976). *The Endocrinologist* 1993; 3(4): 239–41.

CHAPTER 87
Roy Hertz
(1909–2002)
Cure of Choriocarcinoma

Roy Hertz was born in Cleveland, Ohio on June 19, 1909, the fourth of seven children. He was raised in an Orthodox Jewish household, and religion was an important force in Hertz's life. Education claimed primacy in the Hertz family, and Roy was a curious and committed student. Interest in the wonders of the natural world set him on the path to the sciences early in his life. He went to the University of Wisconsin and, to broaden his horizons, studied the humanities. He graduated in 1930 with a degree in comparative literature. The experience, however, had its ups and downs, and he concluded that he did not have the temperament of a scholar. He decided to embark on a life of discovery in the biologic sciences instead. He joined the laboratory of Dr. Frederick Hisaw, who was a leader in the biology of reproduction, considered to be the discoverer of relaxin and the requirement for progesterone in the maintenance of mammalian pregnancy. Hisaw was, at the time, focused on defining the role of pituitary hormones in ovulation, and Hertz was first assigned the task of harvesting pituitary glands at a nearby slaughterhouse. Using these glands as a source of bovine LH and FSH, Hertz successfully demonstrated the dependence of ovulation in the rat on the sequential exposure of the ovary to these hormones. This finding formed the basis of his PhD dissertation, in which he also demonstrated the utility of parabiotic rats in endocrinologic investigation. He was awarded the PhD degree in 1933.

Roy quickly experienced the difficulty of independent research in the pre-National Institutes of Health. He had brief appointments at Howard and then Brown Universities without being able to find the money to sustain his research interest. Discouraged, he returned to the University of Wisconsin and enrolled in medical school, graduating in 1939.

Following a rotating internship at Wisconsin, Hertz joined the U.S. Public Health Service. He was assigned to the Infectious Diseases Division in the Baltimore Public Health Department. In parallel, the Public Health Service subsidized his ongoing education at the Johns Hopkins School of Public Health that led to an MPH degree. Hertz was disturbed by the plight of the poor in receiving the medical treatment of the

---

A Biographical History of Endocrinology, First Edition. D. Lynn Loriaux.

This work is a co-publication between the Endocrine Society and John Wiley & Sons, Ltd.

time and believed that the only solution for the problem was socialized medicine. He wanted to be a part of this solution, and when it did not happen, he turned again to his first love, biology and the study of reproduction. The Public Health Service reassigned Hertz to the nascent NIH in the laboratory of physiology. The date was December 8, 1941.

Hertz began the study of the interrelationships of vitamins and hormones as they affected reproductive function. He studied the relationships among avidin, biotin, progesterone, stilbestrol, and folic acid. In particular, Hertz demonstrated the dependence of the developing female genital tract on relatively high levels of folic acid. In 1944, Hertz was made chief of the Endocrinology Branch.

In 1952, Min Chia Li, a young endocrine fellow at the Presbyterian Hospital in Chicago, applied to Hertz for a position in his laboratory. Rejected, he found a position with Olaf Pearson at the Sloan-Kettering Institute in New York City. Pearson was a leader in the study of the effects of endocrine manipulation on the natural history of cancer. About the same time, a Dr. Van Gilse from the Rotterdam Radiotherapy Institute joined Pearson and Li as a visiting fellow. Her interest was in the development of steroid hormone antagonists that could be used for the treatment of hormone-responsive tumors such as breast and prostate cancer. She knew that Hertz had shown that folate antagonists could block the effects of estrogen on growing chick oviduct. She reasoned that folate antagonists might also be estrogen antagonists. She tested the hypothesis by giving a patient with melanoma daily doses of stilbestrol while being treated with a folate antagonist (methotrexate). Methotrexate had no effect on the cornification of vaginal epithelium and, thus, was not the estrogen antagonist Van Gilse sought. In this regard it was a negative experiment. However, Li, at the same time, was measuring urinary human chorionic gonadotropin (hCG) in daily 24-hour urine collections for no reason other than it was a tumor marker for this patient's tumor. Unexpectedly, methotrexate almost completely suppressed the urinary excretion of hCG. This led Li to speculate that methotrexate might be effective in treating tumors that make hCG, such as choriocarcinoma. Li tucked this information away for future reference. As chance would have it, he made use of the observation sooner rather than later.

Hertz had been given charge of an 18-bed unit in the new clinical center on the NIH Bethesda campus. Not wanting to spend significant time away from his laboratory, he began the search for a clinician to supervise the unit. He rediscovered Li, who took the job. One of Hertz's first projects was to examine the natural history of choriocarcinoma, a malignancy of the trophoblast that was almost uniformly fatal. He monitored the progress of the disease with urinary hCG levels. Within a month of Li's arrival, a new admission with choriocarcinoma promptly died of a cerebral hemorrhage. Li was dismayed with the lack of any rational therapy with which to treat these patients. He approached Hertz with the idea of treating the disease with methotrexate. He related his experience with the effect of methotrexate on the excretion of hCG in the Sloan-Kettering patient with melanoma. Hertz gave Li the go-ahead. Two months later, a 24-year-old woman with widely metastatic choriocarcinoma was transferred to the NIH from the National Naval Medical Center. She promptly developed a large hemopneumothorax, and it appeared she would die in the next few hours. Li gave her 10 mg methotrexate intravenously. She survived the night. The next day he administered 50 mg, and the hemothorax resolved. She was given 10 mg and 15 mg episodically over the next 60 days, leading to the complete disappearance of hCG from her urine. All pulmonary metastasis visible by x-ray disappeared. Therapy was discontinued, and she was found to be well four months later, the first apparent cure of a metastatic cancer with chemotherapy. Two more patients followed closely on this success, both with a similar outcome. The three cases were published in *Proceedings of the Society for Experimental Biology and Medicine* in 1956, a watershed event in cancer chemotherapy [1].

Li tried to take this therapy into the treatment of nongestational choriocarcinoma in men without success. Hertz and Li speculated that the difference in drug sensitivity between men and women was based on the antigenicity of the tumor itself. Choriocarcinoma in women is a "fetal tumor," containing paternal genetic elements that can be recognized and rejected. This is not the case in nongestational choriocarcinoma. Thus, Hertz and Li were among the first to highlight the role of the immune system in tumor surveillance.

Hertz became the scientific director of the National Institute of Child Health and Human Development in 1965, associate director of the Population Council in 1969, professor of pharmacology of George Washington University in 1973, and scientist emeritus at the NIH in 1987, where he remained until the time of his death. He was elected to the National Academy of Sciences in 1972, won the Lasker Award in 1972, and the Koch Award from the Endocrine Society in 1996.

Hertz demonstrated the role of LH and FSH in ovulation, showed the power of parabiotic animals in experimental design, demonstrated the tight binding between biotin and avidin, which paved the way for biotinylated binding assays, developed metyrapone and ortho-para'DDD. He was a guiding force in the development of oral progestins, making possible the birth control pill, and he demonstrated for the first time that a metastatic cancer can be cured with chemotherapy.

Roy Hertz had a fertile mind and an unerring instinct for ideas that could result in clinical utility. He was not an eager physician, but his grounding in medicine served as his scientific compass. He was one of this century's great clinical investigators. He died of stroke on October 28, 2002.

Reference

1. Li M, Hertz R, Spencer DB: Effect of methotrexate therapy upon choriocarcinoma and chorioademona. *Proc Soc Exp Biol Med* 1956; 93: 361–6.

This chapter has been reproduced from Loriaux, D. Lynn: Roy Hertz (1909–2002). *The Endocrinologist* 2004; 14(3): 117–18.

CHAPTER 88

Dorothy Crowfoot Hodgkin (1910–1994)

The Structure of Insulin

Dorothy Mary Crowfoot was born on May 12, 1910, followed by her sisters Joan and Elizabeth in 1912 and 1914. Her father, John, was a well-educated civil servant interested in the Middle East. Her mother, Grace Mary Hood (known as Molly) was the eldest of the six children of Sinclair Hood, squire of Nettleham Hall, a modest estate in Lincolnshire. Molly ultimately became a midwife, and set her heart on a life of service as a medical missionary. Their first child, Dorothy, was born in Cairo. Dorothy and her sisters were largely raised by the family "nurse," Katie Stevens. They never lived with their parents for more than a few months at a time, often in Egypt or Sudan, with long periods between in England with their devoted nurse.

At an early age, Dorothy developed an intense interest in chemistry, largely due to the influence of a family friend, Dr. A.E. Joseph, a government chemist. Impressed by Dorothy's hunger for the subject, he gave her a surveyor's box filled with the following things to do basic chemical experiments: spirit lamp, blow pipe, charcoal blocks, and 48 little bottles of chemicals and minerals. She pursued her passion in an attic laboratory.

It was the intention of Dorothy's father to give her an Oxford or Cambridge education in the same way he would have given for a son. To prepare, she found excellent tutors in Latin, botany, and mathematics. She took the Oxford entrance examination in March of 1928. The interviewer noted her to be "very shy and fragile looking longs to do research or social work." She was accepted to study chemistry in Somerville College.

Chemistry at Oxford was an experimental discipline, in contrast with newer institutions like the California Institute of Technology, where, under Linus Pauling, it was a much more theoretical discipline. Dorothy was interested in crystal structure, and had to create her own crystallographic path at Oxford.

Wilhelm Roentgen discovered x-rays in 1895. In exploring the nature of the x-ray, light was used as an example. It was well known that light of different wavelengths can be "gated" and "diffracted" if passed through a very small aperture. Max von Laue

A Biographical History of Endocrinology, First Edition. D. Lynn Loriaux.

This work is a co-publication between the Endocrine Society and John Wiley & Sons, Ltd.

showed that x-rays were diffracted by passage through the apertures provided by the spaces between atoms in a molecule, leading to the discipline of x-ray diffraction and its use in the study of crystal structure. The BA chemistry honors course at Oxford required a year of original research. This was Dorothy's chance to get involved with crystal structure as revealed by x-ray diffraction. The professor of mineralogy had just purchased an x-ray tube and camera. He appointed Herbert Powell as his research fellow (demonstrator) and Dorothy Hodgkin became Powell's first student. She learned the craft and science of crystallography under his tutelage, mainly with small dimethyl halides as the research focus.

After graduation, Dorothy moved to Cambridge and the fabled laboratory of J.D. Bernal. "John Desmond Bernal was a defiantly unconventional figure, who dazzled almost everyone with whom he came into contact. His brilliant capacity to develop original perspectives on almost any topic, science, politics, esthetics, morality earned him the nickname 'Sage' when he was still an undergraduate. The name stuck." Bernal was a pioneer in applying x-ray diffraction to biologic molecules. Initially, Dorothy worked on the sterols. Her work played an important role in the final elucidation of the structure of calciferol. Another of her papers, however, was to change modern biochemistry. It was the first useful x-ray photograph of a protein, crystalline pepsin. The resulting *Nature* article, co-authored with Bernal, had enormous scientific impact.

Dorothy was invited to return to Oxford as a junior faculty person, which reluctantly she did in 1934. Now she could direct crystallography research as she wished, and she decided to see some crystals through to a complete structural analysis. She continued her work with the sterols, and then, in 1934, she was given 10 mg of a crystalline protein by Boots Pure Drug Company – insulin.

> It worked, but only just. The crystals were less than a quarter of a millimeter across, and shaped more like flowers than perfect crystals, but they were bright and shiny and, unlike pepsin, did not collapse when exposed to air. Sitting in her window, she mounted one of the crystals on a glass fiber under the microscope, and then descended the ladder with her fragile cargo. She set it up in front of the x-ray tube and left it for a 10-hour exposure. The result was all that she could have hoped. "The moment late that evening about 10:00 p.m., when I developed the photograph and saw the central patterns of minute reflections, was probably the most exciting of my life."

She was 24 years old. After 2 years, she was awarded the PhD degree by Cambridge.

Dorothy Hodgkin had almost the whole of her scientific life ahead. The complete structure of insulin was solved in 1969. This scientific tour de force that revealed the chemical structure of the protein was made possible by Hodgkin's pioneering work. It permitted the development of all of the insulin preparations we use to prolong the lives of millions of diabetic patients, to prevent complications, and to "hold the line," until the disease can be prevented and, eventually, cured.

Dorothy married, had three children, won the Nobel Prize, was appointed chancellor of the University of Bristol, became president of the International Union of Crystallography and was a powerful proponent for human rights for all of the world's citizens. I recommend you read the biography by Georgina Ferry. It is a story you will not soon forget.

Source

Ferry G: *Dorothy Hodgkin, A Life*. Cold Spring Harbor, NY: CSH Press, 1998.

This chapter has been reproduced from Loriaux, D. Lynn: Dorothy Crowfoot Hodgkin: 1910–1994. *The Endocrinologist* 2010; 20(5): 207.

CHAPTER 89
Harry F. Klinefelter
(1912–1990)
Genetic Hypogonadism

Harry Klinefelter was born in Baltimore, Maryland on March 20, 1912. He did his undergraduate work at the University of Virginia and went to medical school at Johns Hopkins. He remained at Hopkins as an intern and resident in internal medicine. He next spent a year as a "traveling fellow" with Fuller Albright at the Massachusetts General Hospital. Klinefelter describes this year below:

> I first worked under Dr. Howard Means, measuring oxygen consumption of adrenal gland slices in the Warburg apparatus, but I was so unsuccessful at it, breaking most of the apparatus, that in September, I asked Dr. Means if I might work with Dr. Fuller Albright, since I primarily wanted to learn some clinical endocrinology. Dr. Albright was the most outstanding clinical endocrinologist in the world and Dr. Means readily agreed.
>
> Albright's Saturday morning clinics were famous throughout the Massachusetts General Hospital. At the first one I attended, I saw a tall black boy named George Bland who had gynecomastia and very small testes (1.0–1.5 cm in length). When I asked Dr. Albright what this was all about, he said he did not know but that he would be happy for me to work on it. During the rest of the year, we found 8 other patients with this same condition and reported the series at the endocrine meetings in 1942. Dr. Albright was charitable enough to let me put my name first on the paper that was published later in 1942 in the *Journal of Clinical Endocrinology* [1]. The title, "A syndrome Characterized by Gynecomastia, Aspermatogenesis without Aleydigism, and Increased Excretion of Follicle-stimulating Hormone," was so long that the syndrome came to be known by my name, though it was really just another of Dr. Albright's diseases. Albright had more ideas in a day than most people have in a lifetime, and it was a great pleasure and privilege to work with him. Not only did he have great ideas and theories, but if someone came up with a fact that blasted his current theory, he soon had another one!
>
> These patients tend to be tall, with normal secondary sex characteristics; most have normal sexual function. Figure 2 [not reproduced here] emphasizes that these patients often have an entirely normal appearance save for their small testes, and I am sure many escape detection because the testes are often not examined in a general physical examination. Figure 3 [not reproduced here] illustrates the gynecomastia of several of this group. Figure 4 [not reproduced here], a photomicrograph from a testicular biopsy, shows the atrophy and hyalinization of the seminiferous tubules with preservation of the Leydig interstitial cells.

A Biographical History of Endocrinology, First Edition. D. Lynn Loriaux.

This work is a co-publication between the Endocrine Society and John Wiley & Sons, Ltd.

A few years after the syndrome was described, Heller and Nelson [2] reported that the gynecomastia was not a necessary part of the syndrome, though it occurred in about 75% of the patients. The hallmarks of the syndrome, therefore, are small testes, sterility, and increased excretion of follicle-stimulating hormone.

We thought that this syndrome, which occurs in about one in 500–1,000 male births, indicated there was a second testicular hormone, analogous to estrogen in the female. Figure 5 [not reproduced here] shows diagrammatically the hormone relationships we thought existed. The solid and cross-hatched lines indicate presence of hormones: broken lines indicate absence. Stimulating influences are indicated by solid arrows, and inhibiting influences by open arrows.

There is a good deal of evidence from both animal and human studies to show that a second testicular hormone exists. In the male castrate, testosterone does not control hot flashes, whereas estrogen does. In this syndrome, estrogen decreases the urinary FSH excretion much more readily than testosterone. In animals, testosterone fails to correct all the hypophyseal changes after castration. This second testicular hormone had been labeled inhibin. Despite a great deal of work, it has never been isolated, but we know that it is not a steroid.

We thought the gynecomastia was caused by the action of testosterone on the breast in the absence of this second testicular hormone. Figure 6 [not reproduced here] is a photomicrograph showing the difference in the appearance of the gynecomastia in this syndrome from estrogen-induced gynecomastia, shown on the right. In the latter there is more glandular tissue, and in the former, more peri-acinar fibrous tissue.

Fourteen years after the original description of the syndrome, 2 groups independently discovered that the buccal mucosal cells of these patients contained an extra chromatin mass, or were chromatin positive [3, 4]. A few years later, Jacobs and Strong found that these chromatin-positive patients had 47 chromosomes, and were XXY [5]. The extra X chromosome results from either meiotic non-disjunction, in which a chromosome pair fails to separate during meiosis, or from anaphase lag. Anaphase lag might result in a gamete losing a sex chromosome; a chromosome lags and is not incorporated in the new cell in the next stage of mitosis (anaphase). Such anaphase lag could account for the largest minority of karyotypes, the mosaics XY/XXY and XX/XXY. Eighty percent of these patients have positive sex chromatin, and their karyotypes vary widely with many mosaics.

The syndrome in patients with positive chromatin in the buccal mucosa should probably be called Klinefelter's disease. Although these patients have positive female sex chromatin, they are phenotypic males and should never be considered otherwise. The other 20%, whose testes are not small, have XY chromosomes and should be studied further to determine etiology. These patients often have no complaints, and the condition is discovered in the course of a general physical examination. Sterility and gynecomastia are the most common complaints. It's thought that 5% to 10% of sterile males have this condition. When this disorder is suspected, a buccal smear is the first test to request. If the cells are chromatin positive, the diagnosis is made; testicular biopsy and karyotyping are not necessary. If the buccal mucosa is chromatin negative, further studies are indicated.

The extra X chromosome in these men has stimulated much interest, but its function, if any, has not been determined. Systemic lupus erythematosus, a disorder more common in female patients, has been frequently reported in this syndrome, but the association is not statistically significant. The association with leukemia may also be coincidental. Leg ulcer, osteoporosis, and taurodontism occur with greater frequency in these patents than in control subjects. And dermatoglyphic studies have shown characteristic abnormalities [6].

Following his year with Fuller Albright, Klinefelter served in the U.S. Army for 3 years. Discharged at War's end, he returned to Johns Hopkins and developed an interest in rheumatology, which ultimately he practiced as a member of the Johns Hopkins faculty and in private practice. He rose to the rank of associate professor of medicine in 1966. He retired from practice at 76 years of age, and died in 1990.

The syndrome that Klinefelter described remains one of the commonest causes of primary male infertility, and one of the most "underdiagnosed" of the common syndromes of abnormal sexual differentiation.

References

1. Klinefelter HF, Reifenstein EC, Albright F: Syndrome characterized by gynecomastia, aspermatogenesis with aleydigism, and increased excretion of follicle-stimulating hormone. *J Clin Endocrinol* 1942; 2: 615–27.
2. Heller CG, Nelson WO: Hyalinization of the seminiferous tubules associated with normal or failing Leydig-cell function, discussion of relationship to cunuchoidism, gynecomastia, elevated gonadotropin, depressed 17-ketosteroids and estrogens. *J Clin Endocrinol* 1945; 5: 1–12.
3. Bradbury JT, Bunge RG, Boccabella RA: Chromatin test in Klinefelter's syndrome. *J Clin Endocrinol* 1956; 6: 689.
4. Reis P, Johnson SG, Mosbeck J: Letter to the Editor. *Lancet* 1956; 1: 962.
5. Jacob PA, Strong JA: A case of human intersexuality having a possible having a possible XXY sex-determining mechanism. *Nature* 1959; 183: 302–3.
6. Klinefelter HF: Klinefelter's syndrome: historical background and development. *Southern Med J* 1986; 79: 1089–93.

This chapter has been reproduced from Loriaux, D. Lynn: Harry F. Klinefelter: 1912–1990. *The Endocrinologist* 2009; 19(1): 1–4.

CHAPTER 90

Julius Axelrod (1912–2004)

Epinephrine Synthesis, Secretion, and Reuptake

One of the classic issues in understanding how hormones function is how their action is stopped. Often, in the fervor of trying to see how hormones act (the linear mind at work) scientists can lose sight of the fact that the body must have figured out a way of stopping these actions. The idea of the feedback loop was formalized for hormones in the 1930s. When a rise in a hormone stimulated an action, the action itself shut off the hormone's secretion. But what about the hormone that had already been secreted? Was there no way to stop its action other than by simply waiting for the hormone level to recede? A common answer from the 1930s to about the 1960s was that the hormone got destroyed by one or another enzyme. Enzymatic destruction is, in fact, a real and important factor in the body's management of secreted hormones but is it the only one? What if there is a teleologic need to get rid of a hormone more quickly?

This question came up a bit over 40 years ago for epinephrine (E) and norepinephrine (NE). A solution was needed to pull together ideas about how drugs are metabolized and the exciting and then new disciplines of neuroendocrinology and neurotransmission. That solution also depended on the application of new techniques to a recalcitrant problem, and on the concatenation of curious investigators, good resources, and the right place and right time. One of these curious investigators was Julius Axelrod; the right time was the late 1950s and early 1960s, and the right place with its excellent resources (though sometimes cramped space) was the National Institutes of Health (NIH) in the United States.

Julius Axelrod was not an academic star who moved inexorably from a brilliant youth to a high-performing university to become a professor at an elite institution. His career was the antithesis of this fabled trajectory. Born on the lower East Side of New York City to Polish-Jewish immigrants on May 30, 1912, he attended public schools, but his grades were not good enough to get into one of the city's elite high schools. Still, he did, like many other young men, aspire. He read widely. Along with thousands of others, he was a weekly visitor to the local public library and took out four or five

A Biographical History of Endocrinology, First Edition. D. Lynn Loriaux.

This work is a co-publication between the Endocrine Society and John Wiley & Sons, Ltd.

books at a time (the local public branch libraries were a Godsend in those days when the books had to be close to the reader). Axelrod may not have had this problem but I can recall some of those librarians limiting the number of books that could be taken out or even expressing disbelief that the ones taken out were actually read. Even though he did not make it to an academic high school, he still graduated at age 17 years and planned to become a physician. He thought his chances of entering medical school were better if he went to New York University (NYU) rather than to City College, so he went there in 1929. But it was more than he could afford so he had to transfer to City College after all. He applied to medical school when he graduated in 1933. No medical school took him. He later felt that being Jewish did not help. (Many schools had informal "quotas" for certain groups. More Jews were qualified than were admitted.)

Axelrod was a college graduate in the depths of the Great Depression. Twenty percent of the population was unemployed. Most with a scientific bent took any job that came up and were happy to get it. One did come up and Axelrod took it. He was an assistant in a biochemist's laboratory at NYU and worked on the enzymes of malignant tissues. The salary was $25 per month. Even so, life was not stable. The biochemist's grant ran out in 1935 and Axelrod had to find another job. His experience helped as he then found work as a chemist in New York's non-profit Laboratory of Industrial Hygiene, which was sponsored by the city to assay the vitamin content of foods.

The work was more than routine as the standard vitamin assays had to be adapted to the various foods. Axelrod's mind stayed eager. The laboratory subscribed to the *Journal of Biological Chemistry*, then (and still) the major American biochemical journal, and he read it regularly. He pursued science by attending night school and, after some years, won his master's degree in chemistry in 1942. He did not join the war effort in World War II because he had lost his left eye when a bottle of ammonia exploded in the laboratory. He had clearly settled into his job and his life. He married in 1938, and expected his position to be his life's career. By early 1946, the War was over, he was 33 years old, and he had been at his job for more than 10 years.

Things changed in January 1946. That year Axelrod's boss, the just-retired chairman of NYU's pharmacology department, received a small grant to find out why the analgesics phenacetin and acetanilide caused some people to get methemoglobinemia. He asked Axelrod to work on the problem. Axelrod had little experience in this sort of work, so he was referred to a former department member. Bernard B. Brodie (Brodie's nickname was "Steve," after Steve Brodie, a New York bookmaker who, in 1886, may or may not have jumped into the East River from the Brooklyn Bridge and survived; the publicity served him and his tavern well for years thereafter). Brodie, though only 5 years older than Axelrod, had his PhD from NYU in organic chemistry and was a recognized figure in the world of pharmacology. Brodie had been working during the War years on the Research Service at New York's Goldwater Memorial Hospital, mainly on antimalarials. His chief was James A. Shannon, a renal physiologist trained by Homer Smith and later one of NIH's most powerful figures.

In February, 1946, Axelrod spoke with Brodie about how to attack the analgesic problem. Starting with acetanilide, they wondered whether this drug was converted to aniline, which in turn might cause some of the hemoglobin to be converted to methemoglobin. So, under Brodie's guidance, Axelrod perfected a sensitive assay for aniline and found that it not only appeared in the blood and urine after taking acetanilide, but that it was proportionate to the amount of methemoglobin in the blood. The real issue was, of course, how to prevent this drug from affecting hemoglobin in the red cells. They found that another major metabolite of acetanilide was *N*-acetyl para-aminophenol and that this metabolite did not affect the hemoglobin molecule and was as good an analgesic as acetanilide itself. The metabolite was renamed acetaminophen. We now know it commercially as Tylenol®.

This success changed Axelrod's career: "This was my first taste of real research and I loved it ... and I was determined to continue doing research." A key technical point, essential to Axelrod's future science, was the development of a specific assay for drug-metabolizing enzymes. Brodie asked Axelrod to stay on at Goldwater Memorial and keep on with the study of assays and the metabolism of analgesic and other drugs. He did so for the next 3 years.

In 1949, Shannon, who had left Goldwater later in 1946, became the first director of the newly organized National Heart Institute (NHI). One of his first actions was to recruit many of his co-workers from Goldwater to come to Bethesda, Maryland. This was not as simple then as it is now. The NIH was not a place of prestige and many academics did not think it was a wise move. But the enthusiasm of the Goldwater group persuaded many to join Shannon. Brodie came to be the head of a new Laboratory of Chemical Pharmacology (LCP). Axelrod was invited, too, as a research chemist. He went, in part because the chances of advancement in the academic atmosphere of Goldwater were slim without a doctorate, and Axelrod, at age 37 years, felt he could not afford the time or money to get one. He continued to work with Brodie on drug metabolism, branching out from analgesics to adrenergic blockers and the effects of vitamin C. The LCP group was large and busy. Soon, it had visiting scientists from many parts of the world. Axelrod, uncomfortable working in such a large group, got permission to work independently, though still in the LCP.

His first venture as an independent investigator was to measure caffeine and study its metabolism in humans and dogs. Caffeine was then a commonly used medication. Again, he focused on the assay to make it more specific by using a combination of extraction into benzene and measurement at specific ultraviolet wavelengths with the new Beckman DU spectrophotometer and its valuable quartz-faced cuvettes. He found that caffeine's half-life was about 3.5 hours and that it finds its way rapidly into the brain. He also noted that the average cup of coffee had about 90 mg of caffeine in it.

At about the same time, perhaps stimulated by the work with adrenergic blockers, Axelrod became interested in sympathomimetic methamphetamine and ephedrine. All were then in common medical use, often over-the-counter, and none were then considered as drugs of abuse. An early venture was the analysis, in vivo, of the metabolism of ephedrine. He took advantage of the differential extraction of the two compounds between the nonmiscible mixture of alkaline and water and petroleum ether and showed that ephedrine is rapidly converted to norephedrine. Amphetamine was a different story. Given to rabbits it disappeared quickly and left no measurable material. It must have been metabolized rapidly by a powerful enzyme, Axelrod had to learn about enzymes. He found that amphetamine was deaminated and knew that monoamine oxidase could do this, but the enzyme in question was different. It was located in the microsomal fraction of a liver homogenate and appeared to remove methyl groups as well as amino groups. These studies were an early stage in understanding of how complex cytochrome P-450 enzymes worked. Axelrod thought it "among the best work I did."

This was all very well, but Axelrod remained a research chemist and had difficulty getting promoted. The answer was to get his doctorate. It was going to be a good deal easier than in New York because of an arrangement between the NIH and George Washington University. If one had a master's degree, some courses could be skipped and, if there were substantial publications, they could count toward, and even be written up as, the thesis. Overall, more than a dozen of Brodie's associates took this path to the doctorate. So with a year of classwork, and a thesis on medically related sympathomimetic amines, Axelrod had his degree. It was 1955 and he was 42 years old. This pharmacologic work was the prelude to his neuroendocrine studies over the next few years.

At about this time, Axelrod got an offer to move to a different laboratory and a different Institute at the NIH. He became the head of the Section of Pharmacology in the Laboratory of Clinical Sciences at the National Institute of Mental Health (NIMH). Seymour Kety, the scientific director, was famous for his work on the measurement of local cerebral blood flow and held this position for almost 30 years.

Axelrod knew about drugs and sympathetic amines but little about neuroscience. He was reassured that he had the freedom to study whatever he wanted. So he studied what he knew: drugs and enzymes. In 1957, one of Kety's seminars triggered Axelrod to look at the metabolism of epinephrine which, surprisingly, had been little studied despite a wealth of work in the 1940s and 1950s on the location, synthesis, and secretion of catecholamines. He looked for evidence of oxidation of epinephrine but got nowhere. Later, in 1957, a clinical report of large amounts of an *O*-methylated compound in the urine of patients with pheochromocytoma suggested that a major pathway for epinephrine metabolism might be methylation. Using a system for generating *S*-adenosylmethionine, the methyl donor, he and his colleagues showed that epinephrine was, in fact, converted to 3-*O*-methyl epinephrine. They named this compound metanephrine, which is how we know it today. Going further, they purified the converting enzyme from rat liver, called it catechol-*O*-methyl transferase (COMT), and found it in many other tissues. None of this would have happened were it not for the conjunction of Kety's seminar and help from different colleagues for critical reagents and techniques.

Axelrod now had a firm handle on how epinephrine and its partner in the sympathetic nervous system, norepinephrine, were metabolized. Everyone thought these catecholamines were destroyed by one or another enzyme. Then, an anomaly was found. When the main metabolizing enzymes were blocked from acting, one would expect injected catecholoamine hormones to act for a longer time in vivo. They did not. The physiologic actions disappeared about as quickly as usual. There had to be another way for the body to inactivate these amines. This was not an easy problem to solve. There were plenty of endogenous sympathoamines in the body and there was no way to tell the exogenous from the endogenous. One could give a large amount so that if there were then a large amount at a particular site, one could say there was uptake; but would this be physiologic or simply an artifact of the large dose? There was a technique that would permit the study, the tracer technique. This method, devised in principle some decades earlier had, by 1957, been used since just before the Second World War when radioactive elements were discovered. Possibly, if one could get some radioactive catecholamine, it could trace the path of this hormone through the body.

Axelrod was in luck. As it happened, his chief, Kety, had tritiated epinephrine made to study patients with schizophrenia. He gave some to Axelrod, who, with his colleagues, worked out methods of assaying it and its metabolites, and then gave it to cats. They were able to trace the metabolites in blood and various tissues. At this point, another puzzle came up. The tritium label stayed in certain tissues, such as the heart, spleen, and adrenal gland, for a long time, well past any action of the injected hormone. The same thing happened with norepinephrine, so the finding was no fluke. Possibly these tissues bound the hormone nonspecifically. They were also well-innervated with sympathetic nerves. Maybe the catecholamines were taken up by these nerves. Axelrod noted that "Binding appears to protect these hormones from enzymatic attack." That tissues bound these hormones was not a new idea and was in fact part of a contemporary controversy that was clouded by the inability to tell endogenous from exogenous hormone. There was a claim that uptake had been shown in the early 1930s by J.H. Burns. He did, in fact, have reason to suspect neural uptake, but only by inference rather than by direct demonstration. Even to Axelrod's laboratory, the issue was not settled quickly. It took several years (from 1957 to 1960) to get to this point. But how to tell whether or not the hormones were actually in the sympathetic nerves in these tissues?

Axelrod returned to the tritiated hormones and, at the suggestion of a visiting scientist from Vienna, Georg Hertting, combined them with a well-established sympathetic denervation technique. If one could remove the sympathetic nerves in an area of the body and then show that that tissue no longer bound the hormone, then that would be clear evidence that, when the hormone was bound, it was bound to the nerves in that tissue. The technique was to remove the cat's cervical sympathetic ganglion on one side only and wait a few days. It was known that the neurons from the excised ganglion to the iris and salivary glands would degenerate over this time. Now when tritiated norepinephrine was injected, it showed up clearly in the tissues on the normal side and only a little bound to the tissues on the operated side. The rapid inactivation of the hormone was not enzymatic at all but was in fact due to rapid uptake by the sympathetic nerves themselves. To make it final, the investigators also showed that the hormone taken up was not destroyed but was simply stored because nerve stimulation released the tritiated hormone.

To go down one more level in localizing the taken-up hormone, Axelrod and his associates turned to radioautography combined with electron microscopy. Now with this technique the tritiated hormone could be seen directly over preterminal axons, proving without a doubt that the nerves took up the hormone. The labeled hormone was also suggestively located near granulated vesicles in these nerve endings "strongly suggesting that their granulated vesicles contain norepinephrine." The newly found mechanism was clear: sympathetic nerve endings take up, store, and release norepinephrine. This uptake is rapid and leads to rapid cessation of catecholamine action. There is inactivation by enzymes but it is slower.

Axelrod had many co-workers over his long tenure at NIH and worked in many other areas, such as the synthesis of melatonin and the role of adrenergic compounds in the central nervous system. His laboratory was a lively place with Axelrod actively engaged in his work and bringing a "constant stream of ideas" for others to think about. But his work on the uptake of catecholamines by sympathetic neurons, with its clear and elegant designs, is likely the main reason he received the Nobel Prize in 1970, an award that was shared with Bernard Katz and Ulf von Euler. He "retired" in 1984 at age 72 years but did not really leave the laboratory and continued as an unpaid guest researcher. In 1996, at age 84 years, the NIH named him Scientist Emeritus. His life in science may have been unexpected, but what a run.

Sources

Axelrod J: Nobel Lecture, 1970. In *Nobel Lectures, Physiology or Medicine, 1963–1970*. Amsterdam: Elsevier Publishing, 1972.

Snyder S: *A Biographical Memoir, Julius Axelrod 1912–2004. National Academy of Sciences Biographical Memoirs*, Vol. 87. Washington, DC: National Academies Press, 2005.

This chapter has been reproduced from Sawin, Clark T: Historical Note: What stops the action of norepinephrine? Julius Axelrod, enzymes and neural uptake. *The Endocrinologist* 2000; 10(6): 357–62.

CHAPTER 91

Geoffrey W. Harris (1913–1967)

The Brain's Control of the Pituitary Gland

Today all who deal with hormones and their regulation know that the secretion of the pituitary hormones is controlled by the hypothalamus. The pituitary is not the master gland it once was thought to be.

The idea that the brain controlled the pituitary hormone secretion arose in the minds of serious scientists about 70 years ago. The pituitary hormones were beginning to be recognized and, in the 1930s, defined. The "master gland" took pre-eminence in both the public and scientific mind. In the excitement, few thought to ask, even when it became clear that there was a feedback system that regulated the secretion of these pituitary hormones, just how it was done. For example, everyone knew that reproduction was seasonal or cyclic in many animals, including humans, and in the early 1930s they knew that pituitary hormones affected gonadal function. How were the two connected? How did the seasonal change in ovulation, for instance, fit with the stimulation of ovulation by gonadotropins? Did seasonal change act via the brain and pituitary gland, or did it act via a direct neural effect on the ovary? And if it were via the brain, how did the brain affect the pituitary gland? By the mid-1930s, physiologists began to think that these questions were worth answering.

In 1936, Geoffrey Wingfield Harris was finishing his undergraduate degree at the University of Cambridge and thought he should look into ovulation in the rabbit as a tool to find out how ovulation was controlled. It had been common knowledge for 30 years that female rabbits ovulated only after mating. In contrast to most other animals, the timing of ovulation in rabbits could be precise. That rabbits ovulated only after mating suggested that there had to be a neural component to the ovulatory process. Several studies had shown that removal of the nerves to the ovary or interruption of spinal pathways to the brain completely blocked the ovulatory response to coitus, as did removal of the pituitary gland. Thus the brain was the research focus for the likely location of the neural connection from the vagina and ovary. Wherever the location was, the brain somehow acted to induce ovulation through the pituitary gland because removal of the pituitary gland broke the connection. In 1936, Harris, at the suggestion

A Biographical History of Endocrinology, First Edition. D. Lynn Loriaux.

of his mentor, Professor Francis H.A. Marshall, decided to stimulate both the hypothalamus and the pituitary gland with electricity to see whether he could cause rabbits to ovulate.

Harris was born in London in 1913 to parents who were not well-off but who were determined to educate their children well. His scientific education at school in his "teens" was not, however, particularly good. His father, an expert in ballistics, worked hard to remedy the defect. He began college at the University College in London but, in 1933, after only one semester, moved to Emmanuel College in the University of Cambridge. There he managed to avoid most of his tutors and supervisors who were, he thought, uninspired. That did not stop him from winning several prizes and coming in first in most of his examinations. He may have had an incipient interest in endocrinology before coming to Cambridge, but this interest fully blossomed under the influence of Marshall. He had shown that the environment affected ovulation, presumably through neural pathways, and that these neural pathways operated via the pituitary gland. The high-performing Harris won a studentship in anatomy in his last college year and, on Marshall's suggestion, began to investigate the hypothalamic relationship to ovulation. His hypothesis was that there were nerve fibers going from the brain to the pituitary gland and that these controlled gonadotropin secretion.

The 23-year-old Harris prepared himself for these experiments by learning from others how to cut the pituitary stalk with a small piece of razor blade and how to stimulate the hypothalamus and pituitary areas electrically with the rat's head held steady in a type of Horsley–Clarke apparatus. The stalk section experiments, usually not mentioned in reviews of Harris' career, were singularly unsuccessful. Most of the rabbits died with seizures within a few days. The four females that survived were not interested in mating, nor were the two male survivors. Even worse, after a few months, all had wasted away and died. He found that the pituitaries had atrophied and thought this might be caused by the removal of neural impulses to the gland.

The electrical stimulation experiments were more successful. Harris was following directly in Marshall's footsteps. Marshall had shown that global electrical stimulation of the head stimulated ovulation, but the stimulation and its associated stress might well have been nonspecific. Marshall and Harris thought that they should try to localize the effect to show that it was indeed a specific neural action. They chose to stimulate the hypothalamus directly, mainly because it is the part of the brain closest to the pituitary gland. To stimulate the hypothalamus, Harris used a small steel wire encased in a glass capillary tube; he guided it to the hypothalamus with the stereotactic apparatus. For a stimulus, the usual induction coil did not work because it caused the rabbit's head to move, and the intracranial wire was never in one spot. More testing allowed him to settle on a technique that permitted stimulation over an hour without causing anything more than a flickering of the eyelids in the rest of the animal. He found that stimulation of the lower anterior hypothalamus caused ovulation in 12 of 20 rabbits, at times ranging from 15 to 40 hours after stimulation. He also found that stimulation of the pituitary gland itself caused ovulation in about half the animals. He concluded that electrical stimulation of either the hypothalamus or the pituitary gland could induce ovulation. How then did hypothalamic stimulation cause ovulation? He thought there were several possible functional links between the hypothalamus and the gland: cervical nerves, petrosal nerves, or the pituitary stalk. There was no evidence in favor of the cervical or petrosal nerves and some against. He thought that these were not a good explanation. That left the pituitary stalk. His best guess was that small nerves went from the hypothalamus first to the intermediated lobe and then to the anterior lobe: "it is necessary to suppose either that the nerve fibers seen to enter the pars intermedia eventually pass round the cleft into the anterior lobe, or else that the posterior or intermediate lobe can influence the anterior lobe hormonally. The former supposition is felt to be the more probable of the two."

Harris made an error in attributing ovulation to direct stimulation of the pituitary gland. As he and others found after the Second World War, the effect he saw was due to spread of the stimulus to the brain. He was unable to get decent results from the stalk-sectioned animals. His interpretation of the pathway from the brain to the pituitary was wrong. He did not know that the pituitary portal blood flow was from the hypothalamus to the pituitary, a finding that was described only that year, 1936. The hypothalamic stimulation experiments, however were a major success. They showed that a local stimulus to a reasonably specific area of the brain was able to trigger a major reproductive event, ovulation. The results set the tone for the rest of his career.

Harris published little over the next 4 years for the simple reason that he was attending medical school at St. Mary's Hospital in London. He qualified in 1939 at Cambridge and spent another year in hospital residency. After this, he never again held a clinical appointment. In 1940, as Britain fell deeper into the war, he returned to Cambridge University as a demonstrator in anatomy. While he taught, he continued his laboratory work on the hypothalamus. The posterior pituitary gland became the subject of his MD thesis, awarded in 1944. The title was "Innervation and actions of the neurohypophysis."

Harris continued, through it all, to work on the problem of how the hypothalamus communicated with the pituitary gland. He looked again for nerves to the anterior pituitary and found none. He knew that there were hypophysial portal vessels. They had been well-defined by Gregory T. Popa, a Romanian physician–scientist, while still a medical student. Popa, who had become a professor of anatomy in Romania, had visited and worked with Harris at Cambridge in the late 1930s and had instructed Harris on surgical techniques for the hypothalamus and pituitary gland. Popa, however, thought that blood flowed from the pituitary to the hypothalamus. This made it difficult for them to postulate these portal vessels as a conduit for the connection between the hypothalamus and the pituitary. Others, in the mid-1930s, did think that the blood flow was from the "top down." This direction of flow had been observed in vivo in amphibians. This fact, though published in 1935, was not widely known. A few speculated at the time that the portal system might be a way for the body to connect the hypothalamus and the anterior pituitary gland, but the evidence was skimpy and the idea a subject of controversy. A typical opinion in 1939 was that of the Johns Hopkins physiologist Chandler McC. Brooks, who wrote "I personally feel that ... the hypothalamus exerts some control over the gonadotropic functions of the hypophysis by way of fibers passing to the gland through the hypophysial stalk." But after the War, Harris, still a demonstrator in anatomy at Cambridge, renewed his investigation of the portal vessels. Working particularly with John Green, he began to suspect that the hypothalamic–pituitary connection was indeed vascular.

Harris was becoming well-known for his work and, in 1947, was offered a better position in London. He wanted to stay in Cambridge, however, and went to one of his colleagues in Cambridge's Physiology Department to see if anything could be done. It could, and so Harris made a lateral transfer in 1948 from anatomy to physiology as a university lecturer. He stayed there until 1952.

If the hypothalamic–pituitary connection was vascular, what was the physiologic mechanism by which the hypothalamus regulated the anterior pituitary gland? Perhaps nervous stimulation regulated the pituitary's blood flow and hence its secretion, or perhaps the median eminence "filtered out" varying amounts of circulating hormones and so regulated pituitary secretion. These ideas were pure speculations and had no evidence to support them. The likely solution to the problem would be to show that there were substances in the portal vessels that stimulated the anterior pituitary and that these substances came from the hypothalamus. These were not, however, easy problems to solve and were not, in fact, solved until the late 1960s and 1970s.

An alternative approach was needed, that is, indirect inferential evidence. In the early 1950s, Harris and his visiting colleague Dora Jacobsohn (a refugee from Nazi Germany then in Lund, Sweden) did a key experiment that brought acceptance to the idea that specific pituitary stimulators came to the anterior pituitary from the hypothalamus. They showed that pituitary grafts into hypophysectomized rats that were placed under the hypothalamus or under the temporal lobe had clear differences in function. Only the grafts under the hypothalamus continued to function and secrete pituitary hormones. Because the pituitaries at both sites had a good blood supply and were anatomically intact, and because no nerves grew into either type of graft, the functioning grafts under the hypothalamus had to have been supplied with some hypothalamic material through the newly regrown portal vessels.

About this time, Harris got another offer to move to London, which this time he took up. The move was to the recently built Institute of Psychiatry at the Maudsley Hospital. The attraction was not so much psychiatry as a discipline, but a professorship as the holder of the newly created Fitzmary Chair of Physiology and a funded new laboratory of experimental neuroendocrinology. Harris' quarters in the "Institute" were in fairly primitive prefabricated "huts" that were "temporary." He and his many colleagues and visiting workers remained in the "huts" for the 10 years spent in London. Though a great deal of new work was done, the facilities were frustrating. The heat often would fail in the winter, and the low ambient temperature was a stimulus for all to repair to the local pub, the Fox on the Hill.

To most investigators in the 1950s, the connection between the hypothalamus and the anterior pituitary gland was vascular. There were some hold-outs who felt that the evidence was not good enough. This resistance was a spur to further action by those who had been convinced. Arguments between Harris and Solly Zuckerman, then a powerful scientist, were almost titanic. Zuckerman, would show that the pituitary stalk and its vessels could be completely transected in the ferret and still there would be neurally stimulated ovulation. Harris would then show that Zuckerman's experiments were not reproducible and that the problem was that in Zuckerman's preparations the vessels grew back after they were cut, hence the ovulation. Then Zuckerman would show that his preparations were as good as anyone else's. And so it went, back and forth. As late as 1978, long after many of the hypothalamic releasing factors had been isolated and after the Nobel Prizes for their isolation had been awarded, Zuckerman still held to his now isolated position. The debates with Zuckerman were vigorous, to say the least, but Harris was ever forthright. The difference of opinion with the well-connected Zuckerman could have held up Harris' election to the Royal Society, but it did not. He was elected in 1953.

Major efforts to satisfy everyone began in earnest in the mid-1950s and moved from functional anatomy to physiology and extraction biochemistry. One major stimulus, in addition to the controversies swirling about the field, was Harris' synthesis of the evidence up to 1955 in his only published book, *Neural Control of the Pituitary Gland.* Though now more than 40 years old, it still can be read with profit. At the time, his feeling was that all would be convinced of the roles of the hypothalamus and the pituitary portal vessels in pituitary function if it could be shown that there were extractable substances in the hypothalamus that stimulated the anterior pituitary gland. Others in the United States, influenced by Hans Selye in Montreal, tried to find the factor that enhanced ACTH secretion. Harris went after the one that stimulated LH secretion, and hence ovulation. This choice was a clear follow-up of his rabbit work of 24 years before. He continued this effort at Oxford where he moved in 1962 as professor and chairman of the Anatomy Department and head of a Neuroendocrinology Research Unit funded for him by the Medical Research Council. The work required thousands of hypothalami and so was expensive. Harris managed to raise a fair amount of money to fund the effort. He also had a number of administrative duties and traveled often, all of which may have limited his direct involvement. In addition, the chemistry was not easy, even though he worked with an expert, Harry Gregory.

Through the 1960s, there were many false starts by many investigators, including Harris. For a time in the late 1960s, there was a groundswell among endocrinologists that these presumed hypothalamic factor(s) did not exist and that more funds for chasing this will-o'-the-wisp simply were not warranted. Too many had promised success just around the corner and failed. Harris, in this "race" to isolate a hypothalamic factor, was further handicapped by his insistence on the use of a specific but cumbersome bioassay that permitted the assay of only a few hypothalamic fractions at a time. Further, for whatever reason, he did not trust the new immunoassays when they became available in the 1960s. He tended not to accept things he could not see with his own eyes. One can see a rabbit's ovulation. The result was that his work was slow. Others, looking first for the factor that stimulated ACTH secretion and then for the one that stimulated TSH secretion, used faster and simpler bioassays and so solved the problem first with the isolation and chemical identification of thyrotropin-releasing factor, or TRF, in 1969. (Harris saw no reason to call these factors "hormones" because they really were not effective systemically but acted only a few millimeters from where they were produced.)

Although others found the hypothalamic factors and deduced their chemical structure and Harris did not, there is little question that his intellect and leadership was important for the field. His work helped establish the reality of hypothalamic control of the anterior pituitary. The excitement he generated, at a time when the ideas were not widely accepted, was a major influence in others coming into the field, including Roger Guillemin, who later shared a Nobel Prize for his own work with TRF. In the laboratory, Harris was not an isolated professor but worked with everyone. He performed the difficult maneuvers himself. He was smart, original, and competitive, both in the laboratory and on the squash court. Though he liked new ideas, he was quite stubborn. If another's idea was not to his liking, he would dismiss it, but if it were any good, it would reappear a while later in his discussions as if it were newly minted. Though a clear leader, he always gave credit to other's work, whether recent or in the distant past, and he was generous in the support of those who worked with him. His legacy is not only his pioneering work and the influence he had on others. He made neuroendocrinology respectable, high praise indeed for a man called by one memorialist "the perfect Englishman."

In May 1971, Harris was awarded the Dale Medal of the British Society for Endocrinology, its highest award. The honoree must give a lecture to the assembled Society. He did so on May 27 and gave the audience a survey of his entire career, which, as it happened, coincided with the development of the new field of neuroendocrinology. It was his last lecture and was published posthumously the next year because Harris died on November 29, 1971, only a few months after the lecture. He was only 58 years old. The cause of death was bleeding esophageal varices.

Sources

Brooks CMcC: Relation of the hypothalamus to gonadotropic functions of the hypophysis. *Res Publ Assoc Res Nerv Ment Dis* 1940; 20: 525.

Guillemin R: Pioneering in neuroendocrinology 1952–1969. In *Pioneers in Neuroendocrinology II*, edited by J Meites, BT Donovan, SM McCann. New York: Plenum Press, 1978, p. 221.

Harris GW: The induction of ovulation in the rabbit, by electrical stimulation of the hypothalamo-hypophysial mechanism. *Proc R Soc Lond [Biol]* 1937; 122: 374.

Harris GW: Electrical stimulation of the hypothalamus and the mechanism of neural control of the adenohypophysis. *J Physiol* 1948; 107: 418.

Harris GW: *Neural Control of the Pituitary Gland*. London: Edward Arnold, 1955.

Harris GW: Humours and hormones. The Sir Henry Dale Lecture for 1971. *J Endocrinol* 1972; 53: ii.

Harris GW, Jacobsohn D: Functional grafts of the anterior pituitary gland. *Proc R Soc Lond [Biol]* 1952; 139: 263.

Jensen RL, Stone JL, Hayne RA: Introduction of the human Horsley-Clarke stereotactic frame. *Neurosurgery* 1996; 38: 563.

Marshall FHA, Verney EB: The occurrence of ovulation and pseudo pregnancy in the rabbit as a result of central nervous system stimulation. *J. Physiol* 1936; 86: 327.

Raisman G: An urge to explain the incomprehensible: Geoffrey Harris and the discovery of the neural control of the pituitary gland. *Annu Rev Neurosci* 1997; 20: 533.

Reichlin S: Formative years as an investigator of hypothalamic-pituitary physiology. In *Pioneers in Neuroendocrinology II*, edited by J Meites, BT Donovan, SM McCann. New York: Plenum Press, 1978, p. 313.
Scharrer B: Neurosecretion and neuroendocrinology in historical perspective. In *Hormonal Proteins and Peptides. Hypothalamic Hormones*, edited by CH Li. New York: Academic Press, 1979, p. 279.
Vogt M: Geoffrey Wingfield Harris 1913–1971. *Biogr Mem Fellows R Soc* 1972; 18: 309.
Zuckerman S: A skeptical neuroendocrinologist. In *Pioneers in Neuroendocrinology II*, edited by J Meites, BT Donovan, SM McCann. New York: Plenum Press, 1978, p. 403.

This chapter has been reproduced from Sawin, Clark T: Geoffrey W. Harris and the brain's control of the pituitary gland. *The Endocrinologist* 1998; 8(2): 117–22.

CHAPTER 92

Frederic C. Bartter (1914–1983)

Disorders of "The Pump"

It is not often that a syndrome is named after a person. The major exceptions that come to mind for endocrinologists are the several named after Fuller Albright, the well-known clinical investigator who worked for so many years at Boston's Massachusetts General Hospital (MGH). He was the one who perfected the long-term study of patients with complex diseases on a metabolic ward designed to elucidate the hidden mechanisms of pathophysiology using "balance studies." Metabolic disorders should be studied quantitatively with measurements as precise as possible if the problems are to be solved. This meant that as many variables as possible must be eliminated, which in turn meant that the twists and turns of everyday life, to which the body responds without thought, had to be kept constant so as not to mask the changes of the disease. The basic principle undertaken was that the best "model" of a disease was the patient with that disease, rather than an analogous, but perhaps not quite the same, apparent animal example of the disorder. There was little talk of membranes or genes for the simple reason that such studies were not then possible. The ultimate aim was to use the data gained to treat the disease. What better place to study a condition than in the patient one hoped to help?

No doubt because of Albright's approach, Frederic C. Bartter chose to study with him. He absorbed this mode of attack completely, and eventually had two syndromes named after him. One of these, Bartter's syndrome, is known to most physicians and to all endocrinologists but is quite rare and is usually an inherited disorder. The other, the Schwartz–Bartter syndrome, is more often termed the syndrome of inappropriate secretion of antidiuretic hormone. It is much more common than Bartter's syndrome, but few now remember its eponym. Perhaps this reflects the thinking of those who dislike eponyms: if a disease has a simple name or has a clear pathophysiologically based explanation that lends itself to a specific label or is reasonably common, perhaps it must lose its eponymic quality and be absorbed into the timeless nomenclature of the ICD-10 (International Classification of Diseases). It may thus be suitable to retain an eponym if the entry is rare or has no good explanatory term. Perhaps so, but one

---

A Biographical History of Endocrinology, First Edition. D. Lynn Loriaux.

This work is a co-publication between the Endocrine Society and John Wiley & Sons, Ltd.

loses the historical context and any clue as to why the eponym arose in the first place. There is a place for both.

Bartter was not born to medicine. Quite the contrary, his father was an Anglican missionary to the Philippines (then the Philippine Islands, a possession of the United States) and his mother, an American, was trained in the classics at Smith College. The couple seem to have gotten along well with the local Roman Catholic clergy. The priests shared with the parents in the early education of the two Bartter boys. Both sons, Frederic and George, were born in Manila and were raised in the small town of Baguio, further north on the island of Luzon. Frederic's early education at home ended at age 13 when he and his brother left to go to Massachusetts to attend the Lenox School in the western part of the state. Frederic must have been a bright student, as he finished at Lenox when he was only 15 years old.

Bartter returned home for a year and then went back to Massachusetts, now to its eastern end, to attend Harvard College. He graduated in 1935. The family seems to have had a sufficient income not only to send him to Harvard College but also to cover an extra year in the Department of Physiology at Harvard's School of Public Health. The ongoing Great Depression had little effect on his career. His first paper, in 1935, came from the year at the School. It was on the measurement of glucose in lymph and may have presaged his interest in the burgeoning field of endocrinology.

He then moved on to Harvard's Medical School, from which he graduated in 1940, still quite young at 25 years of age. During his medical school years he would have been exposed to Albright in the course of his clinical rotations through the MGH. Bartter moved to New York for a year's internship in 1941. By then, the Second World War was in full sway and the United States was in it. Bartter did not serve in the military but, instead, served as an officer in the nation's Public Health Service. His main work was on the effects of blood donation on blood volume over time and on parasitic diseases such as onchocerciasis, or "river blindness," a tropical filarial disease. In his last year of service (1945–1946), he was assigned to the Public Health Service's Laboratory of Tropical Diseases at the National Institutes of Health (NIH).

The War slowed down everyone's career. By the time Bartter's service was over, he had gained a wealth of experience but had no training beyond the internship. Today, he would have entered a residency program, probably in internal medicine, and then gone on to decide on fellowship training, and then decided on an academic or clinical pathway, and then found a position somewhere. This lock-step, linear approach to training is a fairly recent development. After the War, and for about two decades thereafter, postgraduate training was far more flexible. For example, Bartter did not return to do a residency in medicine but, rather, went directly into a research fellowship. He chose to go to work with his old teacher, Albright, at the MGH. At first he spent 2 years as a researcher and only then became a resident in medicine, during which he continued his research work. He authored or co-authored a number of papers with his mentor and other colleagues, such as Anne Forbes, Alexander Leaf, and Edward Reifenstein, all of whom became well-known in their fields and two of whom also have a syndrome named after them (Forbes and Reifenstein), in large part because of their association with Albright. The emphasis of Bartter's work at MGH was on various adrenal disorders and salt and water metabolism, although he touched as well on Albright's favorite set of problems: diseases of calcium and the parathyroid glands.

Among Bartter's papers written from work done at MGH, two are of particular interest. The first, published in 1951, established that there was clear clinical relevance to a theoretical analysis of the adrenal dysfunction in virilizing adrenal hyperplasia. The theory was that the apparent hyper-functioning state was actually a deficiency state; the virilization was due to an attempted compensation by the adrenal cortex to make up for the cortisol deficiency that resulted from the cortex's enzymatic defect. The attempted compensation was driven by an increased secretion of adrenocorticotropin (ACTH), which in turn was a result of the low cortisol. The ACTH would try to drive the synthesis of more cortisol but could not; the result was that all the other adrenal steroids were made and secreted in excess. Because some were androgens, the patient became virilized. If this theory was correct, the clinical problem should resolve if one could only block the secretion of the excess ACTH. If one could do this with a replacement for the cortisol deficiency, so much the better. As it happened, synthesized cortisone had just become available in the late 1940s (and a Nobel Prize was awarded in 1950 for its discovery). Bartter was able to show that the new cortisone not only replaced missing endogenous cortisol but also suppressed, as the theory predicted, the raised ACTH levels and so removed the stimulus for the virilizing steroid production. Although there is still today some uncertainty as to the best regimen for treating this disease, Bartter and his colleagues established the principle of the therapy and did so by translating pathophysiologic observations to the clinic.

The other paper, published in 1953, was the demonstration that pitressin-induced water retention caused urinary loss of electrolytes such as sodium and chloride. Bartter later was to turn this physiologic observation into an analysis of a different disease, an unusual form of hyponatremia (see below). This work clearly primed him to recognize a parallel to physiology in a patient.

In 1951, Bartter ended his 5 years with Albright. He was then 36 years old and had established himself with a national reputation. That year he moved from Albright's laboratory and junior position at Harvard's Medical School directly to the NIH (at first in Baltimore but then in Bethesda, Maryland), where he was appointed the chief of the endocrinology branch at the National Heart Institute, a position he held for the next 22 years. In 1973, his title changed to chief of the hypertension and endocrine branch of the same Institute, a position he held until 1978. He ended his NIH career that year when he began another career in Texas, where he became professor of medicine at the relatively new medical school in San Antonio and joined the staff at San Antonio's Veterans Administration (VA) Hospital as the associate chief of staff for research.

At the NIH, aldosterone – its physiological control and its relationship to disease – became his principal focus. The hormone itself had only been discovered in 1953. Bartter was superbly prepared in his years at the MGH to study this new hormone in humans. His work was recognized by an invitation in 1958 to speak at the annual Laurentian Hormone Conference, held in the Laurentian Mountains of Canada. The hope at the time was that, with sufficient energy and resources, one could tease apart all of the many presumed causes of hypertension and then, once the causes were known, devise a therapy for each. We now know that hope was in vain. The cause of hypertension is still an important problem. Our efforts are still inadequate, aimed at lowering the blood pressure by whatever means available. But then, in the 1950s and 1960s, the hope was real and led to major discoveries that included the far less frequent, but very real, treatable causes of hypertension. One of these was primary aldosteronism, which causes hypokalemic alkalosis associated with the hypertension. Bartter became an expert in this area and included himself in some of the studies as a subject. In one such study, he discovered his own hypertension.

It was in this context of detailed study of salt and water balance and its hormonal control that his two syndromes were described. The first, described in 1957, is the Schwartz–Bartter syndrome, the result of a collaboration between him and William Schwartz at Tufts-New England Medical Center in Boston. They observed that two patients with lung cancer had hyponatremia, despite which they lost significant amounts of sodium in their urine. Neither had renal or adrenal disease. Bartter, as noted above, was primed to see the parallel between these patients and his prior work on the physiology of vasopressin (antidiuretic hormone). Bartter and Schwartz reasoned that there was an increase in ADH secretion in these patients with lung cancer and showed that the intuitive therapy (i.e., to give more salt) was not the best approach. The best approach was to restrict water intake, thus removing the renal substrate for the ADH to act on. It should be remembered that there was then no easy assay for ADH in blood and that the disorder was described and treated entirely on physiological reasoning, a remarkable achievement.

The other syndrome, published in 1962, grew out of his work in primary aldosteronism with its characteristic hypokalemic alkalosis but without any of the usual causes of secondary hyperaldosteronism. These patients had excess aldosterone secretion with a high level of renin. Bartter puzzled over the cause of this peculiar condition and thought for a time that it was due to an excess of prostaglandin production. This did not pan out. He did not solve the problem of etiology, nor did he successfully explain why there was no hypertension, but he brought the disorder to everyone's attention and helped us understand it better.

We now know that the disease is a rare, genetic, usually autosomally recessive disorder. It is related to a similar syndrome, Gitelman's syndrome, that presents clinically in almost the exact same fashion. Bartter's syndrome is ultimately usually due to a mutation in the sodium potassium chloride co-transporter molecule in the thick ascending limb of Henle's loop. The mutation results in the inability to resorb sodium at this site. This leads to mild sodium loss, and increased aldosterone secretion, enhanced loss of potassium and hydrogen ions in the more distal collecting tubules. The result is hypokalemic alkalosis. A parallel increase in renal release of vasodilatory prostaglandins, especially prostacyclin, may partially explain why the blood pressure remains in the normal range. There is still no satisfactory treatment. The genetic defect is not treatable and the only approach is to block a part of the abnormal physiology, decrease prostaglandin secretion with an anti-inflammatory drug or lower angiotensin activation with an ACE inhibitor.

Bartter continued to work until he died from a hemorrhagic stroke in 1983 at the age of 68. Honors had come his way. One was his election in 1979 to the National Academy of Sciences, whose meeting he was attending when he was struck down. Although many workers in the field of salt and water phenomena consider themselves nephrologists, Bartter seemed to stay in the camp of endocrinologists. The Endocrine Society awarded him its highest honor, the Fred Koch award, and locally, the VA Medical Center where he worked in Texas perpetuated his memory by naming its clinical study center after him. A good scientist and a good man.

Sources

Bartter FC, Albright F, Forbes AP, et al.: The effects of adrenocorticotropic hormone and cortisone in the adrenogenital syndrome associated with congenital adrenal hyperplasia: an attempt to explain and correct its disordered hormonal pattern. *J Clin Invest* 1951; 30: 237.

Bartter FC, Leaf A, Santos RF, Wrong O: Evidence in man that urinary electrolyte loss induced by pitressin is a function of water retention. *J Clin Invest* 1953; 32: 868.

Bartter FC, Schwartz WB, Bennett W, et al.: A syndrome of renal sodium loss and hypernatremia probably resulting from inappropriate secretion of antidiuretic hormone. *Am J Med* 1957; 33: 529.

Bartter FC, Mills IH, Biglieri EG, Delea C: Studies on the control and physiological actions of aldosterone. *Recent Progr Horm Res* 1959; 15: 311.

Bartter FC, Pronove P, Gill JR, et al.: Hyperplasia of the juxtaglomerular complex with hyperaldosteronism and hypokalemic alkalosis. *Am J Med* 1962; 33: 811.

Wilson JD, Delea CS: Frederic C. Bartter. *Biogr Mem Natl Acad Sci* 1990; 59: 3.

This chapter has been reproduced from Sawin, C.: Frederic C. Bartter (1914–1983). *The Endocrinologist* 2006; 16(4): 187–8.

CHAPTER 93
Earl W. Sutherland
(1915–1974)
Discovery of Cyclic AMP

Education was a high priority in Kansas in the early twentieth century. The largely agricultural state had one of the highest literacy rates in the United States (>99%), higher than any of the states on the eastern seaboard so widely known for their education prowess, despite the fact that Kansans spent no more on public education than did the older states of Massachusetts or Pennsylvania. So, it is no surprise to learn that the parents of Earl Wilbur Sutherland, Jr. both had attended college, although neither had a degree. By the time Sutherland was born in 1915, the family had settled in the small farming town of Burlingame, Kansas, about 25 miles southwest of Topeka. There Sutherland, Sr., owned and ran a prosperous dry goods store. Earl's mother, his father's second wife, encouraged the boy's interest in science and allowed him a high degree of independence from a young age. He was fishing and hunting with his own shotgun when he was 8 years old.

The father's business deteriorated when the Great Depression hit in the 1930s and, to make things worse, Kansas was part of the infamous Dust Bowl. So, when the time came for Earl to go to college, he went to a local school, Washburn College in Topeka. He covered the costs by working as an orderly in a local hospital. He did well as a student and applied for, and was accepted by, Washington University School of Medicine about 300 miles east in St. Louis, Missouri. The austerity of the 1930s clearly affected his view of the world and it is likely that he intended to practice medicine, as do most entering medical students.

However, in his second-year course of pharmacology, Sutherland caught the attention of Carl Ferdinand Cori, then the chairman of the department and later a Nobel Laureate (1947). Cori was impressed enough that he offered Sutherland a student assistantship in the department. Sutherland was enchanted by the idea of research and he joined in the work of the department while he himself was still a student. The setting of Cori's laboratory and the research questions studied were powerful influences on Sutherland's future.

A Biographical History of Endocrinology, First Edition. D. Lynn Loriaux.

This work is a co-publication between the Endocrine Society and John Wiley & Sons, Ltd.

Cori was born in 1896 in Prague into an academic family. His education was classical and, in 1914, just before the outbreak of the First World War, he began medical school with the idea that he would go into some area of the biological sciences. When the War began, he was drafted into the Austrian Army, though still a student, and nearly died. In 1918 he returned to medical school, graduated in 1920, and in that same year, married a classmate, Gerty Radnitz. Cori's Nobel Prize in 1947 was shared equally with his wife and with Bernardo Houssay of Argentina. Some say that Gerty Cori was the real driving force behind the husband and wife. The *Dictionary of Scientific Biography* lists Gerty, but not Carl. They moved to Vienna, where Carl Cori divided his time between the clinic and the laboratory and Gerty worked in a children's hospital. But the postwar times were hard. Funds for research were nonexistent. The food supply was so bad that Gerty Cori developed clinical vitamin A deficiency, and Carl was unhappy with the overtly anti-Semitic ambience of his clinic. They sought a way out and succeeded in 1922, when they were offered positions in Buffalo, New York, at the State Institute for the Study of Malignant Disease (later the Roswell Park Institute). They stayed in Buffalo until 1931, when they went to St. Louis.

In Buffalo, the Coris published dozens of papers, few of which had anything to do with cancer. Their focus was on carbohydrate metabolism, an emphasis stimulated by the discovery of insulin in 1921–1922. They were eager to understand glucose balance and were intrigued by the problems of how insulin and epinephrine worked to affect the metabolism of glucose. Their tools were in vitro studies of rats and rabbits and, importantly, liver slices in vitro. By the time they left for St. Louis, they had achieved a world-wide reputation for the Cori Cycle, in which glucose in muscle is split into two lactate molecules if metabolized anaerobically, and the two lactate molecules are converted to glucose in the liver, and cycled back to muscle again.

In Cori's laboratory, Sutherland, the medical student, teamed with one of Cori's first graduate students, Sidney Colowick. By the time Sutherland graduated in 1942, he had published two papers in the *Journal of Biological Chemistry*. This was his introduction to phosphorylase reactions, which ultimately led to his now well-known discovery. Sutherland later recalled that, even as a student, he was "intrigued and puzzled by the actions of hormones," thoughts that were no doubt instilled by the Coris' work.

As a new medical graduate, Sutherland stayed at his alma mater to do an internship at Barnes Hospital. It is said that he was hard to find as he spent a good deal of time in Cori's laboratory. Cori defended Sutherland's behavior as being to the benefit of mankind. By the end of his internship in 1943, World War II had engulfed most of the "developed" nations of the world. Sutherland, like most new young physicians, went into military service. In his 2 years on active duty in the European theater, he served in General Patton's Army as a battalion surgeon and in a U.S. Army Military Hospital in Germany. When he returned to St. Louis after War's end in 1945, he was not sure whether to stay with research or to practice medicine. Carl Cori's influence led him to stick with the laboratory, and he rose from internship to assistant professor. For the next 8 years, 1945–1953, Sutherland was a member of Washington University's Department of Biochemistry.

By the late 1940s the Coris' laboratory, which was internationally famous, became even more so after both Coris got the Nobel Prize in 1947. One of Sutherland's colleagues in 1947–1948 was Christian de Duve, who came to the Coris' for a year on a Rockefeller Foundation Fellowship. He won a Nobel Prize in 1974 for his work on cell particles and the discovery of the lysosome. Sutherland and de Duve took up the old "insulin contaminant" problem that had puzzled Carl Cori almost two decades earlier. They found that there was indeed a separate factor in commercial "insulin" that was separable and that raised instead of suppressed blood glucose levels. They called it the "hyperglycemic-glycogen lytic factor," an awkward name at best. They thought it came mainly from the pancreatic alpha cells. De Duve returned to Belgium when his fellowship was over, and Sutherland pursued this new "factor."

Sutherland and his colleagues purified the elusive factor in 1949 and he presented his collected results at the Laurentian Hormone Conference that same year. Though preceded by suspicions that dated back to the 1920s, a separate factor, clearly different from insulin, had not been shown before. In fact, Sutherland had defined a new hormone, only later in the 1950s given a discrete and pronounceable name, glucagon. For the rest of his career, Sutherland was to pursue the question of how it was that glucagon and epinephrine broke down hepatic glycogen and released glucose to the blood stream.

One should note that the thinking of the time was that hormones acted directly on enzymes to enhance their activity. How this could occur was not clear, and there were some smatterings of data that suggested that it was not so, but it was the prevailing idea. There was no concept of hormones acting via receptors, specific or otherwise, which is the reigning concept of today. This idea of receptors held some attraction for pharmacologists, but that attraction was seen by others as good for drugs but not for real biology. The concept of hormones acting directly to stimulate enzyme activity was the prevailing idea in the Coris' laboratory and was actively promoted there. Carl Cori thought, at least until 1949 and probably into the early 1950s, that the evidence showed that insulin acted directly on hepatic hexokinase. Although he never withdrew this ultimately incorrect idea, he stopped referring to it after 1955. Nevertheless, the idea was a major influence in the Coris' laboratory and permeated Sutherland's thought as well.

To try to understand how glucagon and epinephrine acted in the liver, Sutherland studied the phosphorylation reaction intensively, using liver slices as the model system. By 1951, he and Carl Cori were able to show that the phosphorylate reaction was the rate-limiting step for hepatic glycogenolysis and that both glucagon and epinephrine stimulated the activation of phosphorylase by converting it from what they now called phosphorylase b (inactive) to phosphorylase a (active). This effect occurred in fresh liver slices but not with liver slices after freezing (which breaks up cellular structure), or with liver extracts, or with semi-purified phosphorylase preparations. There was no explanation that made sense. The theory of direct hormonal action on enzymes was in trouble. Even so, it still seemed that intact cells were necessary for these hormones to act.

Sutherland moved to Cleveland in 1953 as chairman of the Pharmacological Department at Western Reserve University, now known as Case-Western Reserve

University. From his last work in St. Louis, it seems reasonably clear that he thought at least one answer to the problem of why hormones failed to act directly on enzymes lay in better purification of the phosphorylase enzyme. His work in Cleveland was slow for the first 3 years, in part because he needed to set up a new laboratory and run a department. He was back on track by 1955. He and his colleagues found that the phosphorylate reaction was even more complex than they thought. The activation step involved the phosphorylation of the phosphorylate kinase, and the inactivation step required a novel phosphatase, which removed the previously added phosphate residue. Now, with better knowledge of the details, he could pursue the problem of why hormonal effects disappeared in preparations wherein the cells were broken and re-examined the issue of whether or not there was a direct effect of a hormone on the phosphorylase enzyme reaction.

Sutherland was now the chief and leader of the laboratory. Many of the experiments were done by those he attracted to the laboratory. One of these was Theodore W. Rall, whose previous work had mainly been with homogenized rat liver and who was used to preparing the several cell fractions (e.g., mitochondria or endoplasmic reticulum). He thought it would be interesting to apply this technique to Sutherland's problem. Sutherland, still with the mindset that intact cells are needed for his hormones to act, was a bit reluctant but probably knew that something like this approach was necessary to attack the problem. So Rall ground up rat livers – and nothing happened. Then they realized that all of Sutherland's prior work was with liver tissue from dogs, not rats. Maybe this caused the difference. On November 5, 1955, Sutherland was "absolutely ecstatic" when the crude liver homogenate from dogs showed a clear-cut activation of phosphorylase when either epinephrine or glucagon were added. Cells were not needed after all!

The next step was to see whether the effect still happened when they removed the "cellular debris" and studied only the supernatant fluid. The hormones still worked. However, Rall, though an expert on liver fractions, used a fairly crude method of separating one fraction from another; he basically did a simple centrifugation, poured off the supernate, and used it to do the experiment. A Belgian postdoctoral student, Jacques Berthet, who had trained with de Duve and was quite precise as to just how liver homogenates should be made, was "offended" by Rall's technique and wrote a protocol that was precise and eliminated any spillover of particulate material. The supernate was now "clean." The only problem was that now the hormones failed to work. With a truly "clean" preparation, completely free of cellular particles, hormones simply did not activate phosphorylase. Rall was upset with Berthet, but soon realized that the failure of Berthet's method was in fact the answer: the reactions happened in the particulate matter.

They now did a critical experiment; they added back some of the cellular debris to Berthet's "clean" supernate and re-ran the experiment with each hormone. If a critical factor was lost or disintegrated, nothing would happen. What actually happened was that the addition of the centrifuged debris once again allowed the hormones to activate the phosphorylase. There was something in the debris that mediated the reaction.

They next added each hormone to the cellular debris, heated it to kill any enzymes (such as phosphorylase), centrifuged it to remove the debris, and then added this supernate to a separate inactive phosphorylase preparation. Once again, the phosphorylase was activated. Sutherland now had proof that the hormones activated phosphorylase not directly, as thought, but in a two-step process. In the first step, the hormone caused the generation of a heat-stable dialyzable substance that in turn activated the enzyme. They had luck here. It was fortuitous that the substance was not destroyed by the heating. The substance turned out to be made by the fraction of the cellular debris that corresponded to the cell membrane. The theory of direct enzyme activation by hormones was wrong and a new paradigm was in the offing, though how revolutionary this finding would be was not seen by the experimenters.

Sutherland and his co-workers did a great deal of work in the remainder of 1955 and into 1956 to try to delineate the process in more detail, using both glucagon and epinephrine as stimulators. Their major paper in the *Journal of Biological Chemistry* came out in January 1957. While this paper was in press, their main aim was to isolate and identify the heat-stable compound that seemed responsible for mediating the hormone's effect. The work was difficult. They did not know at the time how little of the compound there was or how rapidly it was destroyed. But they did succeed. Their work was advanced by collaboration with a group of chemists who had found the same chemical entity in hydrolyzed adenosine triphosphate (ATP). A mutual colleague of the two groups suggested that they might both be dealing with the same compound. Exchanged samples confirmed that both groups, in fact, had the identical chemical, an adenine ribonucleotide. Both published their preliminary reports in the July issue of the *Journal of the American Chemical Society*.

Variously named by Sutherland himself over the next few years as "cyclic adenine ribonucleotide," "adenosine 3′,5′ phosphate," "cyclic adenylic acid," "cyclic adenylate," or "cyclic 3′,5′ adenosine monophosphate," the compound is usually colloquially called "cyclic AMP." Sutherland was invited back for an almost unprecedented second major presentation at the Laurentian Hormone Conference in 1960. All knew that this was a major discovery. Hormones did not have to act directly on enzymes and did not have to permeate the cell membrane to bring about a cellular response. And one did not need intact cells to show a hormonal effect. Sutherland's work made him famous and laid the groundwork for the imminent rise of the idea of hormone receptors in cell membranes.

But was Sutherland's newly discovered effect a local effect that applied only to the liver? Or was it more general? In fact, the concept and the finding did not immediately cause a great stir nor was it seen early on as a general solution to an entire class of hormonal mechanisms of action. The techniques Sutherland used were difficult and not all could copy them. Further, the idea itself was so disparate from what most scientists thought that it took a while to be accepted as "real." More studies showed that a wide range of hormone actions involved this newcomer, cyclic AMP. Sutherland himself with his colleagues showed its effects in the adrenal cortex, pigeon red cells, cardiac muscle, the toad urinary bladder, the corpus luteum, the rat epididymal fat pad, and even bacteria. Others carried the idea to many other tissues. The concept of an intracellular "second messenger" (the hormone itself is the "first messenger") that mediates the action of a hormone was established. Other second messengers were found later and cyclic AMP may not always be a hormone's only second messenger, even if the hormone is a peptide. Nevertheless, Sutherland's data were a "first"; they separated the cell's "inside" from its "outside," generalized the concept of intracellular mediation of hormonal effects, showed that hormones did not act directly on enzymes, and showed the way for others to define the cell surface, find receptors, and put an entirely new focus on what hormones do.

Sutherland was not particularly happy at Western Reserve. A new curriculum was coming in, later to be followed by many American medical schools, called a "systems-based" curriculum. He did not like it as he would have to play a much larger part in teaching. He personally did not like to give lectures and was not particularly good at it. In addition, the administration of his department was getting him down. He wanted to work full-time on his discovery. He moved to Vanderbilt University in 1963 as professor of physiology, funded by grants and a career Investigator award from the American Heart Association. He knew full well that the next question was to find out how cyclic AMP worked and he pursued this for some years, although in his later years he added to his main focus studies on another cyclic nucleotide, guanosine 3′,5′-monophosphate (cyclic GMP). In 1971, he was awarded the Nobel Prize in Medicine or Physiology, one of the few awardees in recent years to receive an unshared Prize.

For reasons still unclear, in 1973 Sutherland left Vanderbilt to go to the University of Miami in Florida. Though only 57 years of age, his health may have been an issue. He was in Miami less than a year when he died on March 9, 1974, as a result of massive esophageal bleeding.

Sutherland succeeded because of a combination of talent and luck. He did not set out to win a Nobel Prize. The topic he chose was a direct follow-on of his mentor's work. But the Coris' did not direct him. Once started, he led himself. He did not know where he was going, in the sense that he was not seeking a general hormonal mechanism of action. He simply wanted to figure out how phosphorylase worked and how hormones made it work faster. He mastered methods. He once estimated that he spent at least a third of his time in the laboratory on methods. He was persistent, and he had an excellent memory. These seem necessary qualities for a good scientist. He chose problems and their solutions well. But it was more of a lucky stroke rather than careful planning that led him to choose a problem that turned out to be generally applicable and that would change the way we think hormones act. And he died too young. But, in all, he was a good model and did great work; his prizes were well-deserved and his work was truly of lasting value.

Sources

Carnes MC, Garrary JA: *Mapping America's Past.* New York: Henry Holt, 1996, p. 167.

Cori CI: Earl Wilbur Sutherland. 1915–1974. *Biogr Mem Natl Acad Sci* 1978; 49: 319.

Gallagher GL: Getting the message across. *J NIH Res* 1990; 2: 77.

Rall TW, Sutherland EW, Berthet J: The relationship of epinephrine and glucagon to liver phosphorylase. IV. Effect of epinephrine and glucagon on the reactivation of phosphorylase in liver homogenates. *J Biol Chem* 1957; 224: 463.

Randall P: Carl Ferdinand Cori: 5 December 1896–20 October 1984. *Biogr Mem Fellows R Soc* 1986; 32: 67.

Roth J: Receptors: Birth, eclipse, and rediscovery. In *Endocrinology: People and Ideas*, edited by SM McCann. Bethesda, MD: American Physiological Society, 1988, p. 369.

Sherman L: Earl Wilbur Sutherland Jr. 1971. In *Nobel Laureates in Medicine or Physiology, A Biographical Dictionary*, edited by DM Fox, M Meldrum, I Rezak. New York: Garland Press, 1990, p. 509.

Sutherland EW, Rall TW: The properties of an adenine ribonucleotide produced with cellular particles, ATP, Mg^{++}, and epinephrine or glucagon. *J Am Chem Soc* 1957; 79: 3608.

This chapter has been reproduced from Sawin, Clark T: How does a hormone act inside a cell? Earl W. Sutherland (1915–1974) and the discovery of cyclic AMP. *The Endocrinologist* 2000; 10(3): 139–44.

CHAPTER 94
Maurice S. Raben
(1915–1977)
The Treatment of Growth Hormone Deficiency

In late February 1957, Maurice S. Raben saw a boy who was much shorter than he should have been. Even though he was 17 years old, he was only 4 feet and 2 inches tall and had never shown signs of puberty. Raben had seen the boy over the course of the previous year and a half, and he had grown only three-quarters of an inch during that time. The boy, who should have been a man, had the diagnosis of "pituitary dwarf," or "pituitary infantilism." There was no apparent reason for his pituitary hormones to be absent. That February, Raben began to administer injections of an extract of human pituitary glands that contained growth hormone (GH). The hope was that it would cause the boy to grow. It was an experiment. Previous attempts to bring about growth in these patients with pituitary extracts had either failed or provided false hope. To Raben's great satisfaction, the boy did in fact grow. At the end of 10 months of treatment, the boy had grown more than 2 inches in height [1]. The treatment had worked and a new era had begun for these patients.

Raben sent a short letter describing these results to the editor of the principal endocrine clinical journal, the *Journal of Clinical Endocrinology and Metabolism*, and it was printed in the August 1958 issue. The contrast to the July 1958 issue of the same journal was striking. Lawson Wilkins, the premier pediatric endocrinologist of the time, reported his work with 26 such patients. Six had been administered some sort of pituitary GH preparation over the course of the years "without discernible effect," and Wilkins noted that he had to manage his patients "in the absence of an effective GH preparation" [2]. Incidentally, modern endocrinologists need to remember that when Raben performed his work there was no assay for GH in humans and all effects of treatment were based on clinical observation and judgment. In essence, today's current management of children who are short and who grow better with injections of human GH flows directly from Raben's studies more than 40 years ago.

Maurice Raben, "Maury" to all who knew him, was a smart and quiet man who seemed to know almost everything. He was not one to break into a conversation so that his view would be known early. Others would finish what they had to say and

A Biographical History of Endocrinology, First Edition. D. Lynn Loriaux.

This work is a co-publication between the Endocrine Society and John Wiley & Sons, Ltd.

then he would speak. He spoke hesitatingly but thought clearly. He did not hesitate to express his views whether or not they agreed with whoever had just spoken. He would carefully explain why he thought the way he did. He was that seemingly outmoded term, a "gentleman."

Maury was born in 1915 in Port Chester, New York. After Yale and medical school at New York University, he finished an internship and a year of residency and then joined the United States Army (it was the time of World War II). After the military, he trained as a resident at Goldwater Memorial Hospital in New York, then a hotbed of training for academic medicine, and at Boston City Hospital, which was his first year of exposure to Boston medicine. He returned to New York as a junior staff physician in cardiology at Bellevue Hospital, but, in 1948, he decided to go back to Boston as a research fellow in endocrinology. He chose to work with Edwin B. "Ted" Astwood, who at the time was only 6 years Maury's senior, and had become world-famous because of his discovery of the anti-thyroid drug treatment of hyperthyroidism. Maury had stepped into a world highly focused on the thyroid gland and remained there for the rest of his career.

Maury's initial ventures were in the physiology and clinical aspects of the thyroid gland. By the end of 1950, he had published three articles on the effects of anti-thyroid agents on thyroid function in animals and on the use of radioiodine in humans. Characteristically, as was always the case in Astwood's laboratory, Raben was either the sole author or co-author with another fellow on any publication that did not directly involve Ted in the actual work (the result is that Ted's input is not always evident in what was discovered in his laboratory).

But 1949 and 1950 were also years of the adrenal gland in endocrinology. In 1949, the biochemist Edward C. Kendall, working with his clinical colleague Philip S. Hench at the Mayo Clinic in Rochester, Minnesota, reported the remarkable success of "curing" rheumatoid arthritis with injections of cortisone or the pituitary hormone adrenocorticotropin (ACTH). These results so struck the world of science that both Kendall and Hench won the Nobel Prize in 1950.

Ted and Maury, the latter now a senior fellow, became involved with the issue of ACTH in 1950 and aimed for its purification and identification in addition to examining its role in the treatment of human disease. As it happened, this was not really an entirely new venture for Ted. He had already worked on the assay and effects of ACTH during the War as a result of the U.S. Government's interest in adrenal function (this interest itself was the result of rumors that German aviators experienced less fatigue and could fly for more hours if administered adrenal extracts; funds for adrenal research flowed almost instantly). In 1942, Ted found that a low pH level enhanced the extraction of ACTH from pituitary powder (mostly from pigs or cows). But adrenal research in Ted's laboratory lapsed after 1943 when he worked out the use of anti-thyroid drugs.

When Maury arrived and they examined ACTH again, they applied what was an almost heretical extraction medium to porcine pituitary powder, namely glacial acetic acid. Most expected that this would be so destructive that no ACTH would be retrieved. In fact, this turned out to be an ideal extractant. Almost all of the ACTH was extracted into the strong acetic acid. With a few more steps, including the adsorption of ACTH onto oxycellulose, they had a reasonably pure preparation of ACTH suitable for clinical use that was essentially uncontaminated by other pituitary hormones [3, 4]. Thus, pure porcine ACTH was clinically effective in humans.

With this purer preparation of ACTH they thought that they were on the way to its chemical identification. They were confident enough that they placed their names on the program of the Laurentian Hormone Conference (which was co-chaired by Ted in the first place), expecting to announce the structure of ACTH [5]. It was not to be. The structure was not elucidated by the summer of 1951 and the molecular weight of ACTH was still uncertain.

That same year, 1951, Raben performed another experiment with glacial acetic acid extract, apparently out of curiosity. When extracting ACTH, reasonable assurance that the ACTH preparation administered to patients contained little or none of the other pituitary hormones was needed. The bioassays were reassuring. There were almost no thyroid-stimulating hormones or gonadotropins after the initial extraction steps, and the oxycellulose step took the ACTH out of whatever was left in solution. But where was the GH? Somewhat to their surprise, they found that the fractions of porcine pituitary extract used to derive the porcine ACTH, and from which the oxycellulose finally extracted the ACTH, contained a large amount of GH, as assayed in hypophysectomized rats. Fortunately, ACTH was adsorbed by the oxycellulose but GH was not. What Maury and his fellow, Westermeyer, had serendipitously found was a method for the extraction of GH itself [6]. It turned out that, though far from planned, this article was the critical one for the future treatment of hypopituitarism with GH.

Maury was nothing if not versatile. The end of the 1940s and the early 1950s were times of the increasing use of radioisotopes in science. Ted and Maury were familiar with various radioiodine isotopes, but the newly available carbon-14 was not easy to measure with the then-available techniques. Perhaps there was a way to magnify the relatively weak β radiation. Indeed, there was: dissolve the material containing the carbon-14 in a "scintillator." So, working with a colleague at the Nuclear Laboratory at Harvard University, Maury invented liquid scintillation counting with the addition of coincidence counting using two photomultipliers so that what was counted was likely to be a true flash from a radioisotope and not random noise [7]. This was a truly remarkable feat that was the basis for a great deal of the research performed worldwide over the course of the next decades. Today, of course, it would have been patented with royalties flowing to Maury (and perhaps his colleagues and the New England Medical Center where he worked), but I can testify that it was not his way, nor was it the ethic of the time. Physicians, including Ted, simply did not believe one should patent their discoveries made for the benefit of patients, and they did not.

By the early 1950s, Maury was established on the staff of the New England Medical Center and Tufts Medical School. He functioned, in essence, as Ted's major research "arm" (if one could describe anyone in Ted's loosely run laboratory in such terms). Most of the clinical work was performed by others.

During the 1950s, Maury pursued the problems of GH and ACTH and published one or two papers a year on these topics. During this time, GH became even more confusing. Whereas ACTH from pigs worked well in humans, GH from pigs or cows did not. Many thought it was just a matter of purity. The idea was that impure preparations of GH from cows did not work in humans, even though they did in rats, because the preparations were too impure. So the thrust of much work was to purify GH. However, that did not seem to do the trick. The answer came from the field of comparative endocrinology [8]. Data from 1954 showed that fish GH worked in fish but not in rats. This raised the idea that perhaps some hormones had a degree, larger or smaller, of species-specificity. A hormone, even when pure, might work in one species but not in another. This would be, of course, in contrast to the case of ACTH in which purification did make it more effective and there was little species-specificity. Maury hoped this did not apply to GH [9].

In Boston in 1955 at Harvard Medical School's Department of Physiology, Ernst Knobil was puzzled by the inability of both porcine and bovine GH to act in monkeys [10]. He, too, learned of the fish experiments and decided that the answer might be that GH was species-specific in its actions. Knobil arranged for Raben to prepare monkey GH from Knobil's collection of monkey pituitary glands. Maury did so, and gave some of his human GH to colleagues in Canada, one of whom had previously worked with Ted Astwood, to see if this GH had physiologic effects in humans. It did, although the study was not designed to show an effect on growth [11]. Note that Maury still had not published his method for making primate GH, yet he had provided it to other investigators to study–another characteristic of the man.

Maury finally published his method for preparing biologically active human GH in a 2-page paper printed in the same issue of *Science* as the article documenting the effects of human GH in humans [12]. Because the two articles were printed on sequential pages, it seems likely that there was an editorial arrangement.

A few months before his article describing the method of preparing human GH appeared in *Science*, Maury had started treating of the short boy noted at the beginning of this note. The culmination was Maury's article in the *Journal of Clinical Endocrinology and Metabolism* documenting that the boy grew [1]. The first patient treated for short stature with human GH was a success. GH therapy in humans was a reality.

Once he had started, it was difficult for Maury to stop. His laboratory became a place of production of human GH on an industrial scale. Each year, he collected thousands of human pituitaries that had been gathered during autopsies from all over the United States. Stored in acetone until the magical days in the spring when they were converted to human GH, these pituitaries were legendary. Initially, with the help of others in the laboratory and after a few years with the collaboration of Fukashi Matsuzaki from Japan, the odor of glacial acetic acid permeated the air. There were no doors on other laboratories to block the fumes, so many would find other activities to perform on those days. Even more pungent was the next day when Maury used large quantities of ether as a precipitant. Nothing ever blew up, but no one today would be allowed to (or would want to) use that procedure. The product was human GH in such quantities that others all over the country had their supply for experimental use in GH-deficient children. Maury's superb review says it all, and it is still worth a look by modern clinicians [13].

After a few years, it was clear that Maury could not handle production and distribution alone. The Endocrine Study Section of the National Institutes of Health stepped in, and in 1962, with Maury's strong support, devised the National Pituitary Agency that not only supplied human GH to those in need but also made other human pituitary hormones available to investigators. Maury was the stimulus for it all. He had managed to do what most physician–endocrinologists would want to do: combine laboratory investigation with clinical therapy for the direct benefit of patients.

Maury continued to study GH and its actions over the course of the next decade and a half. His responsibilities shifted, however, in the 1960s when he was asked to direct cardiovascular research at the hospital. He focused on metabolic changes in the heart in various experimental models. He took up a few byways as well: the curious growth factor in the *Spirometra* parasite that interacts with GH receptors, and the hypoglycemic effect of the Jamaican "Ackee" bean. By the early 1970s, his mentor, Ted Astwood, had retired to work in general practice in Bermuda where he was born. Maury worked in cardiovascular research, and a new chief of endocrinology, Seymour Reichlin, was recruited to replace Ted. Many will remember the tight funding for research in the 1970s (if one was not studying cancer). But Maury, as always, continued on and published three or four articles each year. Most will recall him, however, as the Master of GH.

For his real contributions, his colleagues in the Endocrine Society awarded him one of its high honors, the Ayerst Award, in 1975. Maury died suddenly on September 19, 1977, when he was only 62 years old. All who knew him felt the loss; I suspect he would not mind being remembered as the one who made short persons grow.

References

1. Raben MS: Treatment of a pituitary dwarf with human growth hormone. *J Clin Endocrinol Metab* 1958; 18: 901.
2. Martin MM, Wilkins L: Pituitary dwarfism: diagnosis and treatment. *J Clin Endocrinol Metab* 1958; 18: 679.
3. Payne RW, Raben MS, Astwood EB: Extraction and purification of corticotropin. *J Biol Chem* 1950; 187: 719.
4. Astwood EB, Raben MS, Payne RW, et al.: Purification of corticotropin with oxycellulose. *J Am Chem Soc* 1951; 73: 2969.
5. Astwood EB, Raben MS, Payne RW: Chemistry of corticotrophin. *Recent Prog Horm Res* 1952; 7: 1.
6. Raben MS, Westermeyer VW: Recovery of growth hormone in purification of corticotropin. *Proc Soc Exp Biol Med* 1951; 78: 550.
7. Raben MS, Bloembergen N: Determination of radioactivity by solution in a liquid scintillator. *Science* 1951; 114: 363.
8. Friesen HG: Raben lecture 1980: A tale of stature. *Endocr Rev* 1980; 1: 309.
9. Raben MS: Discussion. In *Hypophyseal Growth Hormone,* edited by RW Smith, OH Gaebler, CNH Long. New York: McGraw-Hill, 1955, p. 98.
10. Knobil E, Wolf RC, Greep RO: Some physiological effects of primate growth hormone preparations in hypophysectomized rhesus monkeys. *J Clin Endocrinol Metab* 1956; 16: 916.

11. Beck JC, McGarry EE, Dyrenfurth I, et al.: Metabolic effects of human and monkey growth hormone in man. *Science* 1957; 125: 884.
12. Raben MS: Preparation of growth hormone from pituitaries of man and monkey *Science* 1957; 125: 883.
13. Raben MS: Human growth hormone. *Recent Prog Horm Res* 1959; 15: 71.

This chapter has been reproduced from Sawin, Clark T: Maurice S. Raben and the treatment of growth hormone deficiency. *The Endocrinologist* 2002; 12(2): 73–6.

CHAPTER 95

Alfred Jost
(1916–1991)
Sexual Ambiguity

Alfred Jost was born in Strasbourg in 1916 [1]. His father died when Alfred was 13 years old and his mother, unable to care financially for four sons, made plans for Alfred to live with his grandmother. She was planning to apprentice the boy to a local grocer but a neighbor, Madame Oguse, offered instead to let Alfred live with her. Her husband, a professor of Ancient Greek at the University of Strasbourg, was impressed by the boy's intellect and began to tutor him in his studies. He rose from the bottom of his class to the top, paving the way to enrollment in the École Normale Supérieure. His academic career was on its way. In addition, the Oguse family provided Alfred with his wife, their youngest daughter, a union that endured more than 50 years.

Jost went on to become the world's leading scientist in the field of fetal endocrinology. Instead of studying the usual avian models, Jost focused on mammals. Using rabbits, he showed that castration of the male fetus before sexual differentiation led to a female phenotype with persistent Müllerian ducts and no Wolffian structures [2]. Jost then explored the role of testosterone in male genital development and was able to show that testosterone is the stimulus for Wolffian development but has no effect on Müllerian regression. Subsequent studies with implanted testicular fragments showed that the testis produced a "factor" that causes Müllerian inhibition, a factor he termed the "Müllerian inhibiting factor" [3].

Jost's findings were not widely accepted until a meeting with Lawson Wilkins convinced the famous endocrinologist that his work could explain most, if not all congenital abnormalities of sexual development.

The pathophysiology of an "experiment of nature," the freemartin calf, had puzzled endocrinologists for years. It was ultimately understood through Jost's experimental findings. A freemartin calf, the female twin of a male calf, has ambiguous genitalia with Wolffian development and Müllerian regression. This was finally explained by the endocrine effects of testosterone and the anti-Müllerian factor from the male calf on the genital development of the female. These endocrine effects were made possible by the hemochorial placenta of cattle in which the circulations of twin calves are conjoined [4].

A Biographical History of Endocrinology, First Edition. D. Lynn Loriaux.

This work is a co-publication between the Endocrine Society and John Wiley & Sons, Ltd.

"Antimullerian hormone" was subsequently characterized as a dimeric glycoprotein, and the gene has been cloned and localized in the human genome.

Jost held the posts of professor of comparative physiology, Faculty of Science of Paris, and professor and chairman of physiologic development, College of France. He died of a heart attack in 1991 at 74 years of age.

References

1. Remembrance: Dr. Alfred Jost. *Endocrinology* 1991; 129: 2274–6.
2. Jost A: Researches sur la differentiation sexuelle de l'embryon de Lapin. *Arch Anat Microsc Morphol Exp* 1947; 36: 271–315.
3. Jost A: Problems of fetal endocrinology: the gonadal and hypophyseal hormones. *Recent Prog Horm Res* 1953; 8: 379–418.
4. Jost A, Bigier B, Prepin J: Freemartins in cattle: The first steps of sexual organogenesis. *J Reprod Fertil* 1972; 29: 349–79.

This chapter has been reproduced from Loriaux, D. Lynn: Alfred Jost: 1916–1991. *The Endocrinologist* 2010; 20(1): 1.

CHAPTER 96

Robert Burns Woodward (1917–1979)

Synthesis of Cholesterol

Robert Woodward was born April 10, 1917 in Boston, Massachusetts. His parents were both immigrants, his father, Arthur, from England and his mother, Margaret (nee Burns), from Scotland. His father died a year after Robert was born, and he was raised by a single mother. Early on, Robert demonstrated a keen interest in science, especially chemistry. He studied chemistry independently throughout primary and secondary school and, by the time he entered high school, he had performed most of the experiments in a college text of organic chemistry. Woodward was admitted to MIT in 1933 at 16 years of age, but was expelled the following year for neglecting most of the curriculum other than chemistry. Chastised, he was admitted again in 1935 and received the Bachelor of Science degree in 1936 at 19 years of age. One year later, MIT awarded the 19-year-old Woodward a PhD in organic chemistry. He took a fellowship at Harvard in 1937, and remained there for the rest of his scientific career.

Woodward's passion was the complete chemical synthesis of important naturally occurring compounds. His first major advance was the complete synthesis of quinine in 1944. Instead of the usual brute force method, this synthesis was highlighted by a rational "decision tree" approach using the established principles of reactivity and structure. This became his "scientific trademark," as it were.

Woodward won the Nobel Prize in 1965 based on his total synthesis of cephalosporin. Along the way, he had synthesized strychnine, lysergic acid, risperprine, chlorophyll, and colchicine. He was the first to achieve the total synthesis of cholesterol and cortisone. Neither of these syntheses did much to change the availability of the molecules, nor did they alter the approach of the pharmaceutical industry to the commercial preparation of the molecules. They did, however, contribute enormously to the understanding of steroid chemistry and facilitated all of the chemistry that was yet to come in understanding glucocorticoid, mineralocorticoid, estrogen, androgen, and progesterone physiology.

Other contributions include the first synthesis of vitamin B-12, elucidating the correct structure of penicillin and developing, with Roald Hoffmann, the Woodward–Hoffmann

---

A Biographical History of Endocrinology, First Edition. D. Lynn Loriaux.

This work is a co-publication between the Endocrine Society and John Wiley & Sons, Ltd.

rules that are still used for defining the stereochemistry of organic molecules. In 1963, Woodward became the director of the Woodward Research Institute in Basel, Switzerland, and he was a trustee of MIT from 1966 to 1971.

Woodward married Ilja Pullman in 1938 and they had two daughters. His second marriage was to Endoria Miller in 1946, and they had a daughter and a son. The marriage lasted until Woodward's death in 1979.

Woodward was a celebrated lecturer: His lectures could last for 3 or 4 hours, during which he used a blackboard to draw structures with multi-colored chalk. He was a chain smoker and could consume a pack or two during one lecture. He disliked exercise and slept just a few hours a night. He also enjoyed scotch whiskey and a martini or two. He died in his sleep of a myocardial infarction on July 8, 1979.

Reference

1. Blout E: Robert Burns Woodward (1917–1979). A biographical memoir. In *Biographical Memoirs*, Vol. 80. Washington, DC: National Academy Press, 2001.

This chapter has been reproduced from Loriaux, D. Lynn: Robert Burns Woodward: 1917–1979. *The Endocrinologist* 2009; 19(4): 153.

CHAPTER 97

Sylvia Agnes Sophia Tait (1917–2003)

Steroid Metabolism

Sylvia Agnes Sophia Wardropper was born in Tumen, Russia, January 8, 1917. Her father was a British agronomist stationed in Russia, and her mother was a Russian mathematician. With the outbreak of the Russian Revolution, the family returned to the United Kingdom in 1919. Sylvia studied at the University College London between 1935 and 1939. She graduated with a BSc in zoology. She married Flt Lt Anthony Simpson in 1940. He was killed in action near Bergen in 1941.

Sylvia moved to graduate study, first with J.Z. Young at Oxford working on nerve regeneration, and then in 1944, with P.C. Williams who was head of the biological laboratories at the Courtauld Institute of Biochemistry. She became very skilled in the techniques and statistical interpretation of bioassays, in particular bioassays for estrogen.

About this time, it became clear that in the amorphous unfractionated portion of adrenal extracts, a potent salt-retaining "factor" could consistently be demonstrated [1]. The source of this activity in the adrenal gland was localized to the zona glomerulosa by Roy Greep and colleagues [2]. In parallel, Ralph Dorfman and his group in Cleveland described a micro-bioassay for mineralocorticoid activity that could serve as the foundation upon which the effort to isolate the responsible compounds could be based.

Sylvia, working with James Tait and Helen Grundy, quickly simplified and improved the precision of this assay by using as an endpoint the $^{24}Na/^{42}K$ ratio in the urine of "salt-loaded" rats [3]. This advance led naturally to the search for the chemical structure of "electrocortin."

There was already a strong entrant in the race, Edward Kendall's group at the Mayo Clinic. H.L. Mason had been designated as "lead" scientist for the effort. To challenge this formidable group, Sylvia would need a comparable group of strong collaborators. She out did herself. First, she recruited Ian Bush, the world's leader in the development of new chromatographic techniques of liquid/liquid partition chromatography, with a special interest in steroid hormones, working at the Medical

A Biographical History of Endocrinology, First Edition. D. Lynn Loriaux.

Research Council Laboratories at Mill Hill. Next was Tadeus Reichstein, the world's leading steroid chemist working at the CIBA Corporation in Basle. Reichstein had played an instrumental role in elucidating the structure of cortisol with Edward Kendall, ultimately leading to a Nobel Prize in 1950.

Thus began an intense race to isolate, purify, and characterize electrocortin: Simpson–Reichstein–Bush in Europe and Mason–Kendall–Meyers in the United States. This race is serialized in the correspondence between Simpson and Reichstein between the years 1952 and 1954. It describes progress in stark detail; mistakes, blind alleys, misunderstandings, structural analysis, anxieties–it is all there [4]. The structure was published in 1953 [5].

Simpson and Tait were married in 1956. They became lifelong scientific colleagues, and were universally referred to as "The Taits." They had a long and productive career, dominating the "aldosterone" field for three decades. They were leaders in developing "assays" that could measure hormones in picomolar quantities. They, and the Lieberman–Siiteri–Gurpide group at Columbia, essentially developed the discipline of steroid dynamics and the compartment modeling of steroid metabolism.

The Taits were elected Fellows of the Royal Society in 1959. In 1960, they were recruited to the Worcester Foundation of Experimental Biology and Medicine in Shrewsbury, Massachusetts by Gregory Pincus. They remained there for 10 years and then returned to London as co-directors of the Biophysical Endocrine Unit at the Middlesex Hospital Medical School, London University. In 1980, the Taits retired and moved to the country to enjoy their last years together in a comparative peace. Sylvia died on February 28, 2003.

References

1. Kuizenga MH, Cartland GF: Fractionation studies on adrenal cortex extract with notes on the distribution of biological activity among the crystalline and amorphous fractions. *Endocrinology* 1939; 24: 526–35.
2. Deane HW, Shaw JH, Greep RO: The effect of altered sodium or potassium intake on the width and cytochemistry of the zona glomerulosa of the rat's adrenal cortex. *Endocrinology* 1948; 43: 133–53.
3. Simpson SA, Tait JF: A quantitative method for the bioassay of the effect of adrenal cortical steroids on mineral metabolism. *Endocrinology* 1952; 50: 150–61.
4. Tait SAS, Tait JF: The correspondence of S.A.S. Simpson and J.F. Tait with T. Reichstein during their collaborative work on the isolation and elucidation of the structure of electrocortin. (later aldosterone). *Steroids* 1998; 63: 440–53.
5. Simpson SA, Tait JF, Wellstein A, et al.: Isolation from the adrenals of a new crystalline hormone with especially high effectiveness on mineral metabolism. *Experientia* 1953; 9: 333–5.

This chapter has been reproduced from Loriaux, D. Lynn: Sylvia Agnes Sophia Tait: 1917–2003. *The Endocrinologist* 2008; 18(5): 205–6.

CHAPTER 98
Solomon Berson
(1918–1972)
Radioimmunoassay

Solomon Berson was born in New York City on April 22, 1918 [1]. He was the eldest of three children. His father was a Russian immigrant who developed a prosperous fur business in the New World. The Berson family was intellectually inclined. Berson's father was well versed in mathematics and chemistry. Bridge, chess, and music were ever present in the family activities. Sol became an accomplished violinist, played in a number of chamber music groups, and pursued music as an avocation for the duration of his life.

Sol had a quick mind. He was an expert chess player and could win multiple simultaneous games blindfolded. He entered the City College of New York at age 16 and graduated 4 years later with the intention of going to medical school. Interestingly in retrospect, he applied to 21 medical schools and was rejected by all. Discouraged but not dismayed, he applied to New York University's Graduate School and earned a master's degree in biology in 1939 and a fellowship to teach anatomy at the NYU School of Dentistry. This paved the way for his admission to NYU Medical School in 1941. It is said by a student that knew him that "within 48 hours of beginning the freshman classes [everyone] knew that he was the leader of the class" [2]. He led his class academically all 4 years, was elected to the Alpha Omega Alpha honor society in his junior year, and was elected president of the class in the senior year. He graduated in 1945. Along the way, he married Miriam Gittleson. They had two daughters. By all accounts, it was a warm and loving family.

Berson interned at the Boston City Hospital and then served in the Army until 1948. He returned to New York to complete his training in internal medicine at the Bronx Veterans Administration Hospital. In 1950, as his training neared its end, Berson accepted a position at the Bedford VA Hospital in Massachusetts. At the same time, Rosalyn Yalow, a PhD in physics and assistant chief of the Radioisotope Service of the Radiotherapy Department at the Bronx VA Hospital, began searching for a physician colleague. She asked Bernard Strauss, chief of the Medicine Service, whom he might recommend. Knowing that Berson had already accepted the Bedford VA Hospital

A Biographical History of Endocrinology, First Edition. D. Lynn Loriaux.

This work is a co-publication between the Endocrine Society and John Wiley & Sons, Ltd.

position, he still thought it worth while to approach Berson about the opportunity. He told Yalow that Berson's background in mathematics and chemistry made him an ideal candidate for the job. Her interview with Berson apparently was not a smooth one, but, in spite of this, Yalow offered him the position and he accepted. Thus began a scientific collaboration that would fundamentally change the future of endocrinology and much of medicine and biomedical research.

Berson and Yalow's early studies focused on the metabolism of iodine by the thyroid gland, specifically the uptake of radioactive iodine from circulating blood [3, 4]. These studies provide the foundation upon which the measurement of radioactive iodine uptake is used as a clinical test. In addition, it demonstrated the potential power of "tracers" to help in understanding the fundamentals of kinetic processes and their measurement, tools that made possible the insights to come. Subsequent studies focused on the metabolism of iodinated proteins such as albumin [5] and the globins [6]. These were among the earliest studies to characterize the in vivo rates of production, metabolism, and clearance of these molecules.

It was in the context of these studies that Berson and Yalow conceived of a new hypothesis to weave together the known clinical attributes of noninsulin-dependent diabetes mellitus (NIDDM) into a single pathophysiological mechanism. They reasoned that "maturity"-onset diabetes mellitus could best be explained by an increased rate of insulin clearance from the circulation. The hypothesis was approached with the same tools used in the earlier studies with other molecules. The results were unanticipated. Instead of an increased clearance rate for insulin. Berson and Yalow found the clearance rate to be prolonged [7]. This led to the idea that the metabolism of insulin in NIDDM was retarded because insulin was protected from metabolism in this condition, possibly by binding to a larger molecule. This hypothesis led to the discovery of circulating anti-insulin antibodies caused by antecedent insulin treatment [8]. These findings were followed by a careful analysis of the physicochemical characteristics of the binding of insulin to its antibody and revealed that the Michaelis–Menten constant for the reaction was in the nanomolar range, sometimes approaching the picomolar range. This also was unexpected. At the time, the prevailing dogma was that the binding affinity of antibodies for their ligands was in the micromolar range [9]. The stage was set. This constellation of findings, developed against the gradient of prevailing opinion, prepared the way for one of the most important scientific insights of the twentieth century: insulin antibodies could be used to measure insulin in extremely low concentration in biological fluids. Berson and Yalow showed how this could be done in a preliminary publication in *Nature* in 1959 [9], and in a definitive publication in the *Journal of Clinical Investigation* in 1960 [10].

The ability to measure molecules in biological fluids in concentration between 10^{-9} and 10^{-13} molar profoundly altered modern clinical investigation and biomedical science. Phenomena heretofore only implied could now be examined directly with this powerful tool. Berson and Yalow exploited the technique in the study of insulin, growth hormone, ACTH, parathyroid hormone, and gastrin. In parallel, the rest of the world developed radioimmunoassays for all of the known hormones and vitamins, as well as many other biologically important molecules. An explosion of scientific activity ensued. The pace of biomedical research quickened perceptibility. In 1977, Rosalyn Yalow was awarded the Nobel Prize for developing the technique of radioimmunoassay, 5 years after Berson's death.

Sol Berson accepted the chairmanship of the Department of Medicine of the Mount Sinai Hospital of the City University of New York in 1968. Although he continued to conduct research productively at the Radioisotope Laboratory of the Bronx VA Hospital, the bulk of his time and energies were now consumed by the new and demanding position. It was a new kind of life and as far from the ascetic existence of the engaged scientist as can be imagined. It was a constant swirl of administrative controversy, medical student education, house staff training, and patient care; it proved to be a joy to Berson. He never regretted his choice of career change. At the time of his premature death at 53 years of age, he was working as hard to mold medical education into his own image as he had done with clinical science a decade before. But this goal was to remain unfulfilled. He died of a myocardial infarction at the Federation meetings in Atlantic City, April 11, 1972.

References

1. Rall JE: Solomon A. Berson. *Biogr Mem Natl Acad Sci* 1990; 99: 55–70.
2. Graef 1: Solomon A. Berson Memorial Service. *Metabolism* 1973; 22: 966.
3. Berson SA, Yalow RS, Sorrentino J, Roswit B: The determination of thyroidal and renal plasma I^{131}–Clearance rates as a routine diagnostic test of thyroid dysfunction. *J Clin Invest* 1952; 31: 141–58.
4. Berson SA, Yalow RS: The iodide trapping and binding functions of the thyroid. *J Clin Invest* 1955; 34: 186–204.
5. Berson SA, Yalow RS, Schreiber SS, Post J: Tracer experiments with I^{131}-labeled human serum albumin. *J Clin Invest* 1953; 32: 746–68.
6. Berson SA, Yalow RS, Post J, et al.: Distribution and fate of intravenously administered modified human globin and its effects on blood volume: Studies using I^{131} tagged globin. *J Clin Invest* 1953; 32: 22–32.
7. Berson SA, Yalow RS, Bauman A, Rothschild MA, Newerly K: Insulin I^{131} metabolism in human subjects: Demonstration of insulin binding globin in the circulation of insulin-treated subjects. *J Clin Invest* 1953; 35: 170–90.
8. Berson SA, Yalow RS: Quantitative aspects of reaction between insulin and insulin binding antibody. *J Clin Invest* 1959; 39: 1996–2016.
9. Yalow RS, Berson SA: Assay of plasma insulin in human subjects by immunological methods. *Nature* 1959; 184: 1648–9.
10. Yalow RS, Berson SA: Immunoassay of endogenous plasma insulin in man. *J Clin Invest* 1960; 30: 1157.

This chapter has been reproduced from Loriaux, D. Lynn: Solomn Berson April 22, 1918–April 11, 1972. *The Endocrinologist* 1995; 5(1): 1–2.

CHAPTER 99
Rosalyn Sussman Yalow (1921–2011)
Radioimmunoassay

Rosalyn Yalow was born on July 19, 1921 in the Bronx, New York. She attended the New York public school system. It was clear, even in elementary school, that she had a gift for mathematics. In Walton High School, she was encouraged by her chemistry teacher to consider a career in science. Her parents, however, encouraged her to become an elementary school teacher. She went to Hunter College with the goal of a career in science in mind. There she became fascinated by physics after attending a college colloquium on nuclear fission given by Enrico Fermi. She knew, however, that getting into a good graduate program in physics was very unlikely for a Jewish woman. After graduating from Hunter in 1941, she had no offers and took a job as secretary to Dr. Rudolph Schoenheimer, a prominent biochemist at Columbia University's College of Physicians and Surgeons. This was a time when most young men were being drafted into the military and, as a result, graduate schools were having a difficult time recruiting talented young men. Positions began to open up for women. Thus, in February 1942, Yalow received an offer to become a teaching assistant in physics at the University of Illinois at Urbana-Champaign. She was the only woman in a science faculty of almost 400. She married a fellow student, Aaron Yalow, in 1943, and received a PhD in nuclear physics in 1945. Her graduate school performance had been outstanding, and she was given a position as an engineer at the Federal Telecommunications Laboratory. In 1946, she was further offered a full-time teaching position at Hunter College, which she accepted.

During her graduate school years, Yalow became expert in developing and applying precision instruments for measuring radioactivity. The Veterans Administration (VA) had established radioisotope services in several of its hospitals to examine the results of exposure to radioactivity, and to find new uses for radioactivity in medicine. Yalow became a consultant in nuclear physics to the VA Hospital in the Bronx.

Yalow left Hunter College in 1950 and took a full-time position in the radioisotope unit at the Bronx, VA, becoming its chief 4 years later. It was there that Yalow met a young medicine resident, Solomon Berson, interested in potential applications of

A Biographical History of Endocrinology, First Edition. D. Lynn Loriaux.

This work is a co-publication between the Endocrine Society and John Wiley & Sons, Ltd.

radioactivity to endocrinology. Their first collaborations focused on using radioisotopes to study blood volume, and then, using radioactive iodine to study iodine metabolism in thyroid disease. They developed a method to determine the quantity of blood cleared of iodine per minute by the thyroid gland. They began to think about studying other hormone systems, especially those associated with polypeptide hormones. They chose insulin as their first experimental target. Developing techniques for radiolabeling proteins, they began to study metabolic disposition of insulin. It became clear that the clearance of insulin in normal subjects was much faster than in diabetic patients. They hypothesized that patients receiving the relatively crude insulin extracts available were making antibodies to insulin that bound the molecule and markedly retarded its clearance. It was the first proof that small polypeptides could stimulate an immune response. The scientific community was skeptical of the findings, and the article was rejected by several of the leading journals. It was finally accepted for publication in 1959, and the results were quickly confirmed by other workers in the field.

Yalow and Berson soon realized that antibodies to small molecules such as insulin could be used in a novel way as a reagent to measure the concentrations of hormone molecules in biologic fluids. A standard curve could be constructed by incubating a fixed concentration of antibody and radioactive ligand, with increasing concentrations of unlabeled insulin. The radioimmunoassay was born. Molecules in biologic specimens could be measured in never before imagined concentrations: nanograms, picograms, and even femtograms. Again, resistance to the research was intense. I remember, as a young endocrine fellow, attending a lecture in which Yalow began her talk with a slide of the rejection letter she received from the *Journal of Clinical Investigation* for their work on radioimmunoassay. The paper was finally accepted when the words "insulin antibody" were deleted from the paper [2]. The concept, however, was a juggernaut, and was soon expanded to the measurement of hormone receptors, using the receptor in place of the antibody.

The commercial potential of these discoveries was enormous. Yalow and Berson knew this, but refused to patent the method. "We never thought of patenting RIA. Patents are about keeping things away from people for the purpose of making money. We wanted others to be able to use RIA." Riches and celebrity were not a primary concern for either Yalow or Berson, an attitude far different from that which prevails today.

The work of Yalow and Berson was truly transformative. For the first time, biologic molecules could be measured in human beings in amounts that were biologically relevant. RIA transformed biomedical science. For these contributions, Yalow was elected to the National Academy of Sciences in 1975, won the Lasker Award in 1976, and the Nobel Prize in 1977.

Berson died of a myocardial infarction in 1972, and Yalow lost her closest friend and collaborator. However, she continued her work at the Bronx VA and retired from that position in 1991.

Rosalyn Yalow is one of our preeminent role models in translational medical science. She persevered where others had given up, and followed her dreams against substantial social resistance. In the end, she changed the way we see the world.

References

1. Yalow RS, Berson S: Immunoassay of endogenous plasma insulin in man. *J Clin Invest* 1960; 39: 1157–75.
2. Yalow RS: The Nobel Lecture in immunology. *Scand J Immunol* 1992; 35: 1–23.

This chapter has been reproduced from Loriaux, D. Lynn: Rosalyn Sussman Yalow: 1921. *The Endocrinologist* 2010; 20(6): 259.

CHAPTER 100
Mort Lipsett
(1921–1984)
The Syndromes of Adrenal Insufficiency

It was the height of the Vietnam War, 1967. I had my orders to report to Fort Letterman on such and such a date. There was only one way out–the National Institutes of Health (NIH). Thousands applied every year. Fifty were chosen. The chances were poor. Amazingly, a note finally came inviting me to an interview. I needed an airplane ticket to get to Washington, DC. I remember asking my father for a loan for the trip. He asked what the chances were. I said "slim." He said, "Then it's a waste of money. Maybe next time." Thanks a lot. I asked my research mentor and he said "Sure, I'm betting on you!" Perhaps his confidence was unjustified. I don't know, but I took the money. It was a struggle getting to the NIH and finding my way to the first interview with Mort Lipsett. I knew of his work, steroid dynamics, an area that I had dabbled in. The interview was no picnic; it was cold, intimidating, rapid fire. Question upon question about "rho" factors, disequilibrium, models, equilibrium models, radiation dosimetry, steroid structure, reaction mechanisms, and the like. When he asked a question, his pupils would dilate momentarily. This fascinated me and probably accounted for my poor performance. Nonetheless, on July 4, a week before my "report" date, I got the call. I was in! Hallelujah! The way was open for an internship, residency, and fellowship.

I worked with Mort from 1970 until the time of his death in 1984. I think I knew him as well as anybody, and better than most. This is what I wrote about him in another place [1, 2].

> Mort was born in the Bronx of Jewish immigrant parents. His father was a pharmacist on 180th street. The family moved to San Francisco at the beginning of World War II. Mort went to [University of California] "Berkeley" and majored in chemistry. His education was interrupted by the draft. He served as a medic in the 10th Mountain Division and was twice decorated for valor in combat during the Italian campaign. After the war, he went to the USC [University of Southern California] Medical School on the GI bill. An internship at the L.A. [Los Angeles] County Hospital was followed by medicine residency at the Sawtelle, V.A. Hospital. Mort then returned to New York to work with Olaf Pearson at the Sloan Kettering. His interest in the endocrinology of neoplasia led to a position at the NIH with Roy Hertz. That was 1957. Mort

A Biographical History of Endocrinology, First Edition. D. Lynn Loriaux.

This work is a co-publication between the Endocrine Society and John Wiley & Sons, Ltd.

was a genius. He forgot nothing, could beat 3 or 4 competent chess players at a time, was a life master bridge player, and could do differential equations in his head. He read articles vertically, and could toss off whole journals before the rest of us had finished the first few pages. When I tell this to people, they smile and consider it a gross exaggeration. All the more remarkable! Mort loved competition. He was focused on the state of his cardiovascular health. He relished a game of his own design, racing up 10 flights of stairs, and then seeing who could first decelerate their pulse to 60 beats/min or less. The younger the adversary, the better. Some of us never got down to a pulse of 60. Some of us never got to the 10th floor. Mort's taste in music ran to Mozart; in literature, to Thucidides and Gibbon; in art to Miro; in furniture, to Danish Modern; in food, to French; and in drink, the fine reds from the continent. Mort loved books. He used books like an artist uses brushes. He always had a book in hand. He left several of his endocrine texts to me. The gold lettering is worn off the covers by hard use, but the pages are clean; no marginalia, no dog-ears. He treated books with respect, with a caress.

Mort would not spend time in conversation unless it was productively centered about a problem of interest. Even then, he wouldn't give it much effort unless there were new data. If there were, things happened fast. In his impatience to digest the material, he would take data sheets from you. He worked best if you were quiet. This was learned quickly. You could follow Mort's progress through the data by the location of his index finger, which moved with his eye. A quantitative analysis would begin as he approached the end. "This means...," or "remember the table in...," A JCEM or JCI would be pulled from the shelf. Tables and isolated statements would be found with pinpoint accuracy. He would copy numbers out of these references, and make mental calculations. There was some conversation, but it was with himself, not you. Presently, comments and suggestions were made, and you were left to think it over alone in the library, books open everywhere, and a vague impression that instructions had been given. It could take hours to piece it together. The motivation was high, however, since nobody wanted to appear stupid. Twenty years later, I still occasionally "see," for the first time, what Mort was trying to tell me at some of those meetings. Mort was "deductively" hypertrophied. He moved fast with syllogisms, blindingly fast. He had no patience for doing it twice. He cut the path; you made the road.

Mort was free of preconception and bias; freer than any person I have known. He drove the scientific method into every recess of his life and ferreted out the last vestiges of dogma. He was free to see clearly. I well remember my first patient presentation to him. I had been warned to be ready with a thorough understanding of the nuances of the steroid abnormalities that were salient features of the case. I got through the tough part unscathed. In fact, Mort seemed bored by the whole thing. Wrapping up, I mentioned that because of an elevated postprandial glucose, I had instructed the patient on a 1200 calorie diet and prescribed a distribution of calories recommended by the ADA. Mort woke up. "Why did you do that? Is there any evidence that this will help the man? Who does the cooking? His wife? How will this impact upon her? How much will it cost? What about the quality of life?" It went on. At the end, all I could muster was a weak "Well, this is the way that we did it at the Mecca." Mort, who by this time was half out of the door, retraced his steps. "This is the Mecca," he said. Mort wasn't angry (although it took years to understand that), he was merely illustrating an important point about the practice of medicine. He detested appeal to authority. In fact, no issue was too small to be unimportant in this way. Mort weighted facts in "Russelian" isolation where all were given equal weight. This clarity of process gave him great critical power. At the same time, it denied him a certain passion in science. Mort never loved a hypothesis.

Mort tried life away from the NIH for a short time. He had expected, in time, to be appointed director of NICHD. When it failed to happen and the job was given to someone else, Mort decided that his future at the NIH was constricted. He left to head a Cancer Center in Cleveland.

> The Cancer Center never really got off the ground and Mort was expected to be a Professor of Medicine in the traditional sense. His skepticism was misinterpreted as lack of knowledge and his critical approach was misinterpreted as aloofness and Mort found his way back to NIH where he was, by turns, Director of the Clinical Center, Director of NICHD, and Director of NIAMDD.

One day in 1983, I was waiting "in the wings" to give a talk to the Lawson Wilkins Pediatric Endocrine Society when I was paged to a nearby phone. It was Mort. He said that he had been playing tennis earlier in the day and noticed that he was unable to make a certain passing shot that had, in the past, been routine. Upon returning to work, he went down to the x-ray department for a head CT. A cerebellar mass was discovered. His question to me: "Should I have it out here, today, or go elsewhere?" Five minutes to go before the talk. I took a deep breath, and we began the long discussion of the pros and cons of each approach. I was 20 minutes late to start the talk, and Mort went to Boston for neurosurgery. The tumor was removed and followed by whole brain irradiation. It was a lymphoma, and it soon recurred systemically. The radiation predictably began to erode his intellect, and the chemotherapy soon failed to maintain the short remission he had been granted. He called me one day and said he had decided to stop all therapy. I said I would come up to see him. He was thin and weak, jaundiced, and anorectic. He smiled at me and asked if we could take a walk down the hall. "Sure." I had to support him so that he could stand, and we stopped every 20 steps or so to rest. Toward the end of the walk he looked at me, smiled again, and said, "We must do this every day! I just have to get back into shape." It was a remarkable moment. He died within the week.

In his time, Mort Lipsett was the most respected endocrinologist in the world. This was not because of the books or chapters or papers he wrote, and not because everybody knew that he was the smartest person they had ever met. It was Lipsett who gave shape and direction, clinically and scientifically, to the specialty. Charlatans gained no purchase with Mort on the playing field. A reasonable analogue might be George Marshall and the Second World War. It was that kind of thing.

I have had a number of mentors, and all have changed me in one way or another. Mort changed me in this way. For the first time, I understood nothing is so powerful in achieving a meaningful life as clarity of thought energized by a scientific habit of mind. He had this in full measure. I try to emulate, but will never achieve his mastery. Few ever will. We must compensate in other ways. So we beat on, doing our best with what we have, forever on the learning curve that Mort so clearly defined. We progress. That is Mort's gift to humankind. Powerful, clear, effective. That was Mort.

References

1. Loriaux DL: In memoriam. Mortimer B. Lipsett. *Mol Endocrinol* 1987; 1: 195–7.
2. Loriaux DL: Remembrance: Mort and Griff. *Endocrinology* 1992; 131: 1–3.

This chapter has been reproduced from Loriaux, D. Lynn: Mort Lipsett (1921–1984). *The Endocrinologist* 2005; 15(1): 1–3.

CHAPTER 101

Griff Terry Ross (1921–1985)

The β Subunit of hCG

Griff Ross was born in Mount Enterprise, "East" Texas. His father, grandfather, and great grandfather were all general practitioners in that town. Griff's childhood was steeped in the culture of medicine and, not surprisingly, he aspired to perpetuate the tradition. He went to Stephen F. Austin State Teachers College in 1938 and then the University of Texas Medical Branch in Galveston in 1942. On graduation, he entered into the practice of general medicine in Mount Enterprise, the fourth generation in his family to do so.

With the outbreak of the Korean War, Griff was drafted into the Air Force and spent 2 years as a general medical officer at an air base in England. With the cessation of hostilities, Griff decided to specialize and went to the Mayo Clinic as an "internal medicine fellow." He worked with Al Albert, a pioneer in reproductive endocrinology. As part of Griff's work with Albert, he developed an improved urine bioassay for gonadotropin using mouse uterine weight as the endpoint. At the same time, at the National Institutes of Health (NIH), Roy Hertz had found the first effective medical treatment for a metastatic cancer–choriocarcinoma. Treatment success or failure was mirrored in the concentration of urinary human chorionic gonadotropin (hCG). As the number of patients treated at the NIH skyrocketed, Hertz needed someone to manage the huge load of bioassays generated thereby. Ross was recruited to Bethesda.

Mort Lipsett had been recruited by Hertz 3 years before, and when Griff arrived, both men found an ideal scientific collaborator in each other. Mort worked mainly with the steroid "dynamics," secretion rates, metabolic clearance rates, metabolic pathways, interconversions, movements into and out of physiological compartments, and so forth.

Griff worked mainly with the gonadotropins. He used his bioassay to develop one of the first radioimmunoassays for luteinizing hormone (LH), hCG and follicle-stimulating hormone (FSH). His work with Bob Canfield at Columbia on the purified subunits of LH, thyroid-stimulating hormone (TSH), and hCG led to the development of the first specific radioimmunoassay for hCG, the report of which soon became a citation

A Biographical History of Endocrinology, First Edition. D. Lynn Loriaux.

classic [1]. This advance moved the world of "pregnancy tests" out of the rabbit and into the test tube. It did not take long to realize that a really good antibody, immobilized and linked to a color reaction, could be the basis of a dipstick test for pregnancy that could be used in the privacy of one's own home. The societal impact of this advance remains substantial.

Griff always strived to bring some order to the difficult discipline of reproductive endocrinology. His breakthrough in this effort was linked to an invitation to write the chapter on this subject for *Williams Textbook of Endocrinology* with Raymond Vande Wiel as co-author. He went at this with a vengeance, and he would talk of little else for what seemed like years, making many trips to New York City to work out details with Raymond. The product, 50 pages in the 5th edition was, and remains, an organizing force for scholarship and research in reproductive endocrinology. Titled "The ovaries," it is divided into three sections: normal ovary, abnormal ovary, and references. All of the data on the effects of ovarian function on growth and development, and the associated disorders was codified, sifted, weighed, and assembled into one of those rare scholarly contributions in medicine–a true masterpiece. Griff called the chapter his "arbeit" and the book his "plumb" [2]. Along with Mort, Griff rose through the ranks of leadership at the NIH as senior investigator, branch chief, clinical director, associate director of the clinical center, director of the clinical center, and scientific director of NICHD.

Griff was in ill health for the entire period of our association. The main problem was atherosclerotic heart disease with multiple myocardial infarctions. In addition, he had serious hypertension and, later, carcinoma of the prostate gland. He was often in the hospital or back at the Mayo Clinic, looked frail, sometimes unsteady, but never despondent, never "down." There was always a new idea, a new book, a new acquaintance, new things, forward-looking things. Griff could be depressed but never morose.

Griff was as equally renowned for the intensity of his work. In the days of the "Atlantic City Meeting," most academic types would gather there in the spring of the year for the latest scientific information and socialization. Griff loved the meeting. He particularly loved the first night when he and all of his colleagues and fellows would go to dinner at Zaberer's Restaurant. They served a martini there that was easily a pint in volume. Few of us could handle even one of those behemoths. Griff could work his way through several in the course of dinner. He called it "getting Zaberized." It set a certain tone for the proceedings. Griff loved to entertain in his home, always with barbecue, a keg of beer, and a complete wet bar. His drink was bourbon and "branch water." He loved music and played the harmonica by ear with a remarkable level of mastery. If an attendee had any facility with music, that person was immediately dragged into the ensemble, often kicking and screaming, always to the delight of the attendees. Everybody worried about Griff's heart on these occasions. He worked that harmonica hard but he never seemed to get angina in these gatherings, although he would often complain of chest pain if he knew he had a "committee" meeting to attend. He was a warm and enveloping man, bigger than life really, a "once-in-a-lifetime" kind of acquaintance.

Griff loved to read and he was always interested in what those around him were reading. Once he asked me what I was reading, and I told him that I was reading all of Steinbeck's books, currently finishing up *Tortilla Flat*. "What's next?" he asked. "*Sweet Thursday*," I told him [3]. "I never heard of it," he said. "Not surprised," I said, "I think it is his best and, at the same time, least read book."

Approximately 2:00 the next morning, I was awakened from a sound sleep by the urgency of a ringing phone.

"Hello," I said.

"Listen to this!" It was Griff.

> Where does discontent start? You are warm enough, but you shiver. You are fed, yet hunger gnaws you. You have been loved, but your yearning wanders in new fields. And to prod all these there's time, the blasted time. The end of life is now not so terribly far away you can see it the way you see the finish line when you come into the stretch and your mind says, "Have I worked enough? Have I eaten enough? Have I loved enough?" All of these, of course, are the foundation of man's greatest curse, and perhaps his greatest glory. "What has my life meant so far, and what can it mean in the time left to me?" And now we're coming to the wicked, poisoned dart: "What have I contributed in the Great Ledger? What am I worth?" And this isn't vanity or ambition. Men seem to be born with a debt they can never pay no matter how hard they try. It piles up ahead of them. Man owes something to man. If he ignores the debt it poisons him, and if he tries to make payments the debt only increases, and the quality of his gift is the measure of the man.

"Isn't that the grandest thing you have ever heard outside of Richard the Second?"

"Yes it is," I said. He read it to me again.

Griff died with "all of the diseases that kill a man: heart disease, hypertension, a cerebral aneurysm, and cancer." It was a long and heroic struggle. His funeral was in Houston, Texas, thronged by admirers, students, and family. The program contained only a single thing directed to be there by Griff, that passage from *Sweet Thursday* [3]. It hits close to home. Not a dry eye in the place.

References

1. Vaitukaitis JL, Braunstein GD, Ross GT: A radioimmunoassay which specifically measures human chorionic gonadotropin in the presence of human luteinizing hormone. *Am J Obstet Gynecol* 1972; 113: 751–8.
2. *Williams Textbook of Endocrinology* (5th edn.). Philadelphia: W.B. Saunders Co., 1974, p. 368.
3. Steinbeck J: *Sweet Thursday*. New York: Viking Penguin Books, 1954.

This chapter has been reproduced from Loriaux, D. Lynn: Griff Terry Ross (1921–1985). *The Endocrinologist* 2005; 15(3): 133–4.

CHAPTER 102

Grant Liddle (1921–1989)

Differential Diagnosis of Cushing's Syndrome

Grant Liddle was born on a little farm in American Fork, Utah. He graduated from the University of Utah in 1943, valedictorian of his class. He was drafted by the Army, but was sent to medical school at the University of California at San Francisco (UCSF) instead of some theater of war. There, he was a student leader and president of his senior class. He was awarded the Gold Headed Cane at graduation. After an internship and residency, he stayed on at UCSF as a research fellow in the Metabolic Research Unit. In 1953, he went to the National Institutes of Health (NIH) as a clinical associate to work with the legendary Fred Bartter in the National Heart Institute. Three years later, he left the NIH to become head of the endocrine service at Vanderbilt. It was there that his most important contributions to endocrinology were made.

First and foremost was his contribution to the development of a clinical test for the differential diagnosis of Cushing's syndrome. Differentiating ACTH-dependent Cushing's syndrome from adrenal adenoma was very difficult and differentiating Cushing's disease from the ectopic ACTH syndrome virtually impossible. Liddle reasoned that by using a synthetic glucocorticoid such as dexamethasone, he could suppress adrenal function in normal people, but not people with Cushing's syndrome. What he found was that dexamethasone failed to suppress the adrenal axis in patients with an adrenal adenoma or cancer, but suppressed adrenal function in an attenuated way in patients with Cushing's disease [1]. In one study, he determined the cause of Cushing's disease, resistance of the pituitary adenoma to glucocorticoid feedback, and showed that the phenomenon could be used as a clinical test in the differential diagnosis of Cushing's syndrome. This test became the clinician's workhorse in dissecting adrenal pathophysiology. Now long superseded as a clinical test, it is still often used, a testament to its historical importance in clinical endocrinology.

Liddle's second great contribution was the description of Liddle's syndrome [2]. His interest in hypertension was stimulated by his years with Fred Bartter. In the course of his studies, he identified a "familial" form of hypertension. It had all of the clinical manifestations of hypertension associated with mineralocorticoid excess: hypernatremia,

A Biographical History of Endocrinology, First Edition. D. Lynn Loriaux.

hypokalemia, and metabolic alkalosis. No responsible mineralocorticoid, however, could be identified. In fact, the known mineralocorticoids appeared to be suppressed. Liddle reasoned that this form of hypertension was renal in origin and was passed on in families as an autosomal dominant trait. This was confirmed dramatically many years later when the proband of the family received a kidney transplant. Subsequently, all of the clinical stigmata of the hypertensive disorder resolved. Recent studies have localized the defect to a mutation in the renal epithelial sodium channel, thus validating Liddle's early claim that this syndrome was the result of an inborn error in metabolism.

Finally, he was among the first to recognize paraneoplastic endocrine syndromes, and coined the term "ectopic" hormone secretion [3].

As a young endocrinologist, I knew Grant Liddle only from afar. I went to all of his presentations that I could, usually at annual meetings of the Endocrine Society. He was a methodical speaker, reading from his notes, every word carefully chosen, humorless–it was serious business. However, the material was always new, exhaustively analyzed, beautifully synthesized. One left his presentations fatigued and always a little demoralized. He set the bar very high.

The first scientific presentation of my own work away from the NIH was to Grant Liddle and his endocrine division at Vanderbilt. To say that the tension was high understates the situation considerably. I am sure my presentation was hesitant with quavering voice, but I did get my stride with time. He sat immobile throughout and I was sure, with the end the presentation, a withering critique would emerge that would leave me even more shaken. It was not to be. All faces turned to him after a brief period of desultory applause, and he gave a coherent and improved synopsis of the talk, suggested a number of alternate ways to think about the data, and proposed new lines of investigation, all in a most constructive and sympathetic way. I went home with renewed energy for the work and a sense of having passed an important milestone of sorts. He was a remarkable man.

Grant Liddle was appointed chairman of medicine at Vanderbilt in 1968 and served in that capacity until 1983. He suffered a severe and debilitating stroke in 1988 and died of its complications in 1989. He was well-recognized in his lifetime, president of the Endocrine Society, president of the Association of Professors of Medicine, the Robert H. Williams Distinguished Leadership Award, and was elected to the National Academy of Sciences in 1981.

References

1. Liddle GW: Tests of pituitary adrenal suppressibility in the diagnosis of Cushing's Syndrome. *J Clin Endocrinol Metab* 1960; 20: 1539.
2. Liddle GW, Bledsoe T, Coppage WS: A familial renal disorder stimulating primary aldosteronism, but with negligible aldosterone secretion. *Trans Assoc Am Phys* 1963; 76: 199.
3. Liddle GW, Givens JR, Nicholson WE, Island DP: The ectopic ACTH syndrome. *Cancer Res* 1965; 25: 1057–61.

This chapter has been reproduced from Loriaux, D. Lynn: Grant Liddle (1921–1989). *The Endocrinologist* 2005; 15(5): 255–6.

CHAPTER 103
Monte Arnold Greer
(1922–2002)
Thyroid Nodules

Monte Greer, the well-known thyroid investigator and senior member of the faculty at the Oregon Health Sciences University in Portland, Oregon, was killed along with Peggy, his wife of more than 50 years, in a car crash on March 22, 2002. He was 79 years old but certainly did not seem to be of such an age; his sharpness of mind certainly showed no blunting.

Monte had worked in the thyroid field for more than 50 years; his publications spanned this entire time, from his paper on ACTH and platelets in 1947 to his last, published posthumously in 2002, on possibly the oldest known case of exophthalmos. His career, in fact, reflects the field of thyroidology as it developed during the last half-century. But he did not start out to be a thyroid scientist. He landed in the field of endocrinology more by chance than by plan and in his course managed to touch on most of the thyroid problems faced by us all during the past half-century. In doing this he often stimulated or provoked; in his own affable way, he sometimes managed to find results that would question the accepted wisdom, but always welcomed other views to explain the data. He summarized some of his career in 1975 [1].

Born in 1922, Monte was a Portland boy from the start. His stepfather, William Greer, was a food broker (his father, Arnold Cohen, died when Monte was quite young, and his mother, originally Rose Rasmussen, then remarried). Monte was named after one of his father's brothers who had also died. As a child, Monte suffered many fractures, mainly of his wrists and arms, and so missed a fair amount of school. There was no one in his family in medicine or the sciences, but the fractures led to many contacts with doctors who tried to find out what was wrong with the boy's bones. There was never a clear diagnosis, but it probably influenced Monte's childhood goal to become an orthopedic surgeon. In fact, as is often the case, he recalled wanting to be a physician even before going to elementary school and wanting to be a researcher when he was only 7 years old.

He had the usual budding scientist's chemistry set and mixed a number of strange chemicals, but that all stopped when he was age 14 after a home-made flare destroyed

A Biographical History of Endocrinology, First Edition. D. Lynn Loriaux.

This work is a co-publication between the Endocrine Society and John Wiley & Sons, Ltd.

his father's new Christmas sweater. He missed much of his junior year in high school because of a femoral fracture but still managed to graduate in 1940 at age 17 years. The high school course was the standard college course for the times; he had some physics and biology, but he missed chemistry altogether because of the fracture. It was biology that Monte loved. The biology so interested Monte that he took a course in fish biology one summer while trying to get a job in an aquarium.

Monte went to college at Oregon State College, now University. Even though he had been accepted at Stanford, he chose Oregon State mainly because his friends were going there. Also, Oregon State had a bit more science then than did the University of Oregon. The biology-oriented student still had no particular interest but, because he now knew something about fish, he took a course in endocrinology with Clifford Grobstein who had just gotten his PhD in fish endocrinology at UCLA. Monte knew nothing about endocrinology and was not sure exactly what the word meant, but it sounded intriguing. Grobstein seems to have turned Monte on to the field, so much so that Monte not only took the course but went on to do an undergraduate research project on the effect of thyroxine (T4) on leg development in bullfrog tadpoles. Unfortunately all the tadpoles died. He had given them too much T4 and caused the gills to regress before the legs developed; they could not breathe and could not climb out of the water.

By now, it was 1942 and World War II had broken out. Monte took a summer course in physics so he could apply to medical school. He finished his third year of college and immediately went on to Stanford Medical School in 1943. He chose Stanford, in part, because of its close proximity to Peggy, his future wife, but also because Oregon's medical school had turned him down even though he had been accepted to several other medical schools. After a year at Stanford, he got his BA degree and could have it from either his school of origin, Oregon State, or from the school where he finished, Stanford. Monte chose the Stanford degree although he had never attended an undergraduate course there.

Medical school cost nothing then because every student was in the military and in uniform. Monte was not enchanted by Palo Alto or Stanford Medical School. Anatomy was confusing (all dissection and no lectures) and physiology was weak. The clinical years were in San Francisco in an old hospital full of cockroaches. The clinical teaching was often good, but there was little to encourage his nascent interest in endocrinology. One bright spot was the professor of medicine, Arthur Bloomfield, who later wrote a fine bibliography of internal medicine diseases [2]. Because of the war, Monte finished medical school in only 3 years and began his rotating internship at San Francisco General Hospital in 1946. He did not receive his MD degree until 1947 because of the then arcane custom of not granting the degree until completion of an internship. Monte had planned to go on with his childhood goal of becoming an orthopedic surgeon and had won a surgical internship at Stanford. For some reason, at the last minute, he decided that the life of the surgeon was not for him, and he backed out. By that time in the academic year, there were few alternatives for internship, but San Francisco General was amenable. That internship decided him on medicine rather than surgery as a career.

While Monte was an intern, he had a patient with idiopathic thrombocytopenic purpura (ITP) who died. In trying to see what he could have done better, he read that platelet levels could be raised by stress. He reasoned that, if platelets rose with stress, maybe platelets would rise with ACTH because ACTH is a stress-related hormone. And so he began his first research study. Note that there was no fixed protocol, no grant, no review board, and no signed consent form. Nevertheless, at this point, his plan was to do a residency in internal medicine and become a practicing internist. The next step was obvious: go from his internship at San Francisco General to a residency there and learn how to practice medicine. He was turned down for the residency. All the slots had been reserved for physicians returning from military duty. This failure was the direct cause of Monte's decision, colored now by his experience with Grobstein and his attempt at hormonal research, to seek a year's position doing research in endocrinology.

He sought advice from a Stanford physiology professor, who helpfully gave Monte several names to write to and then asked Monte whether he thought a year's study of endocrinology would help him get into medical school. Crushed, Monte went ahead anyway and wrote his letters. He got several offers of an endocrine fellowship, even though he was just out of his internship. But the only offer that had a stipend, and no interview, was one on the other side of the country in Boston with Edwin (Ted) Astwood, professor of medicine at Tufts Medical School and chief of endocrinology at the New England Medical Center. Ted had become known for his invention of anti-thyroid drug therapy for hyperthyroidism, but Monte was only vaguely aware of this and really did not know who Astwood was. Still, the job had a salary. Monte was then 24 years old, had never been to Boston, and had never met Astwood. His first impression of Boston was awful, but he found a nice place to live in the Boston suburb of Waltham and settled in.

As usual, Astwood asked the fledgling scientist what he wanted to do. Monte had no interest in thyroid work. He wanted to pursue his idea of ACTH and platelets. Ted was skeptical but, again as usual, let Monte proceed. Unfortunately, there was no good commercial preparation of ACTH. What Monte had used in San Francisco was, he learned, inert. So, he started to make his own ACTH, which also meant that he would have to set up his own assay with hypophysectomized rats. After all this, a gift came from the Armor Company of an active preparation of ACTH, and he could move directly to the project without making his own ACTH. ACTH had no effect on the number of platelets [3].

At this point, Monte was floundering. Ted suggested that he work on a thyroid project already under way: the investigation of whether foods contain a natural goitrogen. The idea was an attempt to explain how goiter occurred in an iodine-replete area and was an offshoot of older work in rabbits that suggested that cabbage caused goiter. Monte got heavily involved in the project. He recruited volunteers, mostly nurses and technicians in the New England Medical Center, and got them to eat large amounts of raw vegetables, 50 different varieties. Monte looked for an inhibition of thyroid function using radioactive iodine. Monte found that turnip and rutabaga, both of the brassica family, had distinct anti-thyroid activity and helped work out the chemical structure of the new substance, goitrin [4, 5].

Monte's next project grew out of a partnership with another of Ted's fellows. The idea was to see if obesity in rats disrupted the estrous cycle, based on the observation that obesity in women sometimes caused amenorrhea. They were able to make fat rats by simple overfeeding, but it took a long time. Ted thought it could be done faster by making hypothalamic lesions. Monte and his colleague looked into getting a stereotactic device for making hypothalamic lesions, but none was commercially available; they would have to make one themselves, so they dropped the idea. Monte did conceive another project, however, to test the idea that giving thyroid hormone to people should suppress thyroid function.

By now, Monte's 2-year fellowship was about to end. He still had the idea that he might become an internist so sought a residency in Boston. Thus, in 1949, he went a mile south to Boston University's Massachusetts Memorial Hospital for a 2-year residency in internal medicine. There, working with Joseph Ross, he did the study on thyroid suppression just mentioned. It was clear that normal thyroid function was almost abolished if the subject took 1–3 grains of desiccated thyroid per day, 60–80 µg of oral T4. He also showed that no matter how long a person took thyroid hormone, when it was stopped thyroid function returned to normal within two weeks. Although obvious to us now, no one had ever done this before [6].

It was a good experience at Boston University, but he wound up doing more studies rather than learning the medicine he thought he needed. So, in 1950 he decided to stop after 1 year of residency and return to Ted's laboratory, now on a postdoctoral fellowship from the National Cancer Institute. By then Monte had published 11 papers, including a review of foods and goiter in *Physiological Reviews* [7] and a paper in the *Journal of Clinical Investigation* [8], and he was about to begin his last year in Boston back with Astwood.

It was time for Greer to return to the hypothalamus, in part because of his previous idea about hypothalamic obesity and in part because he had read Geoffrey Harris' seminal review on the hypothalamic control of pituitary function [9]. Greer's focus was still on obesity and its possible disruption of the rat's estrous cycle. Although Harris' idea seemed speculative, it was enough for Monte's application for the NIH fellowship. The fellowship application was not only to study the effect of hypothalamic lesions on gonadal function but also on thyroid function. Now the problem was to get a working stereotactic apparatus. Astwood allowed Greer to use his workshop in the basement of his home and wound up making most of the machine himself. All was set. But Astwood, ever generous, then gave the machine away to a visiting colleague who was about to start work on the hypothalamus. Greer started over and after some months managed to overcome a number of stumbling blocks and had a technique for making hypothalamic lesions in rats. The rats did indeed become obese but, unfortunately, there was no direct correlation with disrupted estrus.

Disappointed, Monte moved on to the effects of hypothalamic lesions on the thyroid. This time the experiments worked. He used a standard bioassay for thyrotropin (TSH) that involved giving the rats propylthiouracil (PTU). In a normal rat given PTU, serum thyroxin falls, and TSH rises leading to a goiter. The rat without TSH, such as after hypophysectomy, does not develop a goiter with PTU. One can conclude that the hypothalamic lesion interfered with TSH secretion. This is exactly what Monte found; the conclusion was that the hypothalamus had control over pituitary TSH secretion [10, 11].

By now, it was near the end of 1951 and the Korean War was in full swing. Although dismissed from military service because of asthma at the end of his medical school years, the rules had changed and Monte was now eligible for active duty. So, with Ted's help, he was able to get an appointment at the NIH to fulfill his military obligation. Monte was assigned to the National Cancer Institute to work with Roy Hertz. There was then no Clinical Center on the Bethesda Campus, so Greer did his laboratory and rat studies at the NIH and his clinical work at the DC General Hospital. He built a new stereotactic machine so that he could define more precisely the hypothalamic area responsible for the control of TSH. To his great chagrin he could not repeat his Boston experiment. The rats now had normal thyroid function after a hypothalamic lesion. The smaller lesions had missed the critical hypothalamic area. More carefully placed, and larger, lesions brought the now expected results and the results were expanded to mice as well as rats [12].

For most of the 4 years he spent at the NIH, Monte focused on the anatomy and physiology of the hypothalamus and the thyroid. He finished the study, begun with Astwood, that showed that one could treat goiter with thyroid hormone, basically an offshoot of his study on thyroid suppression in normal person. They also observed that the treatment could work for thyroid nodules as well [13]. The paper was quite controversial. Surgeons were piqued and for others it was new and hard to digest, even though the therapy had been used in the 1890s, it was long since forgotten. Still controversial today, the therapy has now largely been abandoned by many as controlled trials were completed in the last few years, but it remains a useful option for some. Greer used it in some patients until the day he died.

By 1955, the Clinical Center at NIH had been built and the hypothalamus presented still further fascinating problems for the thyroid. Greer pursued the physiology of the hypothalamus and thyroid gland. That work went well but, as often happens in government life, there were rules that might or might not be broken without consequence. When, on several occasions, Monte ran afoul of these rules in taking care of patients who were being treated with radioiodine, he decided to leave. He hoped that he might return to Portland, but there was nothing in the offing. A friend told him that the VA was setting up a number of radioisotope services all around the country and that Monte ought to look into it. He applied and was offered a job as chief of the Radioisotope Service at the Manhattan VA Hospital. He took the job and bought a house in a New York City suburb. Then he got a call from his old friend from Boston University, Joe Ross, who had since moved to UCLA to become associate dean of the medical school. Ross said to come to California. Monte checked with the VA, was able to withdraw from the New York position, and became the first chief of the Radioisotope Service at the Long Beach VA Hospital.

In one of the few papers he wrote while at the VA Hospital, Monte derived data that suggested that patients with Graves' disease have an excess of TSH, again a controversial idea and known now to be incorrect. When challenged on this, he was his affable, gentlemanly self. He said, "I certainly do not feel that it is by any means established" [14].

Monte stayed with the VA for only a year. A job in Portland opened up. He was offered the head of the endocrinology division at the Oregon Health Sciences University, and he immediately accepted. At the age of 33, the young investigator was in charge of a division of endocrinology. He came as an associate professor of medicine and, after a few years, was promoted to professor. Most of his salary during the next 20 years came from an NIH Career Research Award. Having returned home, Greer never left.

His main efforts in Portland were aimed at the hypothalamus, focusing on the relation of the thyroid gland to the adrenal. Dozens of his more than 300 publications were targeted at the understanding of thyroid control. Here he remained a physiologist. He was not a chemist and did not take part in the race for the chemical structure of TRH that occurred in 1960s.

His recognition grew. For example, he presented twice at the prestigious Laurentian Hormone Conference in 1957 and 1962. He was elected to the Association of American Physicians. He became a member of the American Goiter Association (now the American Thyroid Association or ATA) in 1963. In the ATA, he advanced through the ranks. He was one of the vice presidents in the 1960s, and again in the 1970s, during which he was also a director (now councilor), and then president in 1980. He openly regarded his presidency to be the "pinnacle of his career." He was kind to his colleagues and kept his presidential speech short.

He continued with his research on the anti-thyroid turnip substance he had worked on in the early 1950s. Further study showed that it existed in the vegetable in a precursor form, called progoitrin [15]. The effect of giving progoitrin to a person was to block thyroid function for most of the day [16]; Monte got the idea that it could be a "once-a-day" medical therapy for hyperthyroidism. It seemed to be just that. This would have been an advance because the standard therapy with PTU was to give it three times a day. A substantial number of hyperthyroid patents did quite well when they took PTU only once a day. So, instead of having a new medical therapy for Graves' disease, he had a new regimen for using PTU [17]. However, the standard therapy had become so ingrained, plus the fact that a few patients did not need to take it two to three times a day, that most physicians did not use Monte's approach and it never really caught on.

Another variation on this theme, also to become controversial, was his suggestion that one did not need to give prolonged therapy with an anti-thyroid drug (i.e., continue it for a year or more). His idea was that one could simply give it until the patient returned to normal and then just stop [18]. Few liked that idea, either, but in his hands it seems to have worked in selected patients.

Toward the end of his career, Monte became interested in the history of his profession. He had co-authored, with Roy Greep, the biographical memoir of Ted Astwood for the National Academy of Sciences in 1985 [19]. That effort seemed to fuel his historical interest which, in truth, was not new. His presentation that thyroid hormone can shrink both goiter and thyroid nodules was soundly based in thyroid history that dated back to the 1890s [13]. During the last few years, Monte was a valued member of the ATA's History and Archives Committee. To no one's surprise, he was always gently provocative.

Monte's career touched on almost every major thyroid issue of the past 50 years. He always thought clearly about these issues, usually had something of substance to say, and helped to solve many of them. His proudest accomplishments were often his controversial ones: thyroid hormone therapy for goiter and thyroid nodules, and once-a-day treatment with anti-thyroid drug therapy. He was most proud of goitrin and progoitrin, of course, and his early findings on the hypothalamic control of TSH. To me, however, his most important quality was his ability to catch people's attention, with a twinkle in his eye, and make them think. He received a devilish delight in posing a question that may have sounded odd to the listener, but who then might think "odd but what if, after all, Greer is right?"

References

1. Greer MA: Why I am still waiting for a free trip to Stockholm. In *Pioneers in Neuroendocrinology*, Vol. II, edited by J Meites, BT Donovan, SM McCann. New York: Plenum Press, 1975, p. 203.
2. Bloomfield AL: *A Bibliography of Internal Medicine. Selected Diseases*. Chicago, IL: University of Chicago Press, 1960.
3. Greer MA, Brown B: Concerning the relation between pituitary adrenocorticotropin and the circulating blood platelets. *Proc Soc Exp Biol Med* 1948; 69: 361.
4. Astwood EB, Greer, MA, Ettlinger MG: The anti-thyroid factor of yellow turnip. *Science* 1949; 109: 631.
5. Greer MA, Ettinger MG, Astwood EB: Dietary factors in the pathogenesis of simple goiter. *J Clin Endocrinol* 1949; 9: 1069.
6. Greer MA: The effect on endogenous activity of feeding desiccated thyroid to normal human subjects. *New Engl J Med* 1951; 244: 385.
7. Greer MA: Nutrition and goiter. *Physiol Rev* 1950; 30: 513.
8. Greer MA: Correlation of the 24-hour radioiodine uptake of the human thyroid gland with the 6 and 8 hour uptakes and with the "accumulation gradient." *J Clin Invest* 1951; 30: 301.
9. Harris GW: Natural control of the pituitary gland. *Physiol Rev* 1948; 28: 139.
10. Greer MA: Evidence of hypothalamic control of the pituitary release of thyrotrophin. *Proc Soc Exp Biol Med* 1951; 77: 603.
11. Greer MA: The role of the hypothalamus in the control of thyroid function. *J Clin Endocrinol Metab* 1952; 12: 1259.
12. Greer MA, Scow RO, Grobstein C: Thyroid function in hypophysectomized mice bearing intraocular pituitary implants. *Proc Soc Exp Biol Med* 1953; 82: 28.
13. Greer MA, Astwood EB: Treatment of simple goiter with thyroid. *J Clin Endocrinol Metab* 1953; 13: 1312.
14. Greer MA: A quantitative study of the effect of thyrotropin upon the thyroidal secretion rate in euthyroid and thyrotoxic subjects. *Trans Am Goiter Assoc* 1958; (discussion).
15. Greer MA: Isolation from rutabaga seed of progoitrin, the precursor of the naturally occurring anti-thyroid compound, goitrin (L-5-vinyl-2-thiooxazolidone). *J Am Chem Soc* 1956; 78: 1260.
16. Greer MA, Deeney JM: Anti-thyroid activity elicited vy the ingestion of pure progoitrin, a naturally occurring thiooligy-coside of the turnip family. *J Clin Invest* 1959; 38: 1465.

17. Greer MA, Meihoff W, Studer H: Treatment of hyperthyroidism with single daily dose of propylthiouacil. *New Engl J Med* 1965; 272: 888.
18. Greer MA, Kammer H, Bouma DJ: Short-term anti-thyroid drug therapy for the thyrotoxicosis of Grave's disease. *New Engl J Med* 1977; 297: 173.
19. Greep RO, Greer MA: Edwin Bennett Astwood. December 29, 1919–February 17, 1976. *Biogr Mem Natl Acad Sci* 1985; 55: 1.

This chapter has been reproduced from Sawin, Clark T: Monte Arnold Greer and the thyroid gland; A 50-year view. *The Endocrinologist* 2002; 12(6): 477–82.

CHAPTER 104
Jacob Robbins
(1923–2008)
Radiation-Induced Thyroid Cancer

Jacob (Jack) Robbins was an important force for order and thoughtful reflection among the large group of National Institutes of Health (NIH) endocrinologists. His calming nature and broad world-view helped many, if not all, endocrine trainees at the NIH find their "sea legs." You always felt better about life after a meeting with Jack.

Jack was born in Yonkers, New York. He went to Cornell for both an undergraduate degree and his medical degree, which he received in 1947.

> I chose Cornell University in New York City but because of my family's financial position and a scholarship award by Cornell University, I began my career at Cornell in Ithaca, New York, in 1940 and continued it at the Cornell Medical College in New York City. But even that progression was erratic. Admission to medical schools in 1944 was expensive and difficult to achieve, especially if there were restrictions based on gender, race, or religious background. Cornell, at the time, admitted 66 medical students each year of whom no more than 10% could be women and 10% Jewish. I, therefore, chose a practical college course, chemistry, to allow for failure to gain admission. I entered the Army instead of the fourth university year, and ultimately attended medical school in a special accelerated program for soldiers and sailors to supply needed physicians. I graduated just as the war ended, and prepared for a career in medical science instead [1].

Jack then joined Rulon Rawson at the Memorial Hospital-Sloan Kettering Cancer Center and his career in thyroidology was set in motion. Iodine-131 was now available in large quantities and the beginnings of radioactive iodine treatment of Graves' disease were well underway. Jack was encouraged to study the radioactive compounds circulating in the blood of patients treated with I^{131}. It was known that protein-bound iodine in the thyroid gland was different from protein-bound iodine circulating in blood. Using the "new" technique of paper electrophoresis, Jack was able to show that thyroxine in the blood was bound to a minor protein component migrating with the α globulins. He and his lifelong collaborator Ed Rall named the protein thyroid

A Biographical History of Endocrinology, First Edition. D. Lynn Loriaux.

This work is a co-publication between the Endocrine Society and John Wiley & Sons, Ltd.

binding globulin (TBG), as it is still called today. They began an intensive study of the physiology and pathophysiology of TBG.

> We were particularly interested in certain discrepancies that were not well understood. Why is a pregnant woman not hyperthyroid when her protein-bound iodine and serum thyroxine are high? Why is a patient with nephrosis, a protein-losing form of kidney disease, not hypothyroid when his PBI and serum thyroxine are low? And of particular interest, why are the patients with inherited abnormalities in TBG and very low serum thyroxine totally normal in every other way? We postulated that it was the serum concentration of unbound, or free, thyroxine that determined a person's thyroid health status, and we showed by theoretical calculations that it was a reasonable hypothesis. Other scientists then developed methods to measure the very tiny free thyroxine concentration and proved that we were correct. These new methods soon became a better way to test a patient's thyroid function [1].

After 5 years at the Sloan Kettering Center, Jack decided to move to the new "intramural program" at the NIH.

> It was the time of the Korean War and American Physicians were being called to service in the military. An alternative for those who were engaged or interested in biomedical research was to join the United States Public Health Service and seek employment in its research arm, the National Institutes of Health (NIH) in Bethesda, Maryland. The clinical facility, the NIH Clinical Center, had been opened in 1953. Appointment was highly competitive and it attracted many outstanding medical school graduates, even if their research interest was only tentative. NIH then had the pick of the crop, and I was one of the fortunate ones. In later years, I did some of the picking and I can easily list a number of leaders in their field who would surely have been medical practitioners rather than medical researchers without this career incentive.
>
> There were, in fact, 2 incentives. One was the ability to continue doing research, or to sample it and discover whether one was suited for such a career. The other incentive was the fact that American politicians had decided to invest a significant portion of the nation's resources in the medical sciences. This continued after the war and the doctors' draft and NIH grew rapidly in size and scope. Not only did this generous support of research make NIH a marvelous place to build and staff research groups, but it also created opportunities for a return to academia. Although I was one of those who decided to stay at NIH, others formed a pool from which universities and medical schools lured many of their senior staff. A personal incentive for me to stay was the fact that DeWitt Stettin, the research director of my institute (NIAMD), the National Institute of Arthritis and Metabolic Diseases) decided to invite Ed Rall, my New York colleague, to form and lead the Clinical Endocrinology Branch (CEB). In rapid succession beginning in 1955, Ed gathered chemists, biochemists, and medical researchers into the CEB, a core group devoted to thyroid studies. Its members, well known to the thyroidiologists in this room, enjoyed independence and support in designing their research that ranged from thyroxine chemistry and thyroglobulin structure to thyroid cell function and thyroid disease. These men, well suited to lead their own departments, were content to work in a limited space with a few junior scientist in a collegial atmosphere that was conducive to collaboration and exchange of ideas [1].

And thus it remained. The scientists in the CEB worked out the concept of "free hormone," the nature of the TBG molecule and its disorders, the effects, good and bad, of radioactive iodine treatment for hyperthyroidism and, in later years, the epidemiology of radioactive fallout on the incidence of thyroid cancer. They devised a preventative measure; saturate the thyroid with iodine at the first hint of trouble (SSKI).

Jack remained in the CEB until his death at 85 years of age from an apparent myocardial infarction in his office in the building he so loved.

There are many things said of Jack Robbins–solid, focused, thoughtful, thorough, and so on. One thing, however, is on everyone's list–gentleman. He was one of the kindest and most supportive people I have ever known, perhaps the kindest and most supportive. He walked the walk without having to be first in line, and was happy for it. A life lesson for many of his acolytes.

Reference

1. Trimarchi F: Laudatio for the Laurea Honoris Causa of Jacob Robbins, M.D. from the University of Messina, Italy. *Thyroid* 2002; 12: 337–41.

This chapter has been reproduced from Loriaux, D. Lynn: Jacob Robbins, MD: 1923–2008. *The Endocrinologist* 2009; 19(2): 53–4.

CHAPTER 105
Donald S. Fredrickson
(1924–2002)
Lipid Dyscrasiasis

Don Fredrickson was born in Cañon City, Colorado. His father was a lawyer. Fredrickson attended the University of Colorado in Boulder for a year in 1942, and then joined the Army, which sent him to the University of Michigan where he graduated with a BS in 1946. He attended the University of Michigan Medical School and graduated with an MD "with distinction" in 1949. Fredrickson left Michigan for Boston and did his residency at the Peter Bent Brigham hospital with Dr. George Thorn, followed by a year at the Massachusetts General Hospital with Ivan Frantz, a cholesterol biochemist.

Fredrickson moved to the National Institutes of Health (NIH) in 1953. He worked in the laboratory of Christian Anfinsen for several years. Anfinsen was a leading protein chemist who went on to win the Nobel Prize in Medicine in 1972. Fredrickson's focus was the plasma lipoproteins and their role in lipid transport. He was able to separate the Apo lipoproteins A, B, and C into component parts and subsequently sequenced and characterized several of them: A-II, C-I, C-II, and C-III. Along the way, Fredrickson and his growing group of junior colleagues described two diseases of lipid metabolism: Tangier disease, characterized by abnormal lipid storage in a number of organs, especially the tonsils (the orange tonsil sign), and the cholesterol ester storage disease, a lysosome disorder resulting in hyperlipidemia, hepatomegaly, and premature atherosclerosis. During this period, Fredrickson developed the now legendary classification of plasma lipid patterns using paper electrophoresis and ultracentrifugation.

Type I was designated as familial fat-induced hyperlipidemia, also known as familial hyperchylomicronemia. Type II was designated as familial hyperbetalipoproteinemia, also known as familial hypercholesterolemia. Type III was familial hyper-beta and hyper-prebeta lipoproteinemia, also known as familial hypercholesterolemia with hyperlipemia (remembered by students of medicine as a combination of Types I and II, adding up to Type III).

A Biographical History of Endocrinology, First Edition. D. Lynn Loriaux.

This work is a co-publication between the Endocrine Society and John Wiley & Sons, Ltd.

Type IV was familial hyper-prebeta lipoproteinemia, also known as carbohydrate-induced hyperlipemia, and Type V was familial hyperchylomicronemia with hyper-prebeta lipoproteinemia, also known as carbohydrate-induced hyperlipemia (remembered by students as a combination of Type I and Type IV, adding up to Type V).

This classification of the hyperlipidemic disorders was adopted by the World Health Organization as the "standard" classification of these common and complex diseases. It made the Fredrickson name famous the world over. As you would expect, this insight opened the doors to a large new area of scientific investigation–natural history, genetics, pathophysiology, and rational therapy, its success or failure.

The fundamental advance happened in the midst of an unprecedented explosion of knowledge in genetics and in the characterization of hereditary diseases. All of this culminated in the 1960 publication of *The Metabolic Basis of Inherited Disease*, a one-volume text of about 1000 pages edited by John Stanbury, James Wyngaarden, and Donald Fredrickson. The book was a modern continuation of the famous review of *Inborn Errors of Metabolism* by Archibald Garrod in 1908. The book is still with us as *The Metabolic and Molecular Basis of Inherited Disease*. The seventh edition has three volumes and 4605 pages. It is now a four-volume work in its eighth edition. It remains the encyclopedia of the discipline.

Fredrickson moved up through the ranks at the NIH. He became the head of the Section on Molecular Diseases and clinical director of the National Heart Institute in 1961. He was appointed head of the Metabolic Diseases Branch and director of the National Heart Institute in 1966. He left the NIH in 1974 to become the president of the Institute of Medicine of the National Academy of Sciences in Washington, DC. Shortly thereafter, in 1975, he was appointed as the director of the NIH. He resigned from that position in 1981 and, in 1983, was appointed the vice president of the Howard Hughes Medical Institute under George Thorn. One year later, upon George Thorn's retirement, Fredrickson was appointed director. Under Fredrickson's leadership, the Hughes Aircraft Company was sold to General Motors and the Howard Hughes Medical Institute received a 5 billion dollar endowment with which it expanded its fields of research to include neuroscience, structural biology, genetics, immunology, and cell biology. It was now a true powerhouse in biomedical research funding.

Fredrickson left the Hughes Medical Institute in 1987 and returned to the NIH as a scholar at the National Library of Medicine. It so happened that I was an NLM scholar at the same time. I had a small office down in the stacks and had a free rein of the place. It was Nirvana. Nothing was checked out. Anything one wanted was always where the card file said it would be. When you finished with it, you put it on a table near the card file and it was reshelved that night. Next to my office was another just like it. Nobody ever seemed to be there. Then, one day, I heard the door to that office open and close and I decided to meet my neighbor. It was Don Fredrickson.

"Lynn Loriaux," he said. "You are from Santa Fe!"

How could he know that?

"Yes–born and raised."
"I am from Cañon City, on the other side of the Sangre de Cristos."
"Wow, I know the place."

We talked the afternoon away, everything from the Anasazi to Zebra Fish. He was a gentleman, a scholar, and smart as hell. We decided to meet once a week and monitor each other's progress.

I never saw him again. Somehow, we missed each other in passing. He died before he finished his history of the NIH. He died swimming laps in his pool on June 7, 2002. I have never understood why he did not get a Nobel Prize. Perhaps it was because he died before his number came up. Who knows? He should have won. His contributions were more than sufficient.

Sources

Stanbury JB, Wyngaarden JB, Fredrickson DS (Eds.): *The Metabolic Basis of Inherited Disease* (2nd edn.), Chapter 22. New York: The Blakiston Division, McGraw-Hill Book Company, 1966.
Wynngaarden JB: Donald Sharp Fredrickson, a biographical memoir. *Proc Am Phil Soc* 2004; 148(3).

This chapter has been reproduced from Loriaux, D. Lynn: Donald S. Fredrickson: 1924–2002. *The Endocrinologist* 2008; 18(6): 261–2.

CHAPTER 106
John Doppman
(1928–2000)
Interventional Radiology

I met John Doppman at the National Institutes of Health (NIH) in 1973. He had just returned from a brief foray into academic medicine outside of the NIH at San Diego. It was not his cup of tea. Like many first- or second-generation NIH'ers who tried life "outside," John wasted no time in getting back. The NIH offered its people the remarkable job description of studying human disease in a setting that was financially secure, albeit at a relatively low rate of pay, and high on "non-interference." As long as you produced, the money kept coming. It was the ideal setting for a translational investigator, perhaps the only setting that maximized success. John thrived in this setting.

John Doppman was born in Springfield, Massachusetts on June 4, 1928. He attended Holy Cross in Worcester, Massachusetts where he graduated Summa Cum Laude in 1949. He went to medical school at Yale, graduating Cum Laude in 1953. He did a rotating internship at Mercy Hospital in Springfield, Massachusetts and then worked in the U.S. Navy from 1954 to 1957. John did his radiology residency at the Hospital of St. Raphael in New Haven., Connecticut. This was followed by a Fulbright Fellowship in radiology at the Hammersmith Hospital in London and the Karolinska Institute in Stockholm. He came to the NIH in 1964. He remained there until his death in 2000.

John was a pioneer in the new discipline of interventional radiology. He developed the techniques for localizing parathyroid adenomas, for localizing the source of ACTH secretion in Cushing syndrome, and for treating spinal arteriovenous malformations.

The parathyroid work centered around arteriographic imaging and venous sampling coupled with the measurement of PTH before, during, and after surgery. His techniques have become the standard of care in that disease. It is now a rare event to be faced with a patient dying of hypercalcemia in whom the tumor cannot be found. His work was done in collaboration with first-rate endocrinologists and surgeons: Gerry Auerbach, Stephen Marx, Alan Spiegel, and Murray Brennan. None the less,

A Biographical History of Endocrinology, First Edition. D. Lynn Loriaux.

This work is a co-publication between the Endocrine Society and John Wiley & Sons, Ltd.

John would always say that "the most accurate tool for localizing a parathyroid adenoma are the 'fingers' of a skilled and experienced surgeon."

The differential diagnosis of Cushing syndrome in the 1970s and 1980s was complicated by too many tests, none of which were specific or predictive. In the end, knowing the relative incidence of the different causes of Cushing syndrome was the best predictor of the cause in any given case. I remember well the day that John came to my office and told me that he could reliably and safely sample pituitary venous effluent in which we could measure ACTH. This had been done in a small number of cases in San Francisco and the data looked promising for improving the differentiation between ectopic from eutopic ACTH-dependent Cushing syndrome. The problem was that we could not measure ACTH. A visiting fellow at the time, Heinrich Schulte, had visited David Orth's laboratory in Nashville and had seen the radioimmunoassay for the measurement of serum ACTH in action. He offered to go to David Orth's laboratory and learn the assay if I could get Orth's permission. Orth immediately agreed to help and Schulte brought the assay and all of the reagents back to the NIH. With these tools, augmented by CRH generously provided by Wylie Vale at the Salk Institute, we took advantage of John Doppman's offer, and the IPSS test was developed. These tools markedly simplified the differential diagnosis of Cushing syndrome and became the standard approach of today. The main criticism of the technique remains that only Doppman could do the test. "The test could not be generalized." To this criticism, John said, "give me a radiologist of average intelligence, and I can teach him the method in one afternoon, and will do so for all that apply." He was as good as his word.

Toward the end of his career at the NIH, John became ensnared in a particularly dispiriting set of events. During the early years of the AIDS epidemic, several high-profile people suspected of having this disease were admitted to the NIH. One day, a disgruntled clerk in the radiology department revealed an x-ray request on such a patient to a newspaper reporter. The x-ray request noted "suspected AIDS" as the reason for the study. It appeared in the daily newspaper. The backlash was intense. Doppman was ordered, henceforth, to keep all such "sensitive" films in a locked cabinet in his office. He complied. Then, several years later, an "investigative reporter" found out about the "locked files" and trumpeted the story that U.S. government officials were getting "free care" at the NIH and that their files were hidden from public view in a locked file in Doppman's office, or words to that effect. Shortly thereafter, the file was broken into and many of the files stolen. Doppman was hounded by reporters from one of the more "sensational" late night news programs. They followed him to work, on trips to the grocery store, thrusting microphones into his face and illuminating the scene with powerful television lights toted around for the purpose. A new director of the NIH wondered how Doppman could have "allowed this to happen." There was little in the way of explanation forthcoming from the "top" and the saga dragged on. All of this was the result of changing institutional policy, policy Doppman had followed to the letter. In the end, however, Doppman was left to fend for himself. *Sic Simper fidelis*. As a result, one of the most "pure" translational scientists anybody has ever known was vilified in the daily rags without much, if any, support from the institution that had created the situation in the first place.

Interest in the story faded with time, but John never really recovered from the inquisition. Throughout, he was optimistic, forgiving, but diminished in energy and emotional reserve. This was followed by the diagnosis of a hematologic malignancy, from which he died, as so many radiologists of his generation seemed to do.

John was a powerful original thinker and conceived fruitful ideas that crossed most of the traditional boundaries of the day. He was optimistic and supportive, did more than his share, and loved what he did. He did much more for endocrinology than he did for radiology, and in that discipline, his contributions are gauged as transformative. He was a good friend, and a marvelous colleague. Reagan had a little sign on his desk when he was President that said, "it is amazing what you can accomplish if you don't care who gets the credit." That sign was about John Doppman.

Sources

Doppman JL: Regenerative parathyroid surgery: Localization procedures. *Prog Surg* 1986; 18: 117–32.

Nordenström J: *The Hunt for the Parathyroid*. Chichester: Wiley-Blackwell, 2013.

Oldfield E, Doppman JL: Petrosal sinus sampling with and without CRH for differential diagnosis of Cushing's syndrome. *N Engl J Med* 1991; 325: 897–905.

This chapter has been reproduced from Loriaux, D. Lynn: John Doppman (1928–2000). *The Endocrinologist* 2006; 16(6): 301–2.

CHAPTER 107
Gerald Aurbach (1927–1991)
Parathormone

Gerald Aurbach (Gerry) was born in Cleveland, Ohio, March 24, 1927. His family moved to Washington DC, early in his life, where he attended Lafayette Elementary School and graduated from Wilson High School in 1945. He spent one year in the Air Force, and then enrolled as a student at the University of Virginia, graduating with a bachelor's degree in 1950. He was accepted to the University of Virginia Medical School and graduated with the MD degree in 1954. While a medical student, Gerry worked with Dr. William Parson, chief of medicine and a former fellow of Fuller Albright at the Massachusetts General Hospital.

Gerry did his internship at the New England Medical Center, associated with Tufts University, and a residency in internal medicine at the Boston City Hospital. He joined the Ted Astwood Laboratory as a fellow in 1956. With Astwood, he picked up where he had left off with Parson and parathyroid hormone. He quickly succeeded in extracting the "active principle" from the parathyroid gland using phenol to inactivate associated proteolytic enzymes which had, up to then, interfered with the extraction of intact parathormone. Aurbach's extract of parathormone was achieved without requiring further protein purification [1]. It was a major step forward.

Now it became apparent to Gerry that he could really use some training in the rapidly evolving area of protein chemistry and biochemistry. He applied, and was accepted, to the Research Associate Training Program at the National Institutes of Health (NIH). He joined the laboratory of William Jakoby where he worked for 2 years, and then moved to the Metabolic Diseases Branch of the National Institute of Arthritis and Metabolic Disease. He spent his entire research career in that branch, becoming its chief in 1973.

The task that was before Aurbach was the isolation of human parathormone, its purification, and a method to measure parathormone in human plasma so that the disorders of parathormone action could begin to be examined directly.

> Influenced by the classic studies of Earl Sanderland, Gerry reasoned that parathyroid hormone acted on its target tissues, kidney and bone, by raising cyclic adenosinemonophosphate

A Biographical History of Endocrinology, First Edition. D. Lynn Loriaux.

This work is a co-publication between the Endocrine Society and John Wiley & Sons, Ltd.

(AMP) levels. To study the process in animals and humans, he and his fellow, Lew Chase, developed a highly sensitive assay for cyclic AMP. They then used the assay to show that parathormone activated adenylate cyclase and elevated cyclic AMP levels in targeted cells and urine [2].

This property of parathormone was then used as a bioassay to measure parathormone [3], allowing it to be isolated [4] and purified. This led directly to the development of a radioimmunoassay of the molecule [5]. The assay was not as simple as it had been for other peptide hormones. It was found that the bioactivity of PTH was in the first 34 amino acids of the hormone after realizing that assays against the intact molecule did not correlate well with bioactivity.

Once this was clarified, the application of two assays led to the understanding of the pathophysiology of primary, secondary, and tertiary hyperparathyroidism, and familial hypocalciuric hypercalcemia, hypoparathyroidism, pseudohypoparathyroidism, and pseudopseudohypoparathyroidism, vitamin D deficiency and toxicity, tumor-related hypercalcemia, the hypercalcemia of sarcoidosis, and many more of the obscure disorders of calcium metabolism. It was a tour de force.

In the effort, Aurbach benefitted greatly from the NIH Research and Clinical Associate Program. Fondly referred to as the "Yellow Berets," these programs brought the very cream of the crop of graduating MDs and PhDs to the NIH for a 2-year tour of duty [6]. Gerry's association with John T. Potts was transformative. Potts became Aurbach's right-hand man. No one could wish for more! Others include Henry Kentman, Len Deftos, Steve Marx, John Bilezikian, Larry Mallette, Gino Segre, Alan Spiegel, Ed Brown, Maurice Attie, Bob Downs, Michael Levine, John Stock, Roz Lasker, Art Santora, Laurie Fitzpatrick, Mike Bliziotes, and many others in cross-divisional collaborations. This kind of hyperfertile scientific environment is unlikely ever to happen again.

On the afternoon of Saturday, November 4th, 1991, Gerry was parking his car on Main Street in Charlottesville, Virginia. He was preparing to spend the afternoon at one of his favorite pastimes–watching a UVA football game. It was just past noon, and as Gerry got out of his car, a 22-year-old man in the passenger seat of a passing automobile lofted a brick-sized stone high into the air over the roof of the car. The stone fell and hit Gerry in the head. Knocked unconscious, he was taken to his beloved UVA Medical Center, where he had been a student, and where he died of this senseless injury 2 days later.

References

1. Aurbach G: Isolation of parathyroid hormone after extraction with phenol. *J Biol Chem* 1959; 234: 3179–81.
2. Pastan I: *A Biographical Memoir of Gerald Donald Aurbach*. Washington DC: National Academy of Sciences, 2007, p. 5.
3. Marcus R, Aurbach GD: Bioassay of parathyroid hormone in vitro with a stable preparation of adenyl cyclase from rat kidney. *Endocrinology* 1969; 85: 801–81.

4. O'Riordan JLH, Potts JT, Aurbach GD: Isolation of human parathyroid hormone. *Endocrinology* 1971; 89: 234–9.
5. Berson SA, Yalow RS, Aurbach GD, Potts JT: Immunoassay of bovine and human parathyroid hormone. *Proc Natl Acad Sci* 1963; 49: 613–17.
6. Klein MK: *The Vietnam War, the Doctor Draft, and the NIH Associate Training Program – The Legacy of the "Yellow Berets."* Bethesda, MD: NIH History Office, NIH, 1998.

CHAPTER 108

Roger Guillemin and Andrew Schally

(1924–) (1926–)

The Hypothalamic-Releasing Hormones

I began medical school at Baylor College of Medicine in Houston, Texas in 1962. My intention was to be one of the first combined degree (MD/PhD) students in the Baylor program. I started working in the laboratory virtually on my first day. I was interested in the steroid hormones, and Mathew Noall was a recent graduate of the Steroid Chemistry Program at the University of Utah under Leo T. Samuels and Kristin Eik-Nes. Noall was to be my mentor for the following 6 years. Nonetheless, a requirement of the new program was to visit several active and funded labs before a mentor was chosen. I made two visits. The first was to the Noall lab, the second was with a young French scientist, Roger Guillemin, who had just returned to Baylor from the College de France in Paris. It turned out that he had two active laboratories, one in Houston, and one in Paris. His focus, for some years, had been the isolation and characterization of an ACTH releasing factor, CRF (corticotropin-releasing factor) thought to be in the hypothalamus. While Guillemin was in Paris, a young physician scientist, Harry Lipscomb, was in charge of the day-to-day operations of the Houston lab. Lipscomb had been an endocrine fellow at the Peter Bent Brigham Hospital in Boston, and had developed one of the first bioassays for ACTH, using an in vivo perfusion of the rat adrenal gland. It was a cumbersome assay. It was Lipscomb who arranged for me to meet with Roger Guillemin.

The appointment was in the spring of 1963. The Guillemin labs were among the first in a brand new research building. As I entered the suite, I was definitely intimidated. A secretary, who served as a receptionist, was in the main office. There was a waiting room and a conference room, and many modern and well-equipped laboratories. I had never seen anything like it, and never would again. I was escorted into one of the first labs in the hall. It was relatively empty. The whole order of things seemed to be centered around an 8- or 12-inch diameter glass column that reached from sitting level up through the ceiling into the room above. It looked like a giant Sephadex glass column and, as it turned out, that was exactly what it was. There must have been a

A Biographical History of Endocrinology, First Edition. D. Lynn Loriaux.

million dollars worth of Sephadex in that column. Sitting on a stool at the base of the column was a slight, well-groomed man in what appeared to be a tailored lab coat. He was working with the stopcock, probably collecting fractions.

> "Hello," I said.
> "I am Roger Guillemin. What is it that you want?"

I told him a little about myself and that I was looking at several labs before choosing one (although I had already chosen). All through my little talk, he was working with the stopcock. Something was not going well.

After a while, he looked up from the stopcock and said, "Well, as you can see, I am the only one in the lab." He was definitely not happy about that.

> "Do you know anything about peptide chemistry?"
> "Not really," I said.
> "Well, never mind," he said. "You can come if you want to. Tell the secretary what you want to do and when you will start."

That was it. His attention was back on the stopcock. I found my way back into the hall and as I was passing the secretary's door, a young man stood up in the waiting area and strode across the floor toward me with hand extended.

> "Hi! I am Wylie Vale. From Rice, across the street. I am thinking about coming here. You too?"

We shook hands.

> "Hi Wylie," I said. "I am one of the MD/PhD students here. Interested in steroids. This is probably not the right lab for me."
> "How did the interview go?"
> "Well, it was short and to the point. He was sitting at the bottom of what is probably the biggest chromatography column in the world working with the stopcock. He didn't seem too happy. My guess is that if you come here, you will be on that stool collecting those fractions."
> "Wow," he said, "I have to see this."

I believe that was Wylie Vale's first day in the Guillemin Laboratory. He obviously did not take my advice, and, probably as a result, flourished as a scientist. He was the most instantly likeable man I have ever known. Our paths would cross many times in the years to come. He was one of the keys, perhaps the key, to the many successes of the Guillemin lab.

At the time of my introduction to Roger Guillemin, he and Andrew Schally had been working together on the CRF problem for 5 years without much success. About all they had to show at the time was that there was a hypothalamic CRF, perhaps two, and it was uncertain, perhaps unlikely, that is was a polypeptide. The Guillemin–Schally relationship was coming apart. Funding sources, primarily the NIH, were pushing harder for better results, and threatening a reduction in funding. It was a watershed moment. Schally soon left to a new job in the New Orleans VA. With a new group, he initiated a fresh start on the hypothalamic-releasing factor problem as a whole. Guillemin made a new start as well. With Wylie Vale and Roger Burgus filling the key bioassay and protein chemistry slots, Guillemin decided to abandon

CRF, at least for the time being, and focus on TRF (thyrotropin-releasing factor). He had developed the best bioassay for TSH that was available and proposed to take advantage of it [1]. The race was on.

Roger Guillemin was born in Dijon, France, in 1924. His father was a mechanical engineer and, financially, the family was solidly middle class. Roger enrolled in medical school in Dijon when he was 19 years old (1943). His medical studies were interrupted (1944–1945) by his work with the French Resistance forces. He helped French citizens in high political jeopardy to escape the Nazis by getting them across the Jura Mountains into Switzerland. After the War, he received the MD degree from the Faculté de Médecine of Lyon in 1949.

In 1948, Guillemin heard a lecture by Hans Selye on the "general stress response." This led to an introduction to Selye and a job with him in Montreal. Working with a graduate student, Claude Fortier, he decided to focus on the "hypothalamic-releasing" factors as hypothesized by Geoffrey Harris. In 1949, while preparing for his MD thesis examination in Lyon, Guillemin became seriously ill. The diagnosis was tubercular meningitis, in essence, a death sentence. Fortier, taking matters into his own hands, treated Guillemin with intrathecal INH, probably the first such case, and Guillemin lived. He had endured three months of the most intensive treatment in the hospital that one can imagine [2].

In 1953, Guillemin was recruited to the Physiology Department at Baylor College of Medicine by Hebbel Hoff, a Canadian educated in Montreal. Guillemin had better resources in Houston, but was working essentially alone. Soon after his arrival in Houston, he paid a visit to Charles Pomerat in Galveston. Pomerat showed Guillemin tubes of anterior pituitary cells that he was culturing. Pomerat noted that even though the cells looked healthy, they never produced any of the anterior pituitary hormones. Guillemin suggested that Pomerat co-culture his pituitary cells with hypothalamic tissue to see if the stimulus of the hypothalamus could stimulate hormone secretion by the anterior pituitary cells. After a few attempts, Guillemin did the experiment in his Baylor labs and found that the pituitary cells secreted ACTH when co-cultured with hypothalamic tissue. It was one of those times when the delayed gratification of basic science finally pays off. It was a transformational experiment in the quest for the hypothalamic-releasing factors.

Andrew Schally was born in Wilno, Poland in 1926. His father was an officer in the Polish Army. When his father escaped the Nazi Juggernaut in 1939, his wife and two children, Andrew and Halina, moved in with other Polish Army families in Craiova, Romania. It was about this time that Andrew decided to become a chemist.

The family relocated again in 1949, this time to Edinburgh, Scotland. Andrew found his way to the University of London and, after 3 years of chemistry, he was hired as a laboratory technician at the National Institute of Medical Research in Mill Hill. He worked for Donald Elliott, a protein chemist. Schally left Mill Hill for Montreal in 1952, and was hired as a laboratory technician in the Allan Memorial Institute for Psychiatry at McGill University. His new boss, Murray Saffron, was a young biochemist who believed that Geoffrey Harris was right about the "hypothalamic-releasing factors." Saffron and his new laboratory technician decided to focus on the releasing factor(s) for ACTH [3]. They named the factor CRF. Like Guillemin, the course of Schally's scientific career was now set.

At about this time, 1956, Guillemin's protein chemist, Walter Hearn, decided to take a new job at Down State University, and Schally's supervisor, Murray Saffron, was leaving for a sabbatical year, maybe 2. Schally needed another job. The result was that Schally was hired by Roger Guillemin to replace Hearn, and Schally moved to Houston to work with Guillemin. On the surface of it all, it seemed like the perfect solution as Schally and Guillemin settled in together to isolate and characterize CRF.

The relationship lasted 5 years. One of the major problems was the acquisition of massive amounts of hypothalamus. It was expensive and often of dubious quality. Guillemin spent a lot of time in his laboratories in Paris. Progress was stiflingly slow and Guillemin and Schally began to blame one another for the lack of results. The funding institutions began to wonder if there really was a CRF separate from vasopressin. In the end, Schally left for a new and more "supportive" job in the Veterans Administration Hospital in New Orleans. Abba Kastin, an endocrinologist, and Akira Arimura, a physiologist, filled out his new team. Guillemin replaced Schally with Roger Bergus, a protein chemist who had earned his PhD with Hearn, and Wylie Vale who came from Rice University to get his PhD with Guillemin and who became one of the great bioassayists of his time. Both teams were improved. From this point forward, the two groups were in serious competition to be "first." The rift between Guillemin and Schally soon became public, and people began to "take sides" based on "who they knew," not "what they knew."

The structure of TRH was the first to fall. The TRH structure was reported by the Schally group on November 6, 1969, in Volume 37 of *Biochemical and Biophysical Research Communications* [4]. The date of publication of the Schally TRH structure was six days ahead of the November 12th paper by the Guillemin group in *Compte Rendus* [5].

Gonadotropin-releasing hormone, then known as LRII, was next. Again, the Schally group came up with the structure of pig GnRH perhaps a month before the Guillemin group sorted out the structure in sheep. Guillemin and his group were first with somatostatin [6]. In the grand scheme of things, the "race" was a tie. In the years that followed, Guillemin and Schally won the Lasker Award in 1975, and the Nobel Prize in 1977.

Both men continue to be scientifically active–Guillemin at the Salk Institute in San Diego, making contributions to the endorphin story, and in the characterization of inhibin and activin. Schally remains in the VA system, now in Miami, and continues to conceive of, and produce modified neuropeptides that show progress in the ongoing struggle with neoplastic disease.

Everybody has their own ideas about the famous race for the hypothalamic peptides. What most people remember is the public jousting of the two principles, which from time to time could be *ad hominem* and hurtful. What often gets lost is the extraordinary product of this competition to "be first." Many think the competition was unseemly and that it diminished the participants. My view is different. I see it as one of the greatest accomplishments in the history of endocrinology. The clinical impact was, and is, enormous. One of my mentors, Mort Lipsett, once said to me, "You need three things to succeed in science. You have to be smart, you have to work hard, and you must have some luck. Of the three, luck is by far the most important." It certainly characterizes this chapter in endocrinology. And, in my view, a generous dollop of competition did not hurt.

Source

Wade N: *The Nobel Duel.* Garden City, NY: Anchor Press/Doubleday, 1981.

References

1. Yamazaki E, Sakiz E, Guillemin R: An in vivo bioassay for TSH-releasing factor. *Experientia* 1963; 19: 480–1.
2. Fortier C, Fauzz G: Nouvelles Conceptions sur la Pathogenic et le Translucent du Processus Tuberculeux. *Schweizerische Medizinische Wochenschrift* 1952: 82: 953.
3. Saffron M, Schalley AV, Benfey BG: Stimulation of the release of corticotropin from the adenohypophysis by a neurohypophysial factor. *Endocrinology* 1955; 57: 439–44.
4. Boler J, Enzmann F, Folkers K, Bowers CY, Shalley AV: The identity of chemical and hormonal properties of thyrotropin releasing hormone and pyroglutamly-histidyl-proline amide. *Biochem Biophys Res Commun* 1969; 37: 705–10.
5. Burgus R, Dunn TF, Desiderio D, Guillemin R: [Molecular structure of the hypothalamic hypophysiotropic TRF factor of ovine origin: Mass spectrometry demonstration of the PCA-His-Pro-NH2 sequence.] *C R Acad Sci Hebd Seances Acad Sci D* 1969; 269(19): 1870–3.
6. Brazeau P, Vale W, Burgus R, Ling N, Butcher M, Rivier J, Guillemin R. Hypothalamic polypeptide that inhibits the secretion of immunoreactive pituitary growth hormone. *Science* 1973; 179: 77–9.

This chapter has been reproduced from Loriaux, D. Lynn: Schally, Andrew V and Gual, Carlos. Some recollections of early clinical studies on hypothalamic hormones: A tale of a successful international collaboration. *The Endocrinologist* 2001; 11(5): 341–9.

Criticism

A through Z. The author is aware that there has been a goodly sprinkling of metaphysics among this recording of some experimental facts; he is very well aware that the deductions will not stand the test of time; he does hope, however, that thoughts will be stimulated by this presentation–if not by truths, why then by errors; *apologiae* are there none.

Fuller Albright
Harvey Lecture
Series 38, p. 123, 1942–3

A Biographical History of Endocrinology, First Edition. D. Lynn Loriaux.

This work is a co-publication between the Endocrine Society and John Wiley & Sons, Ltd.

Index

Page numbers in **bold** refer to chapters.

A Biographical History of Endocrinology, First Edition. D. Lynn Loriaux.

This work is a co-publication between the Endocrine Society and John Wiley & Sons, Ltd.